ANTIVIRAL DRUG DISCOVERY FOR EMERGING DISEASES AND BIOTERRORISM THREATS

ANTIVIRAL DRUG DISCOVERY FOR EMERGING DISEASES AND BIOTERRORISM THREATS

Edited by

Paul F. Torrence
Northern Arizona University

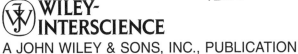

WILEY-INTERSCIENCE

A JOHN WILEY & SONS, INC., PUBLICATION

Published by John Wiley & Sons, Inc., Hoboken, New Jersey.
Published simultaneously in Canada.

For general information on our other products and services please contact our Customer Care Department within the U.S. at 877-762-2974, outside the U.S. at 317-572-3993 or fax 317-572-4002.

Wiley also publishes its books in a variety of electronic formats. Some content that appears in print, however, may not be available in electronic format. For more information about Wiley products, visit our web site at www.wiley.com

Library of Congress Cataloging-in-Publication Data:

Antiviral drug discovery for emerging diseases and bioterrorism threats/edited by Paul F. Torrence.
    p. ; cm.
  Includes bibliographical references and index.
  ISBN-13 978-0-471-66827-5 (cloth : alk. paper)
  ISBN-10 0-471-66827-3 (cloth : alk. paper)
 1. Antiviral Agents. 2. Drug development 3. Bioterrorism.
  [DNLM: 1. Antiviral Agents – therapeutic use. 2. Bioterrorism – prevention & control.
 3. Communicable Diseases, Emerging – drug therapy. 4. Communicable Diseases, Emerging – prevention & control. 5. Drug Design. QV 268.5 A6295 2005] I. Torrence, Paul F. II. Title.

  RM411.A5747 2005
  616.9′1061–dc22   2004019934

Printed in the United States of America

10 9 8 7 6 5 4 3 2 1

◼◼◼ CONTENTS

When I was just beginning my career at the National Institutes of Health as an organic chemist who wished to contribute to medicine in some way, I was advised to stay away from research on the discovery of antiviral agents since viruses were well under control. That was when the World Health Organization nearly had eliminated variola virus, the causative agent of smallpox and the worst killer in human history. Years earlier, Salk, Sabin, and Koprowski had given the world the means to eliminate polio. These were massive accomplishments and optimism was only natural. Of course, the antiviral naysayers could not read the future. And the future contained HIV/AIDS...and Ebola hemorrhagic fever...and West Nile virus. Respiratory syncytial virus, a significant cause of morbidity and mortality among infants and children, expanded its host range to the elderly and the immunosuppressed. Epidemics of herpes and viral hepatitis became commonplace. Cytomegalovirus also took advantage of the biological niche provided by the unfortunate immunosuppressed. Yellow fever continued to attack, along with a host of other diseases, the aspirations and well-being of millions upon millions in the developing world, while simultaneously undermining economies and providing conditions for unrest and extremism. Virus names such as Nipah, Hendra, and the SARS virus became part of the common lexicon. And all the while, waiting like a card up a gamblers shirt sleeve, the influenza virus, wild or bioengineered, remains the ace of spades. The human toll of the 1918–1919 "Spanish" flu will never be known accurately, but best estimates are 20–40 million dead.

We have changed the world dramatically in the past few decades. Indeed the human alterations began in earnest with the introduction of agriculture, which bred a series of formidable viruses, including variola (smallpox) and influenza. Yet the changes wrought by humans over the past 10,000 years may be dwarfed by what we have "accomplished" in the past century or so. We have brought about massive habitat changes, penetrated ecological niches with a speed and thoroughness never known in human history, destroyed ecosystems, contributed substantially to global warming, bred resistance to our best antibiotics, undergone uncontained population expansion, and introduced so much mobility that at any time a great fraction of our number is crossing even the oceans that once provided a barrier to species migration.

If all this were not enough to provide diseases, including those of viral origin, with a strong if not invinceable hand, consider that many of the viruses that threaten *Homo sapiens* are RNA viruses that exist as quasi-species or "swarms," always ready to exploit a new niche, always prepared to meet the challenge of drug therapy with resistance. And then finally the *coup de grace*. As unfathomable as it may seem, there are the extremists and zealots who threaten to use any such agents they can obtain or engineer to carry out their agendas. As enemies of all decent people on earth, their hatred may be directed at the more highly developed nations, but the result of their bioterrorism may set the struggling people of developing countries back a thousand years. Imagine reintroduction of smallpox to a continent already fighting the burden of HIV/AIDS, yellow fever, dengue, Ebola, malaria, river blindness, and on and on.

In spite of the counsel I received to let antivirals alone, I fulfilled my contrary nature. That has led me to know and respect a number of fellow travelers and some of them are, I am pleased to say, contributors to this volume. This volume is intended to provide reasons for optimism in view of the dark and pessimistic picture I just painted above.

The journal *Emerging Infections Diseases* kindly cooperated on the use of certain of their covers throughout the book, and the editior and authors are deeply grateful for this.

Several individuals have been very helpful in the compilation of this effort. Bonnie Johnson provided excellent editorial assistance. Polyxeni Potter of *Emerging Infectious Diseases* provided assistance in garnering permission to reproduce covers from the journal. Amy Romano, Assistant Editor at John Wiley & Sons, provided valuable advice and patience. Rosalyn Farkas, also at John Wiley, helped pull it all together.

PAUL F. TORRENCE
Northern Arizona University
Flagstaff, Arizona

CONTRIBUTORS

Peter Borowski, University Hospital Hamburg-Eppendorf, Institute for Infectious Diseases, 20246 Hamburg, Germany

Alison Boyers, Retroscreen Virology, Ltd., Centre for Infectious Diseases, Bart's and The London Queen Mary's School of Medicine and Dentistry, London E1 4NS UK

Mike Bray, Biodefense Clinical Research Branch, OCR/OD/NIAID, National Institutes of Health, Bethesda, MD 20892 USA

Craig E. Cameron, Department of Biochemistry and Molecular Biology, Pennsylvania State University, University Park, PA 16802 USA

Elsa B. Damonte, Laboratorio de Virología, Departamento de Química Biológica, Facultad de Ciencias Exactas y Naturales, Universidad de Buenos Aires, Ciudad Universitaria, 1428 Buenos Aires, Argentina

Erik De Clercq, Rega Institute for Medical Research, Katholieke Universiteit Leuven, B-3000 Leuven, Belgium

Menashe Elazar, Division of Gastroenterology and Hepatology, Stanford University School of Medicine, Palo Alto, CA 94305 USA

Cybele C. García, Laboratorio de Virología, Departamento de Química Biológica, Facultad de Ciencias Exactas y Naturales, Universidad de Buenos Aires, Ciudad Universitaria, 1428 Buenos Aires, Argentina

Jeffrey S. Glenn, Division of Gastroenterology and Hepatology, Stanford University School of Medicine, and Veterans Administration Medical Center, Palo Alto, CA 94305 USA

Jason D. Graci, Department of Biochemistry and Molecular Biology, Pennsylvania State University, University Park, PA 16802 USA

Ronald N. Harty, Department of Pathobiology, School of Veterinary Medicine, University of Pennsylvania, Philadelphia, PA 19104 USA

Bertram L. Jacobs, School of Life Sciences/Biodesign Institute, Arizona State University, Tempe, AZ 85287 USA

Matthias Kalitzky, University Hospital Hamburg-Eppendorf, Institute for Infectious Diseases, 20246 Hamburg, Germany

Earl R. Kern, Department of Pediatrics, Division of Infectious Diseases, The University of Alabama at Birmingham, Birmingham, AL 35233 USA

R. Lambkin, Retroscreen Virology Ltd., Centre for Infectious Diseases, Bart's and The London Queen Mary's School of Medicine and Dentistry, London E1 4NS UK

Vanessa Lancaster, School of Life Sciences/Biodesign Institute, Arizona State University, Tempe, AZ 85287 USA

Jeffrey O. Langland, School of Life Sciences/Biodesign Institute, Arizona State University, Tempe, AZ 85287 USA

Jillian M. Licata, Department of Pathobiology, School of Veterinary Medicine, University of Pennsylvania, Philadelphia, PA 19104 USA

Lori L. McCoy, Canadian Blood Services and Department of Pathology and Laboratory Medicine, University of British Columbia, Vancouver, BC V6T 2B5 Canada

Alex Mann, Retroscreen Virology, Ltd., Centre for Infectious Diseases, Bart's and The London Queen Mary's School of Medicine and Dentistry, London E1 4NS UK

Krishna Murthy, Center for Biophysical Sciences and Engineering, University of Alabama at Birmingham, Birmingham, AL 35294 USA

Vasu Nair, Department of Pharmaceutical and Biomedical Sciences and The Center for Drug Discovery, The University of Georgia, Athens, GA 30606 USA

John S. Oxford, Retroscreen Virology Ltd., Centre for Infectious Diseases, Bart's and The London Queen Mary's School of Medicine and Dentistry, London E1 4NS UK

Linda Powell, Department of Chemistry and Biochemistry, Northern Arizona University, Flagstaff, AZ 86011 USA

Holger Rohde, University Hospital Hamburg-Eppendorf, Institute for Infectious Diseases, 20246 Hamburg, Germany

Stewart W. Schneller, Department of Chemistry and Biochemistry, Auburn University, Auburn, AL 36849 USA

Mark D. Scott, Canadian Blood Services and Department of Pathology and Laboratory Medicine, University of British Columbia, Vancouver, BC V6T 2B5 Canada

Paul F. Torrence, Department of Chemistry and Biochemistry, Northern Arizona University, Flagstaff, AZ 86011 USA

Christopher K. Tseng, Antiviral Research and Antimicrobial Chemistry, DMID/NIAID, National Institutes of Health, Bethesda, MD 20892 USA

Minmin Yang, Department of Chemistry and Biochemistry, Auburn University, Auburn, AL 36849 USA

EMERGING
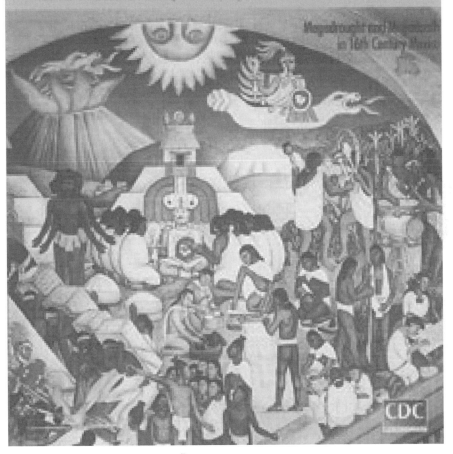

INFECTIOUS DISEASES

A Peer-Reviewed Journal Tracking and Analyzing Disease Trends   Vol.8, No.4, April 2002

EID Online

Megadrought and Megadeath in 16th Century Mexico

CDC

CHAPTER 1

Introduction: Pestilence, Plague, Bioterrorism

PAUL F. TORRENCE

Department of Chemistry and Biochemistry, Northern Arizona University

Ring around the rosie,
Pocket full of posies,
a-tishoo, a-tishoo,
All fall down.

> Old European nursery rhyme about smallpox and the bubonic plague

I have examined Man's wonderful inventions. And I tell you that in the arts of life man invents nothing; but in the arts of death he outdoes Nature herself, and produces by chemistry and machinery all the slaughter of plague, pestilence, and famine.

> The Devil speaking in *Don Juan in Hell*, Act III of *Man and Superman* by George Bernard Shaw, 1902

Human history has been shaped by virus infections. For instance, without the introduction of smallpox, measles, and yellow fever to the New World, it is likely that a significantly different natural, cultural, and governmental landscape may exist in the Americas. Not only are the factors that launched successful emerging viral diseases very much still with us, but modern societies have added multiple facilitating forces that ensure the continued role of viral infectious diseases in the future of *Homo sapiens*. Our response to this challenge will speak to the yet unanswered question: Are we deserving of our species name?

Humans have come to an exaggerated image of their role in the evolution of human history. While stacks of books narrate in detail human acts that molded the

Antiviral Drug Discovery for Emerging Diseases and Bioterrorism Threats. Edited by Paul F. Torrence
Copyright © 2005 John Wiley & Sons, Inc.

fate of nation-states and civilizations, few admit the role of natural elements in shaping human destiny. Among such primal forces as volcanism, earthquakes, floods, drought, and climate change must be counted biogenic forces. Among the latter, infectious diseases of viral origin have writ large upon the chronicle of civilization's development.[1] The mummified remains of Egyptian royalty Ramses V documented his death from smallpox in 1158 BC. Smallpox imported from the East and known as the Plague of Antonius took the lives of millions of Romans in AD 165–180. Variola virus, as the causative agent of smallpox, likely was responsible for the decimation and subsequent defeat of Abyssinian troops in the attack upon the Arabic capital of Mecca in AD 570.

The accidental introduction of smallpox to the New World assumed a central role in the European conquest of Mexico, Peru, Brazil, North America, and Australia.[1] Variola virus was imported to the Americas through the West African slave trade. The Spanish invaders under Hernan Cortes initially were appeased by Aztec Emperor Montezuma, who believed them the embodiment of the god Quetzalcoatl, the prophesized destroyer of the Aztec Empire. Later armed resistance by the Aztecs led by Montezuma's brother Cuitlahuac drove the vastly outnumbered Spanish expeditionary troops to a last enclave, where annihilation would have seemed certain. Yet the arrival near Veracruz of a second expeditionary force that joined ranks with Cortes' vastly diminished army perchance included a slave with smallpox. The disaster that followed was massive and world-shaping. The immunologically and genetically naïve native population of Veracruz was rapidly decimated, and the disease spread quickly to Tenochtitlán (now Mexico City), where it killed as many as half the population in some areas, and eventually took the lives of more than three million Aztecs. Because the disease spared the Spanish soldiers, who possessed both genetic and immunological resistance, but savagely destroyed the Aztecs, the native people came to accept this as punishment by an angry god. The Aztecs therefore accepted Spanish rule as their fate and no longer resisted. Conquest, subjugation, and Christianity followed hard on the heels of smallpox.

A similar fate befell the Inca of Peru. Smallpox's arrival preceded Pizarro's force of 168 men with whom he conquered an Empire of millions of Incas. Variola virus was Pizarro's greatest ally, as it destroyed not only great numbers of Incas but led to social upheaval and civil war. Smallpox, measles, influenza, yellow fever, plague, tuberculosis, typhus, and other European imports effected a 95% decline in North American Indian populations, certainly preparing the path for domination and westward expansion.

The first recognized intentional use of smallpox as a biological weapon was by Sir Geoffery Amherst who, as British Commander-in-Chief in North America during the French and Indian War, authorized provision of variola virus-contaminated blankets to hostile Indian tribes.[1] During the American Revolution, George Washington greatly feared the use of smallpox as a bioweapon by the British. In fact, American troops under Benedict Arnold failed in their mission to conquer Quebec in 1776 when nearly half of the Continental forces died of smallpox, albeit an epidemic of natural origin.

By the conclusion of the eighteenth century, nearly 10% of all humans had been disfigured, crippled, or killed by smallpox. Cosmetics had come into being as a result of a need to hide the scars of smallpox. In the twentieth century alone, approximately 300 million people had perished from smallpox. For comparison, all the wars of the twentieth century killed just one-third the number of humans as did smallpox.

Variolation, the practice of rubbing smallpox pustule exudate into a needle scratch on the arm, provided protection against variola virus, but at a cost of 2 deaths per 100 variolations. Edward Jenner's cowpox vaccination gave smallpox prophylaxis with a dramatic decrease in iatrogenic disease and death and further set the stage for the eradication of smallpox, a hope once advanced both by Jenner himself as well as Thomas Jefferson.

In spite of initial widespread opposition to a program of worldwide smallpox eradication, continued pressure by individuals such as Brock Chisholm of the World Health Organization (WHO), Victor Zhadnov of the Soviet Union, and Marcelino Candau of WHO, saw the worldwide eradication program eventually actualized and financed. Under the direction of Donald A. Henderson from 1966, the WHO smallpox eradication campaign achieved its remarkable goal of worldwide eradication when the last case of smallpox was reported in Somalia in 1977.

The yellow fever virus also has directed the course of human history.[1] This flavivirus was introduced into the New World from Africa by means of the slave trade, which Europeans expanded to replace the human labor lost when smallpox and measles took their ghastly toll of Native American slaves. In a strange turn of fate, the yellow fever virus thwarted the ambitions of at least one European empire builder when it essentially destroyed Napoleon's expeditionary force sent to put down the Haitian rebellion. Thus Haiti won its independence from France. Moreover, Napoleon was so rattled by this empire-defeating disaster wrought by a lowly virus that it was a key factor in his decision to execute the Louisiana Purchase with Jefferson, thereby abandoning France's claims and avoiding a war with the United States. This sequence of events catalyzed the American westward expansion.

It was the yellow fever virus that forced France to abandon the Panama Canal Project. Subsequently, bolstered by the findings of the Yellow Fever Commission that revealed the mosquito as the vector for yellow fever, the United States was able to shoulder the Canal Project.[1]

For most people, measles invokes a childhood disease that, before vaccine was available, was an unpleasant but common occurrence albeit with rare sequelae of encephalitis and, even rarer, subacute sclerosing panencephalitis. Nonetheless, to a totally immunologically isolated and naïve population, measles is a deadly disease. To wit, its introduction to Fiji in 1875 resulted in widespread social disruption and a 40% decrease in the native population.[1] Measles also collaborated with smallpox in the ravaging of the early Native Americans, thereby facilitating European domination. However, even in non-naïve populations, the effects of measles were devastating. Both Union and Confederate Armies in the American Civil War suffered extensively. Although the WHO has proposed steps toward eradication of measles, it remains a major source of morbidity and mortality in developing countries.

No one can debate the effects of influenza virus on the human condition. In recent times, the defeat of Germany in World War I was in part related to an influenza outbreak. At detailed by Oldstone,[1c] Germany's spring 1918 offensive, after the withdrawal of Russia from the war, threatened the Allies with defeat. However, influenza brought about a massive loss of German troops and concurrent breakdown of logistics. German Commander Eric von Ludendorff blamed influenza for cessation of the German Army offensive. This in turn permitted time for the influx of the American Expeditionary Force, the accompanied regain of lost French soil, and an eventual armistice. Yet influenza, not the weapons of war, caused 80% of American casualties and 43,000 deaths. This experience was generalized expertly by Jared Diamond in *Guns, Germs, and Steel*[1a]: "All those military histories glorifying great generals oversimplify the ego-deflating truth: the winners of past wars were not always the armies with the best generals and weapons, but were often merely those bearing the nastiest germs to transmit to their enemies."

Worldwide, the 1918–1919 influenza epidemic (termed the Spanish flu) infected a fifth of the total human population at that time and killed an estimated 20–50 million people.

Other RNA viruses evoke concern. Many of them have been the subject of press accounts over the past few decades and, in various modified embodiments, have become the stuff of novels and stars of films alike.

Presently, human immunodeficiency virus (HIV), with the resultant acquired immune deficiency syndrome (AIDS), is the most infamous example of a modern emerging infectious disease.[2] There were 38 million HIV-infected humans in 2003, and nearly five million people became infected with HIV in 2003, more than any year before. Over 20 million already have died. Over 90% of people living with HIV/AIDS are in the developing world, with sub-Saharan Africa claiming the greatest number (25 million) and the greatest number of deaths (3 million) from AIDS. Nonetheless, Asia now has the fastest-growing HIV/AIDS epidemic on earth, and sadly the advent of antiretroviral drugs has led to an increase in high-risk behavior in high-income countries, resulting in an increase in the number of new HIV infections.

While only time will reveal the full impact of HIV/AIDS on the human story, it is already certain that it has altered the future of Africa. The pandemic has already reduced average national economic growth rates by 2–4% a year across Africa.[2] Some predictions call for even greater impacts.[2] Through increased mortality and morbidity, the HIV/AIDS pandemic impacts labor supply, causing loss of skills in key sectors of the labor market. In South Africa, for example, around 60% of the mining workforce is aged between 30 and 44 years; in 15 years this is predicted to fall to 10%. In the South African healthcare sector, 20% of student nurses are HIV positive. AIDS reduces labor productivity, thereby reducing competitiveness, profits, exports, and balance of payments.

And it must be remembered that HIV/AIDS has released a host of opportunistic infections caused by organisms ranging from other viruses to helminths, some of which are newly recognized taxa or organisms never before identified as serious pathogens of humans. Thus HIV has provided a potential factory for the generation of even more novel emerging pathogens.

Other RNA viruses, emergent or reemergent, already are determining regional futures and may write even more upon the annals of human history. For instance, yellow fever has reemerged to constitute a major public health problem in Africa.[3] Dengue virus and its associated DHF (dengue hemorrhagic fever) is an emergent disease in India and has spread from Asia to most of the tropics.[4] Although rotaviruses already are the cause of extensive morbidity and mortality in children in developing countries, it appears that G serotype 5 is of emerging epidemiological importance in Brazil.[5] West Nile (WN) virus invaded the Western Hemisphere in the summer of 1999 and represented the first introduction in recent history of an Old World flavivirus into the New World.[6] Japanese encephalitis (JE) virus has recently encroached on the northern shores of Australia.[7] As this manuscript is being prepared, another lethal outbreak of Ebola hemorrhagic fever has been reported in southern Sudan.[8] Human-induced landscape alterations and/or climatic changes have caused emerging Hantavirus infections in rodents with resulting lethal spread to humans.[9] Rabies is undergoing geographic expansion due to natural and anthropogenic movements of wild animals.[10] Other emerging viruses, recognized now even by laypeople, include human monkeypox,[11] Nipah virus,[12] Hendra virus,[12] and the coronavirus that causes SARS (severe acute respiratory syndrome).[13]

Of course, at one time during human development, diseases such as smallpox, measles, and influenza were themselves emergent. Their emergence was facilitated greatly by the growing human populations, higher population densities, and domesticated animals.[14] Just as variola arose from cattle poxvirus, measles from rinderpest from pigs, and influenza from ducks and chickens, today's emerging diseases often have their roots in animals. The most infamous example would be HIV origination from chimpanzees. Yet, like our ancestors, we have introduced novel conditions for the emergence of new diseases. This emergence is the result of shifts in human demographics and behavior, changes in technology and industry, economic development, habitat invasion and destruction, increasing and facile international travel and commerce, microbial adaptation, alterations in human immune response and viral evasion, social and governmental disruptions, wars and the generation of great numbers of refugees, and the deterioration of public health measures.[14]

Added to this multifactorial equation are the unknowns of microbial resistance development (as with HIV), insufficient political commitment to control by governments of countries where the disease is endemic and high-income countries where it may not seem a present threat, poor or inadequate disease surveillance, inappropriate disease control measures, and preventable poverty and living conditions that facilitate disease.[14,15] At the least from a purely selfish viewpoint, high-income governments need to educate their populace that emerging microbial infectious diseases, so long as uncontrolled elsewhere on earth, provide an ongoing potential source of new and perhaps even deadlier organisms. This would seem a special threat in the case of RNA viruses, which exist as genetic swarms and can easily mutate.

Finally, added into this witch's cauldron is the unthinkable threat of biological terrorism.[16] The threat was realized in the United States with the anthrax attacks in 2001. Although smallpox was declared to be eradicated on 8 May 1980, during the Thirty-third World Health Assembly, concerns about the possible use of the virus in bioterrorism have grown in the past few years.[16,17] Other viruses, such as those that cause hemorrhagic fevers, have been identified as possible bioterrorism agents by the Centers for Disease Control and Prevention.[16] They have been so designated because large amounts can be generated in cell culture, they are transmissible in aerosol form, and there are limited or nonexistent vaccine and drug strategies for either prevention or treatment of established infection. In addition, these viruses could be modified genetically to enhance their virulence or to promote resistance to vaccines or antivirals.

The purposeful manipulation, introduction, and/or reintroduction of these viruses would represent a wildcard in our future struggle with emerging infectious diseases. Almost certainly, the greatest damage would be borne in developing countries (say, by the reintroduction of smallpox). Imagine the horrific consequences of the added burden of reestablished smallpox in Africa on the existing pandemic of HIV/AIDS, yellow fever, and a host of other microbial and parasitic infections.

A new variant of mousepox virus with increased virulence for mice has been reported.[18] This was created by splicing a gene for interleukin-4 into mousepox virus. Addition of the IL-4 gene apparently suppressed the normal immunological response against the mousepox virus infection, and the new poxvirus was able to evade vaccine-induced protection. Moreover, cidofovir, the only available drug thought to be effective against smallpox, did not protect mice against challenge with the IL-4 mousepox virus.

The threat from emerging diseases, whether of "natural" origin or the introduction of terrorists, cannot be underestimated. There is much that needs to be done in this fertile area for drug discovery. This volume deals with approaches to drug discovery and development for a number of emerging viruses and some of those of bioterrrorism interest. HIV, although still emerging, is not included because of the enormous volume of research that has been well described in many other venues. We trust that the contributions herein will illuminate the path for an increasing number of able investigators to follow.

REFERENCES

1. Material in this introduction has drawn heavily upon the following resources. (a) Diamond, J. *Guns, Germs and Steel: The Fates of Human Societies*, W. W. Norton, New York, 1999. (b) Karlen, A. *Man and Microbes: Disease and Plagues in History and Modern Times*, Simon and Schuster, New York, 1995. (c) Oldstone, M. B. A. *Viruses, Plagues and History*, Oxford University Press, New York, 1998. (d) Garrett, L. *The Coming Plague: Newly Emerging Diseases in a World Out of Balance*, Penguin Books, New York, 1995. (e) Preston, R. *The Hot Zone*, Random House, New York, 1994. (f) Black, F. L. Infectious diseases in primitive societies. *Science* **1975**, *187*(4176), 515–518.

(g) Zinsser, H. *Rats, Lice, and History.* Little, Brown, & Co., Boston, 1935. (h) Smith, G. *A Plague on Us*, Commonwealth Fund, New York, 1941. (i) McNeill, W. *Plagues and Peoples*, Doubleday, Garden City, NY, 1976. (j) Edward, P. *Evolution of Infectious Disease*, Oxford University Press, New York, 1994. (k) Panum, P. *Observations Made During the Epidemic of Measles on the Faroe Islands in the Year 1846*, American Public Health Association, New York, 1940. (l) Cockburn, A.; Cockburn, E. eds., *Mummies, Disease, and Ancient Cultures*, Cambridge University Press, Cambridge, 1983. (m) Dobyns, H. *Their Number Became Thinned*, University of Tennessee Press, Knoxville, 1983. (n) Verano, J.; Ubelaker, B. eds. *Disease and Demography in the Americas*, Smithsonian Institution Press, Washington, DC, 1992. (o) Ramenofsky, A. *Vectors of Death*, University of New Mexico Press, Albuquerque, 1987. (p) Thornton, R. *American Indian Holocaust and Survival*, University of Oklahoma Press, Norman, 1987. (q) Snow, D. Microchronology and demographic evidence relating to the size of the pre-Columbian North American Indian population. *Science* **1995**, *268*, 1601–1604. (r) Curtin, P. *Death by Migration: Europe's Encounter with the Tropical World in the 19th Century*, Cambridge University Press, Cambridge, 1989. (s) Hopkins, D. *Princes and Peasants: Smallpox in History*, University of Chicago Press, Chicago, 1983. (t) Drexler, M. *Secret Agents: The Menace of Emerging Infections*, Joseph Henry Press, Washington, DC, 2002.

2. (a) Dixon, S.; McDonald, S.; Roberts, J. The impact of HIV and AIDS on Africa's economic development. *BMJ* **2002**, *324* (7331), 232–234. (b) Whiteside, A. Demography and economics of HIV/AIDS. *Br. Med. Bull.* **2001**, *58*, 73–88. (c) Piot, P.; Bartos, M.; Ghys, P. D.; Walker, N.; Schwartlander, B. The global impact of HIV/AIDS. *Nature* **2001**, *410* (6831), 968–973. (d) Gayle, H. D.; Hill, G. L. Global impact of human immunodeficiency virus and AIDS. *Clin. Microbiol. Rev.* **2001**, *14* (2), 327–335.

3. Tomori, O. Yellow fever in Africa: public health impact and prospects for control in the 21st century. *Biomedica* **2002**, *22*(2), 178–210.

4. Sharma, S. N.; Raina, V. K.; Kumar, A. Dengue/DHF: an emerging disease in India. *J. Commun. Dis.* **2000**, 175–9.

5. Linhares, A. C.; Bresee, J. S. Rotavirus vaccines and vaccination in Latin America. *Rev. Panam. Salud Publica* **2000**, *8*(5), 305–331.

6. Petersen, L. R.; Roehrig, J. T. West Nile virus: a reemerging global pathogen. *Emerging Infect. Dis.* **2001**, *7*(4), 611–614.

7. Solomon, T. Exotic and emerging viral encephalitides. *Curr. Opin. Neurol.* **2003**, *16*(3), 411–418.

8. Goldrick, B. A. Ebola outbreak in southern Sudan: seven have died, but it's contained—for now. *Am. J. Nurs.* **2004**, *104*(7), 29.

9. Ridel, G. M.; Luis, I. R.; Teja, J. Emerging and reemerging diseases: a health problem in the Americas. *Rev. Panam. Salud Publica* **2004**, *15*(4), 285–287.

10. Williams, E. S.; Yuill, T.; Artois, M.; Fischer, J.; Haigh, S. A. Emerging infectious diseases in wildlife. *Rev. Sci. Tech.* **2002**, *21*(1), 139–157.

11. Di Giulio, D. B.; Eckburg, P. B. Human monkeypox: an emerging zoonosis. *Lancet Infect. Dis.* **2004**, (1), 15–25.

12. Mackenzie, J. S.; Field, H. E. Emerging encephalitogenic viruses: lyssaviruses and henipaviruses transmitted by frugivorous bats. *Arch. Virol. Suppl.* **2004**, (18), 97–111.

13. Vijayanand, P.; Wilkins, E.; Woodhead, M. Severe acute respiratory syndrome (SARS): a review. *Clin. Med.* **2004**, *4*(2), 152–160.

14. (a) Woolhouse, M. E. Population biology of emerging and re-emerging pathogens. *Trends Microbiol.* **2002**, *10*(10 Suppl), S3–7. (b) Peters, W. Novel and challenging infections of man. A brief overview. *Parassitologia* **2002**, *44*(1–2), 33–42. (c) Harvell, C. D.; Mitchell, C. E.; Ward, J. R.; Altizer, S.; Dobson, A. P.; Ostfeld, R. S.; Samuel, M. D. Climate warming and disease risks for terrestrial and marine biota. *Science* **2002**, *296*(5576), 2158–2162. (d) Lee, L. M.; Henderson, D. K. Emerging viral infections. *Curr. Opin. Infect. Dis.* **2001**, *14*(4), 467–480. (e) Bengis, R. G.; Kock, R. A.; Fischer, J. Infectious animal diseases: the wildlife/livestock interface. *Rev. Sci. Tech.* **2002**, *21*(1), 53–65. (f) Kombe, G. C.; Darrow, D. M. Revisiting emerging infectious diseases: the unfinished agenda. *J. Community Health* **2001**, *26*(2), 113–122. (g) Daszak, P.; Cunningham, A. A.; Hyatt, A. D. Anthropogenic environmental change and the emergence of infectious diseases in wildlife. *Acta Trop.* **2001**, *78*(2), 103–116. (h) Mahy, B. W.; Brown, C. C. Emerging zoonoses: crossing the species barrier. *Rev. Sci. Tech.* **2000**, *19*(1), 33–40. (i) Meslin, F. X.; Stohr, K.; Heymann, D. Public health implications of emerging zoonoses. *Rev. Sci. Tech.* **2000**, *19*(1), 310–317. (j) Daszak, P.; Cunningham, A. A.; Hyatt, A. D. Emerging infectious diseases of wildlife—threats to biodiversity and human health. *Science* **2000**, *287*(5452), 443–449. (k) Cohen, M. L. Resurgent and emergent disease in a changing world. *Br. Med. Bull.* **1998**, *54*(3), 523–532. (l) Morse, S. S. Factors in the emergence of infectious diseases. *Emerging Infect. Dis.* **1995**, *1*(1), 7–15. (m) Nichol, S. T.; Arikawa, J.; Kawaoka, Y. Emerging viral diseases. *Proc. Natl. Acad. Sci. USA* **2000**, *97*(23), 12411–12412. (n) Wilson, M. E. The traveller and emerging infections: sentinel, courier, transmitter. *J. Appl. Microbiol.* **2003**, *94* (Suppl.), 1S–11S.

15. (a) Rice, L. B. Emergence of vancomycin-resistant enterococci. *Emerging Infect. Dis.* **2001**, *7*(2), 183–187. (b) Mah, M. W.; Memish, Z. A. Antibiotic resistance. An impending crisis. *Saudi Med. J.* **2000**, *21*(12), 1125–1129. (c) Farmer, P. Social inequalities and emerging infectious diseases. *Emerging Infect. Dis.* **1996**, *2*, 259–269.

16. (a) Fitch, J. P.; Raber, E.; Imbro, D. R. Technology challenges in responding to biological or chemical attacks in the civilian sector. *Science* **2003**, *302*(5649), 1350–1354. (b) Alexander, D. A. Bioterrorism: preparing for the unthinkable. *J. R. Army Med. Corps* **2003**, *149*(2), 125–130. (c) Atlas, R. M. Bioterrorism and biodefence research: changing the focus of microbiology. *Nat. Rev. Microbiol.* **2003**, *1*(1), 70–74. (d) Lane, H. C.; La Montagne, J. R.; Fauci, A. S. Bioterrorism: a clear and present danger. *Nature Medicine* **2001**, *7*(12): 1271–1273. (e) Kwik, G.; Fitzgerald, J.; Inglesby, T. V.; O'Toole, T. Biosecurity: responsible stewardship of bioscience in an age of catastrophic terrorism. *Biosecur. Bioterror.* **2003**, *1*(1), 27–35. (f) Barnaby, W. *The Plague Makers: The Secret World of Biological Warfare*, Vision Paperbacks, London, 1997. (g) Preston, R. *The Demon in the Freezer: The Terrifying Truth About the Threat from Bioterrorism*, Random House, New York, 2002.

17. (a) Guharoy, R.; Panzik, R.; Noviasky, J. A.; Krenzelok, E. P.; Blair, D. C. Smallpox: clinical features, prevention, and management. *Ann. Pharmacother.* **2004**, *38*(3), 440–447. (b) Crotty, S.; Felgner, P.; Davies, H.; Glidewell, J.; Villarreal, L.; Ahmed, R. Cutting edge: long-term B cell memory in humans after smallpox vaccination. *J. Immunol.* **2003**, *171*, 4969–4973. (c) Wright, M. E.; Fauci, A. S. Smallpox immunization in the 21st century: the old and the new. *JAMA* **2003**, *289*, 3306–3308. (d) Lane, J. M.; Goldstein, J. Evaluation of 21st-century risks of smallpox vaccination and policy options. *Ann. Intern. Med.* **2003**, *138*, 488–493. (e) Everett, W. W.; Coffin, S. E.; Zaoutis, T.; Halpern, S. D.; Strom, B. L. Smallpox vaccination: a national survey of emergency health care providers. *Acad. Emerg. Med.* **2003**, *10*, 606–611. (f) Booss, J.; Davis, L. E. Smallpox and smallpox

vaccination: neurological implications. *Neurology* **2003**, *60*, 1241–1245. (g) Blendon, R. J.; DesRoches, C. M.; Benson, J. M.; Herrmann, M. J.; Taylor–Clark, K.; Weldon, K. J. The public and the smallpox threat. *N. Engl. J. Med.* **2003**, *348*, 426–432. (h) Neff, J. M.; Lane, J. M.; Fulginiti, V. A.; Henderson, D. A. Contact vaccinia—transmission of vaccinia from smallpox vaccination. *JAMA* **2002**, *288*, 1901–1905. (i) Halloran, M. E.; Longini, I. M. Jr.; Nizam, A.; Yang, Y. Containing bioterrorist smallpox. *Science* **2002**, *298*, 1428–1432. (j) Committee on Infectious Diseases. Smallpox vaccine. *Pediatrics* **2002**, *110*, 841–845. (k) Poland, G. A.; Neff, J. M. Smallpox vaccine: problems and prospects. *Immunol. Allergy Clin. North Am.* **2003**, *23*(4): 731–743. (l) Henderson, D. A.; Inglesby, T. V.; Bartlett, J. G.; Ascher, M. S.; Eitzen, E.; Jahrling, P. B.; Hauer, J.; Layton, M.; McDade, J.; Osterholm, M. T.; O'Toole, T.; Parker, G.; Perl, T.; Russell, P. K.; Tonat, K. Smallpox as a biological weapon: medical and public health management. Working Group on Civilian Biodefense. *JAMA* **1999**, *281*(22), 2127–2137. (m) Mayr, A. Smallpox vaccination and bioterrorism with pox viruses. *Comp. Immunol. Microbiol. Infect. Dis.* **2003**, *26*(5–6), 423–430.

18. (a) Finkel, E. Australia. Engineered mouse virus spurs bioweapon fears. *Science* **2001** (Jan. 26), *291*(5504), 585. (b) Jackson, R. J.; Ramsay, A. J.; Christensen, C. D.; Beaton, S.; Hall, D. F.; Ramshaw, I. A. Expression of mouse interleukin-4 by a recombinant ectromelia virus suppresses cytolytic lymphocyte responses and overcomes genetic resistance to mousepox. *J. Virol.* **2001**, *75*(3), 1205–1210.

BOOKS

Committee on R&D Needs for Improving Civilian Medical Response to Chemical and Biological Terrorism Incidents. *Chemical and Biological Terrorism: Research and Development to Improve Civilian Medical Response*, Institute of Medicine, National Academy Press, Washington, DC, 1999.

Division of Health Science[s] Policy, Institute of Medicine [and] Board on Environmental Studies and Toxicology, Commission on Life Sciences, National Research Council. *Improving Civilian Medical Response to Chemical or Biological Terrorist Incidents Interim Report on Current Capabilities*, National Academy Press, Washington, DC, 1998.

Ellison, D. H. *Emergency Action for Chemical and Biological Warfare Agents*, CRC Press, Boca Raton, FL, 1999.

Layne, S. P.; Beugelsdijk, T. J.; and Patel, C. K. N. eds. *Firepower in the Lab: Automation in the Fight Against Infectious Diseases and Bioterrorism*, Joseph Henry Press, Washington. DC, 2001.

Miller, J.; Engelberg, S.; Broad, W. *Germs: Biological Weapons and America's Secret War,* Simon & Schuster, New York, 2001.

Osterholm, M. T.; Schwartz, J. *Living Terrors: What America Needs to Know to Survive the Coming Bioterrorist Catastrophe*, Delacorte Press, New York, 2000.

JOURNAL ARTICLES

Anon. How would you handle a terrorist act involving weapons of mass destruction? *ED Management* **1999**, *11*(11), 121–24.

Arnon, S. S. et al. Botulinum toxin as a biological weapon: medical and public health management. *JAMA* **2001**, *285*(8), 1059–1070.

Bravata, D. M. et al. Systematic review: surveillance systems for early detection of bioterrorism-related diseases. *Ann. Intern. Med.* **2004** (Jun 1), *140*(11), 910–922 (review).

Buehler, J.W. et al. Framework for evaluating public health surveillance systems for early detection of outbreaks: recommendations from the CDC Working Group. *MMWR Recomm. Rep.* **2004** (May 7), *53*(RR-5), 1–11.

Dennis, D. T. et al. Tularemia as a biological weapon: medical and public health management. *JAMA* **2001**, *285* (21), 2763–2773.

Franz, D. R. et al. Clinical recognition and management of patients exposed to biological warfare agents. *Clin. Lab. Med.* **2001**, *21*(3), 435–473.

Henderson, D. A. et al. Smallpox as a biological weapon: medical and public health management. *JAMA* **1999**, *281*(22), 2127–2137.

Inglesby, T. V. et al. Plague as a biological weapon: medical and public health management. *JAMA* **2000**, *283*(17), 2281–2290.

Inglesby, T. V. et al. Anthrax as a biological weapon: medical and public health management. *JAMA* **1999**, *281*(18), 1735–1745.

Khan, A. S. et al. Precautions against biological and chemical terrorism directed at food and water supplies. *Public Health Rep.* **2001**, *116*(1), 3–14.

Kortepeter, M. G. et al. Bioterrorism. *J. Environ. Health* **2001**, *63*(6), 21–24.

MacIntyre, A. G. et al. Weapons of mass destruction events with contaminated casualties. Effective planning for health care facilities. *JAMA* **2000**, *283*(2), 242–249.

Moser, R. Jr. et al. Preparing for expected bioterrorism attacks. *Mil. Med.* **2001**, *166*(5), 369–374.

Raber, E. et al. Decontamination issues for chemical and biological warfare agents: how clean is clean enough? *Int. J. Environ. Health Res.* **2001**, *11*(2), 128–148.

Rotz, L. D. et al. Report summary: public health assessment of potential biological terrorism agents. *Emerging Infect. Dis.* **2002** (Feb.), *8*(2), 225–230.

U.S. Department of Health & Human Services, Centers for Disease Control and Prevention. Recommendations and Reports. Biological and chemical terrorism: strategic plan for preparedness and response. Recommendations of the CDC Strategic Planning Workgroup. *MMWR* **2000** (Apr. 21), *49*(RR-4), 1–14.

WWW SITES

Biodefense Digital Library and Collaboratory
    http://www.biodefenseeducation.org/
Center for Infectious Disease Research & Policy, University of Minnesota
    http://www.cidrap.umn.edu/cidrap/content/bt/bioprep/index.html
Center for Nonproliferation Studies. Monterey Institute of International Studies
    http://www.cns.miis.edu/research/cbw/tech.htm
Emerging Infectious Diseases
    http://www.cdc.gov/ncidod/eid/index.htm

Federal Emergency Management Agency

   `http://www.fema.gov/hazards/terrorism/terror.shtm`

General Services Administration. FirstGov®

   `http://www.firstgov.gov/Topics/Usgresponse.shtml`

Health Sciences Library System. University of Pittsburgh

   `http://www.hsls.pitt.edu/bioterrorism/citations.html`

   `http://www.hsls.pitt.edu/guides/internet/terror`

Henry L. Stimson Center

   `http://www.stimson.org/?SN=CB2001112953`

Johns Hopkins University

   `http://www.hopkins-biodefense.org/`

National Institute of Allergy and Infectious Diseases

   `http://www.niaid.nih.gov/`

   `http://www.niaid.nih.gov/publications/bioterrorism.html`

   `http://www2.niaid.nih.gov/biodefense/`

National Technical Information Service

   `http://www.ntis.gov/hs/index.asp`

Occupational Safety and Health Administration

   `http://www.osha-slc.gov/SLTC/emergencypreparedness/biologi-`
     `cal_sub.html`

   `http://www.osha-slc.gov/SLTC/emergencypreparedness/index.html`

Public Broadcasting System. NOVA Online

   `http://www.pbs.org/wgbh/nova/bioterror/`

SIPRI—Stockholm International Peace Research Institute

   `http://projects.sipri.se/cbw/`

St. Louis University. School of Public Health

   `http://www.slu.edu/colleges/sph/bioterrorism/`

Stimson Center Report No. 35

   `http://www.stimson.org/cbw/pubs.cfm?id=12`

U.S. Centers for Disease Control and Prevention

   `http://www.bt.cdc.gov/Agent/Agentlist.asp`

U.S. Department of State. Fact Sheet

   `http://travel.state.gov/cbw.html`

Vector-borne Diseases and Climate Change

   `http://www.ciesin.org/TG/HH/veclev2.html`

Virology Websites

   `http://www.tulane.edu/%7Edmsander/garryfavwebindex.html`

WHO: Emerging and Other Communicable Diseases

   `http://www.who.int/csr/don/en/`

EMERGING
EID Online

INFECTIOUS DISEASES

A Peer-Reviewed Journal Tracking and Analyzing Disease Trends   Vol.8, No.10, October 2002

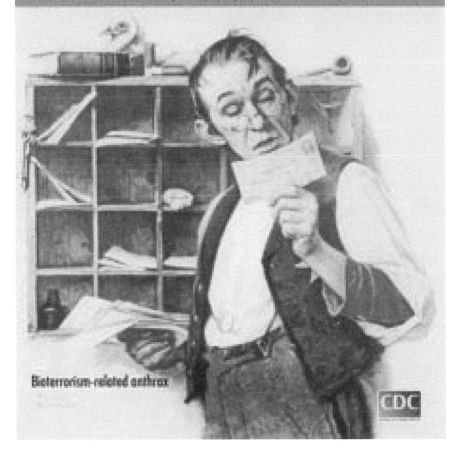

Bioterrorism-related anthrax

CDC

CHAPTER 2

Viral Bioterrorism and Antiviral Countermeasures

MIKE BRAY

Biodefense Clinical Research Branch, Office of Clinical Research, National Institute of Allergy and Infectious Diseases, National Institutes of Health

2.1 INTRODUCTION

Emerging pathogens and the threat of bioterrorism are inherent elements of modern civilization. A variety of activities, including the expansion of human populations into new geographical areas, may result in contact with novel microbes and their rapid distribution by global transportation systems. Modern science has also developed "dual use" technologies that are routinely employed to cultivate microorganisms for benign purposes, such as vaccine development, but could also be used to produce them with malicious intent.[1] Terrorists have not yet released a pathogenic virus, but the potentially devastating consequences of such an event make it essential to recognize our vulnerability and develop effective countermeasures. Since some emerging viruses could potentially be employed as weapons, an enhanced ability to detect and control natural disease outbreaks will also strengthen our defenses against terrorism.

The unpredictable nature of the bioterror threat poses major challenges for antiviral drug discovery. Most of the licensed antiviral medications that have been developed over the past three decades are being used to treat chronic infections, such as those caused by herpesviruses or the human immunodeficiency virus, that are transmitted between humans by pathways other than the respiratory route. By contrast, antiviral drugs are now needed to deal with an entirely different set of viruses that cause acute severe disease and may be deliberately released as infectious aerosols. Fortunately, drug development also provides a model for defense against acute illness caused by airborne viruses, in the form of aerosolized (zanamivir) and oral medications (oseltamivir, amantadine) for the prevention and

Antiviral Drug Discovery for Emerging Diseases and Bioterrorism Threats. Edited by Paul F. Torrence
Copyright © 2005 John Wiley & Sons, Inc.

treatment of influenza.[2] Self-administration of one of these drugs, beginning before or after exposure to a flu patient, can protect against the initiation of infection, restrict viral dissemination, and block further transmission. Similar approaches are being evaluated for smallpox[3] and are needed for defense against other threat agents, particularly those RNA viruses for which we currently lack any effective treatment.

This chapter provides basic information about the threat of viruses as terrorist weapons. It begins with a general description of viruses classified as Category A, B, and C priority pathogens by the National Institute of Allergy and Infectious Diseases (NIAID).[4] It then provides a brief overview of the potential of micro-organisms for use as weapons, based on past military studies, and notes the contrast between biowarfare and bioterrorism. It then examines how viral cytopathic effects, suppression of innate and adaptive immunity, and intense inflammatory responses to infection all contribute to the severity of illness and may be targets for therapeutic intervention. The chapter concludes with a discussion of the potential roles of antiviral drugs and host response modifiers in defense against a bioterror attack.

2.2 CATEGORY A, B, AND C VIRUSES

Until recently, lists of "threat agents" were based on data from military biowarfare research carried out by the United States and other countries beginning in the 1930s.[5,6] Those programs demonstrated that a number of microbes posed a threat as biological weapons, since they could be produced in large quantity and were stable and highly infectious as small-particle aerosols. Because such analyses assumed that biological warfare would be conducted by organized military forces, risk assessments focused on the potential of various microorganisms for use against troops on the battlefield or for broad-area delivery from the air.

The terror attacks of 2001 have now made it clear that military forces do not hold a monopoly on violence, and that civilian populations must also be protected against the deliberate release of biological agents. In particular, the experience of the anthrax-containing letters demonstrated that even a small-scale release of a virulent pathogen can have a massive psychological impact and impose a huge economic cost. Although there is concern that terrorists might be provided with infectious agents by state-sponsored laboratories, or could benefit from the technical expertise of former military biowarfare experts, it is recognized that virulent pathogens could also be obtained from sources in nature or during disease outbreaks. This new perspective has led to the development of revised classification schemes that recognize a broad range of microbial threats. The lists generated by the Centers for Disease Control and Prevention[7] and by NIAID[4] (Table 2.1) include both "traditional" military bioweapons and a variety of emerging pathogens and stratifies them as Category A, B, or C agents.

Category A pathogens are those that would produce the greatest impact if used in a bioterror attack, by having the potential for widespread dissemination, by causing

TABLE 2.1   NIAID Category A, B, and C Priority Viral Pathogens

Category A

Variola major (smallpox) and other poxviruses
Viral hemorrhagic fevers
   Arenaviruses
      Lymphocytic choriomeningitis, Junin, Machupo, Guanarito
      Lassa fever
   Bunyaviruses
      Hantaviruses
      Rift Valley fever
   Flaviviruses
      Dengue
   Filoviruses
      Ebola
      Marburg

Category B

Food-and waterborne pathogens
   Caliciviruses
   Hepatitis A
Additional viral encephalitides
   West Nile virus
   La Crosse virus
   California encephalitis virus
   Venezuelan, eastern, western equine encephalitis virus
   Japanese encephalitis virus
   Kyasanur Forest disease virus

Category C

Emerging infectious disease threats such as Nipah virus and additional
      Hantaviruses
Tickborne hemorrhagic fever viruses
   Crimean-Congo hemorrhagic fever virus
Tickborne encephalitis viruses
Yellow fever
Influenza
Rabies

Source: The NIAID Biodefense Research Agenda for Category B and C Priority Pathogens, available at www2.niaid.nih.gov/biodefense/.

severe disease and death of infected individuals, and by inducing fear, anxiety, and possibly panic in the general population. Variola virus, the agent of smallpox, is widely perceived to pose the greatest danger, since it causes a frightening illness with high mortality, and is the only Category A viral pathogen that is readily transmitted from person to person.[1,8] The group also includes other poxviruses, such as monkeypox, which causes a milder, less contagious disease than smallpox, but still represents a significant threat, because its occurrence as a zoonosis in Africa makes the virus accessible to terrorists. The other Category A viruses are the hemorrhagic fever agents, a heterogeneous group of enveloped RNA viruses that cause severe febrile illness with a high case fatality rate.[9,10] However, even though laboratory studies have shown that these agents are highly infectious when released by aerosol, there is no evidence that they are transmitted among humans by the respiratory route, so they appear to pose little risk of epidemic spread.

The deliberate release of a Category B pathogen would have a lesser public health and social impact than a Category A agent, since even though the former have potential for large-scale dissemination, they generally cause somewhat milder illness with lower mortality rates. The only viruses in this category are a number of positive-sense RNA viruses known as encephalitis agents, since they cause febrile illness accompanied in a variable percentage of cases by infection of the central nervous system. Their natural route of transmission to humans is by mosquito bite, so they would seem to be unlikely bioterror threats, but military research showed that several of them are stable and highly infectious when released by aerosol.[11,12] Their introduction by the respiratory route is expected to cause incapacitating, but generally nonfatal, illness in a high percentage of those exposed. However, aerosol transmission may also result in an increased incidence of neurological complications, since viral infection of the nasal epithelium and olfactory nerve offers a passageway into the central nervous system.

Category C contains a broad variety of pathogens, including a number of emerging disease agents, that pose a bioterror threat both because of their ability to cause moderate to severe illness and because of their potential accessibility to terrorists. Some viruses in this group, such as influenza, are spread naturally from person to person by the airborne route. Others are normally spread by arthropods or through direct contact with virus-containing material but are also infectious when released as aerosols. As noted previously, research aimed at controlling the spread of emerging viruses will help to strengthen defenses against their deliberate release.

2.3   VIRUSES AS WEAPONS

Much of what we know about the potential use of microorganisms as biowarfare agents is derived from military research.[5,6,11] Such studies began in the United States and other countries during the 1920s, but major testing and production efforts did not commence until World War II. As in the case of the atomic bomb, this effort was driven by the suspicion that enemy states were developing biological weapons and the conclusion that the possession of similar armaments was required to deter their use. In fact, only the Japanese army actually released infectious agents during the war (with little apparent effect), but by its end the United States and Great Britain had established extensive research programs, tested a number of pathogens, and prepared and stockpiled large quantities of *Bacillus anthracis*. These programs did not end with the coming of peace, since suspicion was quickly transferred to states on opposite sides of the iron curtain. By the 1950s both the Soviet Union and the United States and its allies had active biowarfare programs.

Military studies focused principally on the preparation and release of aerosolized agents, since this route of attack took advantage of the susceptibility to infection of the immense inner surface of the human respiratory tract and offered the possibility of distributing clouds of invisible microbes across broad areas.[6,11] Most organisms selected for potential use in warfare were bacteria, since their ability to grow in simple medium facilitated bulk preparation. However, a number of viruses, including the agents of Rift Valley fever and Venezuelan equine encephalitis, were already recognized to have potential for offensive use, since they had become notorious for causing outbreaks of illness among laboratory workers following centrifuge accidents or other types of airborne release.[11,12] Their use as weapons was made possible by the discovery that these and other viruses, such as variola, could be grown to high titer in embryonated eggs. Huge incubators were built in preparation for rapid, large-scale production of viruses, but none were ever stockpiled by the U.S. biowarfare program.

Although military research proved that a number of aerosolized microbes could be employed as weapons, it was eventually realized that their use in war would be severely constrained by environmental factors, since adverse winds, rain or snow, rising thermal currents, or other conditions completely beyond the control of military planners could prevent an agent from reaching its intended target. In addition, although the need for a deterrent against enemy bioweapons attacks had been a major justification for the American biowarfare program, by the 1960s the growing arsenal of nuclear weapons was more than capable of performing any retaliatory mission. It was therefore concluded that biological weapons served no useful purpose, and in 1969 the United States ended its biowarfare program. However, offensive research allegedly continued on a large scale in the Soviet Union through the early 1990s[13] and is believed to be continuing at some level in a number of countries.

Although biological weapons were abandoned as impractical by most military forces, they may unfortunately be much better suited to the needs of terrorists. The environmental factors that were a major obstacle to military planning would not be an impediment to a terror attack, since the effects of wind and weather could be avoided, either by carrying pathogens directly to their targets or by releasing them as aerosols in indoor spaces. In addition, terrorist groups may be less interested in attempting to infect a broad target area or causing a large number of deaths than in inducing fear and insecurity through small, unpredictable clandestine attacks. Thus, even if the release of aerosolized Ebola virus into an urban setting, such as a subway station, were to cause only a few cases of disease, such an event might still produce widespread anxiety and extensive social disruption. Countermeasures that would be expected to deter a nation-state from carrying out biological attacks, such as threats of massive retaliation, might be ineffective in dealing with an independent terrorist group or could paradoxically provide an incentive for their use.

2.4   CONTRIBUTIONS OF VIRUS AND HOST TO DISEASE SEVERITY

Effective forms of prophylaxis and therapy are needed for diseases caused by biothreat agents, not only to treat persons exposed in an attack but also to reduce the psychological impact of terrorism by reassuring the public that protective measures are available. Responding to the threat of highly pathogenic viruses will require an understanding of three factors that combine to produce severe illness: (1) viral cytopathic effects, (2) virus-induced suppression or evasion of innate and adaptive immune responses, and (3) intense host inflammatory responses that produce many signs and symptoms of disease and contribute to a fatal outcome.

The first of these factors (direct injury to infected cells) is the most familiar to investigators in antiviral drug development, since most in vitro assays of antiviral activity are based on measuring cytopathic effects. These may result from toxic effects of viral proteins on host cell function, especially protein synthesis; competition for essential metabolites; or injury to the cell membrane caused by the exit of large numbers of nascent virions. Direct damage to cells can be prevented most directly by specific inhibitors of viral replication, which are discussed with respect to individual pathogens in various chapters of this text.

The other two factors that contribute to the severity of illness result from interactions between viruses and the human immune system. The virulence of these agents appears to be based in large part on the fact that they have never adapted to humans but instead have coevolved with various animal species, in which they are maintained through natural chains of transmission. Humans are thus only accidental or "dead-end" hosts, since the outcome of infection is irrelevant to the survival of the pathogen. The progressive adaptation of each virus to its reservoir host has involved accumulated mutations in genes encoding individual viral proteins, which alter the way in which the virus interacts with effectors of innate and adaptive immunity such as macrophages, dendritic cells, and lymphocytes. If such a well-adapted virus happens to enter a human, the same set of viral proteins may interact with corresponding sets of cells in a manner that fortuitously provides it with major advantages over innate and adaptive defenses, allowing it to cause severe or fatal disease.

In addition to their cytotoxicity, the virulence of some bioterror agents results from their ability to overcome initial barriers to infection and spread rapidly to additional cells. Poxviruses, for example, have acquired a battery of genes from their vertebrate hosts over the course of their evolution, and natural selection has retained and modified those that provide a survival advantage.[14] The resulting virus-encoded immunomodulatory proteins suppress innate antiviral responses in a variety of ways. Some are secreted into the extracellular fluid, where they bind cytokines and chemokines, blocking initial stages of the immune response, including the recruitment of inflammatory cells to the site of infection. Other virus-encoded proteins act within the cell to block the production of type I interferon and other cytokines and prevent apoptosis. By contrast, filoviruses encode a much smaller repertoire of proteins but are nonetheless able to suppress type I interferon responses, contributing to their ability to disseminate widely from the site of entry.[15,16] Such strategies have not been defined for most of the other potential bioterror agents, but there is every reason to believe that their virulence results in part from suppression of host antiviral mechanisms.

Once infection has become established, host inflammatory responses may make major contributions to disease severity and, in some instances, may be principally responsible for a fatal outcome. Many viruses that pose a bioterror threat infect monocytes, macrophages, and related cells, causing the release of large quantities of cytokines, chemokines, and other immunological mediators. In the case of Ebola virus, for example, macrophages are the principal target of infection, and their release of interleukin-1, tumor necrosis factor-alpha, and other proinflammatory mediators appears to be the direct cause of the increased vascular permeability, hypotension, and shock seen in severe or fatal illness.[17–19] Infected cells also trigger another major component of hemorrhagic fever—disseminated intravascular coagulation—by producing tissue factor on their surfaces.[20] The fact that a number of other RNA viruses cause a similar syndrome suggests that they evoke similar sets of host responses.

One important pathogen—variola virus, the agent of smallpox—is clearly an exception to the rule that potential bioterror agents do not require human infection for their survival, since the absence of an animal reservoir was an essential factor in its eradication. However, epidemiological considerations indicate that the agent was actually maintained in an animal reservoir until comparatively recent times. Since smallpox is of brief duration and engenders lasting immunity, its continued transmission requires a constant supply of naïve hosts—a condition that could not be met by humans alone until the first cities arose some 5000–10,000 years ago.[14] Smallpox also differs from diseases caused by most other bioterror agents, in that the formation of viral lesions in the respiratory mucosa permits its spread by the airborne route. Transmission is inefficient, however, requiring close (face-to-face) contact, and can be prevented by simple isolation measures. Ultimately, it was the highly accurate poxviral DNA polymerase that made variola virus vulnerable to extinction, since the very low viral mutation rate prevented it from evolving a more secure "survival strategy."

Since host responses to infection are determined by genetically encoded factors, they may not be the same in all individuals. Some persons may thus be able to restrict the replication of a pathogen, while others cannot block its spread and succumb to overwhelming infection. This concept has not yet been widely studied for potential viral bioterror agents, but there is evidence that inherited predispositions affect the outcome of some other infectious processes.[21,22] One of particular relevance is meningococcal infection, which in most persons produces no more than mild illness, but in others causes meningitis, and in a few produces rapidly overwhelming systemic infection (meningococcemia) with severe coagulopathy and shock. Survivors of meningococcemia and close relatives of lethally infected persons respond to challenge with bacterial lipopolysaccharide by producing larger amounts of the anti-inflammatory cytokine interleukin-10 than the proinflammatory cytokine tumor necrosis factor-alpha, while persons who developed only mild infection showed the opposite response.[23] Although Ebola virus infection is less well studied, preliminary evidence suggests that individual variation in cytokine responses may also play a role in determining its outcome.[17,19,24]

Because human infection is not required for the survival of most potential bioterror agents in nature, there has been no evolutionary pressure to ensure their efficient person-to-person transmission. Natural introductions therefore often remain limited to the initial case, and special circumstances may be required to bring about an epidemic. For example, hospitals have played a central role in creating hemorrhagic fever outbreaks, by bringing undiagnosed patients into close physical contact with susceptible individuals. The most dramatic instances have involved Ebola virus, which is transmitted only through direct contact with virus-containing body fluids.[25-27] Large outbreaks have occurred in African medical facilities when doctors, nurses, and family members caring for an Ebola patient transferred virus from their own contaminated hands to their own mouth or eyes and to other persons. In some cases, reuse of contaminated syringes has caused the rapid spread of infection. Other highly virulent viruses, such as the agents of Crimean-Congo hemorrhagic fever and Lassa fever, also spread primarily in hospital settings.[9,10] Once the causative agent has been identified, outbreaks can be brought to an end byinstituting barrier nursing methods and universal precautions in specimen handling.[28]

2.5   POTENTIAL ROLES FOR ANTIVIRAL THERAPY IN BIODEFENSE

Antiviral drugs and host response modifiers could be used in a variety of ways in response to a bioterror attack. The most obvious need is to treat people who have become ill; however, the efficacy of therapy may be limited in persons who have already developed extensive tissue damage and intense host inflammatory responses. By contrast, medications may be much more effective if used to prevent disease in those who have been exposed to a pathogen but have not yet become ill. As noted earlier, such postexposure prophylaxis is highly effective in controlling the spread of influenza. In order for the same approach to be used in biodefense, it will first be necessary to confirm that a pathogen has been released and to identify persons who have been exposed to it. Early recognition of a bioterror attack could occur in several ways: through direct detection of aerosolized material by air monitoring systems, acquisition of information through intelligence methods, or rapid diagnosis of the first persons to become ill. An important prophylactic role for antiviral drugs in such a setting would be to protect health care workers treating victims of the attack.

Efforts are currently under way to develop effective antiviral prophylaxis for smallpox, based on the long-acting antiviral drug cidofovir (Vistide®). Recent studies using murine models of poxviral infection indicate that early prophylactic intervention could supplement vaccination and would be highly effective both in blocking the spread of smallpox and in preventing severe disease. Cidofovir is in clinical use for the treatment of cytomegalovirus retinitis in AIDS patients but is also highly active against poxviruses.[29,30] Although currently administered only by the intravenous route, recent studies suggest that cidofovir could also be delivered by small-particle aerosol to protect the respiratory tract against the initiation of smallpox.[3,31,32] The drug can be made orally available through addition of an alkoxyalkanol side chain, which also markedly enhances its antiviral activity by increasing uptake into cells and prolonging the intracellular half-life from 3 to some 8–10 days.[33,34] A single oral dose of such a compound might provide a prolonged protective effect. Data from mouse experiments suggest that cidofovir treatment would not impair the immune response to simultaneous vaccination,[3,35] but further studies are needed.

The only other licensed antiviral drug with direct application to biodefense is ribavirin (Virazole®), which is active against some arenaviruses and bunyaviruses, but not against the other hemorrhagic fever agents.[36,37] Since ribavirin causes minimal morbidity, its prophylactic administration has been recommended as an initial measure in the management of a bioterror outbreak, when the release of a hemorrhagic fever virus is suspected, but a specific diagnosis has not yet been made.[10] Treatment would be continued or halted once the infectious agent is identified. Similar approaches to pre- or postexposure prophylaxis are needed for other viruses that pose a bioterror threat.

In addition to specific inhibitors of viral replication, medications are also needed to strengthen resistance to infection and prevent the development of damaging host responses. Efforts to bolster resistance have traditionally been based on exogenously administered interferon or its inducers, in the form of double-stranded RNA molecules. However, recent advances in defining the roles of toll-like receptors and other pattern-recognition molecules may help to identify the pathways involved in the action of other immunomodulators, such as CpG oligonucleotides, and facilitate new approaches to antiviral prophylaxis. An especially important target for biodefense is to increase nonspecific resistance to infection in the respiratory tract, so as to block the initiation of viral infection or slow its progression, providing additional time for protective immune mechanisms to come into play.

Since some host responses to viral infection increase the severity of illness, blocking them could be an effective prophylactic or therapeutic strategy. Ebola hemorrhagic fever provides an example of such an approach. As noted, studies in nonhuman primates have shown that the severe coagulopathy seen in this disease results from synthesis of tissue factor by virus-infected macrophages. When an attempt was made to prevent triggering of the coagulation cascade by treating infected monkeys with recombinant nematode anticoagulant protein c2, a number of animals survived this otherwise uniformly lethal infection, and the remainder showed a significant delay in death, compared to controls.[38] Not only did treatment markedly reduce the manifestations of coagulopathy, it also significantly lowered the level of proinflammatory cytokines and decreased peak circulating viral titers in surviving animals by more than 100-fold with respect to the placebo group. The study thus revealed a complex relationship among coagulation, inflammation, and viral replication and demonstrated that the "natural" response of a primate host to Ebola virus permits high levels of viral replication, while modification of that response may lead to more effective control of infection.

2.6   CONCLUSION

New medications are needed to prevent and treat the severe acute infections caused by viral agents of bioterrorism. Not only will development of effective therapy benefit victims of an attack, but it will help to reduce its psychological impact, by reassuring the general public that effective countermeasures are available. Inhibitors of viral replication are needed to block viral cytopathic effects. In addition, because these pathogens are able to overcome innate antiviral mechanisms and elicit damaging inflammatory responses, modification of virus–host interactions may also be an effective therapeutic strategy. Such approaches may prove most beneficial in preventing disease in persons who have been exposed to a bioterror agent but have not yet become ill.

REFERENCES

1. Henderson, D. A. The looming threat of bioterrorism. *Science* **1999**, *283*, 1279–1282.

2. Monto, A. The role of antivirals in the control of influenza. *Vaccine* **2003**, *21*, 1796–1800.

3. Bray, M; Roy, C. J. Antiviral prophylaxis of smallpox. *J. Antimicrob. Chemother.* **2004**, *54*, 1–5.

4. www.niaid.nih.gov/biodefense.

5. Eitzen, E. M. Use of biological weapons. In *Textbook of Military Medicine*, Office of the Surgeon General, Department of the Army, Washington, DC, 1997, pp. 437–450.

6. Eitzen, E. M.; Takafuji, E. Historical overview of biological warfare. In *Textbook of Military Medicine*, Office of the Surgeon General, Department of the Army, Washington, DC, 1997, pp. 415–436.

7. Rotz, L.; Khan, A.; Lillibridge, S. R.; Ostroff, S. M.; Hughes, J. M. Public health assessment of potential biological terrorism agents. *Emerging Infect. Dis.* **2002**, *8*, 225–229.

8. Henderson, D; Inglesby, T.; Bartlett, J. G.; Ascher, M. S.; Eitzen, E.; Jahrling, P. B.; Hauer, J.; Layton, M; McDade, J.; Osterholm, M. T.; O'Toole, T.; Parker, G.; Perl, T.; Russell, P. K.; Tonat, K. Smallpox as a biological weapon: medical and public health management. *JAMA* **1999**, *281*, 2127–2137.

9. Jahrling, P. B. Viral hemorrhagic fevers. In *Textbook of Military Medicine*, Office of the Surgeon General, Department of the Army, Washington, DC, 1997, pp. 591–602.

10. Borio, L.; Inglesby, T.; Peters, C. J.; Schmaljohn, A. L.; Hughes, J. M.; Jahrling, P. B.; Ksiazek, T.; Johnson, K. M.; Meyerhoff, A.; O'Toole, T.; Ascher, M. S.; Bartlett, J.; Breman, J. G.; Eitzen, E. M. Jr.; Hamburg, M.; Hauer, J.; Henderson, D. A.; Johnson, R. T.; Kwik, G.; Layton, M.; Lillibridge, S.; Nabel, G. J.; Osterholm, M. T.; Perl, T. M.; Russell, P.; Tonat, K.; Working Group on Civilian Biodefense. Hemorrhagic fever viruses as biological weapons—medical and public health management. *JAMA* **2002**, *287*, 2391–2405.

11. Franz, D.; Jahrling, P. B; McClain, D. J.; Hoover, D. L.; Byrne, W. R.; Pavlin, J. A.; Christopher, G. W.; Cieslak, T. J.; Friedlander, A. M.; Eitzen, E. M. Jr. Clinical recognition and management of patients exposed to biological warfare agents. *JAMA* **1997**, *278*, 399–411.

12. Smith, J.; Davis, K. Viral encephalitides. In *Textbook of Military Medicine*, Office of the Surgeon General, Department of the Army, Washington, DC, 1997, pp. 561–589.

13. Alibek, J.; Handelman, S. *Biohazard*. Random House, New York, 1999.

14. Bray, M.; Buller, R. M. L. Looking back at smallpox. *Clin. Infect. Dis.* **2004**, *38*, 882–890.

15. Basler, C. F.; Wang, X.; Muhlberger, E.; Volchkov, V.; Paragas, J.; Klenk, H. D.; Garcia-Sastre, A.; Palese, P. The Ebola virus VP35 protein functions as a type I IFN antagonist. *Proc. Natl. Acad. Sci. USA* **2000**, *97*, 12289–12294.

16. Basler, C. F.; Mikulasova, A.; Martinez-Sobrido, L.; Paragas, J.; Muhlberger, E.; Bray, M.; Klenk, H. D.; Palese, P.; Garcia-Sastre, A. The Ebola virus VP35 protein inhibits activation of interferon regulatory factor 3. *J. Virol.* **2003**, *77*, 7945–7956.

17. Bray, M.; Mahanty, S. Ebola hemorrhagic fever and septic shock. *J. Infect. Dis.* **2003**, *188*, 1613–1617.

18. Geisbert, T. W.; Hensley, L. E.; Larsen, T.; Young, H. A.; Reed, D. S.; Geisbert, J. B.; Scott, D. P.; Kagan, E.; Jahrling, P. B.; Davis, K. J. Pathogenesis of Ebola hemorrhagic fever in cynomolgus macaques. *Am. J. Pathol.* **2003**, *163*, 2347–2370.

19. Mahanty, S.; Bray, M. Pathogenesis of filoviral hemorrhagic fevers. *Lancet Infect. Dis.* **2004**, *4*, 487–498.

20. Geisbert, T. W.; Young, H. A.; Jahrling, P. B.; Davis, K. J.; Kagan. E.; Hensley, E. Mechanism underlying coagulation abnormalities in Ebola hemorrhagic fever: over-expression of tissue factor in primate monocytes/macrophages. *J. Infect. Dis.* **2003**, *188*, 1618–1629.

21. Van Dissel, J. T.; van Langevelde, P.; Westendorp, R. G.; Kwappenberg, K.; Frolich, M. Anti-inflammatory cytokine profile and mortality in febrile patients. *Lancet* **1998**, *351*, 950–953.

22. Hill, A. V. The genomics and genetics of human infectious disease susceptibility. *Annu. Rev. Genomics Hum. Genet.* **2001**, *2*, 373–400.

23. Westendorp, R. G.; Langermans, J. A.; Huizinga, T. W.; Verweij, C. L.; Sturk, A. Genetic influence on cytokine production in meningococcal disease. *Lancet* **1997**, *349*, 1912–1917.

24. Baize, S.; Leroy, E. M; Georges, A. J.; Georges-Courbot, M. C.; Capron, M.; Bedjabaga, I.; Lansoud-Soukate, J.; Mavoungou, E. Inflammatory responses in Ebola virus-infected patients. *Clin. Exp. Immunol.* **2002**, *128*, 163–168.

25. Dowell, S. F.; Mukunu, R.; Ksiazek, T. G.; Khan, A. S.; Rollin, P. E.; Peters, C. J. Transmission of Ebola hemorrhagic fever: a study of risk factors in family members, Kikwit, Democratic Republic of the Congo, 1995. Commission de Lutte contre les Epidemies a Kikwit *J. Infect. Dis.* **1999**, *179* Suppl 1, S87–91.

26. Bray, M. Filoviridae. In *Clinical Virology*, 2nd Ed., Richman, D. R.; Whitley, R. J.; Hayden, F. G. (eds.), ASM Press, Washington, DC, 2002, pp. 875–890.

27. Bray, M. Defense against filoviruses used as biological weapons. *Antiviral Res.* **2003**, *57*, 53–60.

28. Anonymous. Infection control for viral hemorrhagic fevers in the African health care setting. Centers for Disease Control and Prevention, Atlanta, 1998.

29. Baker, R. O.; Bray, M.; Huggins, J. W. Potential antiviral therapeutics for smallpox and other orthopoxvirus infections. *Antiviral Res.* **2003**, *57*, 13–23.

30. Neyts, J.; De Clercq, E. Therapy and short-term prophylaxis of poxvirus infections: historical background and perspectives. *Antiviral Res.* **2003**, *57*, 25–33.

31. Bray, M.; Kefauver, D.; Martinez, M.; West, M.; Roy, C. Treatment of aerosolized cowpox virus infection in mice with aerosolized cidofovir. *Antiviral Res.* **2002**, *54*, 129–142.

32. Roy, C.; Baker, R.; Washburn, K.; Bray, M. Aerosolized cidofovir is retained in the respiratory tract and protects mice against intranasal cowpox virus challenge. *Antimicrob. Agents Chemother.* **2003**, *47*, 2933–2937.

33. Kern, E. R.; Hartline, C.; Harden, E.; Keith, K.; Rodriguez, N.; Beadle, J. R.; Hostetler, K. Y. Enhanced inhibition of orthopoxvirus replication in vitro by alkoxyalkyl esters of cidofovir and cyclic cidofovir. *Antimicrob. Agents Chemother.* **2002**, *46*, 991–995.

34. Ciesla, S.; Trahan, J.; Wan, W. B.; Beadle, J. R.; Aldern, K. A.; Painter, G. R.; Hostetler, K. Y. Esterification of cidofovir with alkoxyalkanols increases oral bioavailability and diminishes drug accumulation in kidney. *Antiviral Res.* **2003**, *59*,163–171.

35. Bray. M; Martinez, M.; Smee, D.; Kefauver, D.; Thompson, E.; Huggins, J. W. Cidofovir protects mice against lethal aerosol or intranasal cowpox virus infection. *J. Infect. Dis.* **2000**, *181*, 10–19.

36. Andrei, G.; De Clercq, E. Molecular approaches for the treatment of hemorrhagic fever virus infections. *Antiviral Res.* **1993**, *22*, 45–75.

37. Bray, M.; Paragas, J. Experimental therapy of filovirus infections. *Antiviral Res.* **2002**, *54*, 1–17.

38. Geisbert, T. W.; Hensley, L. E.; Jahrling, P. B.; Larsen, T.; Geisbert, J. B.; Paragas, J.; Young, H. A.; Fredeking, T. M.; Rote, W. E.; Vlasuk, G. P. Treatment of Ebola virus infection with a recombinant inhibitor of factor VIIa/tissue factor: a study in rhesus monkeys. *Lancet* **2003**, *362*, 1953–1958.

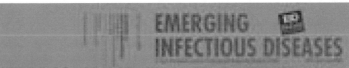

EMERGING
INFECTIOUS DISEASES

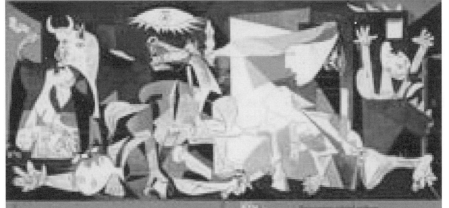

■■■■■■■ CHAPTER 3

Overview of Antiviral Drug Discovery and Development

Christopher K. Tseng

National Institute of Allergy and Infectious Diseases, National Institutes of Health

3.1 INTRODUCTION

The continuous global emergence of new and reemerging/resurging infectious diseases during the last few decades is the cause of serious public health problems. Besides these natural infections, the intentional spread of "deliberately emerging" microbes, such as the 2001 anthrax attack, further complicates the difficult challenge of protecting the public health.[1-4] Although there is no approved antiviral therapy for any of the emerging/reemerging viral diseases, recent advances in biology and chemistry in addition to past drug discovery efforts have provided a promising blueprint for the therapeutic management of these diseases.[5-7]

In the past 30 years, the World Health Organization (WHO) and the Centers for Disease Control and Prevention (CDC) have reported more than 50 new or newly identified pathogens that cause human diseases.[8-10] Table 3.1 shows a list of emerging viral pathogens causing disease in humans and Table 3.2 provides a list of biodefense Category A–C viral pathogens according to the National Institute of Allergy and Infectious Diseases (NIAID) of the National Institutes of Health (NIH). In response to the challenge of biodefense, NIAID has developed a strategic plan to guide the implementation of basic and translational biodefense research and to encourage partners in academia, industry, and other private and public-sector entities to develop biodefense-related diagnostics, therapeutics, and vaccines (see `http://www.niaid.nih.gov/` and `http://www2.niaid.nih.gov/biodefense/`).

Antiviral Drug Discovery for Emerging Diseases and Bioterrorism Threats. Edited by Paul F. Torrence
Copyright © 2005 John Wiley & Sons, Inc.

TABLE 3.1 Emerging Viruses in Humans

1973:	Rotavirus
1975:	Parvovirus B19
1977:	Ebola virus, Hantaan virus
1980:	Human T-lymphotrophic virus (HTLV-I)
1982:	HTLV-II
1983:	Human immunodeficiency virus (HIV)
1988:	Human herpesvirus-6 (HHV-6), hepatitis E virus
1989:	Hepatitis C virus (HCV)
1991:	Guanarito virus
1993:	Sin Nombre virus
1994:	Sabia virus, Hendra virus
1995:	HHV-8
1997:	Avian influenza virus (H5N1)
1999:	Nipah virus, West Nile virus (in U.S.A.)
2001:	Human metapneumovirus
2003:	Severe acute respiratory syndrome coronavirus

3.2 BROAD-SPECTRUM ANTIVIRAL AGENTS

In a series of reviews by De Clercq, compounds with broad-spectrum antiviral activity were classified as follows: inosine monophosphate dehydrogenase (IMPDH) inhibitors, orotidylic acid (OMP) decarboxylase inhibitors, CTP synthetase inhibitors, S-adenosylhomocysteine (SAH) hydrolase inhibitors, immunomodulators, and interferons (IFNs).[11–13]

3.2.1 Ribavirin

In an event of an outbreak of a new emerging viral infection, ribavirin **1** has almost always been the first drug tried. This might be because ribavirin has demonstrated efficacy against a variety of DNA and RNA viruses in cell cultures, in animal models, and in certain clinical cases (see Tables 3.3 and 3.4) since it was first reported in 1972.[14–18] In 1986, it was approved by the U.S. FDA for clinical use only as an aerosol for the treatment of hospitalized infants and young children with

1

TABLE 3.2   NIAID Biodefense Viral Pathogens Categories A–C

NIAID Category A

Variola major (smallpox) and other poxviruses
Viral hemorrhagic fevers
   Arenaviruses
      Lymphocytic choriomeningitis virus, Junin virus, Machupo virus, Guanarito virus
      Lassa virus
   Bunyaviruses
      Hantaviruses
      Rift Valley fever
   Flaviviruses
      Dengue
   Filoviruses
      Ebola
      Marburg

NIAID Category B

Food and waterborne pathogens (caliciviruses, hepatitis A)
Viral encephalitides
   West Nile virus
   La Crosse virus
   California encephalitis
   Venezuelan, eastern, and western equine encephalitis viruses
   Japanese encephalitis virus
   Kysanur Forest virus

NIAID Category C

Nipah virus and additional hantaviruses
Tickborne hemorrhagic fever viruses
   Crimean-Congo hemorrhagic fever virus
Tickborne encephalitis viruses
Influenza
Rabies

severe lower respiratory tract infections due to respiratory syncytial virus (RSV). However, because its clinical effectiveness in the treatment of infants with RSV disease has not been demonstrated conclusively, the American Academy of Pediatrics has recommended that ribavirin therapy may be considered by taking into account the particular clinical situation and the physician's own preference.[19] In 1989, it was approved as an oral formulation in combination with IFN-α in the therapy of chronic hepatitis C virus (HCV).

Inhibition of IMPDH by ribavirin monophosphate was originally identified as the primary mechanism of action of ribavirin.[17,20,21] However, during subsequent studies against various viruses, several possible additional mechanisms have been

TABLE 3.3 In Vitro and In Vivo Activity of Ribavirin

Genus	Virus	In Vitro Activity	Cells	In Vivo Activity	Animal Models
			Arenaviridae		
Arenavirus	Lymphocytic choriomeningitis[54]	Moderate	Vero		
	Lassa[51,55-58]		Vero	Yes	Monkey
	Junin[51,52,59-63]	Yes	Vero	Yes	Monkey, guinea pig
	Machupo[17,51]			Yes	Monkey, guinea pig
	Pichinde[51,54,64-68]	Moderate to yes	Vero	Yes	Guinea pig, hamster
	Tacaribe[59]	Yes	Vero		
			Bunyaviridae		
Bunyavirus	La Crosse[33]	Yes	BHK		
Hantavirus	Hantaan[51,64,67,69-71]	Yes	Vero	Yes	Mouse, suckling mouse
Nairovirus	CCHFV[45,72,73]	Yes	SW-13, CEF, Vero	Yes	Mouse
Phlebovirus	Rift Valley fever[51,64,67,74-77]	Moderate to yes	Vero	Yes	Mouse, monkey, Hamster
	Sandfly fever[64,78]	Moderate	Vero		
	Punta Toro[44,51,54,79]	No to moderate	Vero, LLC-MK2	Yes	Hamster, mouse
			Togaviridae		
Alphavirus	VEE[51,54,64,67]	No to moderate	Vero	No	
	Semliki Forest[51,54,80-84]	No to moderate	Vero	No	

		Flaviviridae			
Flavivirus	Japanese encephalitis[51,64,67,85]	No to moderate	Vero	No	
	Yellow fever[64,67,85-89]	No to yes	Human hepatoma, Vero	Yes (early treatment)	Hamster
	Dengue[46,85,87,90]	No to moderate	Human hepatoma, LLC-MK2, PBL	No	Monkey
	West Nile[47,85,91]	Moderate to yes	Human neural, MA-104, Vero		
		Poxviridae			
Orthopoxvirus	Variola[92,93]	Yes	Vero, LLC-MK2, BSC		
	Vaccinia[49,81,92-95]	No to moderate	HFF, PRK, Vero, LLC-MK2, 3T3, BSC	No	Mouse
	Cowpox[41,49,92-94]	No to yes	HFF, Vero, LLC-MK2, 3T3, BSC	Moderate	Mouse
	Monkeypox[49,92,93]	Moderate to yes	Vero, LLC-MK2, 3T3, BSC		
	Camelpox[93]	Moderate	Vero, BSC		

TABLE 3.4 Experimental Treatments of NIAID Category A–C Viral Agents with Ribavirin

Disease	Virus	Route of Administration	Trial Type	Effectiveness	Site (Year Reported)
Lassa fever	Lassa virus	Intravenous	Open	Effective	Sierra Leone (1986)[55,97]
Bolivian hemorrhagic fever	Machupo virus	Intravenous	Open	Effective (suggested)	Bolivia (1997)[98]
Argentine hemorrhagic fever (AHF)	Junin virus	Intravenous	Open	Effective (suggested)	Argentina (1987)[99]
AHF	Junin virus	Intravenous	Controlled	Effective	Argentina (1994)[62]
Crimean-Congo hemorrhagic fever (CCHF)	CCHFV	Oral	Open	Effective (suggested)	Iran (2003)[100]
CCHF	CCHFV	Oral	Open	Effective (suggested)	Pakistan (1995, 2002)[101,102]
La Crosse encephalitis	La Crosse virus	Intravenous	Open	Effective (suggested)	United States (1997)[103]
Hemorrhagic fever with renal syndrome	Hantaan virus	Intravenous	Controlled	Effective	China (1991)[104]
Hantavirus pulmonary syndrome	Sin Nombre virus	Intravenous	Open	Inconclusive	United States (1999)[105]
Hantavirus cardiopulmonary syndrome	Sin Nombre virus	Intravenous	Controlled	Ineffective (suggested)	United States (2004)[106]
Nipah encephalitis	Nipah virus	Oral, intravenous	Open	Effective (suggested)	Malaysia (2001)[107]

identified.[22–27] These include (1) inhibition of viral capping enzymes by the ribavirin triphosphate (RTP) as illustrated by competitive inhibition against guanylyltransferase mediated 5′-terminal guanylation of vaccinia mRNA[28]; (2) inhibition of viral RNA polymerases in the presence of RTP (e.g., viral polymerases encoded by influenza virus,[20,29,30] HCV,[31, 32] and La Crosse virus[33]); (3) an RNA mutagen that causes a rapidly replicating error-prone RNA virus (e.g., poliovirus[34,35] and Hantaan virus[36]) to experience "error catastrophe,"[37] resulting in reduced overall viral fitness and infectivity; and (4) an immunomodulator to enhance host   T-cell-mediated antiviral immunity through induction of the helper T-cells (CD4$^+$) type 1 (Th1) cytokine expression while suppressing the type 2 (Th2) cytokine response.[38–40] These mechanisms are not mutually exclusive and affect virus-dependent events. It is possible that because of its multiple mechanisms of action, no drug-resistant viral variant has been reported.[17,18] On the other hand, this may result from ribavirin's effect on cellular enzymes that also result in its adverse side effects. In animals treated with ribavirin near its maximum tolerated dosage, immunosuppression (presumably due to IMPDH inhibition) could be induced in the hosts.[41–43] Ribavirin's in vitro antiviral activity varies considerably with the virus and is often dependent on the cell type utilized and the assays/parameters used to measure that activity.[17,44,45] (see Table 3.3). For example, ribavirin markedly reduced the growth of all four types of dengue virus (DENV) in LLC-MK2 cells at concentrations well below cytotoxic levels, whereas it had no effect on DENV replication in peripheral blood lymphocytes (PBLs).[46] When tested against West Nile virus (WNV), it was marginally active using Vero cells, but reasonably active in MA-104 cells.[47,48] It was approximately 40 times more potent in 3T3 cells than in Vero cells against camelpox and cowpox viruses.[49] Differences in the phosphorylation of ribavirin in certain cell types might account for differences in its in vitro activity.[49,50] Like all of the compounds listed in Table 3.5, ribavirin is more toxic to replicating cells than to stationary monolayers.

When administered parenterally to mice, ribavirin had little effect on virus infections of the central nervous system (CNS) induced by Venezuelan equine encephalitis virus (VEEV), Semliki Forest virus (SFV), Japanese encephalitis virus (JEV), and yellow fever virus (YFV).[17,51] Although ribavirin has shown significant in vivo activity in reducing viremia and acute hemorrhagic phase, it was ineffective in treating the encephalitic phase of the diseases due to, for example, Rift Valley fever virus (RVFV), Junin virus, and Machupo virus. These suggested that ribavirin or its active metabolites could not cross the blood–brain barrier (BBB) and reach the brain in adequate concentrations.[17,51,52] However, this situation might be improved by using a lipophilic analogue of ribavirin. For example, intraperitoneal treatment with ribavirin 2′,3′,5′-triacetate significantly increased the survival of mice inoculated intracranially with DENV-2, suggesting that the triacetate analogue may pass through the BBB and act as a prodrug and release ribavirin in the brain.[53]

As summarized in Table 3.4, ribavirin has been used clinically to treat viruses of the Arenaviridae and Bunyaviridae. However, these were not randomized, controlled studies, except the hemorrhagic fever with renal syndrome trial in China and the most recent Hantavirus cardiopulmonary syndrome trial in the United States.

TABLE 3.5 In Vitro Antiviral Activity of Inhibitors of IMPDH, OMP Decarboxylase, CTP Synthetase, and SAH Hydrolase

Genus	Virus	MPA	EICAR	Tiazofurin	Pyrazofurin	6-Azauridine	CPE-C	C³-NPC A	C-c³Ado
				Arenaviridae					
Arenavirus	Lymphocytic choriomeningitis				+[110]				
	Lassa				+[110]				
	Junin			+[59]	+[59]		+[59,82]	+[59]	+[59]
	Pichinde			−[64]	+[110]				
	Tacaribe			+[59]	+[59]		+[59,82]	+[59]	+[59]
				Bunyaviridae					
Bunyavirus	La Crosse			+[64]					
Hantavirus	Hantaan			±[72]		−[72]			
Nairovirus	CCHFV			+[67]	+[110]	+[77]			
Phlebovirus	Rift Valley fever			−[64]	+[110]	+[78]			
	Sandfly fever								
	Punta Toro			+[79]			+[111]		
				Filoviridae					
Filovirus	Ebola	−[86]	−[86]					+[117,118]	+[117,118]

38

Table (rotated in original). Genus/family section headers shown in italics; superscript numbers are reference citations.

Genus	Virus							
Togaviridae								
Alphavirus	VEE							
	Semliki Forest	+[81]	−[81]	+[110]	+[84]	+[82]		
Flaviviridae								
Flavivirus	Japanese encephalitis	+[86,87]	+[86]	+[86,110]	+[85]	+[111]		
	Yellow fever	+[87]	±[64,67]	−[86]	+[85,86]	+[86]		
	Dengue	+[47]	±[64,67,86,119]	+[47]	+[85]	+[47,120]		
	West Nile	+[47]	±[119]	−[47]	+[47,85]			
Poxviridae								
Orthopoxvirus	Variola	+[49]	±[92]		+[85]	+[121]	+[92]	+[92]
	Vaccinia	+[49]	±[81,92,122]	+[122]	+[85,86]	+[82,121,122]	+[92,122–124]	+[92,122]
	Cowpox	+[49]	±[92]	+[92]	+[85]	+[121]	−[92]	±[92]
	Monkeypox	+[49]	±[92]	+[92]	+[85]	+[121]	+[92]	+[92]
	Camelpox	+[49]	+[92]	+[92]		+[121]		+[92]

Activity: +, active; ±, moderate; −, inactive.

Nevertheless, the Working Group on Civilian Biodefense has recommended similar doses of ribavirin to treat patients with clinically evident viral hemorrhagic fever of unknown etiology or secondary to arenaviruses or bunyaviruses.[96]

3.2.2   IMPDH Inhibitors

IMPDH catalyzes the conversion of IMP to XMP, an essential step in the de novo biosynthesis of guanine nucleotides. Inhibition results in lowing intracellular GTP and dGTP pools. Other than ribavirin (a competitive inhibitor), known inhibitors include mycophenolic acid **2** (MPA; an uncompetitive inhibitor), tiazofurin **3**, and EICAR **4**. Their in vitro antiviral activity is summarized in Table 3.5. It was found

that the order and potency of anti-YFV activity of compounds correlates with the activity of the compounds against the enzyme: MPA > EICAR > tiazofurin > ribavirin.[86] MPA is also an immunosuppressant due to its ability to reduce both T and B lymphocyte proliferation via inhibition of IMPDH.[43,108] Combinations of ribavirin and tiazofurin showed synergistic effects in vitro against YFV and JEV but showed additive effects against Korean hemorrhagic fever virus and RVFV.[67] VX-497 **5** is a new reversible uncompetitive IMPDH inhibitor. Its range of activity includes VEEV.[109]

3.2.3 OMP Decarboxylase Inhibitors

This enzyme controls the conversion of OMP to UMP in de novo pyrimidine biosynthesis. Prototypic inhibitors are pyrazofurin **6** and 6-azauridine **7**. Their in vitro activity is summarized in Table 3.5. Despite this activity, pyrazofurin failed to show efficacy against Pichinde virus and VEE in mice and guinea pigs.[110]

6   **7**

3.2.4 CTP Synthetase Inhibitors

This enzyme catalyzes the conversion of UTP to CTP in the last step of de novo pyrimidine biosynthesis. Cyclopentenylcytosine **8** (CPE-C) is a well-known inhibitor of this enzyme.[82, 111] Its in vitro antiviral activity is summarized in Table 3.5.

8

3.2.5 SAH Hydrolase Inhibitors

SAH hydrolase is an intracellular enzyme that regulates biological transmethylation in general. Since many animal viruses require SAH hydrolase in the methylation of the 5′-terminal residue of viral mRNA for forming the cap structure necessary for viral protein translation and replication, this enzyme has been recognized as a suitable antiviral target.[112–116] 3-Deazaneplanocin A **9** (c³-NPC A) and carbocyclic 3-deazaadenosine **10** (C-c³Ado) are two representative inhibitors. Their in vitro activity is summarized in Table 3.5. SAH inhibitors are inactive against togaviruses and flaviviruses.[11] However, they have demonstrated potent activity against Ebola virus in cell cultures and in mice (see Section 3.9).

9   10

3.2.6 Immunomodulators

The antiviral effect elicited by immunomodulators can only be assessed in animal models. 7-Thia-8-oxoguanosine **11** was effective both prophylactically and therapeutically against SFV and Punta Toro virus (PTV) in mice.[79,125–127] 7-Deazaguanosine **12** and 8-chloro-7-deazaguanosine **13** were orally active against SFV in mice.[128–130] IFN induction appears to be the reason for their antiviral activity.

11   12

13

3.3 INHIBITORS OF ORTHOPOXVIRUSES

Variola virus (the causative agent of smallpox) is presumably one of the most attractive pathogens to a potential bioterrorist, as it meets the twin criteria of high transmissibility and high mortality. In addition, survivors are left with disfiguring sequelae. Historically, drugs were tried both for treatment of smallpox and for prophylaxis of contacts but rarely in well-controlled clinical trials. Postexposure

14

prophylaxis with marboran (*N*-methylisatin β-thiosemicarbazone) **14** was hailed as "the most significant advance in smallpox control since the days of Jenner."[131] Yet this influential study was seriously flawed by current standards as most subjects were successfully vaccinated in infancy and revaccinated before receiving therapy. In addition, the study groups were not randomized and subject compliance with the dosing schedule was not adequately ascertained.[132]

Historical data on complication rates from the past will probably not be reliable predictors of future rates should any government undertake the vaccination of large segments of the population to deter or ameliorate the consequences of a potential terrorist use of smallpox. The world's population has changed dramatically since the middle of the twentieth century. Immunocompromised individuals comprise a much larger proportion of the overall population as a result of advances in transplantation and cancer treatment as well as the global devastation caused by HIV. In addition, the incidence of atopic dermatitis has dramatically increased in recent decades. As supplies of vaccinia immune globulin (VIG) are very limited, it may be as or even more important to identify an effective chemotherapeutic agent for the treatment of vaccinia complications as for the treatment of smallpox. Fortunately, as the viruses are closely related, most antiviral agents with activity against one of these viruses is likely to also inhibit the other.

New preclinical data (described below) support use of cidofovir **15** (CDV) for both treatment of smallpox and treatment of complications of vaccination.

15

Accordingly, the Department of Health and Human Services has prepared and sponsors investigational new drugs (INDs) for both potential indications. The U.S. government priority is to have available two smallpox drugs, which operate via distinct mechanisms, and to have two additional drugs in the pipeline.

Concerns about a possible unnatural outbreak of smallpox (such as in a bioterrorist attack) prompted a renewed interest in the search for antiviral agents that might be useful to treat variola, the causative agent of smallpox. However, by an international agreement, any studies involving variola virus can only be performed at CDC and in the former USSR. Because of this restriction as well as the inability of variola (as well as monkeypox) to cause disease in adult mice,[133] routine preclinical assessment of potential anti-variola compounds can only be studied in systems using surrogate viruses, such as vaccinia and cowpox viruses. In 1999, the NIAID and the U.S. Army Medical Research Institute of Infectious Diseases (USAMRIID) established a cooperative relationship in the development of anti-orthopoxvirus agents. In vitro screening is done by both USAMRIID and an NIAID-supported contractor to provide independent confirmation of results. Compounds are further tested in vitro with the collaboration of the CDC against variola itself in their biosafety level four (BSL-4) facility. Compounds with in vitro activity are then studied in rodent models of orthopoxvirus infection. Recently, Huggins and co-workers at USAMRIID described the development of two primate models— monkeypox in cynomolgus monkeys and variola in cynomolgus monkeys—as possible smallpox models to meet the FDA animal efficacy rule for drug licensure.[134] The rule would permit the FDA to rely on animal evidence when a therapeutic agent's safety profile is well understood in humans, the efficacy endpoints in the animal trials are clearly related to comparable benefits in humans, the drug's effect is demonstrated in a species expected to react similarly to humans, and data allow selection of an effective human dose (see http://www.fda. gov/bbs/topics/NEWS/2002/NEW00811.html).

In order to promptly identify an anti-poxvirus drug that could be immediately available in the event of a bioterrorism attack, initial attention focused on currently approved antiviral agents, and CDV was identified as a promising candidate against vaccinia and cowpox viruses.[135,136] CDV was first described in the literature in 1987 by De Clercq and co-workers[137] and was approved in 1996 by the FDA under the licensed name Vistide® as an intravenous treatment for human cytomegalovirus (HCMV) retinitis in AIDS patients.[138,139] Once inside the cells, CDV follows two-step phosphorylation by cellular enzymes: first to CDV monophosphate, CDV-MP (e.g., by pyrimidine nucleoside monophosphate kinase), and then to CDV diphosphate, CDV-DP (e.g., by pyruvate kinase).[140] The latter, structurally analogous to a nucleoside triphosphate, serves as a competitive inhibitor of dCTP and an alternative substrate for HCMV DNA polymerase.[141,142] Incorporation of a single CDV molecule causes a 31% decrease in the rate of DNA elongation by HCMV DNA polymerase; incorporation of two consecutive molecules prevents further elongation.[143] Furthermore, the intracellular CDV metabolites, namely, CDV-MP, CDV-DP, and CDV-MP choline, have very long half-lives and these molecules confer a long-lasting antiviral response of CDV and permit infrequent dosing for antiviral therapy.[144–146]

CDV has broad-spectrum activity against various DNA virus.[138,144,145,147] In cell cultures, it inhibited variola, vaccinia, cowpox, mousepox, camelpox, and monkeypox viruses with EC_{50} values in the range of 6–80 μM.[92,94,135,148–150]

Several different animal models have been used to assess the therapeutic potential of compounds for the treatment of orthopoxvirus infections.[136,151] In earlier studies, tail vein inoculation of vaccinia virus in normal mice or SCID mice was used and drug efficacy was measured by the suppression of tail lesion formation.[122,152] However, inoculation of virus by injection does not simulate the exposure that occurs in natural smallpox infection nor that likely to be encountered in a bioterrorist scenario, namely, infection by the respiratory route. To mimic the natural infection, Bray,[153–155] Smee,[41,95,156–160] and Quenelle[161] demonstrated that aerosol or intranasal infection of BALB/c mice with vaccinia virus or cowpox virus caused the infected animal to develop pneumonia, lose weight, and eventually die from the disease, in many ways mimicking smallpox infection. Collectively, these studies indicated that CDV was highly effective against wild-type virus infections at nontoxic doses when delivered by intraperitoneal, intranasal, or aerosol routes. Mice benefited from as little as a single treatment given a few days before until up to four days after virus exposure. CDV increased the mean day of death in SCID mice but could not protect them from mortality when treatment was discontinued.

SKH-1 hairless mice (immunocompetent or immunosuppressed) readily became infected with either vaccinia or cowpox when virus was applied to abraded skin. Topical treatment with CDV significantly suppressed primary lesion development and satellite lesion formation, whereas parenteral CDV had little impact.[162,163]

Huggins and co-workers reported that cynomolgus monkeys infected with monkeypox either by small-particle aerosol or by intravenous inoculation developed classical poxvirus lesions and pulmonary distress, while one model using intravenous variola produced a similar lesional disease and 33% mortality. CDV prophylaxis was completely protective. CDV treatment initiated as late as 48 hours postinfection still reduced viral load and lesion counts.[134,164]

In a bioterrorist attack the number of exposed individuals is expected to be large; therefore, it may be technically difficult to treat victims with CDV, which requires intravenous administration and careful patient monitoring to avoid toxicity. Because oral bioavailability of CDV is less than 5%, the identification of an orally active prodrug form of CDV is a high priority.

Hostetler and co-workers have shown that the oral bioavailability of nucleosides could be improved by conjugation with long-chain alkoxyalkanols, presumably by increasing oral absorption and cell membrane penetration because of their structural resemblance to lysophosphatidyl choline, a dietary phospholipid.[165] The degree of their antiviral activity against orthopoxviruses in vitro was dependent on the number of atoms in the alkyl or alkoxyalkyl chain, the linker moiety, and the presence of a double bond in the alkoxyalkyl chains linked to the phosphonate moiety of CDV or other nucleoside phosphonates.[148,149,166] HDP-CDV **16** and ODE-CDV **17**, obtained by esterification of CDV with 3-hexadecyloxy-1-propanol and 3-octadecyloxy-1-ethanol, respectively, significantly enhanced both antiviral potency and selective indices over the parent compound in cell cultures.[148–150, 166] Importantly, the potency against variola was also increased by more than 200-fold with the alkoxyalkyl prodrugs.[167] Cellular uptake of ^{14}C-labeled HDP-CDV was many folds greater than that observed with ^{14}C-labeled CDV in human lung

16

17

fibroblast cells.[168] When cells were exposed to HDP-CDV, not only were the levels of CDV-DP (the active metabolite of CDV) more than 100 times greater, but also the intracellular half-life of CDV-DP was much longer than that observed following exposure of cells to CDV.[168]

These alkoxyalkyl esters of CDV have oral bioavailabilities ranging from 88% to 90% in mice and do not concentrate in kidney, the site of the dose-limiting toxicity of CDV.[167,169] They were active orally whether given 3–5 days before or 2–3 days after mice inoculated intranasally with either vaccinia or cowpox virus; even a single dose provided significant protection.[95,170] They also protected mice challenged by aerosol ectromelia virus, the causative agent of mousepox.[150] HDP-CDV and ODE-CDV have been selected for further development supported by an NIAID grant.

Ribavirin **1** is another approved drug whose broad-spectrum antiviral activity also includes orthopoxviruses.[92,122] The anti-vaccinia activity could be attributable, at least in part, to the inhibition of IMPDH by ribavirin 5′-monophosphate,[171] as well as inhibition of the capping of vaccinia mRNA by ribavirin 5′-triphosphate.[28] In one study, ribavirin was a weaker inhibitor than CDV against vaccinia, cowpox, and camelpox in vitro; however, it was comparable to CDV against variola and monkeypox virus.[92] In separate studies, ribavirin showed stronger activity against camelpox, cowpox, monkeypox, or vaccinia viruses in mouse 3T3 cells than in Vero cells. This difference might be related to greater accumulation of ribavirin metabolites in 3T3 cells.[49] It was marginally active against vaccinia and not active against cowpox virus when tested in human foreskin fibroblast (HFF) cells.[148] In animal models, ribavirin protected vaccinia tail lesion formation in mice.[122] However, drug treatment could not protect mice from a high intranasal cowpox virus challenge, although treated animals lived several days longer than those that had received placebos.[41] In the less severe model of cowpox virus infection, a high dose of subcutaneous ribavirin (100 mg/kg/day) completely protected the infected mice from death, and lower doses also improved the survival rate. However, this efficacy in the cowpox model did not translate into similar efficacy in the vaccinia model.[95]

EICAR **4** showed greater anti-poxvirus potency than that of ribavirin.[81,122] However, another IMPDH inhibitor, MPA **2**, was inactive in preventing cowpox respiratory infections in mice, despite its in vitro activity.[49] The failure of MPA to be effective in mice may partly be due to its rapid metabolism to an inactive glucuronide derivative and/or to its immunosuppressive effects.[49] Ultimately, the immune system is needed to clear the virus by the host.[41]

CDV-related acyclic nucleoside phosphonates—HPMPA and PMEG—showed equal or better in vitro anti-orthopoxvirus activity than that of CDV, depending on the cell lines used, whereas PMEA showed inferior activity.[92,94] Other in vitro active nucleoside analogues that presumably target viral DNA synthesis include S2242 **18**, arabinofuranosyl adenine **19** (vidarabine, Ara-A), and certain 5-substituted deoxyuridines (e.g., idoxuridine **20**, IDU).[94,122,172] S2242 was active against vaccinia-induced tail lesions in mice, protected vaccinia-inoculated SCID mice, and effectively treated vaccinia and cowpox respiratory infections in mice,

18   19   20

although it was less potent than CDV.[95,173,174] Ara-A showed efficacy in the vaccinia murine intracranial and tail lesion models.[124] It provided moderate protection to mice infected intranasally with cowpox, but IDU was not effective in this case.[172] However, IDU markedly reduced the number of tail lesions as well as lung viral titers and delayed virus-induced mortality in the vaccinia tail lesion model in immunocompetent mice and in a lethal model for vaccinia infection in SCID mice.[175] 3′-Fluoro-3′-deoxyadenosine **21** also inhibited vaccinia tail lesions in mice.[176]

21

c³-NPC A **9** and C-c³Ado **10**, two potent inhibitors of SAH hydrolase, appeared to have in vitro activity against various poxviruses, except cowpox, in Vero cells.[92,122] Of particular interest, C³-NPC A inhibited several strains of variola virus in submicromolar concentrations.[92] In studies in murine L929 cells, a close correlation was found between these compounds' inhibitory effect on SAH hydrolase and their inhibitory effects on the replication of vaccinia virus.[113,114,177] The combination of SAH inhibitors and ribavirin demonstrated synergistic effects on inhibiting vaccinia virus replication in L929 cells.[178] Pyrazofurin **6** (an OMP decarboxylase inhibitor), CPE-C **8** (a CTP synthetase inhibitor), and trifluridine **22** (a thymidylate synthase inhibitor) showed strong in vitro activity against vaccinia virus.[13,94,121,122]

22

There are some compounds that might target viral RNA rather than DNA. Adenosine N_1-oxide **23** incorporated into the viral mRNA by viral RNA polymerase and selectively blocked vaccinia early gene expression.[179] Marboran **14** possibly caused breakdown of vaccinia virus late mRNA, resulting in a cessation of late protein synthesis.[179,180] Very recently, a series of very potent marboran derivatives has been identified by employing combinatorial library design. Compound **24**, as an example, reduced vaccinia plaques in HFF cells with potency and selectivity 100-fold better than that of CDV.[181]

23

24

Vaccinia DNA topoisomerase has been considered as a potential anti-poxvirus target.[182–184] A topoisomerase inhibitor, novobiocin **25**, inhibited vaccinia replication by blocking virus assembly.[183,185] Other potential antiviral targets include the

25

Z-DNA binding domain of vaccinia virulence factor E3L,[186,187] DNA synthesis processivity factor (A20),[188,189] vaccinia core protein protease,[190] and vaccinia-encoded protein kinases (B1 and F10) and H1 phosphatase.[191,192] For a list of selected poxvirus enzymes that could be potential drug targets, see a review by Harrison et al.[193]

3.4 INHIBITORS OF SEVERE ACUTE RESPIRATORY SYNDROME (SARS)

Recognizing the potentially high mortality and morbidity associated with SARS, in May 2003, NIAID convened a colloquium entitled *SARS: Developing a Research Response* to help identify research needs in SARS research—clinical research, epidemiology, diagnostic, therapeutics, and vaccines—and to help coordinate international research efforts.[194] There are four areas being considered as SARS therapeutic research priorities: (1) drug screening (high throughput screening (HTS) assay and assay of existing compounds), (2) antiviral drug design (identification of viral targets, structural models of viral targets, design and synthesis of candidates), (3) immunomodulation and other therapies, and (4) preclinical (nonhuman primate and small-animal models) and clinical studies. In order to help accelerate the discovery of new leads for effective SARS countermeasures, NIAID offers a "SARS Chip" free to researchers for microarray analysis (see http:// www.niaid.nih.gov). A number of research initiatives and funding opportunities are also published on this website.

In the area of drug screening, NIAID is participating in a project to screen compounds for in vitro activity against SARS associated coronavirus (SARS-CoV). The project was initiated in a collaborative effort with USAMRIID[195] and continued with two domestic institutions under NIAID contracts. At this writing, NIAID is still actively accepting compounds (synthetic compounds and natural products) for screening against SARS-CoV under a confidentiality agreement (see http://www.niaid-aacf.org and http://www.niaid.nih.gov/dmid/viral).

Barnard and co-workers reported that β-D-N^4-hydroxycytidine **26** showed in vitro activity by both cytopathic effect (CPE) inhibition and virus yield reduction assays.[196] Calpain inhibitors, such as calpain inhibitor VI **27**, also were active in the same study. Combined with the data reported in other studies, it appeared that

26

27

28

29

pyrazofurin **6** showed activity in the CPE assay[196–198] but not by using the virus yield reduction assay.[196] Known inhibitors of IMPDH[198] and SAH hydrolase[196,198] were inactive. Other active compounds identified by screening include glycyrrhizin,[197] niclosamide[199] **28**, and valinomycin[200] **29**.

Ribavirin **1** was not active,[196,198,201,202] although some might argue that it would work at high concentrations.[203,204] However, in initial clinical studies, ribavirin offered no apparent benefits.[205–207] Representatives of approved antiviral drugs have also been selected and tested. In one report, except for some IFN preparations, all were shown to be inactive against the SARS-CoV in vitro, including HIV protease inhibitors.[200,204] However, a team in Japan reported that nelfinavir was able to decrease the production of virions from Vero cells.[208] A preliminary uncontrolled open clinical trial in Hong Kong suggested Kaletra (a coformulation of protease inhibitors lopinavir and ritonavir for HIV treatment) might result in a favorable response when administered early.[203,209] A summary of early clinical treatments of SARS can be found in a review by Fujii et al.[207]

Several types of IFN have been used clinically for viral infections; therefore, testing IFNs in vitro and in vivo would potentially lead to the discovery of drugs immediately available for this new disease. However, IFN activity could be species- and cell-specific; therefore, not all of the models are appropriate for evaluation.[201, 202,204,210] As always, in vivo studies might be more predictable for the clinical efficacy in humans.[204] In macaques, it was shown that pegylated IFN-α protected type 1 pneumocytes against SARS-CoV infection.[211] Other than monkeys, potential animal models for general drug evaluation are SARS virus infection in cats, ferrets, hamsters, and mice.[212,213]

The genomic sequence of the SARS-CoV has been published. The initial characterization of the viral genome showed this new virus is not closely related to any of the previously known CoVs,[214–218] but distantly resembles group 2 CoVs.[216,217,219,220] The initial products after translation of the SARS-CoV genome are autoproteolytically processed primarily by the main protease (M^{pro}, also called the 3C-like protease, 3CL^{pro}) to release a number of nonstructural proteins, including the RNA-dependent RNA polymerase[221] (RdRp) and the NTPase/helicase.[218,222] These enzymes are attractive targets for HTS and drug design.[223,224]

Models of SARS-CoV M^{pro} have been constructed based on the crystal structures for group 1 viruses, that is, human coronavirus (HCoV) strain 229E and transmissible gastroenteritis virus (TGEV, a porcine CoV).[225–229] Studies with these models suggested AG7088[225,230] **30** (an inhibitor of HRV 3C^{pro}) and L-700,417[231] **31** (an inhibitor of HIV protease) might be good starting points for drug

30

31

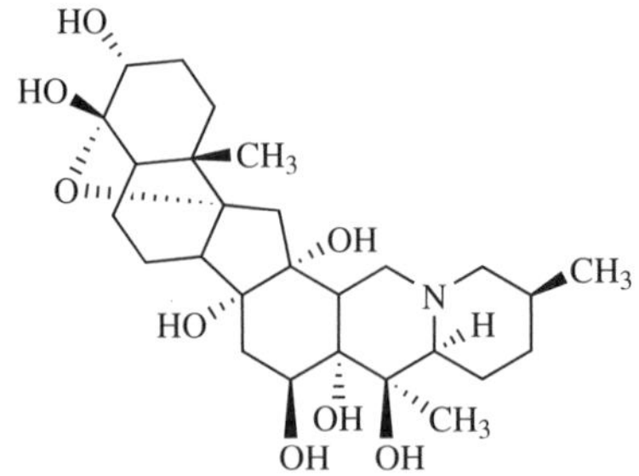

32

design. By employing the CoV M^pro active site in an automatic ligand docking program to map a set of compounds selected from the NCI compound database on a precomputed grid of the protease surface, the nonpeptidyl natural product sabadinine **32** was identified as a hit.[232] Note that selection of these lead compounds relied on homology models based on the structures of HCoV and TGEV. In cells, AG7088 and sabadinine failed to show activity against SARS-CoV[233] and murine hepatitis virus (a mouse CoV),[232] respectively. Molecular models can be improved based on the structural information on the SARS-CoV M^pro, which was published recently.[234, 235] In studies with a cloned full-length M^pro and a truncated form containing only the catalytic domains, a cluster of serine residues near the active site cavity was shown to be susceptible to being targeted by compounds containing boronic acid (exemplified by **33**), providing attractive scaffolds for drug design.[236]

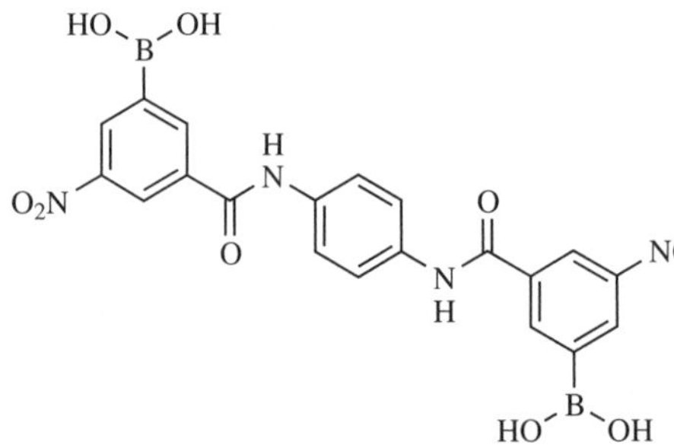

33

A three-dimensional homologue model of the catalytic domain of SARS-CoV RdRp was built based on the polymerases of several RNA viruses.[221] Analysis of the model suggested that active nucleoside analogues would have the C3′ *endo* sugar puckering conformation and contain groups at the 2′ and 3′ positions that are capable of hydrogen bonding.

SARS-CoV entry is mediated by the viral spike (S) protein interacting with a host receptor, angiotensin-converting enzyme 2 (ACE2), leading to membrane fusion and delivery of viral genome to the cytoplasm.[237–239] Recent drug discovery research targeting the S protein includes (1) construction of a three-dimensional homologue model of the ACE2 structure;[240] (2) identification of a peptide, CP-1, derived from the HR2 region in the S2 domain of SARS-CoV S protein to guide the design of fusion inhibitors;[241] (3) identification of human monoclonal antibodies against the S1 domain of S protein;[242] and (4) silencing S protein expression in cultured cells by RNA interference (RNAi).[224,243] Other RNAi approaches targeting different sites on the genome were also reported.[224,244,245]

3.5 INHIBITORS OF FLAVIVIRUSES

JEV, DENV, WNV, Kyasanur Forest virus, and certain tickborne encephalitis viruses are in the *Flavivirus* genus of the Flaviviridae family. In general, the in vitro and in vivo activity of ribavirin against flaviviruses is very weak[119] (see Table 3.3). However, the combination of ribavirin and IFN-α in vitro resulted in significant synergistic interactions against YFV.[89] In hamsters, ribavirin might be effective in the early treatment of YFV.[88] On the other hand, it has been shown to worsen the disease caused by WNV.[246]

IFN-α showed promising results in small open trials,[247] but IFN-α 2a did not affect the outcome in children with JE in a double-blind placebo-controlled trial.[248]

Flaviviral virions are composed of a lipid bilayer with two or more viral glycoproteins, whose fate and functions are governed by the process of *N*-linked glycosylation.[249,250] Blockage of the trimming step of *N*-linked glycosylation by a glucosidase inhibitor, such as *N*-nonyl-deoxynojirimycin **34** (NN-DNJ), has been shown to suppress DENV-2 and JEV in a dose-dependent manner.[251] In addition, in a lethal mouse model of JEV, oral dosing of NN-DNJ reduced the mortality rate.[251]

34

The flavivirus viral genome encodes a polyprotein that is processed into three structural (C, prM, and E) and seven nonstructural (NS1, NS2A, NS2B, NS3, NS4A, NS4B, and NS5) proteins.[119,252,253] NS3 [with serine protease, 5′-RNA triphosphatase (5′-RTPase), nucleoside triphosphatase (NTPase), and RNA helicase activities] and NS5 [with methyltransferase (MTase) and RdRp activities] have been considered to be the optimal targets for antiviral agents.[253,254] The NTPase/helicase associated with NS3 protein of WNV has been purified[255] and assayed, resulting in the identification of several ring systems—imidazo[4,5-*d*]pyridazine (e.g., HMC-HO4[256] **35**), imidazo[4,5-*e*][1,3]diazepine (e.g., **36**[257,258]), benzimidazole (e.g., DRBT[259] **37**), and benzotriazole (e.g., TBBT[259] **38**)—that could serve as starting templates for the development of new helicase-specific antivirals.

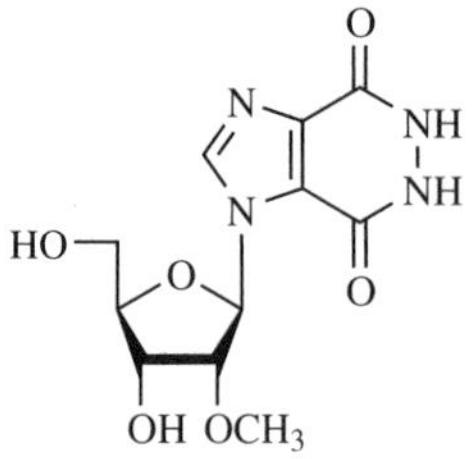

35

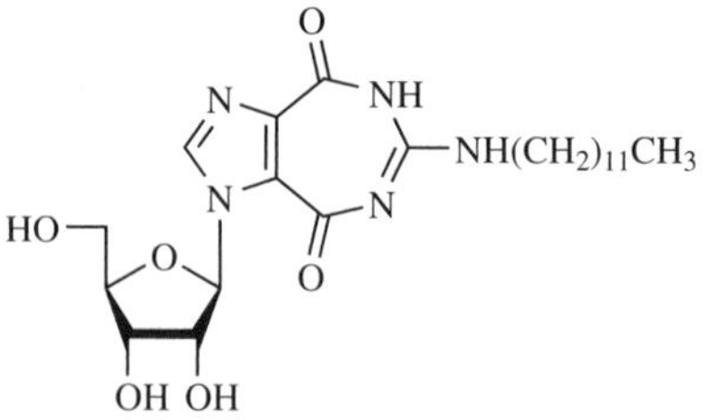

36

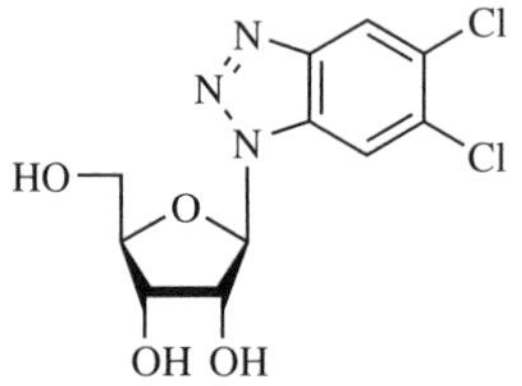

37

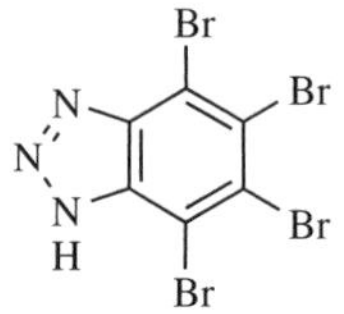

38

Additionally, the crystal structure of DENV NS3 serine protease domain could provide a basis for structure-based drug design.[260]

Utilization of an RdRp assay to evaluate compounds targeted to inhibit RNA synthesis identified POM HPA-23 as having activity.[261] However, this compound has shown significant adverse side effects in clinical trials in AIDS patients. Less toxic derivatives of the drug may have potential for flavivirus infections. Other POMs with in vitro anti-DENV-2 activity were also reported.[262] 2′-Modified nucleoside analogues have been found to inhibit HCV RNA synthesis catalyzed by HCV RdRp. Interestingly, these compounds, exemplified by 2′-C-Me-A **39**, did show in vitro activity against other viruses in the family of Flaviviridae (BVDV, WNV, YFV, and DENV-2).[263]

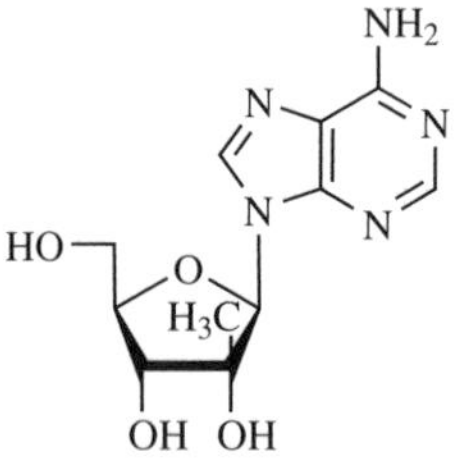

39

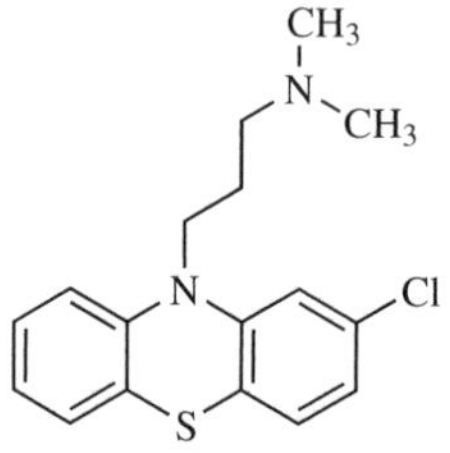

40

JEV is taken up by cells through an endocytic pathway, which was inhibited by pretreatment with chlorpromazine **40**.[264] Bafilomycin A1 **41** (a proton ATPase inhibitor) treatment resulted in the disappearance of acidified compartments in Vero cells and, under such conditions, JEV growth was also inhibited.[265]

Several classes of natural products were reported as having in vitro anti-DENV activity: flavonoids (e.g., glabranine[266] **42**), carrageenans (e.g., 1T1[267] **43**), and

41

42

43

44

45

gymnochrome D[268] **44**. FNQ3 **45** inhibited both JEV RNA and protein synthesis.[269] The antifungal drug amphotericin B **46** was shown to interfere with JEV viral replication and/or the synthesis of viral proteins.[270] The anti-influenza drug amantadine **58** inhibited the replication of DENV in vitro.[271]

46

Antisense oligonucleotides containing modified residues have been employed: modified phosphorothioate oligonucleotides in which the C-5 atoms of uridines and cytidines were replaced by propynyl groups caused a significant inhibition of DENV-2.[272] The antisense oligomer AVI-4020, which contains morpholino backbone, was shown to cross the BBB in infected animals. This drug is currently in a Phase I/II clinical trial for WNV infection.[273]

There have been a number of infectious clones and subgenomic replicons reported in the literature including those of YFV, JEV, DENV (types 2 and 4), tickborne encephalitis virus (TBEV), and WNV.[274,275] (See references cited in a review by Shi.[252]) These reverse genetics systems, full-length infectious cDNA clones, and replicon systems could be utilized to develop cell-based HTS assays to screen chemical libraries for the identification of future novel inhibitors.[252,253,276,277]

3.6 INHIBITORS OF ALPHAVIRUSES

The alphaviruses, eastern (EEE), western (WEE), and Venezuelan (VEE) equine encephalitis virus, of the family of Togaviridae all cause encephalitis in humans. Sindbis and Semliki Forest virus (SFV) have been investigated as models for the study of viral replication. In a review by Sidwell and Smee, the following compounds were listed as having at least moderate efficacy against VEEV and/or SFV-induced encephalitis in mice: ribavirin 5′-sulfamate, 7-thia-8-oxoguanosine **11**, 7-deazaguanosine **12**, poly(ICLC), melatonin, MVE-2, ampligen, and IFNs. IFN-α is currently considered as most useful for therapy in animal models.[278] Ribavirin **1** was somewhat inactive, whereas other IMPDH inhibitors, EICAR **4** and VX-497 **5**, showed in vitro activity against SFV and VEEV, respectively.[81,109] OMP decarboxylase inhibitors, pyrazofurin **6** and 6-azauridine **7**, were also active in vitro against SFV and VEEV, respectively.[84,110] CPE-C **8**, a CTP synthetase inhibitor, was remarkably active against SFV and Sindbis virus in Vero cells.[82] In contrast, adenosine analogues of SAH hydrolase inhibitors are insensitive to togaviruses.[11] 3-Fluoro-3′-deoxyadenosine **21** was inhibitory to SFV and VEEV by an unknown mechanism of action.[54,176]

Entry of SFV into cells requires a pH gradient in the endocytic pathway. This receptor-mediated endocytosis was sensitive to the inhibitors of vacuolar proton-ATPase, for example, bafilomycin A1[279,280] **41** and concanamycin A[281,282] **47**.

47

3.7 INHIBITORS OF ARENAVIRUSES

Arenaviruses are classified as NIAID Category A viruses (see Table 3.2). Ribavirin is the only drug that is known to be of any benefit in the treatment of patients with arenavirus infection (see Table 3.4) but it has been associated with adverse reactions in treated patients.[61,97,99]

Preclinical studies suggested that arenaviruses seemed to be sensitive to inhibitors of IMPDH, OMP decarboxylase, CTP synthetase, and SAH hydrolase[11] (see Table 3.5). Because Pichinde virus infection in humans is not associated with major disease, infection of this virus in cells and in animals have served as safe surrogate systems for the severe human arenavirus hemorrhagic fevers for drug discovery purposes.[65,283,284]

Arenaviruses encode a small (11 kDa) protein with a RING finger motif (Z). Z protein has been shown to drive arenavirus budding[285] and has a strong inhibitory activity on viral transcription and RNA replication.[285–288] Because the Zn-binding domain of several arenaviruses is highly conserved, it has been considered an attractive antiviral target.[289] Several compounds with known activity toward the Zn finger motifs of the HIV p7 nucleocapsid protein were tested in vitro.[289] NSC20625 **48** and NSC624152 **49** were not only able to inactivate both Junin and Tacaribe (a nonpathogenic arenavirus closely related to Junin virus) by direct contact but also were effective in reducing virus yields from infected cells.[289,290] Two azo-based compounds showed different mechanisms of action: ADA **50** was very effective at inactivating both viruses, whereas ANNB **51** inhibited a late maturation stage of the viral replication cycle.[289,291]

Several other antiviral strategies have also been pursued for drug discovery. Because arenaviruses are enveloped viruses, modifications of plasma membrane could affect viral replication. This approach was supported by the demonstration of inhibitory activity exhibited by fatty acids[292] and myristic acids[293] on Junin virus replication. The integrity of the actin microfilaments might be required for optimal arenavirus multiplication as suggested by inhibition of Junin virus in

52

vitro by phenotiazines[294] (exemplified by trifluoroperazine **52**). Lymphocytic choriomeningitis virus (LCMV) was shown to be sensitive to lethal mutagenesis induced by the mutagenic agent 5-fluorouracil[295] and its genome could be cleaved by *trans*-acting ribozymes.[296,297] Recently, α-dystroglycan has been identified as a cellular receptor for LCMV and Lassa virus (both belong to the Old World arenaviruses), suggesting a new target for drug discovery.[298–300] However, New World arenaviruses (Junin, Machupo, and Guanarito) use an as yet unidentified receptor or coreceptor for binding.

Screening in cell cultures identified a variety of classes of compounds with potential antiviral activity: brassinosteroids[301] (e.g., **53**), macrocyclic trichothecenes[302] (e.g., **54**), and 3'-fluoro-3'-deoxyadenosine[54] **21**. Another compound, 2',3'-didehydro-3'-deoxythymidine (stampidine), improved survival in Lassa virus-infected mice.[303]

53

54

3.8   INHIBITORS OF BUNYAVIRUSES

The family of Bunyaviridae is composed of four genera: *Bunyavirus* (La Crosse virus), *Hantavirus* [Hantaan virus, Sin Nombre virus (SNV)], *Nairovirus* [Crimean-Congo hemorrhagic fever virus (CCHFV)], and *Phlebovirus* (RVFV, PTV, sandfly fever virus). These viruses are distributed across the NIAID biodefense categories. As shown in Table 3.4, favorable outcomes were seen when ribavirin was used experimentally to treat CCHFV, La Crosse, and bunyavirus hemorrhagic fever with renal syndrome (HFRS), although the CCHFV and La Crosse trials were not blinded. No definite efficacy was observed in patients with hantavirus pulmonary syndrome (HPS).[105,304] A very recent controlled trial further suggested that ribavirin might not be effective for treatment of hantavirus cardiopulmonary syndrome after onset of the cardiopulmonary phase.[106]

Since these viruses are BSL-3 or -4 agents, this presents a problem for routine antiviral testing. PTV, a phlebovirus related to RVFV, produces nonencephalitic lethal infections in mice. Because this virus presents a lower biohazard (BSL-2), it can serve as substitute in routine drug screening with the caveat that active compounds will have to be checked against the actual target virus eventually.[79,278,305,306] Ribavirin is active against PTV in vitro and is protective when given either parenterally or orally, in single or multiple doses, to PTV-infected mice.[44] In a report by Sidwell et al.,[79] other active compounds included ribamidine, tiazofurin, pyrazofurin, and 3-deazaguanosine. Several immunomodulators, such as poly(ICLC), ampligen, 7-thia-8-oxoguanosine, and IFN-α, were also active.

3.9 INHIBITORS OF EBOLA VIRUS

Ebola virus is classified as a select agent. Because of biosafety and biosecurity concerns, antiviral research has been conducted mainly by USAMRIID investigators. Huggins and co-workers recently established a lethal mouse model suitable for evaluation of prophylaxis and therapy of Ebola virus.[307] Intraperitoneal administration (2.2–20 mg/kg), thrice daily, of C-c^{3}Ado **10** significantly protected BALB/c mice from lethal infection with mouse-adapted Ebola Zaire virus, providing treatment was initiated on day −1, 0, or +1 relative to time of virus challenge.[117,308] Treatment with 2.2 mg/kg initiated on day 3 postinfection still resulted in 40% survival. In another study, a single subcutaneous dose of 80 mg/kg or less of C-c^{3}Ado **10**, or of 1 mg/kg or less of c^3-NPC A **9**, provided equal or better protection, without causing toxicity.[309] One dose of drug given on day 1 or 2 postinfection significantly reduced serum virus titers and resulted in survival of most or all animals. However, drug treatment given within 1 h after infection ("day 0") was less effective. In SCID mice, single or multiple drug treatment suppressed Ebola replication but did not prevent death.[309] The prolonged efficacy of these two SAH hydrolase inhibitors demonstrated a potential useful antiviral strategy in that drug treatment begins early in infection with high but nontoxic doses, in order to hold viral burden below the lethal threshold until the host immune system eliminates the infection.[309] The remarkable antiviral activity observed with these compounds on day 1 or 2 postinfection, but not on the day of viral challenge, suggests that these compounds might have additional mechanisms of action, which contribute to the drug's effect after viral replication has begun, but before widespread dissemination of infection and extensive tissues damage have occurred. c^3-NPC A was shown to induce a massive release of IFN-α when administered to Ebola-infected mice, but not uninfected mice, apparently reversing the virus-induced suppression of the type I

IFN response.[310] However, this effect of IFN stimulation was not observed in similarly treated Ebola-infected monkeys.[118] Treatment delayed the onset of viremia and illness but did not protect the monkeys from death.[311]

In summary, IFN-α is highly effective in cell cultures and in Ebola-infected mice when given as a series of doses beginning on the day of exposure. However, IFN therapy is less effective in primates.[311]

3.10   INHIBITORS OF AVIAN INFLUENZA A VIRUSES

In 1997, an outbreak of H5N1 avian influenza in Hong Kong caused considerable concern about a potential pandemic.[312] Since then, several influenza A viruses of avian origin that cause human disease have been isolated (see Table 3.6). In addition, such a naturally occurring lethal virus as well as recombinant viruses generated in the lab would be potential bioterrorist weapons.[313]

Relenza[TM] **55** (zanamivir for inhalation) and Tamiflu[TM] **56** (oseltamivir phosphate) are two clinically effective anti-influenza therapies approved by the U.S. FDA in 1999. Both drugs are inhibitors of influenza neuraminidase (NA) achieved by structure-based drug design (for further reading, see Tseng and Laughlin[319]). A third structure-based NA inhibitor, peramivir **57** (also known as RWJ-270201 and

55   **56**

BCX-1812), had also been in Phase III trials in Europe. All three compounds showed remarkable antiviral activity in cell cultures and in the mouse model against H5N1, H9N2, and many other avian influenza viruses.[314–317] H5N1 strains are resistant to the traditional influenza drugs amantadine **58** and rimantadine **59**.[312,318]

TABLE 3.6   Recent Human Clinical Isolates of Influenza A Viruses of Avian Origin

1997:	H5N1 from Hong Kong A/HK/156/1997
1999:	H9N2 from Hong Kong A/HK/1074/1999
2002:	H7N2 from Virginia
2003:	H5N1 from Hong Kong A/HK/213/2003; H9N2 from Hong Kong; H7N7 from Netherlands
2004:	H5N1 from Asia; H7N3 from Canada

See http://www.cdc.gov/flu/avian.

57   **58**   **59**

3.11 PERSPECTIVE

Since viral replication closely mimics the host cell's replication machinery, selective drugs should target specific viral events in order to avoid unwanted side effects. Therefore, the complexity inherent in antiviral drug discovery requires interdisciplinary approaches. The toolbox needed for such approaches is outlined in the first major theme of the new NIH Roadmap initiative: New Pathways to Discovery (see `http://nihroadmap.nih.gov/`). It is anticipated that advances in genomics and proteomics (for NIAID bioinformatics resource centers, see `http://www.niaid.nih.gov/dmid/genomes`) should be able to provide new pathways to discover vital targets for rational drug design. Characterization of the targets followed by generation of novel combinatorial chemical libraries coupled with screening assays in high-throughput format should accelerate the discovery of novel potent and selective antiviral agents.

ACKNOWLEDGMENT

The author would like to thank Dr. Catherine Laughlin for her critical reading of the manuscript. Thanks also to Linda Cooney and Darryl Metzler for their assistance in information management.

REFERENCES

1. Morens, D. M.; Folkers, G. K.; Fauci, A. S. The challenge of emerging and re-emerging infectious diseases. *Nature* **2004**, *430*, 242–249.

2. Feldmann, H.; Czub, M.; Jones, S.; Dick, D.; Garbutt, M.; Grolla, A.; Artsob, H. Emerging and re-emerging infectious diseases. *Med. Microbiol. Immunol.* **2002**, *191*, 63–74.

3. Fauci, A. S. Infectious diseases: considerations for the 21st century. *Clin. Infect. Dis.* **2001**, *32*, 675–685.

4. Gomez, L.; Clavel, A.; Castillo, J.; Seral, C.; Rubio, C. Emerging and reemerging pathogens. *Int. J. Antimicrob. Agents* **2000**, *16*, 335–339.

5. Fraser, C. M. A genomics-based approach to biodefence preparedness. *Nat. Rev. Genet.* **2004**, *5*, 23–33.

6. Bronze, M. S.; Greenfield, R. A. Preventive and therapeutic approaches to viral agents of bioterrorism. *Drug Discov. Today* **2003**, *8*, 740–745.

7. Mairuhu, A. T. A.; Brandjes, D. P. M.; van Gorp, E. C. M. Treating viral hemorrhagic fever. *Idrugs* **2003**, *6*, 1061–1066.

8. Kuiken, T.; Fouchier, R.; Rimmelzwaan, G.; Osterhaus, A. Emerging viral infections in a rapidly changing world. *Curr. Opin. Biotechnol.* **2003**, *14*, 641–646.

9. Gubler, D. J. The global emergence/resurgence of arboviral diseases as public health problems. *Arch. Med. Res.* **2002**, *33*, 330–342.

10. Khabbaz, R. F. Emerging viral infections. *Adv. Pediatr. Infect. Dis.* **1999**, *14*, 1–27.

11. Andrei, G.; De Clercq, E. Molecular approaches for the treatment of hemorrhagic fever virus infections. *Antiviral Res.* **1993**, *22*, 45–75.

12. De Clercq, E. Molecular targets for antiviral agents. *J. Pharmacol. Exp. Ther.* **2001**, *297*, 1–10.

13. De Clercq, E. Antiviral agents: characteristic activity spectrum depending on the molecular target with which they interact. *Adv. Virus Res.* **1993**, *42*, 1–55.

14. Huggins, J. W. Prospects for treatment of viral hemorrhagic fevers with ribavirin, a broad-spectrum antiviral drug. *Rev. Infect. Dis.* **1989**, *11* (Suppl. 4), S750–S761.

15. Witkowski, J. T.; Robins, R. K.; Sidwell, R. W.; Simon, L. N. Design, synthesis, and broad spectrum antiviral activity of 1-beta-D-ribofuranosyl-1,2,4-triazole-3-carboxamide and related nucleosides. *J. Med. Chem.* **1972**, *15*, 1150–1154.

16. Sidwell, R. W.; Huffman, J. H.; Khare, G. P.; Allen, L. B.; Witkowski, J. T.; Robins, R. K. Broad-spectrum antiviral activity of virazole: 1-beta-D-ribofuranosyl-1,2,4-triazole-3-carboxamide. *Science* **1972**, *177*, 705–706.

17. Sidwell, R. W. Ribavirin: a review of antiviral efficacy. *Recent Res. Dev. Antimicrob. Agents Chemother.* **1996**, *1*, 219–256.

18. Bray, M.; Huggins, J. Antiviral therapy of haemorrhagic fevers and arbovirus infections. *Antiviral Ther.* **1998**, *3*, 53–79.

19. American Academy of Pediatrics. Reassessment of the indications for ribavirin therapy in respiratory syncytial virus infections. *Pediatrics* **1996**, *97*, 137–140.

20. Wray, S. K.; Gilbert, B. E.; Noall, M. W.; Knight, V. Mode of action of ribavirin—effect of nucleotide pool alterations on influenza virus ribonucleoprotein synthesis. *Antiviral Res.* **1985**, *5*, 29–37.

21. Streeter, D. G.; Witkowski, J. T.; Khare, G. P.; Sidwell, R. W.; Bauer, R. J.; Robins, R. K.; Simon, L. N. Mechanism of action of 1-beta-D-ribofuranosyl-1,2,4-triazole-3-carboxamide (Virazole), a new broad-spectrum antiviral agent. *Proc. Natl. Acad. Sci. U.S.A.* **1973**, *70*, 1174–1178.

22. Tam, R. C.; Lau, J. Y. N.; Hong, Z. Mechanisms of action of ribavirin in antiviral therapies. *Antiviral Chem. Chemother.* **2001**, *12*, 261–272.

23. Reyes, G. R. Ribavirin: recent insights into antiviral mechanisms of action. *Curr. Opin. Drug Discov. Dev.* **2001**, *4*, 651–656.

24. Snell, N. J. C. Ribavirin—current status of a broad spectrum antiviral agent. *Expert Opin. Pharmacother.* **2001**, *2*, 1317–1324.

25. Lau, J. Y. N.; Tam, R. C.; Liang, T. J.; Hong, Z. Mechanism of action of ribavirin in the combination treatment of chronic HCV infection. *Hepatology* **2002**, *35*, 1002–1009.

26. Picardi, A.; Vespasiani Gentilucci, U.; Zardi, E. M.; D'Avola, D.; Amoroso, A.; Afeltra, A. The role of ribavirin in the combination therapy of hepatitis C virus infection. *Curr. Pharm. Des.* **2004**, *10*, 2081–2092.

27. Crotty, S.; Cameron, C.; Andino, R. Ribavirin's antiviral mechanism of action: lethal mutagenesis? *J. Mol. Med.* **2002**, *80*, 86–95.

28. Goswami, B. B.; Borek, E.; Sharma, O. K.; Fujitaki, J.; Smith, R. A. The broad spectrum antiviral agent ribavirin inhibits capping of mRNA. *Biochem. Biophys. Res. Commun.* **1979**, *89*, 830–836.

29. Wray, S. K.; Smith, R. H. A.; Gilbert, B. E.; Knight, V. Effects of selenazofurin and ribavirin and their 5'-triphosphates on replicative functions of influenza A and influenza B viruses. *Antimicrob. Agents Chemother.* **1986**, *29*, 67–72.

30. Wray, S. K.; Gilbert, B. E.; Knight, V. Effect of ribavirin triphosphate on primer generation and elongation during influenza virus transcription in vitro. *Antiviral Res.* **1985**, *5*, 39–48.

31. Maag, D.; Castro, C.; Hong, Z.; Cameron, C. E. Hepatitis C virus RNA-dependent RNA polymerase (NS5B) as a mediator of the antiviral activity of ribavirin. *J. Biol. Chem.* **2001**, *276*, 46094–46098.

32. Hong, Z.; Ferrari, E.; Wright-Minogue, J.; Skelton, A.; Glue, P.; Zhong, W.; Lau, J. Direct antiviral activity of ribavirin: hepatitis C virus NS5B polymerase incorporates ribavirin triphosphate into nascent RNA products. *Hepatology* **1999**, *30*, 773.

33. Cassidy, L. F.; Patterson, J. L. Mechanism of La Crosse virus inhibition by ribavirin. *Antimicrob. Agents Chemother.* **1989**, *33*, 2009–2011.

34. Crotty, S.; Maag, D.; Arnold, J. J.; Zhong, W. D.; Lau, J. Y. N.; Hong, Z.; Andino, R.; Cameron, C. E. The broad-spectrum antiviral ribonucleoside ribavirin is an RNA virus mutagen. *Nat. Med.* **2000**, *6*, 1375–1379.

35. Crotty, S.; Cameron, C. E.; Andino, R. RNA virus error catastrophe: direct molecular test by using ribavirin. *Proc. Natl. Acad. Sci. U.S.A.* **2001**, *98*, 6895–6900.

36. Severson, W. E.; Schmaljohn, C. S.; Javadian, A.; Jonsson, C. B. Ribavirin causes error catastrophe during Hantaan virus replication. *J. Virol.* **2003**, *77*, 481–488.

37. Eigen, M. Error catastrophe and antiviral strategy. *Proc. Natl. Acad. Sci. U.S.A.* **2002**, *99*, 13374–13376.

38. Braun, M.; Vierling, J. M. The clinical and immunologic impact of using interferon and ribavirin in the immunosuppressed host. *Liver Transplant.* **2003**, *9*, S79–S89.

39. Tam, R. C.; Pai, B.; Bard, J.; Lim, C.; Averett, D. R.; Phan, U. T.; Milovanovic, T. Ribavirin polarizes human T cell responses towards a Type 1 cytokine profile. *J. Hepatol.* **1999**, *30*, 376–382.

40. Hultgren, C.; Milich, D. R.; Weiland, O.; Sallberg, M. The antiviral compound ribavirin modulates the T helper (Th)1/Th2 subset balance in hepatitis B and C virus-specific immune responses. *J. Gen. Virol.* **1998**, *79*, 2381–2391.

41. Smee, D. F.; Bailey, K. W.; Sidwell, R. W. Treatment of cowpox virus respiratory infections in mice with ribavirin as a single agent or followed sequentially by cidofovir. *Antiviral Chem. Chemother.* **2000**, *11*, 303–309.

42. Heagy, W.; Crumpacker, C.; Lopez, P. A.; Finberg, R. W. Inhibition of immune functions by antiviral drugs. *J. Clin. Invest.* **1991**, *87*, 1916–1924.

43. Pankiewicz, K. W. Inhibitors of inosine monophosphate dehydrogenase as potential chemotherapeutic agents. *Exp. Opin. Ther. Patents* **1999**, *9*, 55–65.

44. Sidwell, R. W.; Huffman, J. H.; Barnett, B. B.; Pifat, D. Y. In vitro and in vivo Phlebovirus inhibition by ribavirin. *Antimicrob. Agents Chemother.* **1988**, *32*, 331–336.

45. Watts, D. M.; Ussery, M. A.; Nash, D.; Peters, C. J. Inhibition of Crimean-Congo hemorrhagic-fever viral infectivity yields in vitro by ribavirin. *Am. J. Trop. Med. Hyg.* **1989**, *41*, 581–585.

46. Koff, W. C.; Elm, J. L.; Halstead, S. B. Antiviral effects of ribavirin and 6-mercapto-9-tetrahydro-2-furylpurine against dengue viruses in vitro. *Antiviral Res.* **1982**, *2*, 69–79.

47. Morrey, J. D.; Smee, D. F.; Sidwell, R. W.; Tseng, C. Identification of active antiviral compounds against a New York isolate of West Nile virus. *Antiviral Res.* **2002**, *55*, 107–116.

48. Morrey, J. D.; Sidwell, R. W.; Smee, D. L.; Day, C. W. Cell line-dependent antiviral activity of ribavirin for West Nile virus. *Antiviral Res.* **2002**, *53*, A49.

49. Smee, D. F.; Bray, M.; Huggins, J. W. Antiviral activity and mode of action studies of ribavirin and mycophenolic acid against orthopoxviruses in vitro. *Antiviral Chem. Chemother.* **2001**, *12*, 327–335.

50. Doerr, H. W.; Michaelis, M.; Preiser, W.; Cinatl, J. In vitro investigation of potential therapeutics for the severe acute respiratory syndrome (SARS). *Antiviral Res.* **2004**, *62*, A59.

51. Canonico, P. G.; Kende, M.; Luscri, B. J.; Huggins, J. W. In vivo activity of antivirals against exotic RNA viral infections. *J. Antimicrob. Chemother.* **1984**, *14*, 27–41.

52. Kenyon, R. H.; Canonico, P. G.; Green, D. E.; Peters, C. J. Effect of ribavirin and tributylribavirin on Argentine hemorrhagic fever (Junin virus) in guinea pigs. *Antimicrob. Agents Chemother.* **1986**, *29*, 521–523.

53. Koff, W. C.; Pratt, R. D.; Elm, J. L.; Venkateshan, C. N.; Halstead, S. B. Treatment of intracranial dengue virus infections in mice with a lipophilic derivative of ribavirin. *Antimicrob. Agents Chemother.* **1983**, *24*, 134–136.

54. Smee, D. F.; Morris, J. L. B.; Barnard, D. L.; Vanaerschot, A. Selective inhibition of arthropod-borne and arenaviruses in vitro by 3′-fluoro-3′-deoxyadenosine. *Antiviral Res.* **1992**, *18*, 151–162.

55. McCormick, J. B.; King, I. J.; Webb, P. A.; Scribner, C. L.; Craven, R. B.; Johnson, K. M.; Elliott, L. H.; Belmont-Williams, R. Lassa fever—effective therapy with ribavirin. *N. Engl. J. Med.* **1986**, *314*, 20–26.

56. Jahrling, P. B.; Hesse, R. A.; Eddy, G. A.; Johnson, K. M.; Callis, R. T.; Stephen, E. L. Lassa virus infection of rhesus monkeys: pathogenesis and treatment with ribavirin. *J. Infect. Dis.* **1980**, *141*, 580–589.

57. Stephen, E. L.; Jahrling, P. B. Experimental Lassa fever virus infection successfully treated with ribavirin. *Lancet* **1979**, 268–269.

58. Jahrling, P. B.; Peters, C. J.; Stephen, E. L. Enhanced treatment of Lassa fever by immune plasma combined with ribavirin in cynomolgus monkeys. *J. Infect. Dis.* **1984**, *149*, 420–427.

59. Andrei, G.; De Clercq, E. Inhibitory effect of selected antiviral compounds on arenavirus replication in vitro. *Antiviral Res.* **1990**, *14*, 287–300.

60. Weissenbacher, M. C.; Calello, M. A.; Merani, M. S.; McCormick, J. B.; Rodriguez, M. Therapeutic effect of the antiviral agent ribavirin in Junin virus-infection of primates. *J. Med. Virol.* **1986**, *20*, 261–267.

61. McKee, K. T.; Huggins, J. W.; Trahan, C. J.; Mahlandt, B. G. Ribavirin prophylaxis and therapy for experimental Argentine hemorrhagic fever. *Antimicrob. Agents Chemother.* **1988**, *32*, 1304–1309.

62. Enria, D. A.; Maiztegui, J. I. Antiviral treatment of Argentine hemorrhagic fever. *Antiviral Res.* **1994**, *23*, 23–31.

63. Weissenbacher, M. C.; Avila, M. M.; Calello, M. A.; Merani, M. S.; McCormick, J. B.; Rodriguez, M. Effect of ribavirin and immune serum on Junin virus infected primates. *Med. Microbiol. Immunol.* **1986**, *175*, 183–186.

64. Kirsi, J. J.; North, J. A.; Mckernan, P. A.; Murray, B. K.; Canonico, P. G.; Huggins, J. W.; Srivastava, P. C.; Robins, R. K. Broad-spectrum antiviral activity of 2-beta-D-ribofuranosylselenazole-4-carboxamide, a new antiviral agent. *Antimicrob. Agents Chemother.* **1983**, *24*, 353–361.

65. Lucia, H. L.; Coppenhaver, D. H.; Baron, S. Arenavirus infection in the guinea pig model: antiviral therapy with recombinant interferon-alpha, the immunomodulator CL246,738 and ribavirin. *Antiviral Res.* **1989**, *12*, 279–292.

66. Smee, D. F.; Gilbert, J.; Leonhardt, J. A.; Barnett, B. B.; Huggins, J. H.; Sidwell, R. W. Treatment of lethal Pichinde virus infections in weanling LVG/Lak hamsters with ribavirin, ribamidine, selenazofurin, and ampligen. *Antiviral Res.* **1993**, *20*, 57–70.

67. Huggins, J. W.; Robins, R. K.; Canonico, P. G. Synergistic antiviral effects of ribavirin and the C-nucleoside analogs tiazofurin and selenazofurin against togaviruses, bunyaviruses, and arenaviruses. *Antimicrob. Agents Chemother.* **1984**, *26*, 476–480.

68. Burns, N. J.; Barnett, B. B.; Huffman, J. H.; Dawson, M. I.; Sidwell, R. W.; De Clercq, E.; Kende, M. A newly developed immunofluorescent assay for determining the Pichinde virus inhibitory effects of selected nucleoside analogs. *Antiviral Res.* **1988**, *10*, 89–98.

69. Murphy, M. E.; Kariwa, H.; Mizutani, T.; Yoshimatsu, K.; Arikawa, J.; Takashima, I. In vitro antiviral activity of lactoferrin and ribavirin upon hantavirus. *Arch. Virol.* **2000**, *145*, 1571–1582.

70. Murphy, M. E.; Kariwa, H.; Mizutani, T.; Tanabe, H.; Yoshimatsu, K.; Arikawa, J.; Takashima, I. Characterization of in vitro and in vivo antiviral activity of lactoferrin and ribavirin upon hantavirus. *J. Vet. Med. Sci.* **2001**, *63*, 637–645.

71. Huggins, J. W.; Kim, G. R.; Brand, O. M.; McKee, K. T. Ribavirin therapy for Hantaan virus-infection in suckling mice. *J. Infect. Dis.* **1986**, *153*, 489–497.

72. Paragas, J.; Whitehouse, C. A.; Endy, T. P.; Bray, M. A simple assay for determining antiviral activity against Crimean-Congo hemorrhagic fever virus. *Antiviral Res.* **2004**, *62*, 21–25.

73. Tignor, G. H.; Hanham, C. A. Ribavirin efficacy in an in vivo model of Crimean-Congo hemorrhagic fever virus (CCHF) infection. *Antiviral Res.* **1993**, *22*, 309–325.

74. Peters, C. J.; Reynolds, J. A.; Slone, T. W.; Jones, D. E.; Stephen, E. L. Prophylaxis of Rift Valley fever with antiviral drugs, immune serum, an interferon inducer, and a macrophage activator. *Antiviral Res.* **1986**, *6*, 285–297.

75. Kende, M.; Alving, C. R.; Rill, W. L.; Swartz, G. M.; Canonico, P. G. Enhanced efficacy of liposome-encapsulated ribavirin against Rift Valley fever virus infection in mice. *Antimicrob. Agents Chemother.* **1985**, *27*, 903–907.

76. Kende, M.; Lupton, H. W.; Rill, W. L.; Levy, H. B.; Canonico, P. G. Enhanced therapeutic efficacy of poly(ICLC) and ribavirin combinations against Rift Valley fever virus infection in mice. *Antimicrob. Agents Chemother.* **1987**, *31*, 986–990.

77. Garcia, S.; Crance, J. M.; Billecocq, A.; Peinnequin, A.; Jouan, A.; Bouloy, M.; Garin, D. Quantitative real-time PCR detection of Rift Valley fever virus and its application to evaluation of antiviral compounds. *J. Clin. Microbiol.* **2001**, *39*, 4456–4461.

78. Crance, J. M.; Gratier, D.; Guimet, J.; Jouan, A. Inhibition of sandfly fever Sicilian virus (Phlebovirus) replication in vitro by antiviral compounds. *Res. Virol.* **1997**, *148*, 353–365.

79. Sidwell, R. W.; Huffman, J. H.; Barnard, D. L.; Smee, D. F.; Warren, R. P.; Chirigos, M. A.; Kende, M.; Huggins, J. Antiviral and immunomodulating inhibitors of experimentally induced Punta Toro virus infections. *Antiviral Res.* **1994**, *25*, 105–122.

80. Smee, D. F.; Alaghamandan, H. A.; Kini, G. D.; Robins, R. K. Antiviral activity and mode of action of ribavirin 5′-sulfamate against Semliki Forest virus. *Antiviral Res.* **1988**, *10*, 253–262.

81. De Clercq, E.; Cools, M.; Balzarini, J.; Snoeck, R.; Andrei, G.; Hosoya, M.; Shigeta, S.; Ueda, T.; Minakawa, N.; Matsuda, A. Antiviral activities of 5-ethynyl-1-beta-D-ribofuranosylimidazole-4-carboxamide and related-compounds. *Antimicrob. Agents Chemother.* **1991**, *35*, 679–684.

82. De Clercq, E.; Murase, J.; Marquez, V. E. Broad-spectrum antiviral and cytocidal activity of cyclopentenylcytosine, a carbocyclic nucleoside targeted at CTP synthetase. *Biochem. Pharmacol.* **1991**, *41*, 1821–1829.

83. van Tiel, F. H.; Harmsen, M.; Kraaijeveld, C. A.; Snippe, H. Inhibition of Semliki Forest virus multiplication by ribavirin—a potential method for the monitoring of antiviral agents in serum. *J. Virol. Methods* **1986**, *14*, 119–125.

84. Briolant, S.; Garin, D.; Scaramozzino, N.; Jouan, A.; Crance, J. M. In vitro inhibition of Chikungunya and Semliki Forest viruses replication by antiviral compounds: synergistic effect of interferon-alpha and ribavirin combination. *Antiviral Res.* **2004**, *61*, 111–117.

85. Crance, J. M.; Scaramozzino, N.; Jouan, A.; Garin, D. Interferon, ribavirin, 6-azauridine and glycyrrhizin: antiviral compounds active against pathogenic flaviviruses. *Antiviral Res.* **2003**, *58*, 73–79.

86. Neyts, J.; Meerbach, A.; McKenna, P.; De Clercq, E. Use of the yellow fever virus vaccine strain 17D for the study of strategies for the treatment of yellow fever virus infections. *Antiviral Res.* **1996**, *30*, 125–132.

87. Diamond, M. S.; Zachariah, M.; Harris, E. Mycophenolic acid inhibits dengue virus infection by preventing replication of viral RNA. *Virology* **2002**, *304*, 211–221.

88. Sbrana, E.; Xiao, S. Y.; Guzman, H.; Ye, M. G.; Travassos da Rosa, A. P. A.; Tesh, R. B. Efficacy of post-exposure treatment of yellow fever with ribavirin in a hamster model of the disease. *Am. J. Trop. Med. Hyg.,* **2004**, *71*, 306–312.

89. Buckwold, V. E.; Wei, J. Y.; Wenzel-Mathers, M.; Russell, J. Synergistic in vitro interactions between alpha interferon and ribavirin against bovine viral diarrhea virus and yellow fever virus as surrogate models of hepatitis C virus replication. *Antimicrob. Agents Chemother.* **2003**, *47*, 2293–2298.

90. Malinoski, F. J.; Hasty, S. E.; Ussery, M. A.; Dalrymple, J. M. Prophylactic ribavirin treatment of dengue type 1 infection in rhesus monkeys. *Antiviral Res.* **1990**, *13*, 139–149.

91. Jordan, I.; Briese, T.; Fischer, N.; Lau, J. Y. N.; Lipkin, W. I. Ribavirin inhibits West Nile virus replication and cytopathic effect in neural cells. *J. Infect. Dis.* **2000**, *182*, 1214–1217.

92. Baker, R.; Bray, M.; Huggins, J. W. Potential antiviral therapeutics for smallpox, monkeypox and other orthopoxvirus infections. *Antiviral Res.* **2003**, *57*, 13–23.

93. Jahrling, P. B.; Zaucha, G. M.; Huggins, J. W. Countermeasures to the reemergence of smallpox virus as an agent of bioterrorism. In *Emerging Infections 4*, Scheld, W. M.; Craig, W. A.; Hughes, J. M. (Eds.). ASM Press, Washington, DC, 2000, pp 187–200.

94. Kern, E. R. In vitro activity of potential anti-poxvirus agents. *Antiviral Res.* **2003**, *57*, 35–40.

95. Smee, D. F.; Wong, M. H.; Bailey, K. W.; Beadle, J. R.; Hostetler, K. Y.; Sidwell, R. W. Effects of four antiviral substances on lethal vaccinia virus (IHD strain) respiratory infections in mice. *Int. J. Antimicrob. Agents* **2004**, *23*, 430–437.

96. Borio, L.; Inglesby, T.; Peters, C. J.; Schmaljohn, A. L.; Hughes, J. M.; Jahrling, P. B.; Ksiazek, T.; Johnson, K. M.; Meyerhoff, A.; Toole, T.; Ascher, M. S.; Bartlett, J.; Breman, J. G.; Eitzen, E. M.; Hamburg, M.; Hauer, J.; Henderson, D. A.; Johnson, R. T.; Kwik, G.; Layton, M.; Lillibridge, S.; Nabel, G. J.; Osterholm, M. T.; Perl, T. M.; Russell, P.; Tonat, K. Hemorrhagic fever viruses as biological weapons: medical and public health management. *JAMA* **2002**, *287*, 2391–2405.

97. Fisher-Hoch, S. P.; Gborie, S.; Parker, L.; Huggins, J. Unexpected adverse reactions during a clinical trial in rural West Africa. *Antiviral Res.* **1992**, *19*, 139–147.

98. Kilgore, P. E.; Ksiazek, T. G.; Rollin, P. E.; Mills, J. N.; Villagra, M. R.; Montenegro, M. J.; Costales, M. A.; Paredes, L. C.; Peters, C. J. Treatment of Bolivian hemorrhagic fever with intravenous ribavirin. *Clin. Infect. Dis.* **1997**, *24*, 718–722.

99. Enria, D. A.; Briggiler, A. M.; Levis, S.; Vallejos, D.; Maiztegui, I.; Canonico, P. G. Tolerance and antiviral effect of ribavirin in patients with Argentine hemorrhagic fever. *Antiviral Res.* **1987**, *7*, 353–359.

100. Mardani, M.; Jahromi, M. K.; Naieni, K. H.; Zeinali, M. The efficacy of oral ribavirin in the treatment of Crimean-Congo hemorrhagic fever in Iran. *Clin. Infect. Dis.* **2003**, *36*, 1613–1618.

101. Fisher-Hoch, S. P.; Khan, J. A.; Rehman, S.; Mirza, S.; Khurshid, M.; McCormick, J. B. Crimean-Congo hemorrhagic fever treated with oral ribavirin. *Lancet* **1995**, *346*, 472–475.

102. Athar, M. N.; Baqai, H. Z.; Ahmad, M.; Khalid, M. A.; Bashir, N.; Ahmad, A. M.; Balouch, A. H.; Bashir, K. Short report: Crimean-Congo hemorrhagic fever outbreak in Rawalpindi, Pakistan, February 2002. *Am. J. Trop. Med. Hyg.* **2003**, *69*, 284–287.

103. McJunkin, J. E.; Khan, R.; de Los, R.; Parsons, D. L.; Minnich, L. L.; Ashley, R. G.; Tsai, T. F. Treatment of severe La Crosse encephalitis with intravenous ribavirin following diagnosis by brain biopsy. *Pediatrics* **1997**, *99*, 261–267.

104. Huggins, J. W.; Hsiang, C. M.; Cosgriff, T. M.; Guang, M. Y.; Smith, J. I.; Wu, Z. O.; LeDuc, J. W.; Zheng, Z. M.; Meegan, J. M.; Wang, Q. N.; Oland, D. D.; Gui, X. E.; Gibbs, P. H.; Yuan, G. H.; Zhang, T. M. Prospective, double-blind, concurrent, placebo-

controlled clinical trial of intravenous ribavirin therapy of hemorrhagic fever with renal syndrome. *J. Infect. Dis.* **1991**, *164*, 1119–1127.

105. Chapman, L. E.; Mertz, G. J.; Peters, C. J.; Jolson, H. M.; Khan, A. S.; Ksiazek, T. G.; Koster, F. T.; Baum, K. F.; Rollin, P. E.; Pavia, A. T.; Holman, R. C.; Christenson, J. C.; Rubin, P. J.; Behrman, R. E.; Bell, L. J. W.; Simpson, G. L.; Sadek, R. F. Intravenous ribavirin for hantavirus pulmonary syndrome: safety and tolerance during 1 year of open-label experience. *Antiviral Ther.* **1999**, *4*, 211–219.

106. Mertz, G. J. ; Miedzinski, L.; Goade, D.; Pavia, A. T.; Hjelle, B.; Hansbarger, C. O.; Levy, H.; Koster, F. T.; Baum, K.; Lindemulder, A.; Wang, W. Q.; Riser, L.; Fernandez, H.; Whitley, R. J. Placebo-controlled, double blind trial of intravenous ribavirin for hantavirus cardiopulmonary syndrome in North America. *Clin. Infect. Dis.*, **2004**, *39*, 1307–1313.

107. Chong, H. T.; Kamarulzaman, A.; Tan, C. T.; Goh, K. J.; Thayaparan, T.; Kunjapan, R.; Chew, N. K.; Chua, K. B.; Lam, S. K. Treatment of acute Nipah encephalitis with ribavirin. *Ann. Neurol.* **2001**, *49*, 810–813.

108. Goldstein, B. M.; Colby, T. D. IMP dehydrogenase: structural aspects of inhibitor binding. *Curr. Med. Chem.* **1999**, *6*, 519–536.

109. Markland, W.; McQuaid, T. J.; Jain, J.; Kwong, A. D. Broad-spectrum antiviral activity of the IMP dehydrogenase inhibitor VX-497: a comparison with ribavirin and demonstration of antiviral additivity with alpha interferon. *Antimicrob. Agents Chemother.* **2000**, *44*, 859–866.

110. Canonico, P. G.; Jahrling, P. B.; Pannier, W. L. Antiviral efficacy of pyrazofurin against selected RNA viruses. *Antiviral Res.* **1982**, *2*, 331–337.

111. Marquez, V. E.; Lim, M. I.; Treanor, S. P.; Plowman, J.; Priest, M. A.; Markovac, A.; Khan, M. S.; Kaskar, B.; Driscoll, J. S. Cyclopentenylcytosine—a carbocyclic nucleoside with antitumor and antiviral properties. *J. Med. Chem.* **1988**, *31*, 1687–1694.

112. De Clercq, E. Carbocyclic adenosine analogues as *S*-adenosylhomocysteine hydrolase inhibitors and antiviral agents: recent advances. *Nucleosides Nucleotides* **1998**, *17*, 625–634.

113. Hasobe, M.; Liang, H.; Aultriche, D. B.; Borcherding, D. R.; Wolfe, M. S.; Borchardt, R. T. (1′R,2′S,3′R)-9-(2′,3′-Dihydroxycyclopentan-1′-yl)-adenine and 3-deazaadenine analogs of aristeromycin which exhibit potent antiviral activity with reduced cytotoxicity. *Antiviral Chem. Chemother.* **1993**, *4*, 245–248.

114. Hasobe, M.; Mckee, J. G.; Borchardt, R. T. Relationship between intracellular concentration of *S*-adenosylhomocysteine and inhibition of vaccinia virus replication and inhibition of murine L-929 cell growth. *Antimicrob. Agents Chemother.* **1989**, *33*, 828–834.

115. Yuan, C. S.; Saso, Y.; Lazarides, E.; Borchardt, R. T.; Robins, M. J. Recent advances in *S*-adenosyl-L-homocysteine hydrolase inhibitors and their potential clinical applications. *Expert Opin. Ther. Patents* **1999**, *9*, 1197–1206.

116. Wolfe, M. S.; Borchardt, R. T. *S*-Adenosyl-L-homocysteine hydrolase as a target for antiviral chemotherapy. *J. Med. Chem.* **1991**, *34*, 1521–1530.

117. Huggins, J.; Zhang, Z. X.; Bray, M. Antiviral drug therapy of filovirus infections: *S*-adenosylhomocysteine hydrolase inhibitors inhibit Ebola virus in vitro and in a lethal mouse model. *J. Infect. Dis.* **1999**, *179*, S240–S247.

118. Bray, M.; Paragas, J. Experimental therapy of filovirus infections. *Antiviral Res.* **2002**, *54*, 1–17.

119. Leyssen, P.; De Clercq, E.; Neyts, J. Perspective for the treatment of infections with Flaviviridae. *Clin. Microbiol. Rev.* **2000**, *13*, 67–82.

120. Song, G. Y.; Paul, V.; Choo, H.; Morrey, J.; Sidwell, R. W.; Chu, C. K. Enantiomeric synthesis of D- and L-cyclopentenyl nucleosides and their antiviral activity against West Nile virus. *J. Med. Chem.* **2001**, *44*, 3985–3993.

121. Chu, C. K.; Jin, Y. H.; Baker, R. O.; Huggins, J. Antiviral activity of cyclopentenyl nucleosides against orthopox viruses (smallpox, monkeypox and cowpox). *Bioorg. Med. Chem. Lett.* **2003**, *13*, 9–12.

122. De Clercq, E. Vaccinia virus inhibitors as a paradigm for the chemotherapy of poxvirus infections. *Clin. Microbiol. Rev.* **2001**, *14*, 382–397.

123. De Clercq, E.; Cools, M.; Balzarini, J.; Marquez, V. E.; Borcherding, D. R.; Borchardt, R. T.; Drach, J. C.; Kitaoka, S.; Konno, T. Broad-spectrum antiviral activities of neplanocin-A, 3-deazaneplanocin-A, and their 5′-nor derivatives. *Antimicrob. Agents Chemother.* **1989**, *33*, 1291–1297.

124. Tseng, C. K. H.; Marquez, V. E.; Fuller, R. W.; Goldstein, B. M.; Haines, D. R.; Mcpherson, H.; Parsons, J. L.; Shannon, W. M.; Arnett, G.; Hollingshead, M.; Driscoll, J. S. Synthesis of 3-deazaneplanocin-A, a powerful inhibitor of *S*-adenosylhomocysteine hydrolase with potent and selective in vitro and in vivo antiviral activities. *J. Med. Chem.* **1989**, *32*, 1442–1446.

125. Smee, D. F.; Alaghamandan, H. A.; Cottam, H. B.; Jolley, W. B.; Robins, R. K. Antiviral activity of the novel immune modulator 7-thia-8-oxoguanosine. *J. Biol. Response Mod.* **1990**, *9*, 24–32.

126. Smee, D. F.; Alaghamandan, H. A.; Jin, A.; Sharma, B. S.; Jolley, W. B. Roles of interferon and natural killer cells in the antiviral activity of 7-thia-8-oxoguanosine against Semliki Forest virus infections in mice. *Antiviral Res.* **1990**, *13*, 91–102.

127. Smee, D. F.; Huffman, J. H.; Gessaman, A. C.; Huggins, J. W.; Sidwell, R. W. Prophylactic and therapeutic activities of 7-thia-8-oxoguanosine against Punta Toro virus infections in mice. *Antiviral Res.* **1991**, *15*, 229–239.

128. Smee, D. F.; Alaghamandan, H. A.; Gilbert, J.; Burger, R. A.; Jin, A.; Sharma, B. S.; Ramasamy, K.; Revankar, G. R.; Cottam, H. B.; Jolley, W. B.; Robins, R. K. Immunoenhancing properties and antiviral activity of 7-deazaguanosine in mice. *Antimicrob. Agents Chemother.* **1991**, *35*, 152–157.

129. Smee, D. F.; Alaghamandan, H. A.; Ramasamy, K.; Revankar, G. R. Broad-spectrum activity of 8-chloro-7-deazaguanosine against RNA virus infections in mice and rats. *Antiviral Res.* **1995**, *26*, 203–209.

130. Revankar, G. R.; Rao, T. S.; Ramasamy, K.; Smee, D. F. Synthesis and broad-spectrum antiviral activity in mice of certain alkyl, alkenyl and ribofuranosyl derivatives of 7-deazaguanine. *Nucleosides Nucleotides* **1995**, *14*, 671–674.

131. Bauer, D. J.; St.Vincent, L.; Kempe, C. H.; Downie, A. W. Prophylactic treatment of small pox contacts with *N*-methylisatin beta-thiosemicarbazone (compound 33T57, marboran). *Lancet* **1963**, 494–496.

132. Fenner, F.; Henderson, D. A.; Arita, I.; Jezek, Z.; Ladnyi, I. D. *Smallpox and Its Eradication*, World Health Organization, Bethesda, MD, 1988.

133. Bauer, D. J. A history of the discovery and clinical application of antiviral drugs. *Br. Med. Bull.* **1985**, *41*, 309–314.

134. Huggins, J. W.; Martinez, M. J.; Hartmann, C. J.; Hensley, L. E.; Jackson, D. L.; Kefauver, D. L.; Kulesh, D. A.; Larsen, T.; Miller, D. M.; Mucker, E. M.; Shamblin, J. D.; Tate, M. K.; Whitehouse, C. A.; Zwiers, S. H.; Jahrling, P. B. Successful cidofovir treatment of smallpox-like disease in variola and monkeypox primate models. *Antiviral Res.* **2004**, *62*, A57–A58.

135. De Clercq, E. Cidofovir in the treatment of poxvirus infections. *Antiviral Res.* **2002**, *55*, 1–13.

136. De Clercq, E. Cidofovir in the therapy and short-term prophylaxis of poxvirus infections. *Trends Pharmacol. Sci.* **2002**, *23*, 456–458.

137. De Clercq, E.; Sakuma, T.; Baba, M.; Pauwels, R.; Balzarini, J.; Rosenberg, I.; Holy, A. Antiviral activity of phosphonylmethoxyalkyl derivatives of purine and pyrimidines. *Antiviral Res.* **1987**, *8*, 261–272.

138. Safrin, S.; Cherrington, J.; Jaffe, H. S. Clinical uses of cidofovir. *Rev. Med. Virol.* **1997**, *7*, 145–156.

139. Plosker, G. L.; Noble, S. Cidofovir: a review of its use in cytomegalovirus retinitis in patients with AIDS. *Drugs* **1999**, *58*, 325–345.

140. Cihlar, T.; Chen, M. S. Identification of enzymes catalyzing two-step phosphorylation of cidofovir and the effect of cytomegalovirus infection on their activities in host cells. *Mol. Pharmacol.* **1996**, *50*, 1502–1510.

141. Xiong, X.; Smith, J. L.; Kim, C.; Huang, E. S.; Chen, M. S. Kinetic analysis of the interaction of cidofovir diphosphate with human cytomegalovirus DNA polymerase. *Biochem. Pharmacol.* **1996**, *51*, 1563–1567.

142. Hitchcock, M. J. M.; Jaffe, H. S.; Martin, J. C.; Stagg, R. J. Cidofovir, a new agent with potent anti-herpesvirus activity. *Antiviral Chem. Chemother.* **1996**, *7*, 115–127.

143. Xiong, X.; Smith, J. L.; Chen, M. S. Effect of incorporation of cidofovir into DNA by human cytomegalovirus DNA polymerase on DNA elongation. *Antimicrob. Agents Chemother.* **1997**, *41*, 594–599.

144. De Clercq, E. Towards an effective chemotherapy of virus infections: therapeutic potential of cidofovir [(*S*)-1-[3-hydroxy-2-(phosphonomethoxy)propyl]cytosine, HPMPC] for the treatment of DNA virus infections. *Collect. Czech. Chem. Commun.* **1998**, *63*, 480–506.

145. Naesens, L.; Snoeck, R.; Andrei, G.; Balzarini, J.; Neyts, J.; De Clercq, E. HPMPC (cidofovir), PMEA (adefovir) and related acyclic nucleoside phosphonate analogues: a review of their pharmacology and clinical potential in the treatment of viral infections. *Antiviral Chem. Chemother.* **1997**, *8*, 1–23.

146. Cundy, K. C. Clinical pharmacokinetics of the antiviral nucleotide analogues cidofovir and adefovir. *Clin. Pharmacokinet.* **1999**, *36*, 127–143.

147. De Clercq, E. Therapeutic potential of HPMPC as an antiviral drug. *Rev. Med. Virol.* **1993**, *3*, 85–96.

148. Kern, E. R.; Hartline, C.; Harden, E.; Keith, K.; Rodriguez, N.; Beadle, J. R.; Hostetler, K. Y. Enhanced inhibition of orthopoxvirus replication in vitro by alkoxyalkyl esters of cidofovir and cyclic cidofovir. *Antimicrob. Agents Chemother.* **2002**, *46*, 991–995.

149. Keith, K. A.; Hitchcock, M. J. M.; Lee, W. A.; Holy, A.; Kern, E. R. Evaluation of nucleoside phosphonates and their analogs and prodrugs for inhibition of orthopoxvirus replication. *Antimicrob. Agents Chemother.* **2003**, *47*, 2193–2198.

150. Buller, R. M.; Owens, G.; Schriewer, J.; Melman, L.; Beadle, J. R.; Hostetler, K. Y. Efficacy of oral active ether lipid analogs of cidofovir in a lethal mousepox model. *Virology* **2004**, *318*, 474–481.

151. Smee, D. F.; Sidwell, R. W. A review of compounds exhibiting anti-orthopoxvirus activity in animal models. *Antiviral Res.* **2003**, *57*, 41–52.

152. Neyts, J.; De Clercq, E. Efficacy of (*S*)-1-(3-hydroxy-2-phosphonylmethoxypropyl)-cytosine for the treatment of lethal vaccinia virus-infections in severe combined immune-deficiency (SCID) mice. *J. Med. Virol.* **1993**, *41*, 242–246.

153. Bray, M.; Martinez, M.; Smee, D. F.; Kefauver, D.; Thompson, E.; Huggins, J. W. Cidofovir protects mice against lethal aerosol or intranasal cowpox virus challenge. *J. Infect. Dis.* **2000**, *181*, 10–19.

154. Bray, M.; Martinez, M.; Kefauver, D.; West, M.; Roy, C. Treatment of aerosolized cowpox virus infection in mice with aerosolized cidofovir. *Antiviral Res.* **2002**, *54*, 129–142.

155. Roy, C. J.; Baker, R.; Washburn, K.; Bray, M. Aerosolized cidofovir is retained in the respiratory tract and protects mice against intranasal cowpox virus challenge. *Antimicrob. Agents Chemother.* **2003**, *47*, 2933–2937.

156. Smee, D. F.; Bailey, K. W.; Wong, M. H.; Sidwell, R. W. Intranasal treatment of cowpox virus respiratory infections in mice with cidofovir. *Antiviral Res.* **2000**, *47*, 171–177.

157. Smee, D. F.; Bailey, K. W.; Sidwell, R. W. Treatment of lethal vaccinia virus respiratory infections in mice with cidofovir. *Antiviral Chem. Chemother.* **2001**, *12*, 71–76.

158. Smee, D. F.; Bailey, K. W.; Wong, M. H.; Sidwell, R. W. Effects of cidofovir on the pathogenesis of a lethal vaccinia virus respiratory infection in mice. *Antiviral Res.* **2001**, *52*, 55–62.

159. Smee, D. F.; Bailey, K. W.; Sidwell, R. W. Comparative effects of cidofovir and cyclic HPMPC on lethal cowpox and vaccinia virus respiratory infections in mice. *Chemotherapy* **2003**, *49*, 126–131.

160. Smee, D. F.; Sidwell, R. W.; Kefauver, D.; Bray, M.; Huggins, J. W. Characterization of wild-type and cidofovir-resistant strains of camelpox, cowpox, monkeypox, and vaccinia viruses. *Antimicrob. Agents Chemother.* **2002**, *46*, 1329–1335.

161. Quenelle, D. C.; Collins, D. J.; Kern, E. R. Efficacy of multiple- or single-dose cidofovir against vaccinia and cowpox virus infections in mice. *Antimicrob. Agents Chemother.* **2003**, *47*, 3275–3280.

162. Quenelle, D. C.; Collins, D. J.; Kern, E. R. Cutaneous infections of mice with vaccinia or cowpox viruses and efficacy of cidofovir. *Antiviral Res.* **2004**, *63*, 33–40.

163. Smee, D. F.; Bailey, K. W.; Sidwell, R. W. Vaccinia skin lesions in immunosuppressed hairless mice can be treated topically but not parenterally with cidofovir. *Antiviral Res.* **2003**, *57*, A79.

164. Huggins, J. W.; Smee, D. F.; Martinez, M. J.; Bray, M. Cidofovir (HPMPC) treatment of monkeypox. *Antiviral Res.* **1998**, *37*, A73.

165. Beadle, J. R.; Valiaeva, N.; Brad Wan, W.; Hostetler, K. Y. Direct synthesis of acyclic nucleoside phosphonate alkoxyalkyl monoesters. *Antiviral Res.* **2004**, *62*, A66–A67.

166. Keith, K. A.; Wan, W. B.; Ciesla, S. L.; Beadle, J. R.; Hostetler, K. Y.; Kern, E. R. Inhibitory activity of alkoxyalkyl and alkyl esters of cidofovir and cyclic cidofovir against orthopoxvirus replication in vitro. *Antimicrob. Agents Chemother.* **2004**, *48*, 1869–1871.

167. Huggins, J. W.; Baker, R. O.; Beadle, J. R.; Hostetler, K. Y. Orally active ether lipid prodrugs of cidofovir for the treatment of smallpox. *Antiviral Res.* **2002**, *53*, A66.

168. Aldern, K. A.; Ciesla, S. L.; Winegarden, K. L.; Hostetler, K. Y. Increased antiviral activity of 1-*O*-hexadecyloxypropyl-[2-^{14}C]cidofovir in MRC-5 human lung fibroblasts is explained by unique cellular uptake and metabolism. *Mol. Pharmacol.* **2003**, *63*, 678–681.

169. Ciesla, S. L.; Trahan, J.; Wan, W. B.; Beadle, J. R.; Aldern, K. A.; Painter, G. R.; Hostetler, K. Y. Esterification of cidofovir with alkoxyalkanols increases oral bioavailability and diminishes drug accumulation in kidney. *Antiviral Res.* **2003**, *59*, 163–171.

170. Quenelle, D. C.; Collins, D. J.; Wan, W. B.; Beadle, J. R.; Hostetler, K. Y.; Kern, E. R. Oral treatment of cowpox and vaccinia virus infections in mice with ether lipid esters of cidofovir. *Antimicrob. Agents Chemother.* **2004**, *48*, 404–412.

171. Katz, E.; Margalith, E.; Winer, B. Inhibition of vaccinia virus growth by the nucleoside analogue 1-β-D-ribofunanosyl-1,2,4-triazole-3-carboxamide (Virazole, ribavirin). *J. Gen. Virol.* **1976**, *32*, 327–330.

172. Smee, D. F.; Sidwell, R. W. Anti-cowpox virus activities of certain adenosine analogs, arabinofuranosyl nucleosides, and 2′-fluoro-arabinofuranosyl nucleosides. *Nucleosides Nucleotides Nucleic Acids* **2004**, *23*, 375–383.

173. Smee, D. F.; Bailey, K. W.; Sidwell, R. W. Treatment of lethal cowpox virus respiratory infections in mice with 2-amino-7-[(1,3-dihydroxy-2-propoxy)methyl]purine and its orally active diacetate ester prodrug. *Antiviral Res.* **2002**, *54*, 113–120.

174. Neyts, J.; De Clercq, E. Efficacy of 2-amino-7-(1,3-dihydroxy-2-propoxymethyl)purine for treatment of vaccinia virus (Orthopoxvirus) infections in mice. *Antimicrob. Agents Chemother.* **2001**, *45*, 84–87.

175. Neyts, J.; Verbeken, E.; De Clercq, E. Effect of 5-iodo-2′-deoxyuridine on vaccinia virus (Orthopoxvirus) infections in mice. *Antimicrob. Agents Chemother.* **2002**, *46*, 2842–2847.

176. Van Aerschot, A.; Herdewijn, P.; Janssen, G.; Cools, M.; De Clercq, E. Synthesis and antiviral activity evaluation of 3′-fluoro-3′-deoxyribonucleosides: broad-spectrum antiviral activity of 3′-fluoro-3′-deoxyadenosine. *Antiviral Res.* **1989**, *12*, 133–150.

177. Keller, B. T.; Borchardt, R. T. Adenosine dialdehyde—a potent inhibitor of vaccinia virus multiplication in mouse L929 cells. *Mol. Pharmacol.* **1987**, *31*, 485–492.

178. Ishii, H.; Hasobe, M.; Mckee, J. G.; Aultriche, D. B.; Borchardt, R. T. Synergistic antiviral activity of inhibitors of *S*-adenosylhomocysteine hydrolase and ribavirin. *Antiviral. Chem. Chemother.* **1993**, *4*, 127–130.

179. Kane, E. M.; Shuman, S. Adenosine *N*-1-oxide inhibits vaccinia virus replication by blocking translation of viral early messenger RNAs. *J. Virol.* **1995**, *69*, 6352–6358.

180. Rada, B.; Zgorniak-Nowosielska, I. Site of action of *N,N′*-bis(methylisatin-beta-thiosemicarbazone)-2-methylpiperazine in the vaccinia virus replication cycle. *Acta Virol.* **1984**, *28*, 428–432.

181. Pirrung, M. C. Combinatorial Discovery of Novel Anti-poxvirus Isatin-β-Thiosemicarbazones. (personal communication).

182. Hwang, Y.; Wang, B. B.; Bushman, F. D. Molluscum contagiosum virus topoisomerase: purification, activities, and response to inhibitors. *J. Virol.* **1998**, *72*, 3401–3406.

183. Sekiguchi, J.; Stivers, J. T.; Mildvan, A. S.; Shuman, S. Mechanism of inhibition of vaccinia DNA topoisomerase by novobiocin and coumermycin. *J. Biol. Chem.* **1996**, *271*, 2313–2322.

184. Da Fonseca, F.; Moss, B. Poxvirus DNA topoisomerase knockout mutant exhibits decreased infectivity associated with reduced early transcription. *Proc. Natl. Acad. Sci. U.S.A.* **2003**, *100*, 11291–11296.

185. Sekiguchi, J.; Shuman, S. Novobiocin inhibits vaccinia virus replication by blocking virus assembly. *Virology* **1997**, *235*, 129–137.

186. Kim, Y. G.; Muralinath, M.; Brandt, T.; Pearcy, M.; Hauns, K.; Lowenhaupt, K.; Jacobs, B. L.; Rich, A. A role for Z-DNA binding in vaccinia virus pathogenesis. *Proc. Natl. Acad. Sci. U.S.A.* **2003**, *100*, 6974–6979.

187. Kim, Y. G.; Lowenhaupt, K.; Oh, D. Y.; Kim, K. K.; Rich, A. Evidence that vaccinia virulence factor ER binds to Z-DNA in vivo: implications for development of a therapy for poxvirus infection. *Proc. Natl. Acad. Sci. U.S.A.* **2004**, *101*, 1514–1518.

188. Klemperer, N.; McDonald, W.; Boyle, K.; Unger, B.; Traktman, P. The A20R protein is a stoichiometric component of the processive form of vaccinia virus DNA polymerase. *J. Virol.* **2001**, *75*, 12298–12307.

189. McDonald, W. F.; Klemperer, N.; Traktman, P. Characterization of a processive form of the vaccinia virus DNA polymerase. *Virology* **1997**, *234*, 168–175.

190. Byrd, C. A.; Bolken, T. C.; Hruby, D. E. Molecular dissection of the vaccinia virus 17L core protein proteinase. *J. Virol.* **2003**, *77*, 11279–11283.

191. Derrien, M.; Punjabi, A.; Khanna, R.; Grubisha, O.; Traktman, P. Tyrosine phosphorylation of A17 during vaccinia virus infection: involvement of the H1 phosphatase and the F10 kinase. *J. Virol.* **1999**, *73*, 7287–7296.

192. Nichols, R. J.; Traktman, P. Characterization of three paralogous members of the mammalian vaccinia related kinase family. *J. Biol. Chem.* **2004**, *279*, 7934–7946.

193. Harrison, S. C.; Alberts, B.; Ehrenfeld, E.; Enquist, L. ; Fineberg, H.; McKnight, S. L.; Moss, B.; O'Donnell, M.; Ploegh, H.; Schmid, S. L.; Walter, K. P.; Theriot, J. Discovery of antivirals against smallpox. *Proc. Natl. Acad. Sci. U.S.A.* **2004**, *101*, 11178–11192.

194. La Montagne, J. R.; Simonsen, L.; Taylor, R. J.; Turnbull, J.; Severe acute respiratory syndrome: developing a research response. *J. Infect. Dis.* **2004**, *189*, 634–641.

195. Yarnell, A. In search of SARS therapeutics. *Chem. Eng. News* **2003**, *81*, 13.

196. Barnard, D. L.; Hubbard, V. D.; Burton, J.; Smee, D. F.; Morrey, J. D.; Otto, M. J.; Sidwell, R. W. Inhibition of severe acute respiratory syndrome-associated coronavirus (SARS-CoV) by calpain inhibitors and β-D-N^4-hydroxycytidine. *Antiviral Chem. Chemother.* **2004**, *15*, 15–22.

197. Cinatl, J.; Morgenstern, B.; Bauer, G.; Chandra, P.; Rabenau, H.; Doerr, H. W. Glycyrrhizin, an active component of liquorice roots, and replication of SARS-associated coronavirus. *Lancet* **2003**, *361*, 2045–2046.

198. Morgenstern, B.; Cinatl, J.; Neyts, J.; Bauer, G.; Rabenau, H.; Doerr, H. W. Evaluation of compounds against a novel coronavirus from patients with severe acute respiratory syndrome (SARS). *Antiviral Res.* **2003**, *57*, A92.

199. Wu, C. J.; Jan, J. T.; Chen, C. M.; Hsieh, H. P.; Hwang, D. R.; Liu, H. W.; Liu, C. Y.; Huang, H. W.; Chen, S. C.; Hong, C. F.; Lin, R. K.; Chao, Y. S.; Hsu, J. T. A. Inhibition of severe acute respiratory syndrome coronavirus replication by niclosamine. *Antimicrob. Agents Chemother.* **2004**, *48*, 2693–2696.

200. Wu, C. Y.; Jan, J. T.; Ma, S. H.; Kuo, C. J.; Juan, H. F.; Cheng, Y. S. E.; Hsu, H. H.; Huang, H. C.; Wu, D. ; Brik, A.; Liang, F. S.; Liu, R. S.; Fang, J. M.; Chen, S. T.; Liang, P. H.; Wong, C. H. Small molecules targeting severe acute respiratory syndrome human coronavirus. *Proc. Natl. Acad. Sci. U.S.A.* **2004**, *101*, 10012–10017.

201. Hensley, L. E.; Fritz, E. A.; Jahrling, P. B.; Karp, C. L.; Huggins, J. W.; Geisbert, T. W. Interferon-beta 1a and SARS coronavirus replication. *Emerging Infect. Dis.* **2004**, *10*, 317–319.

202. Stroher, U.; DiCaro, A.; Li, Y.; Strong, J. E.; Aoki, F.; Plummer, F.; Jones, S. M.; Feldmann, H. Severe acute respiratory syndrome related coronavirus is inhibited by interferon-alpha. *J. Infect. Dis.* **2004**, *189*, 1164–1167.

203. Chu, C. M.; Cheng, V. C. C.; Hung, I. F. N.; Wong, M. M. L.; Chan, K. H.; Chan, K. S.; Kao, R. Y. T.; Poon, L. L. M.; Wong, C. L. P.; Guan, Y.; Peiris, J. S. M.; Yuen, K. Y. Role of lopinavir/ritonavir in the treatment of SARS: initial virological and clinical findings. *Thorax* **2004**, *59*, 252–256.

204. Tan, E. L. C.; Ooi, E. E.; Lin, C. Y.; Tan, H. C.; Ling, A. E.; Lim, B.; Stanton, L. W. Inhibition of SARS coronavirus infection in vitro with clinically approved antiviral drugs. *Emerging Infect. Dis.* **2004**, *10*, 581–586.

205. Knowles, S. R.; Phillips, E. J.; Dresser, L.; Matukas, L. Common adverse events associated with the use of ribavirin for severe acute respiratory syndrome in Canada. *Clin. Infect. Dis.* **2003**, *37*, 1139–1142.

206. van Vonderen, M. G. A.; Bos, J. C.; Prins, J. M.; Wertheim-van Dillen, P.; Speelman, P. Ribavirin in the treatment of severe acute respiratory syndrome (SARS). *Neth. J. Med.* **2003**, *61*, 238–241.

207. Fujii, T.; Nakamura, T.; Iwamoto, A. Current concepts in SARS treatment. *J. Infect. Chemother.* **2004**, *10*, 1–7.

208. Yamamoto, N.; Yang, R. G.; Yoshinaka, Y.; Amari, S.; Nakano, T.; Cinatl, J.; Rabenau, H.; Doerr, H. W.; Hunsmann, G.; Otaka, A.; Tamamura, H.; Fujii, N.; Yamamoto, N. HIV protease inhibitor nelfinavir inhibits replication of SARS-associated coronavirus. *Biochem. Biophys. Res. Commun.* **2004**, *318*, 719–725.

209. Chan, K. S.; Lai, S. T.; Chu, C. M.; Tsui, E.; Tam, C. Y.; Wong, M. M.; Tse, M. W.; Que, T. L.; Peiris, J. S.; Sung, J.; Wong, V. C.; Yuen, K. Y. Treatment of severe acute respiratory syndrome with lopinavir/ritonavir: a multicentre retrospective matched cohort study. *Hong Kong Med. J.* **2003**, *9*, 399–406.

210. Cinatl, J.; Morgenstern, B.; Bauer, G.; Chandra, P.; Rabenau, H.; Doerr, H. W. Treatment of SARS with human interferons. *Lancet* **2003**, *362*, 293–294.

211. Haagmans, B. L.; Kuiken, T.; Martina, B. E.; Fouchier, R. A. M.; Rimmelzwaan, G. F.; van Amerongen, G.; van Riel, D.; de Jong, T.; Itamura, S.; Chan, K. H.; Tashiro, M.; Osterhaus, A. D. M. E. Pegylated interferon-alpha protects type 1 pneumocytes against SARS coronavirus infection in macaques. *Nat. Med.* **2004**, *10*, 290–293.

212. Martina, B. E. E.; Haagmans, B. L.; Kuiken, T.; Fouchier, R. A. M.; Rimmelzwaan, G. F.; van Amerongen, G.; Peiris, J. S. M.; Lim, W.; Osterhaus, A. D. M. E. SARS virus infection of cats and ferrets. *Nature* **2003**, *425*, 915.

213. Enserink, M. Infectious diseases—SARS researchers report new animal models. *Science* **2003**, *302*, 213.

214. Rota, P. A.; Oberste, M. S.; Monroe, S. S.; Nix, W. A.; Campagnoli, R.; Icenogle, J. P.; Penaranda, S.; Bankamp, B.; Maher, K.; Chen, M. H.; Tong, S. X.; Tamin, A.; Lowe, L.;

Frace, M.; DeRisi, J. L.; Chen, Q.; Wang, D.; Erdman, D. D.; Peret, T. C. T.; Burns, C.; Ksiazek, T. G.; Rollin, P. E.; Sanchez, A.; Liffick, S.; Holloway, B.; Limor, J.; McCaustland, K.; Olsen-Rasmussen, M.; Fouchier, R.; Gunther, S.; Osterhaus, A. D. M. E.; Drosten, C.; Pallansch, M. A.; Anderson, L. J.; Bellini, W. J. Characterization of a novel coronavirus associated with severe acute respiratory syndrome. *Science* **2003**, *300*, 1394–1399.

215. Marra, M. A.; Jones, S. J. M.; Astell, C. R.; Holt, R. A.; Brooks-Wilson, A.; Butterfield, Y. S. N.; Khattra, J.; Asano, J. K.; Barber, S. A.; Chan, S. Y.; Cloutier, A.; Coughlin, S. M.; Freeman, D.; Girn, N.; Griffin, O. L.; Leach, S. R.; Mayo, M.; McDonald, H.; Montgomery, S. B.; Pandoh, P. K.; Petrescu, A. S.; Robertson, A. G.; Schein, J. E.; Siddiqui, A.; Smailus, D. E.; Stott, J. E.; Yang, G. S.; Plummer, F.; Andonov, A.; Artsob, H.; Bastien, N.; Bernard, K.; Booth, T. F.; Bowness, D.; Czub, M.; Drebot, M.; Fernando, L.; Flick, R.; Garbutt, M.; Gray, M.; Grolla, A.; Jones, S.; Feldmann, H.; Meyers, A.; Kabani, A.; Li, Y.; Normand, S.; Stroher, U.; Tipples, G. A.; Tyler, S.; Vogrig, R.; Ward, D.; Watson, B.; Brunham, R. C.; Krajden, M.; Petric, M.; Skowronski, D. M.; Upton, C.; Roper, R. L. The genome sequence of the SARS-associated coronavirus. *Science* **2003**, *300*, 1399–1404.

216. Ruan, Y. J.; Wei, C. L.; Ee, L. A.; Vega, V. B.; Thoreau, H.; Yun, S. T. S.; Chia, J. M.; Ng, P.; Chiu, K. P.; Lim, L.; Tao, Z.; Peng, C. K.; Ean, L. O. L.; Lee, N. M.; Sin, L. Y.; Ng, L. F. P.; Chee, R. E.; Stanton, L. W.; Long, P. M.; Liu, E. T. Comparative full-length genome sequence analysis of 14 SARS coronavirus isolates and common mutations associated with putative origins of infection. *Lancet* **2003**, *361*, 1779–1785.

217. Snijder, E. J.; Bredenbeek, P. J.; Dobbe, J. C.; Thiel, V.; Ziebuhr, J.; Poon, L. L. M.; Guan, Y.; Rozanov, M.; Spaan, W. J. M.; Gorbalenya, A. E. Unique and conserved features of genome and proteome of SARS-coronavirus, an early split-off from the coronavirus group 2 lineage. *J. Mol. Biol.* **2003**, *331*, 991–1004.

218. Thiel, V.; Ivanov, K. A.; Putics, A.; Hertzig, T.; Schelle, B.; Bayer, S.; Weissbrich, B.; Snijder, E. J.; Rabenau, H.; Doerr, H. W.; Gorbalenya, A. E.; Ziebuhr, J. Mechanisms and enzymes involved in SARS coronavirus genome expression. *J. Gen. Virol.* **2003**, *84*, 2305–2315.

219. Liu, S. Q.; Guo, T.; Li, X. L.; Sun, Z. R. Bioinformatical study on the proteomics and evolution of SARS-CoV. *Chin. Sci. Bull.* **2003**, *48*, 1277–1287.

220. Holmes, K. V. SARS coronavirus: a new challenge for prevention and therapy. *J. Clin. Invest.* **2003**, *111*, 1605–1609.

221. Xu, X.; Liu, Y. Q.; Weiss, S.; Arnold, E.; Sarafianos, S. G.; Ding, J. P. Molecular model of SARS coronavirus polymerase: implications for biochemical functions and drug design. *Nucleic Acids Res.* **2003**, *31*, 7117–7130.

222. Tanner, J. A.; Watt, R. M.; Chai, Y. B.; Lu, L. Y.; Lin, M. C.; Peiris, J. S. M.; Poon, L. L. M.; Kung, H. F.; Huang, J. D. The severe acute respiratory syndrome (SARS) coronavirus NTPase/helicase belongs to a distinct class of $5'$ to $3'$ viral helicases. *J. Biol. Chem.* **2003**, *278*, 39578–39582.

223. Yan, L.; Velikanov, M.; Flook, P.; Zheng, W. J.; Szalma, S.; Kahn, S. Assessment of putative protein targets derived from the SARS genome. *FEBS Lett.* **2003**, *554*, 257–263.

224. Zhang, Y.; Xu, J. Y.; Deng, W.; Zhang, N.; Cai, L.; Zhao, Y.; Bu, D.; Chen, R. S. siRNA designs to the crucial proteins of SARS coronavirus. *Prog. Biochem. Biophys.* **2003**, *30*, 335–338.

225. Anand, K.; Ziebuhr, J.; Wadhwani, P.; Mesters, J. R.; Hilgenfeld, R. Coronavirus main proteinase (3CL^pro) structure: basis for design of anti-SARS drugs. *Science* **2003**, *300*, 1763–1767.

226. Xiong, B.; Gui, C. S.; Xu, X. Y.; Luo, C.; Chen, J.; Luo, H. B.; Chen, L. L.; Li, G. W.; Sun, T.; Yu, C. Y.; Yue, L. D.; Duan, W. H.; Shen, J. K.; Qin, L.; Shi, T. L.; Li, Y. X.; Chen, K. X.; Luo, X. M.; Shen, X.; Shen, J. H.; Jiang, H. L. A 3D model of SARS-CoV 3CL proteinase and its inhibitors design by virtual screening. *Acta Pharmacol. Sin.* **2003**, *24*, 497–504.

227. Gao, X. F.; Xi, Z.; Huang, X. R.; Sun, C. C. 3D modeling of SARS virus proteinase and study of imaginable peptide inhibitor. *Chem. J. Chin. Univ.-Chin.* **2003**, *24*, 2279–2281.

228. Takeda-Shitaka, M.; Takaya, D.; Chiba, C.; Tanaka, H.; Umeyama, H. Protein structure prediction in structure based drug design. *Curr. Med. Chem.* **2004**, *11*, 551–558.

229. Takeda-Shitaka, M.; Nojima, H.; Takaya, D.; Kanou, K.; Iwadate, M.; Umeyama, H. Evaluation of homology modeling of the severe acute respiratory syndrome (SARS) coronavirus main protease for structure based drug design. *Chem. Pharm. Bull.* **2004**, *52*, 643–645.

230. Chou, K. C.; Wei, D. Q.; Zhong, W. Z. Binding mechanism of coronavirus main proteinase with ligands and its implication to drug design against SARS. *Biochem. Biophys. Res. Commun.* **2003**, *308*, 148–151.

231. Jenwitheesuk, E.; Samudrala, R. Identifying inhibitors of the SARS coronavirus proteinase. *Bioorg. Med. Chem. Lett.* **2003**, *13*, 3989–3992.

232. Toney, J. H.; Navas-Martin, S.; Weiss, S. R.; Koeller, A. Sabadinine: a potential non-peptide anti-severe acute respiratory-syndrome agent identified using structure-aided design. *J. Med. Chem.* **2004**, *47*, 1079–1080.

233. Clarke, T. *Nature* **2003**, *(Science Update)*, `http://www.nature.com/nsu/030512-030512-11.html`.

234. Yang, H. T.; Yang, M. J.; Ding, Y.; Liu, Y. W.; Lou, Z. Y.; Zhou, Z.; Sun, L.; Mo, L. J.; Ye, S.; Pang, H.; Gao, G. F.; Anand, K.; Bartlam, M.; Hilgenfeld, R.; Rao, Z. H. The crystal structures of severe acute respiratory syndrome virus main protease and its complex with an inhibitor. *Proc. Natl. Acad. Sci. U.S.A.* **2003**, *100*, 13190–13195.

235. Fan, K. Q.; Wei, P.; Feng, Q.; Chen, S. D.; Huang, C. K.; Ma, L.; Lai, B.; Pei, J. F.; Liu, Y.; Chen, J. G.; Lai, L. H. Biosynthesis, purification, and substrate specificity of severe acute respiratory syndrome coronavirus 3C-like proteinase. *J. Biol. Chem.* **2004**, *279*, 1637–1642.

236. Bacha, U.; Barrila, J.; Velazquez-Campoy, A.; Leavitt, S. A.; Freire, E. Identification of novel inhibitors of the SARS coronavirus main protease 3CL^pro. *Biochemistry* **2004**, *43*, 4906–4912.

237. Xiao, X. D.; Chakraborti, S.; Dimitrov, A. S.; Gramatikoff, K.; Dimitrov, D. S. The SARS-CoV S glycoprotein: expression and functional characterization. *Biochem. Biophys. Res. Commun.* **2003**, *312*, 1159–1164.

238. Li, W. H.; Moore, M. J.; Vasilieva, N.; Sui, J. H.; Wong, S. K.; Berne, M. A.; Somasundaran, M.; Sullivan, J. L.; Luzuriaga, K.; Greenough, T. C.; Choe, H.; Farzan, M. Angiotensin-converting enzyme 2 is a functional receptor for the SARS coronavirus. *Nature* **2003**, *426*, 450–454.

239. Simmons, G.; Reeves, J. D.; Rennekamp, A. J.; Amberg, S. M.; Piefer, A. J.; Bates, P. Characterization of severe acute respiratory syndrome-associated coronavirus

(SARS-CoV) spike glycoprotein-mediated viral entry. *Proc. Natl. Acad. Sci. U.S.A.* **2004**, *101*, 4240–4245.

240. Prabakaran, P.; Mao, X. D.; Dimitrov, D. S. A model of the ACE2 structure and function as a SARS-CoV receptor. *Biochem. Biophys. Res. Commun.* **2004**, *314*, 235–241.

241. Liu, S. W.; Xiao, G. F.; Chen, Y. B.; He, Y. X.; Niu, J. K.; Escalante, C. R.; Xiong, H. B.; Farmar, J.; Debnath, A. K.; Tien, P.; Jiang, S. B. Interaction between heptad repeat 1 and 2 regions in spike protein of SARS-associated coronavirus: implications for virus fusogenic mechanism and identification of fusion inhibitors. *Lancet* **2004**, *363*, 938–947.

242. Sui, J. H.; Li, W. H.; Murakami, A.; Tamin, A.; Matthews, L. J.; Wong, S. K.; Moore, M. J.; Tallarico, A. S. C.; Olurinde, M.; Choe, H.; Anderson, L. J.; Bellini, W. J.; Farzan, M.; Marasco, W. A. Potent neutralization of severe acute respiratory syndrome (SARS) coronavirus by a human mAb to S1 protein that blocks receptor association. *Proc. Natl. Acad. Sci. U.S.A.* **2004**, *101*, 2536–2541.

243. Zhang, Y. J.; Li, T. S.; Fu, L.; Yu, C. M.; Li, Y. H.; Xu, X. L.; Wang, Y. Y.; Ning, H. X.; Zhang, S. P.; Chen, W.; Babiuk, L. A.; Chang, Z. J. Silencing SARS-CoV spike protein expression in cultured cells by RNA interference. *FEBS Lett.* **2004**, *560*, 141–146.

244. He, M. L.; Zheng, B. J.; Peng, Y.; Peiris, J. S. M.; Poon, L. L. M.; Yuen, K. Y.; Lin, M. C. M.; Kung, H. F.; Guan, Y. Inhibition of SARS-associated coronavirus infection and replication by RNA interference. *JAMA* **2003**, *290*, 2665–2666.

245. Elmen, J.; Wahlestedt, C.; Brytting, M.; Wahren, B.; Ljungberg, K. SARS virus inhibited by siRNA. *Preclinica* **2004**, *2*, 135–142.

246. Morrey, J. D.; Day, C. W.; Julander, J. G.; Blatt, L. M.; Smee, D. F.; Sidwell, R. W. Effect of Interferon-alpha and interferon-inducers on West Nile virus in mouse and hamster animal models. *Antiviral Chem. Chemother.* **2004**, *15*, 67–75.

247. Solomon, T. Recent advances in Japanese encephalitis. *J. Neurovirol.* **2003**, *9*, 274–283.

248. Solomon, T.; Dung, N. M.; Wills, B.; Kneen, R.; Gainsborough, M.; Diet, T. V.; Thuy, T. T. N.; Loan, H. T.; Khanh, V. C.; Vaughn, D. W.; White, N. J.; Farrar, J. J. Interferon alpha-2a in Japanese encephalitis: a randomized double-blind placebo-controlled trial. *Lancet* **2003**, *361*, 821–826.

249. Block, T. M.; Jordan, R. Iminosugars as possible broad spectrum anti hepatitis virus agents: the glucovirs and alkovirs. *Antiviral Chem. Chemother.* **2001**, *12*, 317–325.

250. Mehta, A.; Zitzmann, N.; Rudd, P. M.; Block, T. M. α-Glucosidase inhibitors as potential broad based antiviral agents. *FEBS Lett.* **1998**, *430*, 17–22.

251. Wu, S. F.; Lee, C. J.; Liao, C. L.; Dwek, R. A.; Zitzmann, N.; Lin, Y. L. Antiviral effects of an iminosugar derivative on flavivirus infections. *J. Virol.* **2002**, *76*, 3596–3604.

252. Shi, P. Y. Genetic systems of West Nile virus and their potential applications. *Curr. Opin. Invest. Drugs* **2003**, *4*, 959–965.

253. Woodmansee, A. N.; Shi, P. Y. Recent developments in West Nile virus vaccine and antiviral therapy. *Expert Opin. Ther. Patents* **2003**, *13*, 1113–1125.

254. Borowski, P.; Niebuhr, A.; Schmitz, H.; Hosmane, R. S.; Bretner, M.; Siwecka, M. A.; Kulikowski, T. NTPase/helicase of Flaviviridae: inhibitors and inhibition of the enzyme. *Acta Biochim. Pol.* **2002**, *49*, 597–614.

255. Borowski, P.; Niebuhr, A.; Mueller, O.; Bretner, M.; Felczak, K.; Kulikowski, T.; Schmitz, H. Purification and characterization of West Nile virus nucleoside triphosphatase (NTPase)/helicase: evidence for dissociation of the NTPase and helicase activities of the enzyme. *J. Virol.* **2001**, *75*, 3220–3229.

256. Borowski, P.; Lang, M.; Haag, A.; Schmitz, H.; Choe, J.; Chen, H. M.; Hosmane, R. S. Characterization of imidazo[4,5-*d*]pyridazine nucleosides as modulators of unwinding reaction mediated by West Nile virus nucleoside triphosphatase/helicase: evidence for activity on the level of substrate and/or enzyme. *Antimicrob. Agents Chemother.* **2002**, *46*, 1231–1239.

257. Zhang, N.; Chen, H. M.; Koch, V.; Schmitz, H.; Liao, C. L.; Bretner, M.; Bhadti, V. S.; Fattom, A. I.; Naso, R. B.; Hosmane, R. S.; Borowski, P. Ring-expanded ("fat") nucleoside and nucleotide analogues exhibit potent in vitro activity against Flaviviridae NTPases/helicases, including those of the West Nile virus, hepatitis C virus, and Japanese encephalitis virus. *J. Med. Chem.* **2003**, *46*, 4149–4164.

258. Zhang, N.; Chen, H. M.; Koch, V.; Schmitz, H.; Minczuk, M.; Stepien, P.; Fattom, A. I.; Naso, R. B.; Kalicharran, K.; Borowski, P.; Hosmane, R. S. Potent inhibition of NTPase/helicase of the West Nile virus by ring-expanded ("fat") nucleoside analogues. *J. Med. Chem.* **2003**, *46*, 4776–4789.

259. Borowski, P.; Deinert, J.; Schalinski, S.; Bretner, M.; Ginalski, K.; Kulikowski, T.; Shugar, D. Halogenated benzimidazoles and benzotriazoles as inhibitors of the NTPase/helicase activities of hepatitis C and related viruses. *Eur. J. Biochem.* **2003**, *270*, 1645–1653.

260. Murthy, H. M. K.; Clum, S.; Padmanabhan, R. Dengue virus NS3 serine protease—crystal structure and insights into interaction of the active site with substrates by molecular modeling and structural analysis of mutational effects. *J. Biol. Chem.* **1999**, *274*, 5573–5580.

261. Bartholomeusz, A.; Tomlinson, E.; Wright, P. J.; Birch, C.; Locarnini, S.; Weigold, H.; Marcuccio, S.; Holan, G. Use of a flavivirus RNA-dependent RNA polymerase assay to investigate the antiviral activity of selected compounds. *Antiviral Res.* **1994**, *24*, 341–350.

262. Shigeta, S.; Mori, S.; Kodama, E.; Kodama, J.; Takahashi, K.; Yamase, T. Broad spectrum anti-RNA virus activities of titanium and vanadium substituted polyoxotungstates. *Antiviral Res.* **2003**, *58*, 265–271.

263. Olsen, D. B.; Bhat, B.; Bosserman, M.; Carroll, S. S.; Colwell, L.; De Francesco, R.; Eldrup, A. B.; Flores, O.; Getty, K.; LaFemina, R.; MacCoss, M.; Migliaccio, G.; Simcoe, A. L.; Rutkowski, C. A.; Stahlhut, M. W.; Tomassini, J. E.; Wolanski, B. 2′-Modified nucleoside analogs as inhibitors of hepatitis C RNA replication. *Antiviral Res.* **2003**, *57*, A76.

264. Nawa, M.; Takasaki, T.; Yamada, K. I.; Kurane, I.; Akatsuka, T. Interference in Japanese encephalitis virus infection of Vero cells by a cationic amphiphilic drug, chlorpromazine. *J. Gen. Virol.* **2003**, *84*, 1737–1741.

265. Andoh, T.; Kawamata, H.; Umatake, M.; Terasawa, K.; Takegami, T.; Ochiai, H. Effect of bafilomycin A1 on the growth of Japanese encephalitis virus in Vero cells. *J. Neurovirol.* **1998**, *4*, 627–631.

266. Sanchez, I.; Gomez-Garibay, F.; Taboada, J.; Ruiz, B. H. Antiviral effect of flavonoids on the dengue virus. *Phytother. Res.* **2000**, *14*, 89–92.

267. Damonte, E. B.; Pujol, C. A.; Noseda, M.; Ciancia, N.; Matulewicz, M. C.; Cerezo, A. S. Potent and selective inhibition of dengue virus by carrageenans. *Antiviral Res.* **2002**, *53*, A49.

268. Laille, M.; Gerald, F.; Debitus, C. In vitro antiviral activity on dengue virus of marine natural products. *Cell. Mol. Life Sci.* **1998**, *54*, 167–170.

269. Takegami, T.; Simamura, E.; Hirai, K. I.; Koyama, J. Inhibitory effect of furanonaphtho-quinone derivatives on the replication of Japanese encephalitis virus. *Antiviral Res.* **1998**, *37*, 37–45.

270. Kim, H.; Kim, S. J.; Park, S. N.; Oh, J. W. Antiviral effect of amphotericin B on Japanese encephalitis virus replication. *J. Microbiol. Biotechnol.* **2004**, *14*, 121–127.

271. Koff, W. C.; Elm, J. L.; Halstead, S. B. Inhibition of dengue virus replication by amantadine hydrochloride. *Antimicrob. Agents Chemother.* **1980**, *18*, 125–129.

272. Raviprakash, K.; Liu, K.; Matteucci, M.; Wagner, R.; Riffenburgh, R.; Carl, M. Inhibition of dengue virus by novel, modified antisense oligonucleotides. *J. Virol.* **1995**, *69*, 69–74.

273. Iversen, P. L.; Stein, D.; Kroeker, A.; Arora, V.; Barklis, E.; Hill, A.; Smith, A.; Wallace, R. Rapid development of an antisense phosphorodiamidate morpholino oligomer for the treatment of West Nile virus. *Antiviral Res.* **2004**, *62*, A32–A33.

274. Shi, P. Y.; Tilgner, M.; Lo, M. K. Construction and characterization of subgenomic replicons of New York strain of West Nile virus. *Virology* **2002**, *296*, 219–233.

275. Shi, P. Y.; Tilgner, M.; Lo, M. K.; Kent, K. A.; Bernard, K. A. Infectious cDNA clone of the epidemic West Nile virus from New York City. *J. Virol.* **2002**, *76*, 5847–5856.

276. Lo, M. K.; Tilgner, M.; Shi, P. Y. Potential high-throughput assay for screening inhibitors of West Nile virus replication. *J. Virol.* **2003**, *77*, 12901–12906.

277. Shi, P. Y. Strategies for the identification of inhibitors of West Nile virus and other flaviviruses. *Curr. Opin. Invest. Drugs* **2002**, *3*, 1567–1573.

278. Sidwell, R. W.; Smee, D. F. Viruses of the Bunya- and Togaviridae families: potential as bioterrorism agents and means of control. *Antiviral Res.* **2003**, *57*, 101–111.

279. Perez, L.; Carrasco, L. Involvement of the vacuolar H^+-ATPase in animal virus entry. *J. Gen. Virol.* **1994**, *75*, 2595–2606.

280. Perez, L.; Carrasco, L. Entry of poliovirus into cells does not require a low-pH step. *J. Virol.* **1993**, *67*, 4543–4548.

281. Guinea, R.; Carrasco, L. Concanamycin-A—a powerful inhibitor of enveloped animal-virus entry into cells. *Biochem. Biophys. Res. Commun.* **1994**, *201*, 1270–1278.

282. Irurzun, A.; Nieva, J. L.; Carrasco, L. Entry of Semliki Forest virus into cells: effects of concanamycin A and nigericin on viral membrane fusion and infection. *Virology* **1997**, *227*, 488–492.

283. Jahrling, P. B.; Hesse, R. A.; Rhoderick, J. B.; Elwell, M. A.; Moe, J. B. Pathogenesis of a Pichinde virus strain adapted to produce lethal infections in guinea pigs. *Infect. Immun.* **1981**, *32*, 872–880.

284. Liu, C. T.; Griffin, M. J.; Jahrling, P. B.; Peters, C. J. Physiologic and pharmacologic treatments of Pichinde virus infection in strain 13 guinea pigs. *Fed. Proc.* **1985**, *44*, 1836.

285. Perez, M.; Craven, R. C.; de la Torre, J. C. The small RING finger protein Z drives arenavirus budding: implications for antiviral strategies. *Proc. Natl. Acad. Sci. U.S.A.* **2003**, *100*, 12978–12983.

286. Lopez, N.; Jacamo, R.; Franze-Fernandez, M. T. Transcription and RNA replication of Tacaribe virus genome and antigenome analogs require N and L proteins: Z protein is an inhibitor of these processes. *J. Virol.* **2001**, *75*, 12241–12251.

287. Jacamo, R.; Lopez, N.; Wilda, M.; Franze-Fernandez, M. T. Tacaribe virus Z protein interacts with the L polymerase protein to inhibit viral RNA synthesis. *J. Virol.* **2003**, *77*, 10383–10393.

288. Cornu, T. I.; de la Torre, J. C. Characterization of the arenavirus RING finger Z protein regions required for Z-mediated inhibition of viral RNA synthesis. *J. Virol.* **2002**, *76*, 6678–6688.

289. Garcia, C. C.; Candurra, N. A.; Damonte, E. B. Antiviral and virucidal activities against arenaviruses of zinc-finger active compounds. *Antiviral Chem. Chemother.* **2000**, *11*, 231–237.

290. Garcia, C. C.; Candurra, N. A.; Damonte, E. B. Mode of inactivation of arenaviruses by disulfide-based compounds. *Antiviral Res.* **2002**, *55*, 437–446.

291. Garcia, C. C.; Candurra, N. A.; Damonte, E. B. Differential inhibitory action of two azoic compounds against arenaviruses. *Int. J. Antimicrob. Agents* **2003**, *21*, 319–324.

292. Bartolotta, S.; Garcia, C. C.; Candurra, N. A.; Damonte, E. B. Effect of fatty acids on arenavirus replication: inhibition of virus production by lauric acid. *Arch. Virol.* **2001**, *146*, 777–790.

293. Cordo, S. M.; Candurra, N. A.; Damonte, E. B. Myristic acid analogs are inhibitors of Junin virus replication. *Microbes Infect.* **1999**, *1*, 609–614.

294. Candurra, N. A.; Maskin, L.; Damonte, E. B. Inhibition of arenavirus multiplication in vitro by phenotiazines. *Antiviral Res.* **1996**, *31*, 149–158.

295. Ruiz-Jarabo, C. M.; Ly, C.; Domingo, E.; de la Torre, J. C. Lethal mutagenesis of the prototypic arenavirus lymphocytic choriomeningitis virus (LCMV). *Virology* **2003**, *308*, 37–47.

296. Xing, Z.; Whitton, J. L. Ribozymes which cleave arenavirus RNAs—identification of susceptible target sites and inhibition by target site secondary structure. *J. Virol.* **1992**, *66*, 1361–1369.

297. Xing, Z.; Whitton, J. L. An anti-lymphocytic choriomeningitis virus ribozyme expressed in tissue culture cells diminishes viral RNA levels and leads to a reduction in infectious virus yield. *J. Virol.* **1993**, *67*, 1840–1847.

298. Kunz, S.; Borrow, P.; Oldstone, M. B. A. Receptor structure, binding, and cell entry of arenaviruses. *Arenaviruses I* **2002**, *262*, 111–137.

299. Spiropoulou, C. F.; Kunz, S.; Rollin, P. E.; Campbell, K. P.; Oldstone, M. B. A. New World arenavirus clade C, but not clade A and B viruses, utilizes alpha-dystroglycan as its major receptor. *J. Virol.* **2002**, *76*, 5140–5146.

300. Cao, W.; Henry, M. D.; Borrow, P.; Yamada, H.; Elder, J. H.; Ravkov, E. V.; Nichol, S. T.; Compans, R. W.; Campbell, K. P.; Oldstone, M. B. A. Identification of alpha-dystroglycan as a receptor for lymphocytic choriomeningitis virus and Lassa fever virus. *Science* **1998**, *282*, 2079–2081.

301. Wachsman, M. B.; Lopez, E. M. F.; Ramirez, J. A.; Galagovsky, L. R.; Coto, C. E. Antiviral effect of brassinosteroids against herpes virus and arenaviruses. *Antiviral Chem. Chemother.* **2000**, *11*, 71–77.

302. Garcia, C. C.; Rosso, M. L.; Bertoni, M. D.; Maier, M. S.; Damonte, E. B. Evaluation of the antiviral activity against Junin virus of macrocyclic trichothecenes produced by the hypocrealean epibiont of *Baccharis coridifolia. Planta Med.* **2002**, *68*, 209–212.

303. Uckun, F. M.; Petkevich, A. S.; Vassilev, A. O.; Tibbles, H. E.; Titov, L. Stampidine prevents mortality in an experimental mouse model of viral hemorrhagic fever caused by Lassa virus. *BMC Infect. Dis.* **2004**, *4*, art-1.

304. Khan, A. S.; Young, J. C. Hantavirus pulmonary syndrome: at the crossroads. *Curr. Opin. Infect. Dis.* **2001**, *14*, 205–209.

305. Sidwell, R. W.; Huffman, J. H.; Barnard, D. L.; Pifat, D. Y. Effects of ribamidine, a 3-carboxamidine derivative of ribavirin, on experimentally induced Phlebovirus infections. *Antiviral Res.* **1988**, *10*, 193–207.

306. Fisher, A. F.; Tesh, R. B.; Tonry, J.; Guzman, H.; Liu, D. Y.; Xiao, S. Y. Induction of severe disease in hamsters by two sandfly fever group viruses, Punta Toro and Gabek Forest (Phlebovirus, Bunyaviridae), similar to that caused by Rift Valley fever virus. *Am. J. Trop. Med. Hyg.* **2003**, *69*, 269–276.

307. Bray, M.; Davis, K.; Geisbert, T.; Schmaljohn, C.; Huggins, J. A mouse model for evaluation of prophylaxis and therapy of Ebola hemorrhagic fever. *J. Infect. Dis.* **1998**, *178*, 651–661.

308. Smee, D. F.; Bray, M.; Huggins, J. W. Intracellular phosphorylation of carbocyclic 3-deazaadenosine, an anti-Ebola virus agent. *Antiviral Chem. Chemother.* **2001**, *12*, 251–258.

309. Bray, M.; Driscoll, J.; Huggins, J. W. Treatment of lethal Ebola virus infection in mice with a single dose of an *S*-adenosyl-L-homocysteine hydrolase inhibitor. *Antiviral Res.* **2000**, *45*, 135–147.

310. Bray, M.; Raymond, J. L.; Geisbert, T.; Baker, R. O. 3-Deazaneplanocin A induces massively increased interferon-alpha production in Ebola virus-infected mice. *Antiviral Res.* **2002**, *55*, 151–159.

311. Bray, M. Defense against filoviruses used as biological weapons. *Antiviral Res.* **2003**, *57*, 53–60.

312. Trampuz, A.; Prabhu, R. M.; Smith, T. F.; Baddour, L. M. Avian influenza: a new pandemic threat. *Mayo Clin. Proc.* **2004**, *79*, 523–530.

313. Krug, R. M. The potential use of influenza virus as an agent for bioterrorism. *Antiviral Res.* **2003**, *57*, 147–150.

314. Gubareva, L. V.; Penn, C. R.; Webster, R. G. Inhibition of replication of avian influenza viruses by the neuraminidase inhibitor 4-guanidino-2,4-dideoxy-2,3-dehydro-*N*-acetylneuraminic acid. *Virology* **1995**, *212*, 323–330.

315. Gubareva, L. V.; McCullers, J. A.; Bethell, R. C.; Webster, R. G. Characterization of influenza A/HongKong/156/97 (H5N1) virus in a mouse model and protective effect of zanamivir on H5N1 infection in mice. *J. Infect. Dis.* **1998**, *178*, 1592–1596.

316. Leneva, I. A.; Roberts, N.; Govorkova, E. A.; Goloubeva, O. G.; Webster, R. G. The neuraminidase inhibitor GS4104 (oseltamivir phosphate) is efficacious against A/Hong Kong/156/97 (H5N1) and A/Hong Kong/1074/99 (H9N2) influenza viruses. *Antiviral Res.* **2000**, *48*, 101–115.

317. Govorkova, E. A.; Leneva, I. A.; Goloubeva, O. G.; Bush, K.; Webster, R. G. Comparison of efficacies of RWJ-270201, zanamivir, and oseltamivir against H5N1, H9N2, and other avian influenza viruses. *Antimicrob. Agents Chemother.* **2001**, *45*, 2723–2732.

318. Brooks, M. J.; Sasadeusz, J. J.; Tannock, G. A. Antiviral chemotherapeutic agents against respiratory viruses: where are we now and what's in the pipeline? *Curr. Opin. Pulm. Med.* **2004**, *10*, 197–203.

319. Tseng, C.; Laughlin, C. Antiviral agents, RNA (viruses other than HIV), and orthopoxviruses. In *Burger's Medicinal Chemistry and Drug Discovery*, 6th ed., V.5, Abraham, D. (Ed.). John Wiley & Sons, Hoboken, NJ, 2003, pp 359–457.

CHAPTER 4

Antiviral Drug Targets and Strategies for Emerging Viral Diseases and Bioterrorism Threats

Erik De Clercq

Rega Institute for Medical Research, Katholieke Universiteit Leuven

4.1 INTRODUCTION

Interest in the development of new antivirals depends primarily on the answers to two questions (1) What is the need for having at hand a specific antiviral drug against the viral disease concerned (and could it be reasonably expected that the virus infection would be controlled by using the antiviral drug)? (2) Which antiviral drugs are currently available to treat or prevent the virus infection concerned, or, if not, which antiviral strategies should be pursued to meet the demands? This chapter examines how different virus infections, depending on the virus species involved, should be approached from a therapeutic viewpoint, especially for those virus infections that may emerge anew, or reemerge after having disappeared, or (re)emerge as part of a bioterrorist scenario. Basic strategies in the design of antiviral drugs have been described previously.[1] Here, I evaluate antiviral drug targets and strategies that would be of primary importance in the case of an advertent or inadvertent virus outbreak or attack. In particular, I focus on the virus infections reviewed in Table 4.1. Of the viral agents listed in Table 4.1, poxviruses such as variola (smallpox), arenaviruses such as Lassa, and filoviruses such as Ebola and Marburg belong to Category A or highest priority agents [according to Centers for Disease Control and Prevention (CDC)] because they can easily be disseminated or transmitted from person to person, result in high mortality rates and have the potential for major public health impact, may cause public panic and social disruption, and require special action for public health preparedness. The alphaviruses western, eastern, and Venezuelan equine encephalitis belong to Category B

Antiviral Drug Discovery for Emerging Diseases and Bioterrorism Threats. Edited by Paul F. Torrence
Copyright © 2005 John Wiley & Sons, Inc.

TABLE 4.1 Virus Infections that Could (Re-)emerge from Nature or Be Used as Bioterrorism Weapons

Poxviruses	Variola, vaccinia, monkeypox, cowpox, camelpox, molluscum contagium, orf (sheep-pox)
Flaviviruses	Yellow fever, dengue fever, West Nile fever, Japanese encephalitis, tickborne encephalitis
Arenaviruses	Lassa, Junin, Machupo, Guanarito, Sabia
Bunyaviruses	Nairo: Crimean-Congo hemorrhagic fever
	Phlebo: Rift Valley fever
	Hanta: Hantaan and other hantaviruses
Togaviruses (Alphaviruses)	Venezuelan equine encephalitis, eastern equine encephalitis, and western equine encephalitis
Rhaboviruses	Rabies
Filoviruses	Marburg, Ebola
Orthomyxoviruses	Influenza A
Paramyxoviruses	Parainfluenza, measles, mumps, RSV (respiratory syncytial virus), metapneumovirus, Nipah, Hendra
Coronaviruses	SARS (severe acute respiratory syndrome)-associated coronavirus

or second highest priority agents because they are moderately easy to disseminate and result in moderate morbidity rates and low mortality rates. Category C or third highest priority agents include emerging infectious pathogens such as Nipah and hantaviruses, which could be made available for mass dissemination in the future and have the potential for high morbidity and mortality.

As background information it may be useful to know which antiviral agents have been formally approved (licensed) and are thus currently available for medical use. These antiviral drugs are listed in Table 4.2 and

TABLE 4.2 Approved Antiviral Drugs

For the treatment of human immunodeficiency virus (HIV) infections

Nucleoside Reverse Transcriptase Inhibitors (NRTIs)

- Zidovudine: 3′-azido-2′,3′-dideoxythymidine (AZT)
- Didanosine: 2′,3′-dideoxyinosine (ddI)
- Zalcitabine: 2′,3′-dideoxycytidine (ddC)
- Stavudine: 2′,3′-dideoxy-2′,3′-didehydrothymidine (d4T)
- Lamivudine: (−)-β-L-3′-thia-2′,3′-dideoxycytidine (3TC)
- Abacavir (ABC): 2-amino-6-cyclopropylaminopurin-9-yl-2-cyclopentene
- Emtricitabine: (−)-β-L-3′-thia-2′,3′-dideoxy-5-fluorocytidine [(−)-FTC]

Nucleotide Reverse Transcriptase Inhibitors (NtRTIs)

- Tenofovir disoproxil: bis(isopropoxycarbonyloxymethyl)ester of (R)-9-(2-phosphonyl-methoxypropyl)adenine

TABLE 4.2 (*Continued*)

Non-nucleoside Reverse Transcriptase Inhibitors (NNRTIs)

- Nevirapine
- Delavirdine
- Efavirenz

Protease Inhibitors (PIs)

- Saquinavir
- Ritonavir
- Indinavir
- Nelfinavir
- Amprenavir
- Lopinavir
- Atazanavir

Fusion Inhibitors (FIs)

- Enfuvirtide: Pentafuside (T-20)

For the treatment of hepatitis B virus (HBV) infections

- Lamivudine (see above)
- Adefovir dipivoxil: bis(pivaloyloxymethyl)ester of 9-(2-phosphonylmethoxy-ethyl)adenine

For the treatment of herpes simplex virus (HSV) and varicella-zoster virus (VZV) infections

- Acyclovir and its oral prodrug, valaciclovir
- Penciclovir and its oral prodrug, famciclovir
- Idoxuridine: 5-iodo-2′-deoxyuridine (IDU)
- Trifluridine: 5-trifluoro-2′-deoxythymidine (TFT)
- Brivudin: (*E*)-5-(2-bromovinyl)-2′-deoxyuridine (BVDU)

For the treatment of cytomegalovirus (CMV) infections

- Ganciclovir and its oral prodrug, valganciclovir
- Foscarnet: phosphonoformic acid (PFA) trisodium salt
- Cidofovir: (*S*)-1-(3-hydroxy-2-phosphonylmethoxypropyl)cytosine (HPMPC)
- Fomivirsen: antisense (phosphorothioate) oligonucleotide

For the treatment of influenza virus infections

- Amantadine
- Rimantadine
- Zanamivir
- Oseltamivir

For the treatment of hepatitis C virus (HCV) infections

- (Pegylated) interferon-α
- Ribavirin

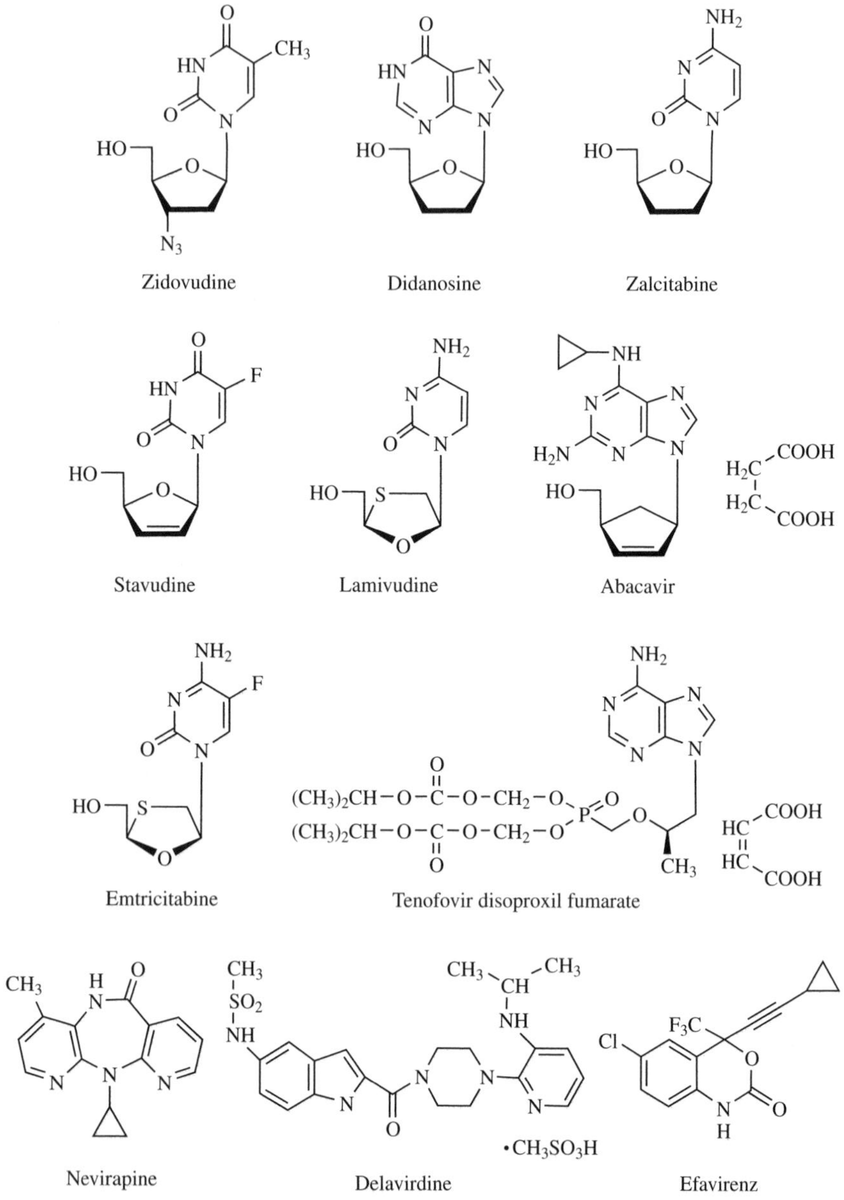

SCHEME 4.1   Structures of licensed antiviral drugs.

their chemical formulas are presented in Scheme 4.1. New compounds (under development) are presented in Scheme 4.2, and general strategies for approaching the therapy of the virus infections concerned are indicated in Figures 4.1–4.5.

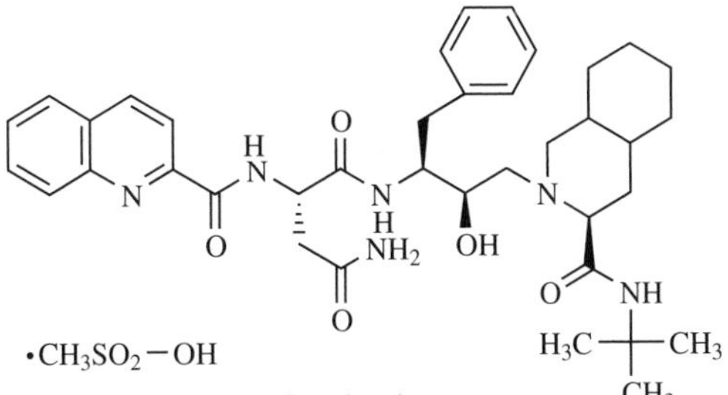

Saquinavir

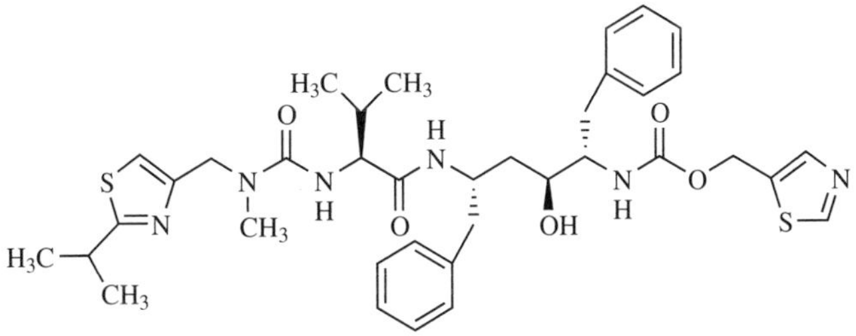

Ritonavir

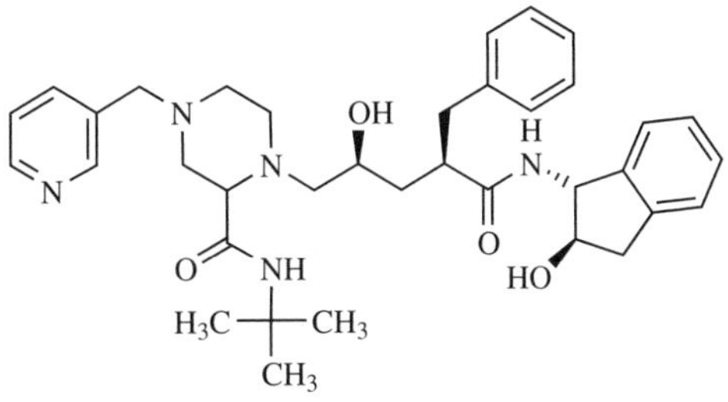

Indinavir

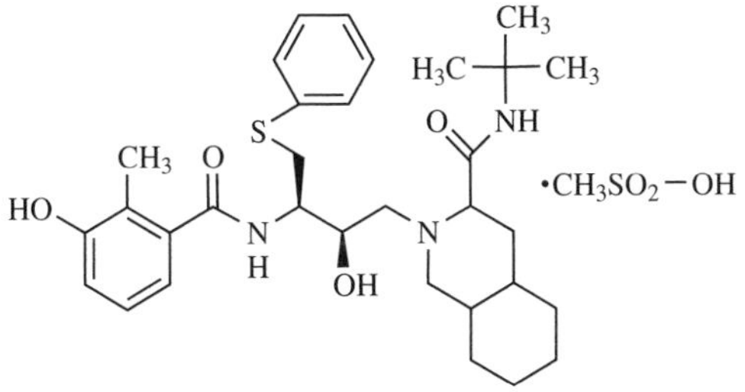

Nelfinavir

SCHEME 4.1 (*Continued*)

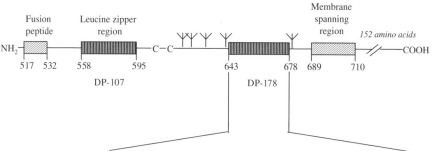

Amprenavir

Lopinavir

Atazanavir

YTSLIHSLIEESQNQQEKNEQELLELDKWASLWNWF

Enfuvirtide

Adefovir dipivoxil

Acyclovir

SCHEME 4.1 (*Continued*)

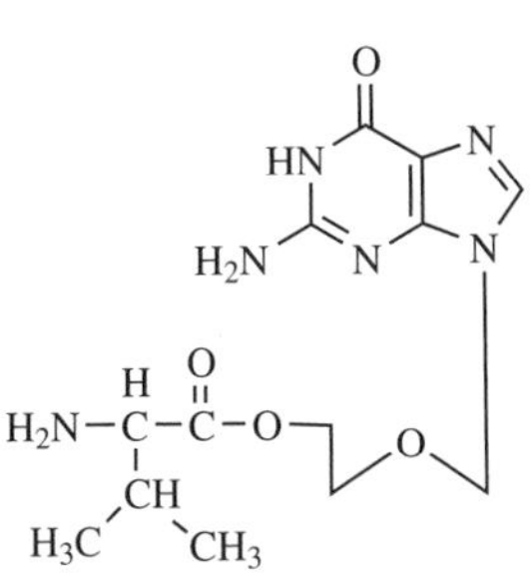

Valaciclovir

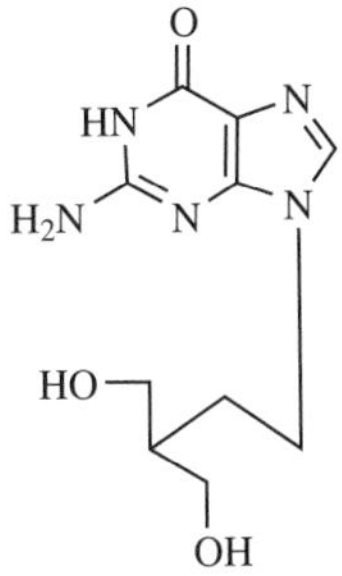

Penciclovir

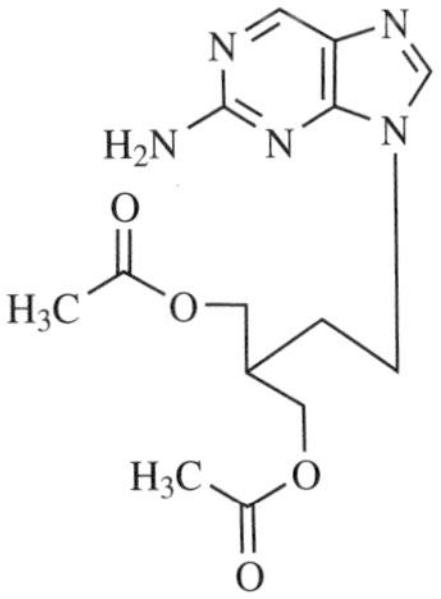

Famciclovir

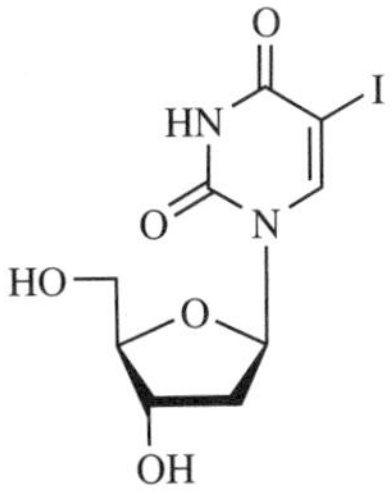

Idoxuridine

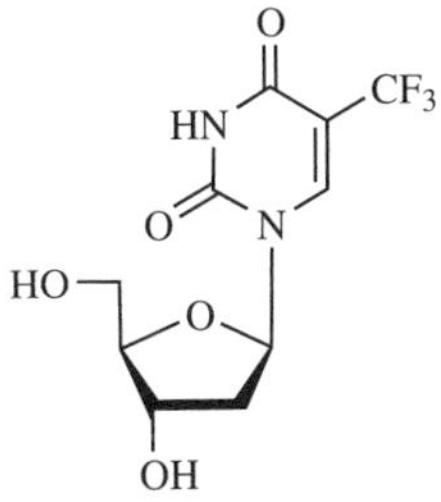

Trifluridine

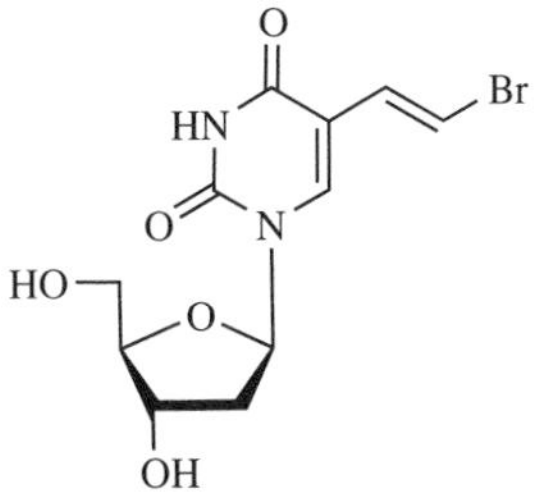

Brivudin

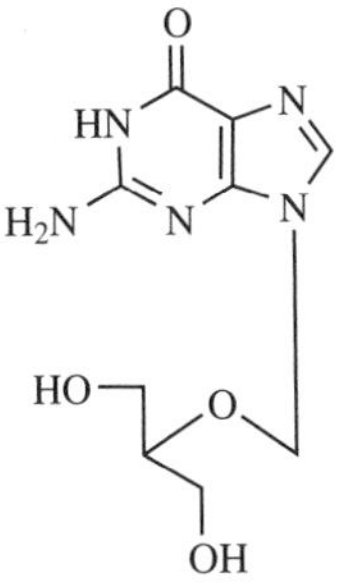

Ganciclovir

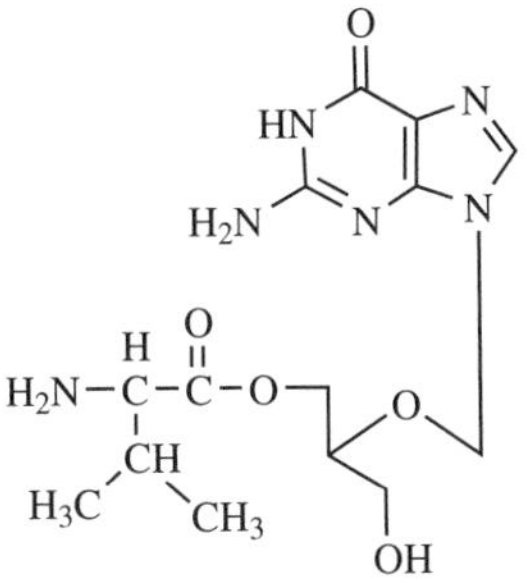

Valganciclovir

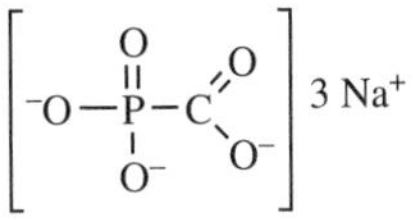

Foscarnet

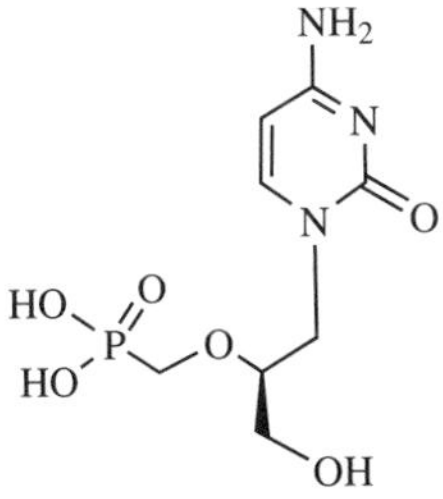

Cidofovir

5′-d-[G*C*G*T*T*T*G*C*T*C*T*T*C*T*T*C*T*T*G*C*G]-3′
sodium salt

* = racemic phosphorothioate

Fomivirsen

SCHEME 4.1 (*Continued*)

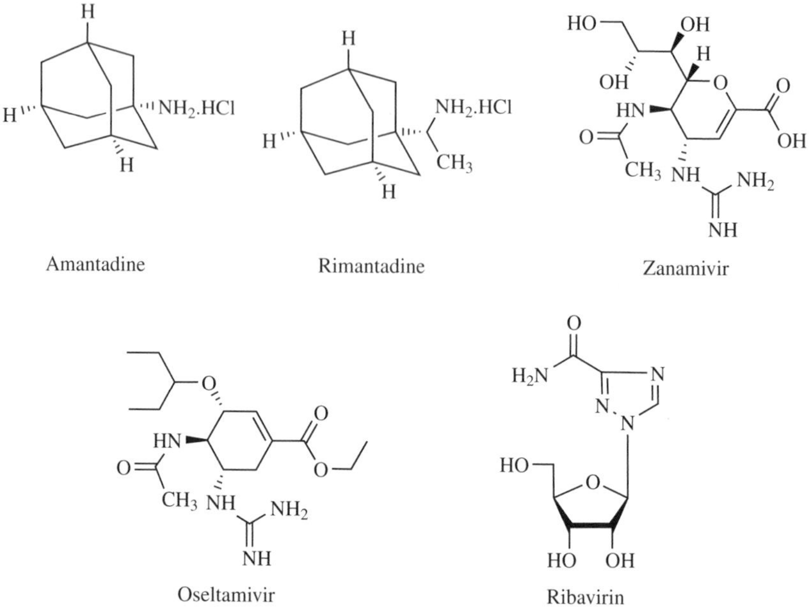

Amantadine   Rimantadine   Zanamivir

Oseltamivir   Ribavirin

SCHEME 4.1 (*Continued*)

4.2 POXVIRUS INFECTIONS

The family of Poxviridae encompasses orthopoxviruses (such as variola, vaccinia, cowpox, monkeypox, and camelpox), parapoxviruses [such as orf (contagious ecthyma)] and molluscipoxviruses (i.e., molluscum contagiosum virus). The last natural case of smallpox, the disease caused by variola virus, occurred in 1977 in Somalia and marked the end of the most successful public health campaign ever undertaken. In 1980 the World Health Organization (WHO) declared global eradication of smallpox. Since then the only known stocks of variola virus have been held in Atlanta (United States) at the Centers for Disease Control and Prevention (CDC) and at the State Research Center of Virology and Biotechnology (VECTOR) in Koltsovo (Russia). If illegally preserved stocks of variola virus were to be used for biological and/or terrorist purposes, in a highly mobile and susceptible population, it would cause a real catastrophe. Variola virus could indeed be considered as an "ideal" bioterrorist weapon for a number of reasons[2]: it is highly transmissible by the aerosol route from infected to susceptible persons; the civilian populations of most countries contain a high proportion of susceptible (unvaccinated) persons; smallpox is associated with high morbidity and about 30%; mortality; initially, diagnosis of a disease that has not been seen for 25 years would be difficult; and, at present, other than the vaccinia-based vaccine, which may be effective in the first few days postinfection, there is no formally approved drug for the treatment of smallpox.[2]

Whereas variola virus is transmissible from human to human, the closely related monkeypox virus is not. The latter can be considered as a zoonosis in that it is transmitted from animals to humans, as was recently demonstrated in an outbreak of monkeypox in the United States, where the virus was imported by the gambian rat (*Cricetomys gambiansis*) and transmitted to humans via prairie dogs. Otherwise, monkeypox virus may lead to clinical manifestations that in humans and monkeys very much resemble the clinical symptoms of smallpox (fever, rash, pustules, etc.).

Yet, quite a variety of potential antiviral therapeutics have proved to be active against orthopoxvirus infections, both in vitro in cell culture,[3] and in vivo in animal models.[4] Therapeutic strategies could be envisaged that are targeted at such cellular enzymes as IMP dehydrogenase (the enzyme responsible for the conversion of IMP

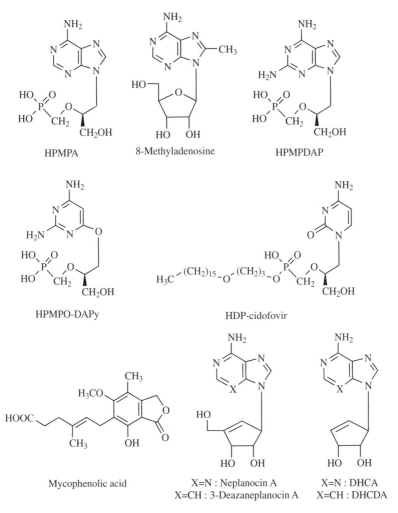

SCHEME 4.2   Structures of antiviral compounds in (pre)clinical development.

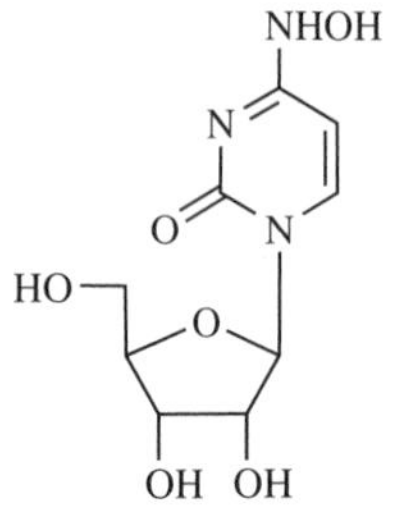

N^4-Hydroxycytidine

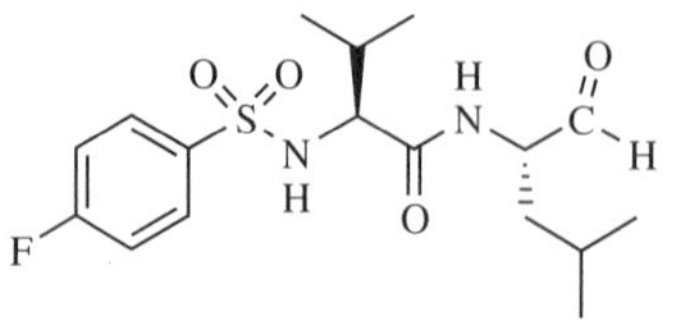

N-(4-Fluorophenylsulfonyl)-L-valyl-L-leucinal

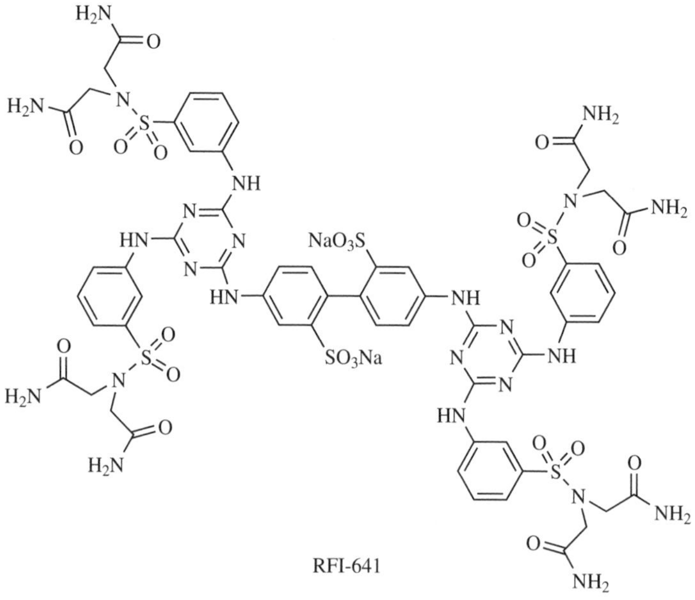

RFI-641

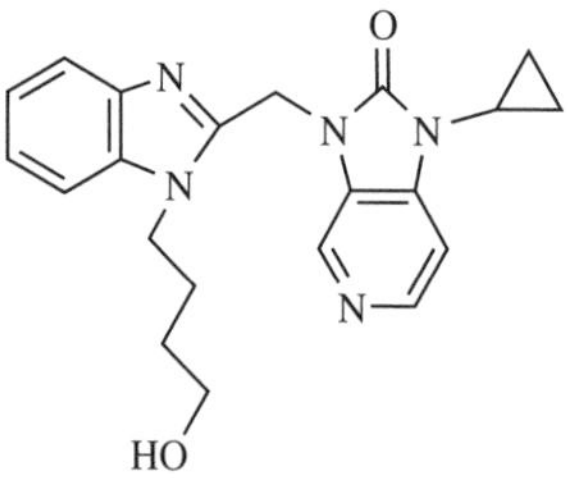

BMS-433771

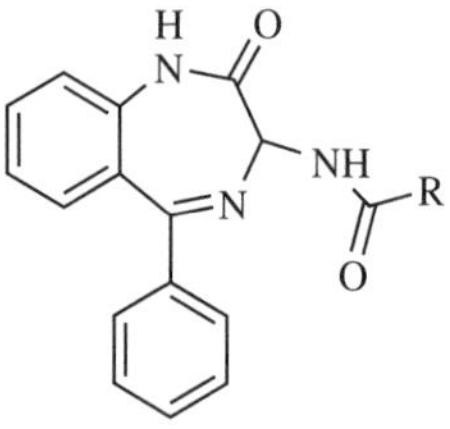

A-33903
A-60444

SCHEME 4.2 (*Continued*)

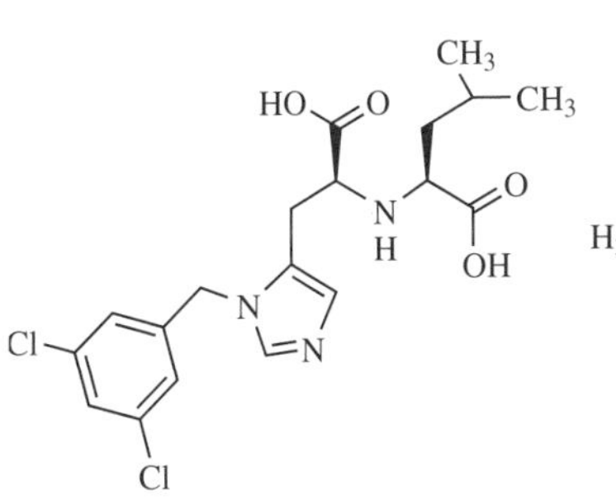

MLN-4760

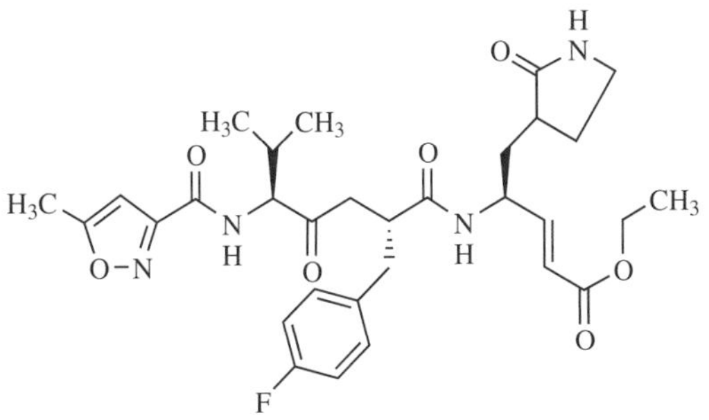

AG7088

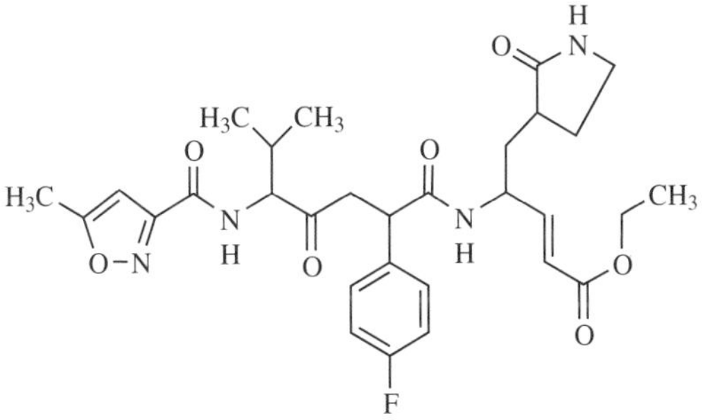

KZ7088

SCHEME 4.2 *(Continued)*

to XMP, a key step in the de novo biosynthesis of GTP), SAH hydrolase [the enzyme responsible for the hydrolysis of *S*-adenosylhomocysteine, the product-inhibitor of *S*-adenosylmethionine (SAM)-dependent methylation reactions, such as those involved in the maturation of viral mRNAs], OMP decarboxylase (the enzyme responsible for the conversion of OMP to UMP, a key reaction in the de novo biosynthesis of UTP), and CTP synthetase (which converts UTP to CTP), as well as viral enzymes such as the poxviral DNA polymerase.[5]

In fact, several nucleoside and nucleotide analogues have been identified as potent anti-poxvirus agents: among the nucleoside analogues are 2-amino-7-[(1,3-dihydroxy-2-propoxy)methyl]purine (S2242) and 8-methyladenosine; among the nucleotide analogues are (*S*)-1-(3-hydroxy-2-phosphonylmethoxypropyl)cytosine (HPMPC, cidofovir), (*S*)-9-(3-hydroxy-2-phosphonylmethoxypropyl)-2,6-diaminopurine (HPMPDAP), and (*S*)-6-(3-hydroxy-2-phosphonylmethoxypropyl)oxy-2,4-diaminopyrimidine (HPMPO-DAPy). These compounds have proved to be effective in various animal models for poxvirus infections.[6] In particular, cidofovir has demonstrated high efficacy, even when administered as a single systemic (intraperitoneal) or intranasal (aerosolized) dose, in protecting mice from a lethal respiratory infection with either vaccinia or cowpox (as reviewed).[7] Cidofovir has also demonstrated high effectiveness in the treatment of lethal vaccinia virus infections in SCID (severe combined immune deficiency) mice.[8] Cidofovir has been shown to

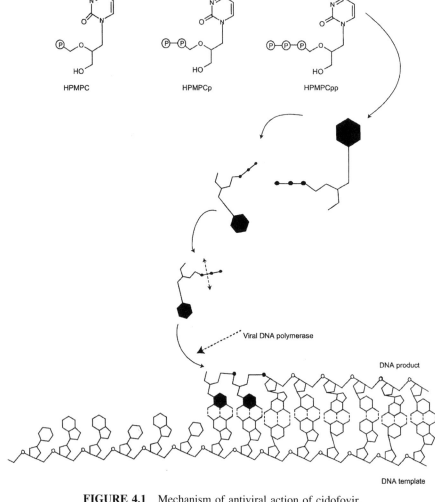

FIGURE 4.1   Mechanism of antiviral action of cidofovir.

protect cynomolgus monkeys against smallpox-like disease induced by either variola or monkeypox.[9] In these experiments, cidofovir effected a significant reduction in viral load, lesion count, and mortality rate, both for variola and monkeypox, and so fulfilled the FDA Animal Efficacy Rule for evaluation of drug efficacy.[9] This is as close as one can get experimentally to predict efficacy in the treatment of smallpox (or monkeypox) in humans.

Cidofovir (in its diphosphate form) appears to specifically interfere with the pox vaccinia virus DNA polymerase; when incorporated into the DNA (opposite a G in the template strand), it would lead to chain termination immediately following the incorporation of one more nucleotide (dNMP).[10] Not surprisingly, vaccinia virus

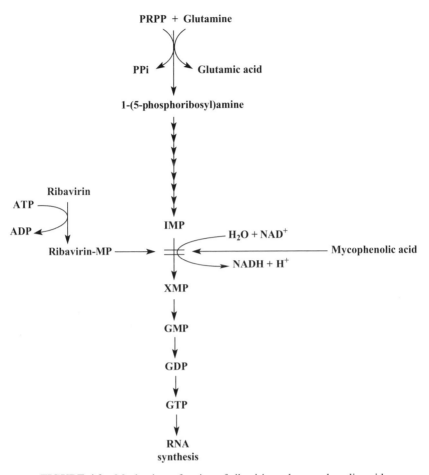

FIGURE 4.2 Mechanism of action of ribavirin and mycophenolic acid.

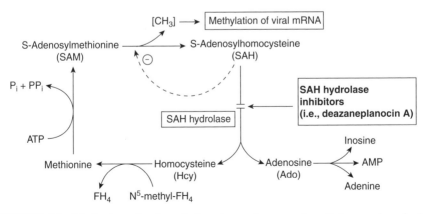

FIGURE 4.3 Mechanism of action of adenosine analogues such as 3-deazaneplanocin A.

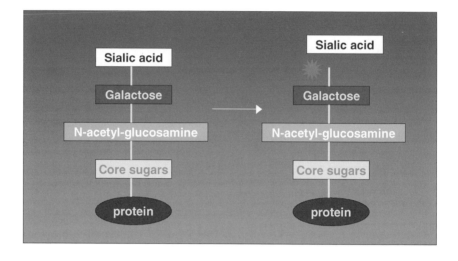

Sialyl α-glycoside
R = glycoprotein

Sialic acid + R-OH

FIGURE 4.4   Mechanism of action of neuraminidase (NA): NA cleaves sialic acid from cell-surface glycoprotein.

mutants have been obtained that are resistant to cidofovir and other acyclic nucleoside phosphonate analogues,[11,12] but the procedure (repeated passages in the presence of the compound) involved in the development of vaccinia virus resistance to cidofovir leads to a marked attenuation of virus virulence, as has been shown in mice.[12]

In humans, cidofovir has been used successfully in the treatment, by both topical and intravenous routes, of recalcitrant molluscum contagiosum and orf in immunocompromised patients (as reviewed).[7] Cidofovir has been formally licensed for clinical use (by intravenous injection) in the treatment of CMV retinitis in AIDS patients. However, it could also be formulated for topical administration (e.g., as a gel or cream), or for oral administration, in prodrug form. Under current investigation is the oral prodrug 1-O-hexadecyloxypropyl derivative (HDP-cidofovir), which has been shown to possess increased anti-poxvirus activity relative to cidofovir,[13] due to facilitated uptake by the cells.[14]

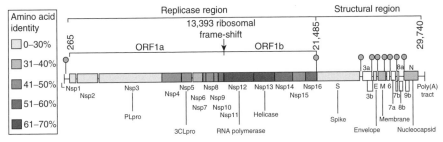

FIGURE 4.5 Genome structure of SARS coronavirus.[62] Replicase and structural regions are shown together with the predicted cleavage products in ORF1a and ORF1b. The position of the leader sequence (L), the 3' poly(A) tract, and the ribosomal frameshift site between ORF1a and ORF1b are also indicated. Each box represents a protein product (Nsp, nonstructural protein). Shading indicates the level of amino acid identity with the best-matching protein of other coronaviruses. The SARS-CoV accessory genes are white. Filled circles indicate the positions of the nine transcription-regulatory sequences (TRSs) that are specific for SARS-CoV (5'ACGAAC3').

Although the ultimate (proof i.e., activity against smallpox in humans) has not (and, for obvious reasons, cannot) be provided, from the foregoing it can be deduced that cidofovir should be effective in the therapy and short-term prophylaxis of smallpox and related poxvirus infections (i.e., monkeypox) in humans, as well as the treatment of the complications of vaccinia that may arise in immunocompromised patients inadvertently inoculated with the smallpox vaccine (vaccinia). We have recently elaborated a murine model that mimics progressive/disseminated vaccinia in humans.[15] In this model (athymic-nude mice inoculated intracutaneously with vaccinia virus), systemic treatment with cidofovir, initiated at the time that disseminated vaccinia had developed, caused the lesions to heal and regress: in most of the animals thus treated, lesions completely (or almost completely) disappeared within 10–15 days after the start of therapy.[15] Obviously, these observations have far-reaching implications for the therapy of complications of vaccination against smallpox.

4.3 FLAVIVIRUS INFECTIONS

The genus *Flavivirus* contains over 70 species, many of which cause disease in humans. Severe flavivirus infections are primarily characterized by encephalitis or hemorrhagic symptoms. Mortality rates may vary from 1–2%; (e.g., for the Central European encephalitis virus) up to 30–40% (e.g., for the Japanese encephalitis virus and the Russian spring-summer encephalitis virus). For yellow fever virus infections, over 5000 fatal cases are reported annually worldwide, despite the availability of an effective (live) vaccine. For dengue virus, each year over 500,000 cases are reported—over 25,000 of which are fatal due to the development of dengue hemorrhagic fever or dengue shock syndrome. Also, West Nile virus, St. Louis encephalitis virus, and Murray Valley encephalitis virus can cause human fatalities. Tickborne encephalitis virus, previously known as Russian spring-summer ence-phalitis virus, is believed to cause annually at least 11,000 human cases of encephalitis in Russia and about 3000 cases in the rest of Europe. Related viruses such as louping ill virus, Langat virus, and Powassan virus also cause human encephalitis but rarely on an epidemic scale. Three other viruses within the same group—Omsk hemorrhagic fever virus, Kyasanur Forest disease virus, and Alkhurma virus—tend to cause fetal hemorrhagic fevers rather than encephalitis.[16] Although feared as a possible bioterroristic weapon, tickborne flavivirus infections may not seem practical, as very large numbers of infected ticks would be required, and it would be extremely difficult to arrange for them to be infected and ready to feed when delivered as biological weapons.[16]

Prospects for the therapy of flavivirus infections look rather meager.[17] Ribavirin has only weak activity against flaviviruses. Interferon and interferon inducers seem to be a valuable option, but, as a rule, treatment with interferon (inducers) should be initiated before or very shortly following infection to yield any beneficial effect. An experimental flavivirus encephalitis model, based on infection of hamsters with the murine Modoc virus, has been elaborated:[18] during the acute phase, the infection is associated with flaccid paralysis, as has also been observed in patients with West Nile virus encephalitis, and neurological sequelae that may develop thereafter are reminiscent of those observed, for example, in survivors of Japanese encephalitis.[18] This model should be highly suitable to evaluate antiviral therapies. At present, interferon (i.e., interferon-α 2b, whether pegylated or not) and interferon inducers [i.e., poly(I)•poly(C) and Ampligen] offer the greatest potential for activity in this model, as they have been shown to significantly delay virus-induced morbidity (paralysis) and mortality (due to progressive encephalitis) in a related model of Modoc virus-induced encephalitis in SCID mice.[19] High-titered immunoglobulins are considered as a possible approach in the containment of West Nile virus infections. Of note, ribavirin did not offer any beneficial effect in this model, whether it was given alone or in combination with interferon, whereas in previous studies (as reviewed,[19] poly(I)•poly(C) was shown to be efficacious in mice against experimental infections with tickborne encephalitis virus, Japanese encephalitis virus, or West Nile virus.

Of a variety of compounds, targeted at either IMP dehydrogenase (ribavirin, EICAR, tiazofurin, selenazofurin, and mycophenolic acid), OMP decarboxylase (pyrazofurin and 6-azauridine), CTP synthetase (carbodine and cyclopentenyl cytosine), dihydrofolate reductase (methotrexate), or sulfated polymers (dextran sulfate and PAVAS), mycophenolic acid, EICAR, and methotrexate proved the most active against yellow fever virus in cell culture.[20] These compounds therefore deserve further evaluation for their potential usefulness in the treatment of yellow fever virus and other flavivirus (i.e., West Nile virus)[21] infections.

Also worthy of further evaluation is the antisense phosphorodiamidate morpho-lino oligomer (PMO) approach designed to inhibit the translation of the single polyprotein in West Nile virus, and which could readily be extended to other flaviviruses.[22] Preliminary data indicate that such an approach might work in vivo (mice, penguins, and humans) in reducing virus titers as well as symptoms,[22] but obviously these data need further corroboration.

4.4 ARENAVIRUS INFECTIONS

Among the 23 arenavirus species known, five are associated with viral hemorrhagic fevers: Lassa, Junin, Machupo, Guanarito, and Sabia. They are included (together with variola, *Bacillus anthracis*, *Yersinia pestis*, *Clostridium botulinum*, *Francisella tularensis*, and filoviruses) in the Category A Pathogen List established by the Centers for Disease Control and Prevention that groups agents with the greatest potential for adverse public health impact and mass casualties in an ill-intentioned abuse situation.[23] Of the (many) hemorrhagic fever viruses brought into the Western world, Lassa virus may certainly be one of the more prominent.[24]

It is gratifying to note that, as demonstrated with Tacaribe virus and an attenuated Junin virus strain, arenavirus replication (in vitro) is highly susceptible to a number of compounds, including adenosine analogues (i.e., SAH hydrolase inhibitors such as 3-deazaneplanocin A), cytidine analogues (i.e., cyclopentenyl cytosine), guanosine analogues (i.e., IMP dehydrogenase inhibitors such as ribavirin), and sulfated polysaccharides such as dextran sulfate.[25]

Why are arenaviruses good candidates for weaponization? As explained before,[23] large quantities of arenaviruses can be produced by propagation in cell culture; contamination of large human populations is likely since infection occurs via the respiratory pathway and virus-containing aerosols may be dispersed through a bioterrorist attack; secondary human-to-human (airborne) transmissions are to be expected; diagnostic capacities are very limited, as there are no commercially available diagnostic kits based on either serologic or molecular techniques; and arenavirus genomes display remarkable plasticity, giving rise to reassortants that may be suspected of being capable of infecting humans (as reviewed).[23]

Ribavirin has proved to be effective in the postexposure prophylaxis and therapy of experimental arenavirus infections in animal models, and anecdotal reports, as mentioned by Charrel and de Lamballerie,[23] suggest that ribavirin might also be effective in the treatment of arenavirus (i.e., Machupo, Sabia) infections in humans.[23] The most convincing evidence for the efficacy of ribavirin was obtained in the case of Lassa fever, where ribavirin was shown to significantly reduce the case-fatality rate, irrespective of the time point in the illness when treatment was started.[26]

4.5 BUNYAVIRUS AND TOGAVIRUS INFECTIONS

Among the togaviruses, Venezuelan equine encephalitis virus, eastern equine encephalitis virus, and western equine encephalitis virus, and among the bunyaviruses, Rift Valley fever, Crimean-Congo hemorrhagic fever, and hantaviruses (i.e., Hantaan virus) are most often cited as potential tools for bioterrorism.[27] However, hantaviruses are unlikely candidates for biological warfare purposes: they are very difficult to isolate (and grow) in cell culture, they are not transmitted between humans, and there is no evidence that they are truly infectious by aerosol.[28] Crimean-Congo hemorrhagic fever virus, however, seems much better suited as a biological weapon: it can readily be cultivated, is highly infective (although so far not documented by aerosol), and is easily transmitted between humans, giving rise to local epidemics and even nosocomial infections. The case-fatality rate associated with Crimean-Congo hemorrhagic virus is about 30%, which is much higher than that of most other viral hemorrhagic fevers.[28]

Bunyaviruses are generally sensitive to ribavirin, and this has also been proved in experimental animal models.[27] Interferon and interferon inducers have also proved efficacious in the treatment of experimental bunyavirus infection if, as usual for interferon (inducers), administered as early as possible after the infection. As for flavivirus infections, ribavirin is of no use in the treatment of togavirus infections. Here, interferon (whether pegylated or not) and interferon inducers (i.e., Ampligen) would appear to currently be the recommended therapy.[27]

4.6 RHABDOVIRUS AND FILOVIRUS INFECTIONS

Rhabdoviruses (i.e., rabies) and filoviruses (i.e., Ebola and Marburg) belong to the most deadly viruses with which humankind can be confronted. Rabies is almost invariably fatal, as illustrated by a recent case report.[29] Rabies can be sufficiently contained by repeated administration of specific immunoglobulin and (killed) rabies vaccine, as soon as possible after the infection has taken place. No such vaccine is available for either Ebola or Marburg. The latter, as indicated above, have been classified as Category A biowarfare agents. Filoviruses are highly infectious by the airborne route but can also be transmitted between humans through direct contact with virus-containing body fluids. Terrorists may have greater difficulty acquiring filoviruses than, say, more easily accessible biological agents such as *B. anthracis*, but this may be offset by the viruses' reputation for causing a horrifying illness.[30]

The threat of Ebola virus for humans and animals should not be underestimated. Its danger to humans is compounded by limited knowledge of its pathogenesis, its unknown natural reservoir (fruit bats?), and limited preventive or therapeutic measures.[31] In addition, Ebola virus infection threatens the survival of gorillas and chimpanzees in their last stronghold in western equatorial Africa, where declines in population of more than 50% in the past two decades have partly been blamed on Ebola outbreaks.[32]

Specific immunoglobulin or interferon-α 2b are only of limited value in the treatment of experimental Ebola virus infections: rhesus macaques, treated from the day of infection with Ebola (Zaire) virus, experienced only a 1-day delay in the onset of illness, viremia, and death.[33] No antiviral drugs currently in clinical use, including ribavirin, provide any protection against filoviruses.[30] The most promising therapeutic strategy may be based on the use of SAH hydrolase inhibitors, such as 3-deazaneplanocin A. As already indicated above, SAH hydrolase inhibitors interfere with SAM-dependent methylation reactions (see Figure 4.3) such as those involved in the maturation ("capping") of viral mRNA.

Apparently, rhabdoviruses, which includes vesicular stomatitis virus, as well as poxviruses (e.g., vaccinia virus), paramyxoviruses (e.g., parainfluenza virus), reoviruses, and some plant viruses heavily rely on such "capping," as they are particularly sensitive to inhibition by SAH hydrolase inhibitors.[34] Filoviruses behave biochemically very much like rhabdoviruses, with regard to the necessity for 5'-capping of their mRNAs, and therefore it could be logically deduced that SAH hydrolase inhibitors such as neplanocin A and 3-deazaneplanocin A, 9-(*trans*-2', *trans*-3'-dihydroxycyclopent-4'-enyl)adenine (DHCA) and 9-(*trans*-2', *trans*-3'-dihydroxycyclopent-4'-enyl)-3-deazaadenine (DHCDA), which are highly active in vitro and in vivo against the rhabdovirus vesicular stomatitis virus,[35] would also be effective in the treatment of filovirus (i.e., Ebola and Marburg) infections.

In fact, 3-deazaneplanocin A, administered as a single dose of 1 mg/kg on the first or second day after a lethal Ebola (Zaire) virus infection in mice, reduced peak viremia by more than 1000-fold, compared with mock-treated controls, and resulted in survival of most or all animals.[36] This protective effect was accompanied, and probably mediated, by a massive production of interferon -α in the Ebola virus-infected mice.[37] It could be hypothesized that 3-deazaneplanocin A, by blocking the 5'-capping of the nascent (+)RNA viral strands, prevented the dissociation of these strands from the viral (−)RNA template, thus leading to an accumulation of the replicative intermediates. Being composed of double-stranded RNA stretches, these replicative intermediates may then engender the mass production of interferon, following an "old" therapy proposed by Carter and De Clercq.[38]

Viral surface glycoproteins of Ebola virus (and other filoviruses) should be considered as potential targets for chemotherapeutic intervention, as, for example, cyanovirin-N[39] and other compounds have been shown to bind to viral glycoproteins, such as the glycopeptide antibiotics (teicoplanin, vancomycin)[40] and plant lectins.[41]

4.7 ORTHOMYXOVIRUS INFECTIONS

Of the orthomyxoviruses, influenza A and B viruses cause epidemics in humans; influenza A viruses, which have been isolated from a wide variety of avian and mammalian species, are responsible for widespread human epidemics (or pandemics) with high mortality rates. Epidemics and pandemics occur because influenza A virus is readily and rapidly transmitted from humans to humans by aerosol. Whereas influenza B virus undergoes only antigenic drift, based on relatively minor changes (transition and/or transversion mutations) in the viral surface glycoproteins, hemagglutinin (H), and neuraminidase (N), influenza A virus is prone to both antigenic drift and antigenic shift, the latter resulting from major antigenic changes due to reassortment (recombination) of genomic fragments between influenza viruses of different animal species.

Most currently circulating influenza A viruses correspond to the H_3N_2 subtype, but in 1997, an avian influenza virus (H_5N_1) emerged in Hong Kong that was directly transmitted from chickens to humans. Rapid slaughter of the poultry in Hong Kong prevented further spread of the virus to humans, but the H_5N_1 virus has continued to circulate in Asian poultry markets, which implies a continuous risk for transmission to humans. This was recently (2003–2004) demonstrated by poultry-to-human transmissions of the avian H_5N_1 influenza in some Asian countries (China, Vietnam, and Thailand).

The high virulence of some influenza A virus strains such as H_5N_1, and the fact that such lethal influenza A viruses can be generated in the laboratory, utilizing the recently developed reverse genetics technique, have accentuated the fear of influenza A viruses being used as a bioterrorist weapon.[42] Additionally, highly pathogenic avian influenza A viruses, of subtype H_7N_7, which are responsible for fowl plaque in poultry, may be transmitted to people directly involved in handling infected poultry and be further transmitted from person to person.[43] A fatal course of pneumonia in association with acute respiratory distress syndrome has been noted in an individual[44] infected with the avian influenza A virus H_7N_7.

Given their specificity for influenza virus strains that are already circulating (i.e., H_3N_2, H_1N_1, and B strains), influenza vaccines are likely to be of limited value against a newly emerging influenza strain, whether occurring naturally or launched as a bioterrorist weapon. In this case, antiviral drugs that are directed at functions shared by as many influenza strains as possible would constitute the best line of defense.[42] The neuraminidase inhibitors zanamivir[45] and oseltamivir[46] meet these requirements. By virtue of their unique mode of action—preventing the removal of the sialic acid ($= N$-acetylneuraminic acid) residue from the glycopeptide receptor (see Figure 4.4) by the viral neuraminidase, which would otherwise allow the virus particles to be released from the infected cell (and to spread to neighboring cells)—the neuraminidase inhibitors are able to suppress the further course and spread of the disease. Both zanamivir and oseltamivir have been formally licensed for the treatment (and prophylaxis) of influenza virus infections, and it would be advisable to have these compounds, particularly oseltamivir (because it can conveniently be administered as capsules, whereas zanamivir has to be inhaled by mouth), at hand and stockpiled, so that they could be used prophylactically [following a strategy that has been provisionally dubbed "tamifluation" (Tamiflu being the marketed name for oseltamivir)] in case of an influenza virus outbreak or attack.

4.8 PARAMYXOVIRUS INFECTIONS

The paramyxoviruses encompass parainfluenza 1, 2, 3, 4a, and 4b, Sendai virus, mumps virus, measles virus, Hendra virus, and Nipah virus as well as the pneumovirus respiratory syncytial virus (RSV) and human metapneumovirus (hMPV). Parainfluenza has not received much attention from either a preventive (vaccination) or curative (therapy) viewpoint. Mumps and measles, like rubella, are now sufficiently contained by vaccination, which makes Nipah (and the related Hendra) as well as RSV and hMPV the paramyxoviruses that are most in need of antiviral approaches.

Nipah was isolated during an outbreak of viral encephalitis in Malaysia, five years ago. The Nipah virus has many of the physical attributes needed to serve as a potential bioterrorist weapon.[47] The outbreak caused widespread panic and fear because of the high mortality and the inability to control the disease initially. There were considerable social disruptions, accompanied by a tremendous economic loss to the important pig-rearing industry. The highly virulent Nipah virus, believed to be introduced into pig farms by fruit bats, spread easily among pigs and was transmitted to humans who came into close contact with infected animals; and from pigs, the virus was also transmitted to other animals such as dogs, cats, and horses.[47] There is no specific antiviral treatment for Nipah virus infections.

The human metapneumovirus (hMVP) was first isolated (in 2001) from young children with respiratory tract disease.[48] The clinical symptoms caused by hMVP are similar to those caused by RSV, ranging from upper respiratory tract disease to severe bronchiolitis and pneumonia. hMVP is similar to RSV in that infection usually occurs during winter months and is common in young children, elderly people, and immunocompromised individuals. In a study carried out on hospitalized patients with respiratory tract illness, hMVP was the second-most-detected viral pathogen (RSV being the first-most-detected) during two successive winter seasons.[49] hMVP infections are certainly a more frequent cause of acute respiratory tract disease than originally thought,[50] and should be considered as a potential cause of respiratory illnesses in hematopoietic stem cell transplant (HSCT) recipients.[51]

A majority part of the patients diagnosed with influenza-like illness harbor RSV, and as influenza and RSV occur roughly at the same time (winter season), there is a need to distinguish between the two, if specific antiviral treatment is to be prescribed.[52] As mentioned earlier, specific treatment for influenza consists of the neuraminidase inhibitors (zanamivir, oseltamivir), whereas for RSV infections the only approved drug is ribavirin (as an aerosol). In practice, however, ribavirin is rarely applied because of the technical burden delivery by aerosol inhalation. Attempts have been made at developing RSV inhibitors that target the viral F (fusion) protein and thus block virus–cell fusion and syncytium formation. An example is 4,4′-bis-{4,6-bis-[3-(bis-carbamoylmethyl-sulfamoyl)-phenylamino]-(1,3,5)triazin-2-ylamino}-biphenyl-2′,2′-disulfonic acid RFI-641, which has proved to be efficacious, when administered prophylactically (or up to 24 hours postinfection) by the intranasal route, in mice, cotton rats, or African green monkeys intranasally infected with RSV.[53]

Recently, two other compounds have been reported to inhibit RSV infection: BMS-433771 and A-33903. The former[54] is targeted at the F-protein (involved in virus–cell fusion), whereas the latter[55] is targeted at the N-protein (function essentially unknown). Both compounds may have potential for the treatment and/or prevention of RSV infections.[54,55]

4.9 CORONAVIRUS INFECTIONS

Human coronaviruses (i.e., 229E and OC43) have in the past not been considered sufficiently serious to be controlled by either vaccination or specific antiviral therapy. This view has now been dramatically changed with the advent of severe acute respiratory syndrome (SARS). SARS, which first emerged in the Guangdong province of southern China in November 2002, from where it spread to Hong Kong, other Asian countries, North America, and Europe, has now unequivocally been associated with a newly discovered coronavirus, SARS-associated coronavirus (SCV).[56–60] The disease is mainly characterized by flu-like symptoms, high fever, myalgia, dyspnea, lymphopenia, and lung infiltrates (pneumonia) leading to acute breathing problems with an overall mortality rate of about 10% (in the elderly as high as 50%). All Koch's postulates are fulfilled for SCV to qualify as the primary etiological agent of SARS: (1) isolation of virus from diseased hosts, (2) cultivation in host cells, (3) proof of filterability, (4) production of comparable disease in the original species (human) or a related one (monkeys), (5) reisolation of the virus, and (6) detection of a specific immune response to the virus.[61]

The genomic structure (see Figure 4.5) of SCV as compared to other coronaviruses, their life cycle, and phylogenetic relationships have been addressed previously.[62] There are a number of proteins, encoded by the SCV genome, that could be considered as targets for chemotherapeutic intervention: namely, the spike (S) protein, the coronavirus main proteinase (3CL^{pro}), the NTPase/helicase, the (RNA-dependent) RNA polymerase, and, possibly, other viral protein-mediated processes. 3CL^{pro} has especially been considered a promising target for the design of potential SCV inhibitors.[63]

The coronavirus spike (S) protein mediates infection of permissive cells through interaction of its S1 domain with angiotensin-converting enzyme 2 (ACE2), a functional receptor for the SARS coronavirus.[64] A 193 amino acid fragment of the S protein (corresponding to residues 318–510) bound ACE2 more efficiently than did the full S1 domain (residues 12–672), and, in fact, the 193 residue fragment was found to block S protein-mediated infection with an IC$_{50}$ of less than 10 nM (IC$_{50}$ of the full S1 domain: ~50 nM).[65] Also, human monoclonal antibodies to the S1 protein have been found to block association of SCV with its receptor ACE2, suggesting that the ACE2 binding site of S1 may be an attractive target for drug development.[66] A first small-molecular-weight inhibitor that interacts with the ACE2 active catalytic site, that is (*S,S*)-2-{1-carboxy-2-[3-(3,5-dichlorobenzyl)-3*H*-imidazol-4-yl]-ethylamino}-4-methyl-pentanoic acid (MLN-4760), has already been described.[67] Whether MLN-4760 inhibits SCV infection, however, remains to be demonstrated.

The coronavirus main proteinase, M^{pro}, also called 3CL^{pro} (3C-like, to indicate a similarity of its cleavage-site specificity to that for picornavirus 3C proteinases), has also been considered as an attractive target for the design of anti-SCV drugs.[68] Here it was proposed that compounds such as AG7088, which have proved to be active against the rhinovirus 3C proteinase, may be modified to make them active against coronaviruses.[68] A first modification of AG7088 yielded KZ7088, which, in comparison with AG7088, is missing the methylene group of the p-fluoropheny-lalanine residue. KZ7088 has been docked into the SCV 3CL^{pro},[69] and further work along these lines may provide a solid footing for structure-based drug design against SARS.[70]

Another potential target for the development of anti-SARS agents is the SCV-associated NTPase/helicase.[71] Inhibitors of the primase-helicase have been successfully pursued in the case of herpes simplex virus, and inhibitors of the NTPase/helicase are being tested for hepatitis C as well.

The SARS coronavirus-associated (RNA-dependent) RNA polymerase represents yet another potential target for anti-SARS therapy.[72] SCV RNA polymerase would not contain a hydrophobic pocket for non-nucleoside inhibitors such as those that have proved active against HCV polymerase or HIV-1 reverse transcriptase.[72] Of the (many) nucleoside analogues that have so far been evaluated against SCV and that may be expected to be targeted at the RNA polymerase, only N^4-hydroxycytidine, showed an, albeit modest, activity ($EC_{50} = 10\ \mu M$; selectivity index ≥ 10) against SCV replication in cell culture.[73]

In addition to N^4-hydroxycytidine, some calpain inhibitors [i.e., N-(4-fluoro-phenylsulfonyl)-L-valyl-L-leucinal][73] were found to inhibit SCV replication ($EC_{50} = 1\ \mu M$) with a selectivity index of ≥ 100. The mode (target) of anti-SCV action of the calpain inhibitors remains to be elucidated.

Inhibitory effects on SCV, again with selectivity indexes up to about 100 (and EC_{50} values as low as 1 μg/mL), have been noted for a variety of compounds—for example, vancomycin, eremomycin and teicoplanin aglycon derivatives[74] and mannose-specific plant lectins derived from *Galanthus nivalis* or *Hippeastrum* hybrid[75] or *Allium porrum*[76]—which may all owe their antiviral activity to an interaction with viral entry. Glycyrrhizin has also been shown to inhibit the replication of SCV,[77] but only at concentrations ($EC_{50} = 300$–600 μg/mL) that are therapeutically unrealistic (i.e., could not be achieved at the target tissue or organs).

There are numerous other approaches that may be considered for inhibiting SCV infections, such as small interfering RNAs (siRNAs),[78] namely, double-stranded RNAs that direct sequence-specific degradation of messenger RNA in mammalian cells. Also, antisense oligonucleotides may be designed so as to inhibit SCV genome expression, a prominent example being the antisense morpholino oligomers.[79]

In addition, monoclonal antibodies against the SCV glycoprotein S have been found to neutralize SCV in vitro and to protect mice from SARS in vivo.[80] Also there are a number of other, non-antiviral drugs (e.g., pentoxifylline) that have been used for other purposes and have been recommended for use in the treatment of SARS.[81]

An effective agent, at least for prophylaxis and early postexposure management of SARS, would seem to be human interferon, whether α, β, or γ.[82] A number of interferons have been found effective against SCV,[83] although there is clearly a differential activity: IFN-β being more effective than IFN-γ, and the latter being more effective than IFN-α.[84] Various subtypes of IFN-α have, in fact, been found to be inactive against SCV.[84] According to these authors' observations, the best choice would be the combination of IFN-β with IFN-γ, as this combination proved to be synergistic against the SARS virus.[84] Pegylated IFN-α was recently shown to significantly reduce viral replication and excretion, viral antigen expression by type 1 pneumocytes, and the attendant pulmonary damage in cynomolgus macaques infected experimentally with SCV.[85] These preliminary results warrant further studies with pegylated IFN-α, which is commercially available, in the prophylactic or early postexposure treatment of SARS, should it reemerge.

As recently attested to by the identification of yet another, previously unde-scribed coronavirus associated with respiratory illness in humans,[86,87] the search for antiviral agents effective against coronaviruses at large may be well vested.

4.10   CONCLUSION

Although there are at present almost 40 compounds formally licensed as antiviral drugs, few of them are directed toward virus infections other than herpes, HIV, or hepatitis (B or C). Only a limited number of compounds are available that may cope with acute virus infections that may suddenly arise in an epidemic or bioterrorist context. Neuraminidase inhibitors such as zanamivir and oseltamivir should be advocated for the prophylaxis and therapy of influenza virus infections. Ribavirin may be considered in the treatment of arenavirus and bunyavirus infections and (pegylated) interferon in the prevention (and early therapy) of paramyxovirus and coronavirus infections. For the prophylaxis and therapy of poxvirus infections, whether variola, vaccinia, or any other poxvirus infections, cidofovir, or, in the future, an oral prodrug derivative thereof or a related acyclic nucleoside phospho-nate counterpart, may be an obvious choice. For rhabdovirus and filovirus infec-tions, there is, at present, no established antiviral treatment, but SAH hydrolase inhibitors such as 3-deazaneplanocin A should be pursued as possible therapeutic options.

REFERENCES

1. De Clercq, E. Strategies in the design of antiviral drugs. *Nat. Rev. Drug Discov.* **2002**, *1*, 13–25.

2. Mahy, B. W. J. An overview on the use of a viral pathogen as a bioterrorism agent: why smallpox? *Antiviral Res.* **2003**, *57*, 1–5.

3. Baker, R. O.; Bray, M.; Huggins, J. W. Potential antiviral therapeutics for smallpox, monkeypox and other orthopoxvirus infections. *Antiviral Res.* **2003**, *57*, 13–23.

4. Smee, D. F.; Sidwell, R. W. A review of compounds exhibiting anti-orthopoxvirus activity in animal models. *Antiviral Res.* **2003**, *57*, 41–52.

5. Neyts, J.; De Clercq, E. Therapy and short-term prophylaxis of poxvirus infections: historical background and perspectives. *Antiviral Res.* **2003**, *57*, 25–33.

6. De Clercq, E.; Neyts, J. Therapeutic potential of nucleoside/nucleotide analogues against poxvirus infections. *Rev. Med. Virol.* **2004**, *14*, 289–300.

7. De Clercq, E. Cidofovir in the treatment of poxvirus infections. *Antiviral Res.* **2002**, *55*, 1–13.

8. Neyts, J.; De Clercq, E. Efficacy of (*S*)-1-(3-hydroxy-2-phosphonylmethoxypropyl)-cytosine for the treatment of lethal vaccinia virus infections in severe combined immune deficiency (SCID) mice. *J. Med. Virol.* **1993**, *41*, 242–246.

9. Huggins, J. W.; Martinez, M. J.; Hartmann, C. J.; Hensley, L. E.; Jackson, D. L.; Kefauver, D. F.; Kulesh, D. A.; Larsen, T.; Miller, D. M.; Mucker, E. M.; Shamblin, J. D.; Tate, M. K.; Whitehouse, C. A.; Zwiers, S. H; Jahrling, P. B. Successful cidofovir treatment of smallpox-like disease in variola and monkeypox primate models. Abstracts of the 17th International Conference on Antiviral Research, Tucson, AZ, USA, 2–6 May 2004. *Antiviral Res.* **2004**, *62*, A57, no. 76.

10. Evans, D. H.; Magee, W.; Hostetler, K. Y. Inhibition of orthopoxvirus DNA polymerases by cidofovir diphosphate: in vitro enzymatic studies using highly purified vaccinia virus DNA polymerase. Abstracts of the 17th International Conference on Antiviral Research, Tucson, AZ, USA, 2–6 May 2004. *Antiviral Res.* **2004**, *62*, A57, no. 74.

11. Andrei, G.; Holý, A.; Fiten, P.; Opdenakker, G.; De Clercq, E.; Snoeck, R. Isolation of vaccinia virus (VV) mutants resistant to different acyclic nucleoside phosphonate analogues (ANPs). Abstracts of the 17th International Conference on Antiviral Research, Tucson, AZ, USA, 2–6 May 2004. *Antiviral Res.* **2004**, *62*, A72, no. 111.

12. Smee, D. F.; Bailey, K. W.; Holý, A.; Sidwell, R. W. A cidofovir-resistant form of the highly virulent WR strain of vaccinia virus is cross-resistant to related antiviral agents and is highly attenuated for virulence in mice. Abstracts of the 17th International Conference on Antiviral Research, Tucson, AZ, USA, 2–6 May 2004. *Antiviral Res.* **2004**, *62*, A57, no. 75.

13. Kern, E. R.; Hartline, C.; Harden, E.; Keith, K.; Rodriguez, N.; Beadle, J. R.; Hostetler, K. Y. Enhanced inhibition of orthopoxvirus replication in vitro by alkoxyalkyl esters of cidofovir and cyclic cidofovir. *Antimicrob. Agents Chemother.* **2002**, *46*, 991–995.

14. Aldern, K. A.; Ciesla, S. L.; Winegarden, K. L.; Hostetler, K. Y. Increased antiviral activity of 1-*O*-hexadecyloxypropyl-[2-^{14}C]cidofovir in MRC-5 human lung fibroblasts is explained by unique cellular uptake and metabolism. *Mol. Pharmacol.* **2003**, *63*, 678–681.

15. Neyts, J.; Leyssen, P.; Verbeken, E.; De Clercq, E. Efficacy of cidofovir in a murine model for disseminated/progressive vaccinia. *Antimicrob. Agents Chemother.* **2004**, *48*, 2267–2273.

16. Gritsun, T. S.; Lashkevich, V. A.; Gould, E. A. Tick-borne encephalitis. *Antiviral Res.* **2003**, *57*, 129–146.

17. Leyssen, P.; Charlier, N.; Paeshuyse, J.; De Clercq, E.; Neyts, J. Prospects for antiviral therapy. *Adv. Virus Res.* **2003**, *61*, 511–553.

18. Leyssen, P.; Croes, R.; Rau, P.; Heiland, S.; Verbeken, E.; Sciot, R.; Paeshuyse, J.; Charlier, N.; De Clercq, E.; Meyding-Lamadé, U.; Neyts, J. Acute encephalitis, a poliomyelitis-like syndrome and neurological sequelae in a hamster model for flavivirus infections. *Brain Pathol.* **2003**, *13*, 279–290.

19. Leyssen, P.; Drosten, C.; Paning, M.; Charlier, N.; Paeshuyse, J.; De Clercq, E.; Neyts, J. Interferons, interferon inducers, and interferon-ribavirin in treatment of flavivirus-induced encephalitis in mice. *Antimicrob. Agents Chemother.* **2003**, *47*, 777–782.

20. Neyts, J.; Meerbach, A.; McKenna, P.; De Clercq, E. Use of the yellow fever virus vaccine strain 17D for the study of strategies for the treatment of yellow fever virus infections. *Antiviral Res.* **1996**, *30*, 125–132.

21. Morrey, J. D.; Smee, D. F.; Sidwell, R. W.; Tseng, C. Identification of active antiviral compounds against a New York isolate of West Nile virus. *Antiviral Res.* **2002**, *55*, 107–116.

22. Iversen, P. L.; Stein, D.; Kroeker, A.; Arora, V.; Barklis, E.; Hill, A.; Smith, A.; Wallace, R. Rapid development of an antisense phosphorodiamidate morpholino oligomer for the treatment of West Nile virus. Abstracts of the 17th International Conference on Antiviral Research, Tucson, AZ, USA, 2–6 May 2004. *Antiviral Res.* **2004**, *62*, A32, no. 15.

23. Charrel, R. N.; de Lamballerie, X. Arenaviruses other than Lassa virus. *Antiviral Res.* **2003**, *57*, 89–100.

24. Drosten, C.; Kümmerer, B. M.; Schmitz, H.; Günther, S. Molecular diagnostics of viral hemorrhagic fevers. *Antiviral Res.* **2003**, *57*, 61–87.

25. Andrei, G.; De Clercq, E. Inhibitory effect of selected antiviral compounds on arenavirus replication in vitro. *Antiviral Res.* **1990**, *14*, 287–300.

26. McCormick, J. B.; King, I. J.; Webb, P. A.; Scribner, C. L.; Craven, R. B.; Johnson, K. M.; Elliott, L. H. Belmont-Williams, R. Lassa fever. Effective therapy with ribavirin. *N. Engl. J. Med.* **1986**, *314*, 20–26.

27. Sidwell, R. W.; Smee, D. F. Viruses of the Bunya- and Togaviridae families: potential as bioterrorism agents and means of control. *Antiviral Res.* **2003**, *57*, 101–111.

28. Clement, J. P. Hantavirus. *Antiviral Res.* **2003**, *57*, 121–127.

29. Case records of the Massachusetts General Hospital. Weekly clinicopathological exercises. Case 21-1998. A 32-year-old woman with pharyngeal spasms and paresthesias after a dog bite. *N. Engl. J. Med.* **1998**, *339*, 105–112.

30. Bray, M. Defense against filoviruses used as biological weapons. *Antiviral Res.* **2003**, *57*, 53–60.

31. Kuiken, T.; Fouchier, R.; Rimmelzwaan, G.; Osterhaus, A. Emerging viral infections in a rapidly changing world. *Curr. Opin. Biotechnol.* **2003**, *14*, 641–646.

32. Walsh, P. D.; Abernethy, K. A.; Bermejo, M.; Beyers, R.; De Wachter, P.; Akou, M. E.; Huijbregts, B.; Mambounga, D. I.; Toham, A. K.; Kilbourn, A. M., Lahm, S. A.; Latour, S.; Maisels, F.; Mbina, C.; Mihindou, Y.; Obiang, S. N.; Effa, E. N.; Starkey, M. P.; Teifer, P.; Thibault, M.; Tutin, C. E. G.; White, L. J. T.; Wilkie, D. S. Catastrophic ape decline in western equatorial Africa. *Nature* **2003**, *422*, 611–614.

33. Jahrling, P. B.; Geisbert, T. W.; Geisbert, J. B.; Swearengen, J. R.; Bray, M.; Jaax, N. K.; Huggins, J. W.; LeDuc, J. W.; Peters, C. J. Evaluation of immune globulin and recombinant interferon-α2b for treatment of experimental Ebola virus infections. *J. Infect. Dis.* **1999**, *179* (Suppl. 1), S224–S234.

34. De Clercq, E., S-Adenosylhomocysteine hydrolase inhibitors as broad-spectrum antiviral agents. *Biochem. Pharmacol.* **1987**, *36*, 2567–2575.

35. De Clercq, E.; Cools, M.; Balzarini, J.; Marquez, V. E.; Borcherding, D. R.; Borchardt, R. T.; Drach, J. C.; Kitaoka, S.; Konno, T. Broad-spectrum antiviral activities of neplanocin A, 3-deazaneplanocin A, and their 5′-nor derivatives. *Antimicrob. Agents Chemother.* **1989**, *33*, 1291–1297.

36. Bray, M.; Driscoll, J.; Huggins, J. W. Treatment of lethal Ebola virus infection in mice with a single dose of an *S*-adenosyl-L-homocysteine hydrolase inhibitor. *Antiviral Res.* **2000**, *45*, 135–147.

37. Bray, M.; Raymond, J. L.; Geisbert, T.; Baker, R. O. 3-Deazaneplanocin A induces massively increased interferon-alpha production in Ebola virus-infected mice. *Antiviral Res.* **2002**, *55*, 151–159.

38. Carter, W. A.; De Clercq, E. Viral infection and host defense (many aspects of viral infection and recovery can be explained by the modulatory role of double-stranded RNA). *Science* **1974**, *186*, 1172–1178.

39. Barrientos, L. G.; O'Keefe, B. R.; Bray, M.; Sanchez, A.; Gronenborn, A. M.; Boyd, M. R. Cyanovirin-N binds to the viral surface glycoprotein, GP1,2 and inhibits infectivity of Ebola virus. *Antiviral Res.* **2003**, *58*, 47–56.

40. Balzarini, J.; Pannecouque, C.; De Clercq, E.; Pavlov, A. Y.; Printsevskaya, S. S.; Miroshnikova, O. V.; Reznikova, M. I.; Preobrazhenskaya, M. N. Antiretroviral activity of semisynthetic derivatives of glycopeptide antibiotics. *J. Med. Chem.* **2003**, *46*, 2755–2764.

41. Balzarini, J.; Schols, D.; Neyts, J.; Van Damme, E.; Peumans, W.; De Clercq, E. α-(1-3)- and α-(1-6)-D-Mannose-specific plant lectins are markedly inhibitory to human immunodeficiency virus and cytomegalovirus infections in vitro. *Antimicrob. Agents Chemother.* **1991**, *35*, 410–416.

42. Krug, R. M. The potential use of influenza virus as an agent for bioterrorism. *Antiviral Res.* **2003**, *57*, 147–150.

43. Koopmans, M.; Wilbrink, B.; Conyn, M.; Natrop, G.; van der Nat, H.; Vennema, H.; Meijer, A.; van Steenbergen, J.; Fouchier, R.; Osterhaus, A.; Bosman, A. Transmission of H7N7 avian influenza A virus to human being during a large outbreak in commercial poultry farms in the Netherlands. *Lancet* **2004**, *363*, 587–593.

44. Fouchier, R. A. M.; Schneeberger, P. M.; Rozendaal, F. W.; Broekman, J. M.; Kemink, S. A. G.; Munster, V.; Kuiken, T.; Rimmelzwaan, G. F.; Schutten, M.; van Doornum, G. J. J.; Koch, G.; Bosman, A.; Koopmans, M.; Osterhaus, A. D. M. E. Avian influenza A virus (H7N7) associated with human conjunctivitis and a fatal case of acute respiratory distress syndrome. *Proc. Natl. Acad. Sci. USA* **2004**, *101*, 1356–1361.

45. von Itzstein, M.; Wu, W. Y.; Kok, G. B.; Pegg, M. S.; Dyason, J. C.; Jin, B.; Van Phan, T.; Smythe, M. L.; White, H. F.; Oliver, S. W.; Colman, P. M.; Varghese, J. N.; Ryan, D. M.; Woods, J. M.; Bethell, R. C.; Hotham, V. J.; Cameron, J. M.; Penn, C. R. Rational design of potent sialidase-based inhibitors of influenza virus replication. *Nature* **1993**, *363*, 418–423.

46. Kim, C. U.; Lew, W.; Williams, M. A.; Liu, H.; Zhang, L.; Swaminathan, S.; Bischofberger, N.; Chen, M. S.; Mendel, D. B.; Tai, C. Y.; Laver, W. G.; Sevens, R. C. Influenza neuraminidase inhibitors possessing a novel hydrophobic interaction in the enzyme active site: design, synthesis, and structural analysis of carbocyclic sialic acid analogues with potent anti-influenza activity. *J. Am. Chem. Soc.* **1997**,*119*, 681–690.

47. Lam, S.-K. Nipah virus—a potential agent of bioterrorism? *Antiviral Res.* **2003**, *57*, 113–119.

48. van den Hoogen, B. G.; de Jong, J. C.; Groen, J.; Kuiken, T.; de Groot, R.; Fouchier, R. A. M.; Osterhaus, A. D. M. E. A newly discovered human pneumovirus isolated from young children with respiratory tract disease. *Nat. Med.* **2001**, *7*, 729–724.

49. van den Hoogen, B. G.; van Doornum, G. J. J.; Fockens, J. C.; Cornelissen, J. J.; Beyer, W. E. P.; de Groot, R.; Osterhaus, A. D. M. E.; Fouchier, R. A. M. Prevalence and clinical symptoms of human metapneumovirus infection in hospitalized patients. *J. Infect. Dis.* **2003**, *188*, 1571–1577.

50. Peret, T. C. T.; Boivin, G.; Li, Y.; Couillard, M.; Humphrey, C.; Osterhaus, A. D. M. E.; Erdman, D. D.; Anderson, L. J. Characterization of human metapneumoviruses isolated from patients in North America. *J. Infect. Dis.* **2002**, *185*, 1660–1663.

51. Cane, P. A.; van den Hoogen, B. G.; Chakrabarti, S.; Fegan, C. D.; Osterhaus, A.D.M.E. Human metapneumovirus in a haematopoietic stem cell transplant recipient with fatal lower respiratory tract disease. *Bone Marrow Transplant.* **2003**, *31*, 309–310.

52. Zambon, M. C.; Stockton, J. D.; Clewley, J. P.; Fleming, D. M. Contribution of influenza and respiratory syncytial virus to community cases of influenza-like illness: an observational study. *Lancet* **2001**, *358*, 1410–1416.

53. Huntley, C. C.; Weiss, W. J.; Gazumyan, A.; Buklan, A.; Feld, B.; Hu, W.; Jones, T. R.; Murphy, T.; Nikitenko, A. A.; O'Hara, B.; Prince, G.; Quartuccio, S.; Raifeld, Y. E.; Wyde, P.; O'Connell, J. F. RFI-641, a potent respiratory syncytial virus inhibitor. *Antimicrob. Agents Chemother.* **2002**, *46*, 841–847.

54. Cianci, C.; Yu, K.-L.; Combrink, K.; Sin, N.; Pearce, B.; Wang, A.; Civiello, R.; Voss, S.; Luo, G.; Kadow, K.; Genovesi, E. V.; Venables, B.; Gulgeze, H.; Trehan, A.; James, J.; Lamb, L.; Medina, I.; Roach, J.; Yang, Z.; Zadjura, L.; Colonno, R.; Clark, J.; Meanwell, N.; Krystal, M. Orally active fusion inhibitor of respiratory syncytial virus. *Antimicrob. Agents Chemother.* **2004**, *48*, 413–422.

55. Alber, D.; Wilson, L.; Baxter, B.; Henderson, E.; Dowdell, V.; Kelsey, R.; Keegan, S.; Harris, R.; McNamara, D.; Bithell, S.; Weerasekera, N.; Harland, R.; Stables, J.; Cockerill, S.; Powell, K.; Carter, M. A novel respiratory syncytial virus inhibitor. Abstracts of the 17th International Conference on Antiviral Research, Tucson, AZ, USA, 2–6 May 2004. *Antiviral Res.* **2004**, *62*, A60, no. 82.

56. Peiris, J. S.; Lai, S. T.; Poon, L. L.; Guan, Y.; Yam, L. Y.; Lim, W.; Nicholls, J.; Yee, W. K.; Yan, W. W.; Cheung, M. T.; Cheng, V. C.; Chan, K. H.; Tsang, D. N.; Yung, R. W.; Ng, T. K.; Yuen, K. Y.; SARS Study Group. Coronavirus as a possible cause of severe acute respiratory syndrome. *Lancet* **2003**, *361*, 1319–1325.

57. Lee, N.; Hui, D.; Wu, A.; Chan, P.; Cameron, P.; Joynt, G. M.; Ahuja, A.; Yung, M. Y.; Leung, C. B.; To, K. F.; Lui, S. F.; Szeto, C. C.; Chung, S.; Sung, J. J. A major outbreak of severe acute respiratory syndrome in Hong Kong. *N. Engl. J. Med.* **2003**, *348*, 1986–1994.

58. Ksiazek, T. G.; Erdman, D.; Goldsmith, C. S.; Zaki, S. R.; Peret, T.; Emery, S.; Tong, S.; Urbani, C.; Comer, J. A.; Lim, W.; Rollin, P. E.; Dowell, S. F.; Ling, A. E.; Humphrey, C. D.; Shieh, W. J.; Guarner, J.; Paddock, C. D.; Rota, P.; Fields, B.; DeRisi, J.; Yang, J. Y.; Cox, N.; Hughes, J. M.; LeDuc, J. W.; Bellini, W. J.; Anderson, L. J.; SARS Working Group. A novel coronavirus associated with severe acute respiratory syndrome. *N. Engl. J. Med.* **2003**, *348*, 1953–1966.

59. Drosten, C.; Gunther, S.; Preiser, W.; van der Werf, S.; Brodt, H. R.; Becker, S.; Rabenau, H.; Panning, M.; Kolesnikova, L.; Fouchier, R. A.; Berger, A.; Burguiere, A. M.; Cinatl, J.; Eickmann, M.; Escriou, N.; Grywna, K.; Kramme, S.; Manuguerra, J. C.; Muller, S.; Rickerts, V.; Sturmer, M.; Vieth, S.; Klenk, H. D.; Osterhaus, A. D.; Schmitz, H.; Doerr, H. W. Identification of a novel coronavirus in patients with severe acute respiratory syndrome. *N. Engl. J. Med.* **2003**, *348*, 1967–1976.

60. Kuiken, T.; Fouchier, R. A. M.; Schutten, M.; Rimmelzwaan, G. F.; van Amerongen, G.; van Riel, D.; Laman, J. D.; de Jong, T.; van Doornum, G.; Lim, W.; Ling, A. E.; Chan, P. K. S.; Tam, J. S.; Zambon, M. C.; Gopal, R.; Drosten, C.; van der Werf, S.; Escriou, N.; Manuguerra, J.-C.; Stöhr, K.; Peiris, J. S. M.; Osterhaus, A. D. M. E. Newly discovered coronavirus as the primary cause of severe acute respiratory syndrome. *Lancet* **2003**, *362*, 263–270.

61. Fouchier, R. A.; Kuiken, T.; Schutten, M.; van Amerongen, G.; van Doornum, G. J. J.; van den Hoogen, B.; Peiris, M.; Lim, W.; Stöhr, K.; Osterhaus, A. D. M. E. Koch's postulates fulfilled for SARS virus. *Nature* **2003**, *423*, 240.

62. Stadler, K.; Masignani, V.; Eickmann, M.; Becker, S.; Abrignani, S.; Klenk, H.-D.; Rappuoli, R. SARS—beginning to understand a new virus. *Nat. Rev. Microbiol.* **2003**, *1*, 209–218.

63. Thiel, V.; Ivanov, K. A.; Putics, A.; Hertzig, T.; Schelle, B.; Bayer, S.; Weissbrich, B.; Snijder, E. J.; Rabenau, H.; Doerr, H. W.; Gorbalenya, A. E.; Ziebuhr, J. Mechanisms and enzymes involved in SARS coronavirus genome expression. *J. Gen. Virol.* **2003**, *84*, 2305–2315.

64. Li, W.; Moore, M. J.; Vasilieva, N.; Sui, J.; Wong, S. K.; Berne, M. A.; Somasundaran, M.; Sullivan, J. L.; Luzuriaga, K.; Greenough, T. C.; Choe, H.; Farzan, M. Angiotensin-converting enzyme 2 is a functional receptor for the SARS coronavirus. *Nature* **2003**, *426*, 450–454.

65. Wong, S. K.; Li, W.; Moore, M. J.; Choe, H.; Farzan, M. A 193-amino acid fragment of the SARS coronavirus S protein efficiently binds angiotensin-converting enzyme 2. *J. Biol. Chem.* **2004**, *279*, 3197–3201.

66. Sui, J.; Li, W.; Murakami, A.; Tamin, A.; Matthews, L. J.; Wong, S. K.; Moore, M. J.; St. Clair Tallarico, A.; Olurinde, M.; Choe, H.; Anderson, L. J.; Bellini, W. J.; Farzan, M.; Marasco, W. A. Potent neutralization of severe acute respiratory syndrome (SARS) coronavirus by a human mAb to S1 protein that blocks receptor association. *Proc. Natl. Acad. Sci. U.S.A.* **2004**, *101*, 2536–2541.

67. Towler, P.; Staker, B.; Prasad, S. G.; Menon, S.; Tang, J.; Parsons, T.; Ryan, D.; Fisher, M.; Williams, D.; Dales, N. A.; Patane, M. A.; Pantoliano, M. W. ACE2 X-ray structures reveal a large hinge-bending motion important for inhibitor binding and catalysis. *J. Biol. Chem.* **2004**, *279*, 17996–18007.

68. Anand, K.; Ziebuhr, J.; Wadhwani, P.; Mesters, J. R.; Hilgenfeld, R. Coronavirus main proteinase (3CL^{pro}) structure: basis for design of anti-SARS drugs. *Science* **2003**, *300*, 1763–1767.

69. Chou, K.-C.; Wei, D. Q.; Zhong, W.-Z. Binding mechanism of coronavirus main proteinase with ligands and its implication to drug design against SARS. *Biochem. Biophys. Res. Commun.* **2003**, *308*, 148–151.

70. Yang, H.; Yang, M.; Liu, Y.; Lou, Z.; Zhou, Z.; Sun, L.; Mo, L.; Ye, S.; Pang, H.; Gao, G. F.; Anand, K.; Bartlam, M.; Hilgenfeld, R.; Rao, Z. The crystal structures of severe acute respiratory syndrome virus main protease and its complex with an inhibitor. *Proc. Natl. Acad. Sci. U.S.A.* **2003**, *100*, 13190–13195.

71. Tanner, J. A.; Watt, R. M.; Chai, Y.-B.; Lu, L.-Y.; Lin, M. C.; Peiris, J. S. M.; Poon, L. L. M.; Kung, H.-F.; Huang, J.-D. The severe acute respiratory syndrome (SARS) coronavirus NTPase/helicase belongs to a distinct class of 5′ to 3′ viral helicases. *J. Biol. Chem.* **2003**, *278*, 39578–39582.

72. Xu, X.; Liu, Y.; Weiss, S.; Arnold, E.; Sarafianos, S. G.; Ding, J. Molecular model of SARS coronavirus polymerase: implications for biochemical functions and drug design. *Nucleic Acids Res.* **2003**, *31*, 7117–7130.

73. Barnard, D. L.; Hubbard, V. D.; Burton, J.; Smee, D. F.; Morrey, J. D.; Otto, M.-J.; Sidwell, R. W. Inhibition of severe acute respiratory syndrome-associated coronavirus (SARSCoV) by calpain inhibitors and β-D-N^4-hydroxycytidine. *Antiviral Chem. Chemother.* **2004**, *15*, 15–22.

74. Balzarini, J.; Keyaerts, E.; Vijgen, L.; De Clercq, E.; Printsevskaya, S. S.; Preobrazhens-kaya, M.; Van Ranst, M. Inhibitory activity of vancomycin, eremomycin and teicoplanin aglycon derivatives against feline and human (i.e., SARS) coronaviruses. Abstracts of the 17th International Conference on Antiviral Research, Tucson, Arizona, USA, 2–6 May 2004. *Antiviral Res.* **2004**, *62*, A59, no. 78.

75. Balzarini, J.; Vijgen, L.; Keyaerts, E.; Van Damme, E.; Peumans, W.; De Clercq, E.; Egberink, H.; Van Ranst, M. Mannose-specific plant lectins are potent inhibitors of coronavirus infection including the virus causing SARS. Abstracts of the 17th International Conference on Antiviral Research, Tucson, AZ, USA, 2–6 May 2004. *Antiviral Res.* **2004**, *62*, A76, no. 122.

76. Vijgen, L.; Keyaerts, E.; Van Damme, E.; Peumans, W.; De Clercq, E.; Balzarini, J.; Van Ranst, M. Antiviral effect of plant compounds of the Alliaceae family against the SARS coronavirus. Abstracts of the 17th International Conference on Antiviral Research, Tucson, AZ, USA, 2–6 May 2004. *Antiviral Res.* **2004**, *62*, A76, no. 123.

77. Cinatl, J.; Morgenstern, B.; Bauer, G.; Chandra, P.; Rabenau, H.; Doerr, H. W. Glycyrrhizin, an active component of liquorice roots, and replication of SARS-associated coronavirus. *Lancet* **2003**, *361*, 2045–2046.

78. He, M.-L.; Zheng, B.; Peng, Y.; Peiris, J. S. M.; Poon, L. L. M.; Yuen, K.Y.; Lin, M. C. M.; Kung, H.-F.; Guan, Y. Inhibition of SARS-associated coronavirus infection and replication by RNA interference. *JAMA.* **2003**, *290*, 2665–2666.

79. Neuman, B.; Stein, D.; Kroeker, A.; Kim, A.; Paulino, A.; Abma, J.; Bestwick, R.; Moulton, H.; Iversen, P.; Buchmeier, M. Rational mechanistic design of antisense morpholino oligomers to inhibit SARS coronavirus proliferation and growth. Abstracts of the 17th International Conference on Antiviral Research, Tucson, AZ, USA, 2–6 May 2004. Late Breakers, p. 11, LB-2.

80. Babcock, G. J.; Greenough, T. C.; Hernandez, H. J.; Thomas, W. D.; Lowy, I.; Graziano, R.; Finberg, R.; Subbarao, K.; Roberts, A.; Vogel, L.; Somasundaran, M.; Luzuriaga, K.; Ambrosino, D. M.; Sullivan, J. L. Human monoclonal antibodies against S glycoprotein neutralize SARS coronavirus (CoV) in mice. Abstracts of the 17th International Conference on Antiviral Research, Tucson, AZ, USA, 2–6 May 2004. Late Beakers, p. 12, LB-3.

81. Marti, J. F. B.; Jiménez, J. L.; Munoz-Fernández, M. A. Pentoxifylline and severe acute respiratory syndrome (SARS): a drug to be considered. *Med. Sci. Monit.* **2003**, *9*, SR41–SR46.

82. Cinatl, J.; Morgenstern, B.; Bauer, G.; Chandra, P.; Rabenau, H.; Doerr, H. W. Treatment of SARS with human interferons. *Lancet* **2003**; *362*, 293–294.

83. Tan, E. L. C.; Ooi, E. E.; Lin, C.-Y.; Tan, H. C.; Ling, A. E.; Lim, B.; Stanton, L. W. Inhibition of SARS coronavirus infection in vitro with clinically approved antiviral drugs. *Emerging Infect. Dis.* **2004**, *10*, 581–586.

84. Dianzani, F.; Scagnolari, C.; Vincenzi, E.; Bellomi, F.; Clementi, M.; Antonelli, G. Antiviral action of interferons on human coronavirus. Abstracts of the 17th International Conference on Antiviral Research, Tucson, AZ, USA, 2–6 May 2004. *Antiviral Res.* **2004**, *62*, A87, no. 152.

85. Haagmans, B. L.; Kuiken, T.; Martina, B. E.; Fouchier, R. A. M.; Rimmelzwaan, G. F.; van Amerongen, G.; van Riel, D.; de Jong, T.; Itamura, S.; Chan, K.-H.; Tashiro, M.; Osterhaus, A. D. M. E. Pegylated interferon-α protects type 1 pneumocytes against SARS coronavirus infection in macaques. *Nat. Med.* **2004**, *10*, 290–293.

86. Fouchier, R. A. M.; Hartwig, N. G.; Bestebroer, T. M.; Niemeyer, B.; de Jong, J. C.; Simon, J. H. Osterhaus, A. D. M. E. A previously undescribed coronavirus associated with respiratory disease in humans. *Proc. Natl. Acad. Sci. U.S.A.* **2004**, *101*, 6212–6216.

87. Van der Hoek, L.; Pyrc, K.; Jebbink, M. F.; Vermeulen-Oost, W.; Berkhout, R. J. M.; Wolthers, K. C.; Wertheim-Van Dillen, P. M.; Kaandorp, J.; Spaargaren, J.; Berkhout, B. Identification of a new human coronavirus. *Nat. Med.* **2004**, *10*, 368–373.

CHAPTER 5

Perspectives for the Therapy Against Arenavirus Infections

ELSA B. DAMONTE and CYBELE C. GARCÍA

Laboratorio de Virología, Departamento de Química Biológica, Facultad de Ciencias Exactas y Naturales, Universidad de Buenos Aires

5.1   INTRODUCTION

The family Arenaviridae comprises 23 viruses, 19 species recognized by the International Committee for Virus Taxonomy[1] and 4 new tentative species, all included in a single genus, *Arenavirus*. The genus is divided into two groups, based on geographic distribution and antigenic cross-reactivity: the Old World group or lymphocytic choriomeningitis–Lassa complex and the New World group or Tacaribe complex.[2,3] The Old World group includes the lymphocytic choriomeningitis virus (LCMV),[4] the prototype species of the family and the only almost worldwide present arenavirus, and four African arenaviruses,[5–8] whereas the New World group comprises fifteen viruses distributed in South America[9–23] and three North American arenaviruses[24–26] (Table 5.1). The results of phylogenetic analyses of genome RNA sequence data are consistent with the serological New World–Old World division of the family and have allowed the classification of New World arenaviruses into three phylogenetic lineages, designated A, B, and C.[23,27–30]

As shown in Table 5.1, there is no obvious correlation between New World arenavirus phylogeny and their geographical distribution, which is determined by the habitat of its reservoir species. With two exceptions, these viruses have been all isolated from rodents of the family Muridae:[31] Tacaribe virus (TCRV) was originally isolated from fruit-eating bats of the genus *Artibeus* in Trinidad,[10] while Sabia virus (SABV) has no known wild reservoir.[18] Characteristically, arenaviruses induce a persistent infection in their rodent reservoirs, and humans may be accidental hosts who become infected by contact with the carrier rodents or their excreta. As summarized in Table 5.1, five members of the family are able to cause

Antiviral Drug Discovery for Emerging Diseases and Bioterrorism Threats. Edited by Paul F. Torrence

TABLE 5.1   Arenaviridae Family Members

Virus (Acronym)	Location	Human Disease	Isolation Reference
Old World Arenavirus			
Ippy (IPPYV)	Central African Republic	No	8
Lassa (LASV)	West Africa	Lassa fever	5
Lymphocytic choriomeningitis (LCMV)	Europe, Asia, Americas	Febrile syndrome, aseptic meningitis	4
Mobala (MOBV)	Central African Republic	No	7
Mopeia (MOPV)	Mozambique, Zimbabwe	No	6
New World Arenavirus			
CLADE A			
Allpahuayo (ALLV)[a]	Peru	No	22
Bear Canyon (BCNV)[a]	United States	No	26
Flexal (FLEV)	Brazil	Yes[b]	16
Parana (PARV)	Paraguay	No	13
Pichinde (PICV)	Colombia	No	14
Pirital (PIRV)	Venezuela	No	20
Tamiami (TAMV)	United States	No	24
Whitewater Arroyo (WWAV)	United States	Yes[c]	25
CLADE B			
Amapari (AMAV)	Brazil	No	12
Cupixi (CPXV)[a]	Brazil	No	23
Guanarito (GTOV)	Venezuela	HF	17
Junin (JUNV)	Argentina	Argentine HF[d]	9
Machupo (MACV)	Bolivia	Bolivian HF	4
Sabia (SABV)	Brazil	HF	18
Tacaribe (TCRV)	Trinidad	Yes[b]	10
CLADE C			
Latino (LATV)	Bolivia	No	15
Pampa (PAMV)[a]	Argentina	No	21
Oliveros (OLVV)	Argentina	No	19

[a]Virus species to be recognized by the International Committee for Virus Taxonomy.
[b]Associated only with single, nonfatal laboratory-acquired infection.
[c]Recently implicated as a possible agent of human infection.
[d]HF, hemorrhagic fever.

severe hemorrhagic fever (HF) in humans. The highly pathogenic arenaviruses include four South American viruses in clade B (Junin virus, JUNV, agent of Argentine HF; Machupo virus, MACV, agent of Bolivian HF; Guanarito virus, GTOV, agent of Venezuelan HF; and Sabia virus, SABV, in Brazil) and Lassa virus (LASV), responsible for Lassa fever in Africa.

The danger of pathogenic arenaviruses for human health, linked to their increased emergence in recent years, and the lack of a totally effective chemotherapy for treatment support their inclusion in the Category A Pathogen List of the Centers for Disease Control and Prevention (CDC) as potential agents of bioterrorism.[32] This chapter describes the historical background and present treatment of arenavirus hemorrhagic fevers and the perspectives for therapy, mainly focused on new possible targets in early and late stages of the replicative cycle.

5.2 THE VIRUS

The virions are pleomorphic particles with a size range from 50 to 300 nm, having an average diameter of 90–110 nm, and composed of two helical nucleocapsids enclosed in a lipid envelope. In the interior, a variable number of electron-dense granules that have been identified as host cell ribosomes were observed in most particles.[33] This unique granular structure accounts for the prefix *arena* given to the family name (*arenosus*, Latin for sandy).[34] However, the virion associated ribosomes are not required for virus multiplication.[35]

The genome consists of two single-stranded RNA molecules known as L (large, average 7100 nucleotides) and S (small, average 3400 nucleotides). In addition, abundant 28S and 18S RNAs from ribosomal origin as well as heterogeneous host and virus derived RNA species of 4–6S are found in virion RNA preparations. The L and S genome RNAs are not present in equimolar amounts, since S is present in excess, suggesting the formation of virions either with multiple copies of viral nucleocapsids or with the S nucleocapsid alone.[36–38]

Each genome segment presents an ambisense coding strategy, with two genes arranged in opposite orientations and separated by an intergenic noncoding region. The S segment encodes the nucleocapsid protein (NP) at its 3′ half from a mRNA in the genome-complementary sense and the glycoprotein precursor (GPC) at the 5′ half from a mRNA in the genome sense. GPC undergoes post-translational cleavage to generate the two envelope glycoproteins, GP1, the most exposed protein on the virion surface, and the transmembrane protein GP2. Similarly, the L RNA encodes the RNA-dependent RNA polymerase (L) in the genome-complementary sense, and a small protein with a RING finger motif (Z) in the opposite sense. Although both genome segments contain protein-coding sense sequences at their 5′ regions, they are not directly translated, and thus arenaviruses behave at this point like true negative-strand viruses with transcription as the first biosynthetic process. The noncoding intergenic region contains one or two sets of self-complementary nucleotide sequences, depending on the virus species, which form very stable hairpin loop structures.[39] The 5′-terminal noncoding sequence of each fragment is complementary to the 3′-end sequence, producing a panhandle structure responsible for the circular forms of nucleocapsids observed by electron microscopy.[33]

5.3   THE HUMAN DISEASE AND PRESENT TREATMENT

From the recognized highly pathogenic arenaviruses, only LASV and JUNV generate periodic annual outbreaks of hemorrhagic fever with high mortality rate and, consequently, are the main focus for antiviral therapies. MACV emerged in human epidemics of Bolivian HF in the 1960s as a result of the invasion of villages by *Calomys callosus*, the MACV reservoir.[11] The disease was controlled by rodent trapping and since then only occasional cases have occurred.[40] Similarly, GTOV emerged as the agent of Venezuelan HF in the 1990s[17] and subsequently the disease incidence was irregular.[41] SABV was only isolated from a fatal case of HF in Brazil[18] and two nonfatal laboratory infections.[42]

LASV is enzootic in the peridomestic rodent *Mastomys natalensis* and is distributed throughout West Africa. There is a spectrum of disease associated with LASV in humans from a mild, almost asymptomatic condition to the serious and often fatal hemorrhagic illness known as Lassa fever. Among arenaviruses, Lassa fever affects the largest number of humans: over 200,000 infections are estimated to occur annually, with an overall mortality of 15–30%.[43] Initially, the infection may present insidious development of fever, headache, and malaise, progressing to a very sore throat, pains in the back, chest, and joints, vomiting, and proteinuria.[43,44] In severe cases, conjuctivitis, pneumonitis, carditis, hepatitis, encephalopathy, nerve deafness, and/or hemorrhages are seen, and death occurs, usually following cardiovascular collapse.

With respect to JUNV, the main natural reservoir is *Calomys musculinus* but it can also infect other wild rodents. Human infection often occurs through cuts or skin abrasions, or inhalation of dust contaminated with infected rodent secretions during farming activities. The disease is geographically restricted to the humid pampa, the most fertile farming land of Argentina, and since it was first recognized in 1958,[9] annual outbreaks have been registered with incidence peaks in coincidence with the harvest times of maize crops (April–July), and with the presentation of an occupational disease affecting mostly 15- to 60-year-old male agricultural workers.[45] During the last two decades, the number of notified cases per year was in the range of 100–1000. As with LASV, the clinical spectrum of the human disease ranges from mild to severe and includes patients presenting neurological manifestations, hemorrhagic signs, or both. The initial symptoms in humans are nonspecific and among the first findings are marked asthenia, muscular pain, dizziness, skin and mucosal rashes, lymph node enlargement, cutaneous petechiae, and retroocular pain. At 7–10 days after onset, cardiovascular, digestive, renal, or neurological involvement becomes more severe, together with hematological and clotting alterations. At 10–15 days, over 80% of the patients improve noticeably, whereas the remainder are prone to worsen. The case-fatality rate ranges between 15% and 20% in the absence of treatment, and the most consistently found pathological lesion in fatal cases is widespread necrosis in the lymphatic tissue and cell depression in bone marrow.

The current treatment of Argentine HF is the early administration of standardized doses of convalescent plasma. The immune plasma therapy attenuates disease severity and significantly reduces mortality from 15–20% to less than 1%, and its efficacy is directly related to the concentration of neutralizing antibodies.[46,47] However, this therapy is not efficient when it is initiated after 8 days of illness and a late neurological syndrome is observed in 10% of the treated patients.[47,48] By contrast, convalescent plasma failed to improve recovery from Lassa fever.[49]

With respect to drug therapy, ribavirin (1-β-D-ribofuranosyl-1,2,4-triazole-3 carboxamide) is the only compound that has shown partial efficacy against arenavirus infections in studies performed in experimental animals and humans. Ribavirin is a guanosine analogue with broad spectrum of antiviral activity against RNA viruses. Three different mechanisms for the in vitro antiviral activity of ribavirin have been proposed. After phosphorylation to ribavirin 5′-monophosphate, the main interaction is a competitive inhibition of inosine monophospate dehydrogenase (IMPDH); by blocking the conversion of IMP to xanthosine monophosphate (XMP), a precursor molecule in the biosynthesis of GTP and dGTP, ribavirin depleted the intracellular GTP pool.[50] But ribavirin can also be phosphorylated to its 5′-triphosphate and in this form can affect either the initiation of viral mRNAs or the elongation of viral RNAs by competitive inhibition of mRNA-capping enzymes or viral polymerases, respectively.[51,52] Another recently proposed mechanism of action for ribavirin is its action as a mutagen, pushing RNA viruses to a critically high mutation rate and driving the virus population into the "error catastrophe."[53] The high error rate of RNA viruses due to the low fidelity of RNA polymerases has been proposed as an evolutionary advantage, but a small increase in the error rate, produced by ribavirin, may lead to a lethal loss of genome viability and virus infectivity. For instance, it was shown that the anti-poliovirus activity of the drug correlated with its mutagenic effect supporting the theory that the mechanism termed "lethal mutagenesis" may be the primary mode of action of the drug in this system.[54] However, a recent report has demonstrated that the inhibitory effect of ribavirin on multiplication of the arenavirus LCMV was not associated with a significant increase in mutation frequencies in the virus genome, but rather with the abrogation of RNA synthesis mediated by the viral polymerase.[55] The multiple mechanisms of action of ribavirin also include in vivo indirect immune-mediated activities.[56]

Ribavirin has been used to treat human patients infected with respiratory syncytial virus[57] and, in combination with interferon-α, is one of the current therapies approved for treatment of chronic or acute hepatitis C virus infections.[58] The first experiments in animal models to test the efficacy of ribavirin against arenaviruses were successfully carried out with LASV in primates.[59] Later, a controlled trial in Sierra Leone, West Africa, proved that ribavirin was very effective when administered intravenously during the first 6 days after the onset of Lassa fever, significantly decreasing case-fatality rates from 50% to 5–9%.[49] Currently, ribavirin is the recommended treatment for patients diagnosed with Lassa fever and is also advised as a prophylactic agent in cases of possible exposure to LASV. However, the drug is not effective for the treatment of advanced LASV infections. It must also be remarked that undesirable secondary reactions such as thrombocytosis and anemia have been recorded for ribavirin treatment in animal models and in humans.[48,60]

For experimental Argentine HF, ribavirin therapy was assayed in guinea pigs and primates. The drug was not effective in guinea pigs, since JUNV replication and mean time of death were delayed but mortality was not affected.[61] In the marmoset *Callithrix jacchus*, ribavirin lowered viremia and increased survival, although late neurological alterations appeared in JUNV-infected animals.[62] The most successful results were obtained in rhesus macaques, since treatment with ribavirin at the time of infection protected the animals from clinical disease; a delay in the drug administration improved the course of the disease but survivor animals developed a neurological infection.[60] In spite of these promising results in primates, the clinical evaluation of ribavirin in Argentine HF patients did not show efficacy in reducing mortality,[48,63] and consequently the treatment in use for this South American HF is the administration of immune plasma in a defined dose of specific anti-JUNV neutralizing antibodies per kilogram of body.[46]

5.4 NEW TARGETS FOR THERAPY IN THE VIRAL CYCLE

Knowledge of the viral life cycle is essential to elucidate potential targets of antiviral therapy, and thus to obtain key information for the rational design of antiviral drugs. The main steps of the arenavirus multiplication cycle are outlined in Figure 5.1. Each point in this cycle may be considered as a possible target for selective attack by chemotherapeutic agents. However, attempts to find antiviral substances able to block the intracellular multiplication of arenaviruses have focused mainly on the screening of probable inhibitors of RNA transcription and/ or replication, as it has occurred for most RNA viruses. These studies led to the above-mentioned clinical use of ribavirin for Lassa fever therapy. Given the low selectivity of the drug and the disadvantages recorded for human treatment, a continuous screening of several other nucleoside analogues has been performed to obtain more selective agents targeted to arenavirus RNA synthesis. The list of substances assayed in vitro and, occasionally, in animal models includes compounds chemically related to ribavirin such as its 3-carboxamide derivative ribamidine and the C-nucleoside analogues tiazofurin, selenazofurin, and pyrazofurin,[64–67] acyclic and carbocyclic adenosine analogues,[67,68] thioadenosine derivatives,[69] cytosine analogues,[67] isocarbonucleosides,[70] and stavudine derivatives.[71] In fact, these agents act through the inhibition of cellular enzymes or factors required for RNA synthesis, and consequently the selectivity indices (ratio between cytotoxic concentration and effective antiviral concentration) for most of them were not very promising and were highly dependent on the method used to evaluate cellular toxicity (DNA synthesis, cell growth, or cell morphology). Thus, at present, this line of antiviral research has not produced successful results.

As occurs with other viruses leading the field of antiviral chemotherapy, such as human immunodeficiency virus (HIV) and herpesviruses, new targets in the viral

1. Adsorption

    Binding GP1- receptor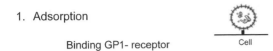

    Cell

2. Entry

    Endocytosis and low pH-dependent fusion ➔ free RNPs

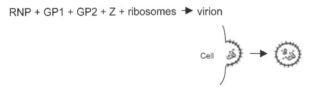

3. Transcription-Translation-Replication

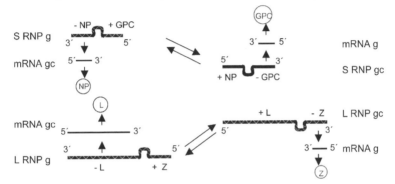

4. Maturation and Transport of GPC (GP1 + GP2) and Z

5. Assembly and Budding

    RNP + GP1 + GP2 + Z + ribosomes ➔ virion

    Cell

FIGURE 5.1   Scheme of the main steps in the replicative cycle of Arenaviridae. RNP, ribonucleoprotein; g, genome sense; gc, genome-complementary sense.

cycle different from nucleic acid synthesis are becoming more attractive candidates. With this in mind, the following sections analyze the actual knowledge and the antiviral possibilities investigated at early and late steps of the arenavirus multiplication cycle, viral entry into the cell, and virus maturation and budding, respectively.

5.4.1 Early Steps: Adsorption and Entry

Adsorption The virus envelope spikes, formed by noncovalently linked homotetramers of the peripheral protein GP1 and the transmembrane protein GP2,[72] participate in both processes of virion attachment and fusion with cell membranes leading to internalization of the viral nucleocapsid. The adsorption of enveloped viruses to their host cell is often a complex process with sequential binding of the virion to various receptors and coreceptors, linked to conformational alterations in the involved glycoproteins.

Several lines of evidence suggest that presumably GP1 is the envelope glycoprotein responsible for arenavirus adsorption to the host cell. GP1 was the target of neutralizing antibodies able to block LCMV infectivity.[73,74] Concomitantly, GP1-specific antibodies blocked LCMV binding to cells and antibodies against GP2 did not disturb virion binding.[75] Additionally, a host range mutant of JUNV unable to bind to murine cells showed an altered GP1 peptide mapping.[76]

With respect to the cell receptor, the high molecular weight glycoprotein α-dystroglycan has been identified as a major receptor for Old World arenaviruses.[77] Dystroglycan is encoded as a glycoprotein precursor and post-translationally processed to form the peripheral protein α-dystroglycan and the membrane-spanning protein β-dystroglycan, a complex highly expressed in a variety of cells and reported as a molecular link between the extracellular matrix and the actin-based cytoskeleton.[78] The situation with the New World arenaviruses is less clear: the assay of virus entry into mouse cells expressing or lacking α-dystroglycan together with a virus overlay protein blot assay demonstrated that only clade C viruses (OLV and LATV) used α-dystroglycan as a major receptor.[79] By contrast, New World clade A and B arenaviruses appeared to use a different receptor or coreceptor for cell binding. The protein nature of the cell receptor for JUNV, a clade B arenavirus, was demonstrated by enzymatic treatment, but the cellular protein was not identified.[80] The use of different receptors by viruses of the same family is not a surprising finding and may be related to biological differences in cell tropism or pathogenicity among viruses.[81] In fact, LCMV strains presenting point mutations in GP1 and differing in their pathogenic potential for mice also exhibited a differential binding affinity to α-dystroglycan: those strains with a high affinity of binding to α-dystroglycan invariably established a persistent infection in mice, whereas the mouse infection with LCMV variants with low level or no binding to α-dystroglycan was rapidly cleared.[82] These results are indicative of the association between receptor usage and pathogenesis and point out the need for the identification of the additional receptors or coreceptors utilized by arenaviruses, particularly those highly pathogenic members of the New World clade B associated to HF such as JUNV, MACV, SABV, and GTOV (see Table 5.1).

The blockade of virus binding is very valuable as an antiviral therapeutic strategy because it allows us to establish a first barrier to suppress infection. For LCMV and LASV, two Old World arenaviruses that utilize α-dystroglycan as the cell receptor, it has been reported that the addition of the soluble α-dystroglycan blocked virus infection in vitro.[77] In another type of experimental approach,

TABLE 5.2   In Vitro Antiviral Activity of Early and Late Inhibitors of Arenaviruses

Compound	Viruses	Target	References
Polysulfates	JUNV, TCRV	Early	67,83
Soluble α-dystroglycan	LCMV, LASV	Early	77
Procaine, chlorpheniramine, ammonium chloride	JUNV	Early	85
Trifluoperazine, chlorpromazine	JUNV, TCRV, PICV	Early/late	95
Caffeine	JUNV	Early	96
Meliacine	JUNV, TCRV	Early/late	99,100
Myristic acid analogues	JUNV, TCRV	Late	112
Lauric acid	JUNV, TCRV	Late	113
Aromatic disulfides, dithianes, azodicarboamide	JUNV, TCRV, PICV	Late/virion	134,138,139
Brassinosteroids	JUNV, TCRV, PICV	Late	142
Macrocyclic trichothecenes	JUNV, TCRV	Late	144
Thiosemicarbazone derivatives	JUNV	Late	145
Cecropin A	JUNV, TCRV, PICV	Late	146

different classes of polysulfates, including sulfated polysaccharides (dextran sulfate, heparin, pentosan polysulfate), polyacetal polysulfate, and polyvinylalcohol sulfate and its copolymer with acrylic acid, were found to be highly selective inhibitors of JUNV and TCRV replication (Table 5.2).[67,83] For other enveloped viruses, including HIV, herpesviruses, and papillomaviruses, the antiviral activity of these negatively charged molecules has been attributed to an interference with virus adsorption by blockade of the interaction between the cellular receptor and the virion external glycoprotein.[83] However, potential clinical application of these kinds of agents against viral hemorrhagic fevers has not been investigated.

Entry   After binding to the cell receptor, arenaviruses enter into the host cell through an endocytic pathway. The complete process includes virion uptake into vesicles followed by a low pH-dependent fusion of viral envelope and endosome membranes, and finally the nucleocapsid is released into the cytoplasm. The mode of entry of arenaviruses by endocytosis relied on results provided by different experimental approaches. The sensitivity of early events in the arenavirus replicative cycle to lysosomotropic compounds was the first evidence of an endosomal route of entry. Weak bases, such as ammonium chloride and chloroquine, as well as carboxylic ionophores, such as nigericin and monensin, were effective inhibitors of the internalization of several arenaviruses, including LASV, MOPV, PICV, JUNV, and LCMV.[84–86] Both classes of compounds raise the endosomal pH either by protonization of the base in the acidic vesicle or by exchange of H^+ for Na^+/K^+, respectively, and under these conditions arenavirus internalization is inhibited. Accordingly, the blockade in JUNV infection induced by weak bases could be overcome by buffering the extracellular medium at a pH below 6.0, a treatment that allowed direct fusion of virus envelope with the cell membrane.[85] Lysosomotropic compounds have side effects on other cellular functions, which can affect virus multiplication; but the mechanism of entry of arenaviruses was confirmed using agents targeted specifically to the components of the endocytic pathway. The macrolide antibiotics bafilomycin A1 and concanamycin A, which are specific inhibitors of the vacuolar proton ATPase, the enzyme responsible for maintaining the low pH of endosomes, inhibited simultaneously JUNV penetration and vesicle acidication.[87] Furthermore, the presence of LCMV particles inside vesicles during virus entry into the cell was visualized by immunoelectronmicroscopy.[86]

The role of the glycoproteins GP1 and GP2 in the acid pH-dependent fusion determinant of arenavirus internalization was also demonstrated. After exposure to acid pH, the LCMV spike glycoprotein complex constituted by GP1 and GP2 undergoes conformational changes characterized by alterations in the antibody binding ability of both glycoproteins and an irreversible dissociation of GP1 from the virions.[88,89] After a brief acid treatment, JUNV-infected cells expressing viral glycoproteins on their surface were able to induce the formation of syncytia by fusion with adjacent cells, providing evidence that conformational changes on the viral glycoproteins have occurred at low pH.[90] For LASV, a fusion activity is triggered by acid pH in a synthetic peptide homologous to an internal sequence of GP2.[91] Altogether, these results allow one to assume that the interaction between GP1 and GP2 is altered under the acidic environment of the endosome, and, in consequence, a fusogenic peptide in GP2, which at neutral pH is located in a hidden position, becomes exposed and triggers the fusion between the viral envelope and the endosomal membrane.

Among probably early inhibitors of the replicative cycle of arenaviruses with therapeutic perspectives, one of the initial compounds studied more than three decades ago was amantadine, known as a blocker of influenza virus uncoating. Amantadine was an effective in vitro inhibitor of LCMV and several New World arenaviruses, but when it was assayed in vivo the results were discouraging because the administration of amantadine shortened the survival of guinea pigs and mice infected with JUNV and LCMV, respectively.[92–94] More recent works have evaluated several pharmacological agents, licensed for clinical use and known to affect the endocytic pathway, for use against arenaviruses. The list of selective inhibitors of JUNV, TCRV, and PICV multiplication by blockade of an early stage included anesthetics like procaine, antihistaminics like chlorpheniramine, and compounds with antiemetic, neuroleptic, and neurostimulating action such as trifluoperazine, chlorpromazine, and caffeine (see Table 5.2).[85,95,96] Chlorpromazine has been employed extensively for studies of virus entry to demonstrate the role of clathrin-mediated endocytosis.[97] The study on the effect of chlorpromazine and trifluoperazine on JUNV multiplication proved that these drugs acted on this virus through their interaction with calmodulin, a structural protein in the cytoskeleton and modulator of many Ca-dependent enzymes in the cell.[95] Based on these in vitro results, it can be considered promising to assay any of these substances, widely applied for medical use, in an experimental model of arenavirus HF to evaluate their usefulness as a therapy.

The integrity of the cytoskeleton is also a requisite for JUNV entry, since agents disrupting the microfilament and microtubule networks, such as EGTA, nifedipine, colchicine, and nocodazole, were also inhibitors of JUNV multiplication at early stages.[98] By contrast, virus uptake in LCMV infection was reported to be a microfilament-independent process, because it was not blocked by cytochalasins.[86] This discrepancy may be due to a technical artifact or probably, as occurs with the above-mentioned differences between the cell receptor for LCMV and New World clade B arenaviruses, is indicative of a different behavior in the mode of internalization of these viruses.

The search for compounds with antiviral activity against arenaviruses has also focused on products obtained from natural sources. This strategy developed in recent years with interesting results. In particular, a cyclic peptide purified from the leaves of the plant *Melia azedarach* L., called meliacine, was a very effective inhibitor of the in vitro replication of the arenaviruses JUNV and TCRV (see Table 5.2).[99] Analysis of the early events after infection demonstrated that meliacine blocked virus penetration into Vero cells by preventing JUNV uncoating due to interference with vacuolar acidification.[100] Furthermore, the administration of partially purified leaf extracts of *M. azedarach* L. to suckling mice infected with TCRV protected them from encephalitis, with a degree of protection from 66% to 100%, depending on the virus dose.[101]

5.4.2 Late Steps: Maturation, Assembly, and Budding

The late steps of the viral cycle comprise the diverse maturation processes leading to virion formation and release: processing and exocytic transport of viral proteins, followed by assembly of the viral particle and budding from the cell. These events are only partially known in the arenavirus life cycle.

The maturation process of viral proteins as well as their transport to the proper cellular location for virion assembly represent interesting antiviral targets. Both genome segments of Arenaviridae encode a total of five mature proteins, which are all structural components of the virion. The NP, the most abundant viral protein in infected cells, and the polymerase L are tightly associated to viral RNA when it is replicated in the genome complementary sense as well as in the genomic sense. This RNA–protein complex known as viral ribonucleoprotein (RNP) is the template for virus transcription and replication (see Figure 5.1) and, as occurs with other negative-strand RNA viruses, is the minimum infectious unit of arenaviruses.[39] In the late stages of the life cycle, this structure must incorporate the small Z protein and both glycoproteins GP1 and GP2, inserted in the host plasma membrane, where viral particles are assembled and released from the cell by budding.[33,102] Assembly of arenaviruses is not a very accurate process, as indicated by the packaging of ribosomes and variable proportions of S and L genomes as well as small virus derived RNAs.

Glycoprotein Maturation   GP1 and GP2 are synthesized as the GPC precursor at the endoplasmic reticulum. Post-translational processing to obtain mature proteins at the plasma membrane involves transition of the oligosaccharide chains from the high mannose type to the complex form, cleavage of GPC, and transport and insertion into the membrane. The progression of this maturation pathway is not uniform for all arenaviruses studied. For LASV and LCMV, GPC is cleaved to generate GP1 at the N-end and GP2 at the C-end by the cellular protease subtilase SKI-1/S1P.[103–105] But, whereas cleavage of LASV GPC occurs in the endoplasmic reticulum,[105] cleavage of LCMV GPC occurs later in the secretory pathway, in a late Golgi or post-Golgi compartment.[106] Cleavage of JUNV GPC also takes place late in transit through or exit from the trans-Golgi.[107] In any case, proteolytic cleavage of GPC is a prerequisite for the formation of infectious particles during JUNV,[107,108] LASV,[104] and LCMV[109] infections. The use of trimming glucosidase and mannosidase inhibitors such as 1-deoxynojirimycin, castanospermine, 1-deoxymannojirimycin, and swainsonine, demonstrated that, although the addition of the oligosaccharide chains was essential for glycoprotein cleavage, transport, and virion infectivity, acquisition of a complex structure of the carbohydrate chains was not required for these events to occur.[106,110] Glycosylation inhibitors are not selective in their antiviral inhibitory action, but the elucidation of the cleavage motif of LASV GPC offers the possibility of a rational design of substrate analogues to block this cleavage and may have meaningful therapeutic potential for treatment of Lassa fever.

Formation of infectious virions not only depends on glycosylation and proteolytic cleavage of the glycoproteins, but also on myristoylation of GPC, a protein modification catalyzed by the enzyme *N*-myristoyltransferase that links myristic acid to the penultimate glycine residue in the N-terminal corresponding consensus sequence, previously reported in JUNV S RNA.[111] Myristic acid analogues, such as 2-hydroxymyristic acid and 13-oxamyristic acid, were found to inhibit JUNV and TCRV production (see Table 5.2) without apparent toxicity to the cells.[112] The cleavage and cell membrane expression of JUNV glycoproteins were not affected by the analogues, suggesting that myristoylation is not essential for the intracellular exocytic transport of the envelope proteins from the site of synthesis to the cell surface, but it may have an important role in their interaction with the plasma membrane during virion assembly and /or budding.

The exocytic pathway of viral glycoproteins may also be affected by agents producing alterations in the properties of the cell membrane. On this basis, compounds disturbing the lipid composition have been analyzed as potential antivirals. Lauric acid, a saturated fatty acid with 12 C, was the most effective inhibitor of JUNV and TCRV multiplication, due to a blockade in the insertion of the viral glycoproteins into the plasma membrane.[113] This antiviral activity appeared to be correlated with an estimulation of the triacylglycerol cell content, since both effects were dependent on the continued presence of the fatty acid.

Z Protein as a Late Target   Z is an 11-kDa protein of about 90–100 amino acids containing a zinc-binding RING finger domain conserved in the members of the family.[114–117] Biochemical and immunological studies demonstrated that LCMV Z is a structural component of the virion, closely associated to NP.[118] Although its precise role is poorly understood, the importance of Z in the arenavirus life cycle is now recognized.

Different investigators have proposed regulatory–structural functions for this protein during virus infection. Early studies based on in vitro transcription combined with immunodepletion of Z from TCRV-infected cells suggested that Z was required for both mRNA synthesis and genome replication.[119] More recently, discrepant results were obtained using a reverse genetics system in which RNA synthesis was reconstituted by intracellular coexpression of a virus minigenome and viral proteins produced from transfected plasmids. With this system, it was shown for two arenaviruses, LCMV and TCRV, that Z was not required for RNA synthesis mediated by the viral polymerase, but rather Z exerted a dose-dependent inhibitory effect on both viral transcription and RNA replication.[120–122] Through this inhibitory activity, Z might contribute to the known restricted replicative ability and noncytopathic properties of many arenaviruses. In natural infection with LCMV, the expression of Z was undetectable during the initial 24 h following infection,[121] precisely avoiding a strong negative effect on viral RNA synthesis and allowing virus multiplication to occur.

Furthermore, Z has also been shown to interact with several cellular proteins. The LCMV Z protein was found to bind to the promyelocytic leukemia protein (PML), leading to the relocation of PML nuclear bodies to the cytoplasm.[123,124] Z has also been reported to interact with the nuclear fraction of the ribosomal protein P0 and with the eukaryotic translation initiation factor eIF4E.[125,126] These cellular interactions of Z may provide mechanisms to elucidate a viral strategy for the establishment of chronic infections, a typical property of arenaviruses.

In addition to its regulatory role during virus replication, the Z protein was also suggested as a virion component with structural functions. Based on the segregation of Z as hydrophobic protein associated with viral membranes upon nonionic detergent extraction of LCMV virions,[118] Z has been proposed as the arenavirus counterpart of the matrix (M) protein, found in most enveloped negative-strand viruses.[33,127] The M proteins interact with membranes and are involved in the organization of viral components during assembly and budding, providing a link between the cytoplasmic tail of the glycoproteins and the nucleocapsid that contains the RNA genome.[128] Further evidence supporting the idea that Z functions as a matrix protein during arenavirus budding was provided by recent studies showing that LCMV and LASV Z proteins are strongly membrane-associated and are sufficient, in the absence of all other viral proteins, to release enveloped virus-like particles.[129,130] The membrane-targeting properties of Z are supported by the presence of a conserved myristoylation motif at the N-terminal portion of the protein. The interaction of Z with NP, previously reported for LCMV,[118] was recently confirmed for LASV proteins, allowing one to assume that Z is responsible for driving arenavirus budding through the recruitment of NP, complexed in the ribonucleoprotein, to the patches in the cellular membranes enriched in GP1/GP2 where virus assembly takes place.[131]

Analysis of the linear amino acid structure for the Z gene in sequenced arenaviruses has shown that this protein is conformed by a RING domain of 37 aa flanked by an N-terminal portion and a C-terminal portion. The C-termini contain proline-rich motifs found in the so-called late (L) domains, which were identified in matrix proteins of enveloped viruses.[132] These late domains mediate protein–protein interactions and play a critical role in the virus budding process. It was found that the integrity of the late motifs and the RING finger domain is necessary for the Z-mediated regulatory and structural functions,[129,130,133] turning this protein into a very promising target for arenavirus chemotherapy.

In the search for agents reactive with the Z protein, a series of compounds with diverse chemical structures, including aliphatic and aromatic disulfides and azoic and hidrazide derivatives, were evaluated and found to be very effective inhibitors of arenaviruses (see Table 5.2).[134] These compounds were targeted to the retroviral zinc-finger motifs of the HIV-1 nucleocapsid protein NCp7, causing Zn ejection from the protein, loss of its native structure, and inhibition of HIV multiplication.[135–137] According to their mode of action against JUNV, TCRV, PICV, and LCMV, these compounds could be classified into two categories: (1) virucidal agents able to inactivate cell-free virions, and (2) antiviral agents that blocked the intracellular viral multiplication cycle. The most effective inactivating agents included intermolecular aromatic disulfides, dithianes, and azodicarbonamide, compounds that quickly inactivate arenaviruses in a concentration- and time-dependent manner.[138,139] Inactivated virions maintained the conformational and functional integrity of the viral glycoproteins, since they were able to bind and enter into the host cell as well as to induce anti-arenavirus neutralizing antibodies in adult mice.[140] By contrast, the treatment of a recombinant Z protein with the virucidal compounds showed the formation of multimers of Z, confirming that this protein is the main target (C. C. García, unpublished results).[141] Accordingly, with the proposed role of Z as an analogue to a matrix protein, the azoic compounds included in the second class of arenavirus inhibitors appeared to block the process of intracellular virus assembly.[139] These investigations evidence, for the first time, the potential of Z as a new and promising target in arenavirus therapy.

Other Late Inhibitors of Assembly/Budding   From time-related inhibition experiments, several natural and synthetic compounds have been found as inhibitors of late stages in the replicative cycle (see Table 5.2), but their precise target is still not elucidated. Some examples of these active compounds include: a natural brassinosteroid and a series of synthetic derivatives, with plant growth promoting properties, that affected the multiplication of JUNV, PICV, and TCRV;[142] sulfated polyhydroxy-steroids isolated from marine organisms and their synthetic derivatives and analogues, active against JUNV;[143] macrocyclic trichothecenes produced by the hypocrealean epibiont of *Baccharis coridifolia*, inhibitors of JUNV and TCRV;[144] thiosemicarbazone derivatives synthesized from aromatic ketones and terpenones, particularly the tetralone thiosemicarbazone, which inhibited a late stage after protein synthesis in the replicative cycle of JUNV;[145] and the antimicrobial cationic peptide cecropin A, active against JUNV, TCRV, and PICV, mainly preventing viral morphogenesis and egress from the cell.[146]

5.5 CONCLUSION

Arenaviruses possess the attributes necessary to serve as potential agents of bioterrorism. Five members of the family are able to produce severe HF and only limited strategies are available for treatment of infection. An attenuated live vaccine named Candid 1 has been developed against JUNV and has been successfully evaluated in the human population of the endemic area of Argentine HF.[147] However, it is not known if this vaccine has the ability to cross-protect against other pathogenic arenaviruses. Furthermore, vaccines probably will never be the complete answer to the control of arenavirus infections, because occasional outbreaks are expected to occur due to the virus characteristics; for example, if ecological changes occur in the habits of the natural rodent reservoir. An even greater threat for arenaviruses is the possibility of inter- or intrasegmental recombination that may originate virus variants with enhanced virulence. The present treatment of arenavirus HF, mainly based on the administration of immune plasma or the drug ribavirin, has important drawbacks and undesirable side effects. Thus, the development and evaluation of effective antiviral agents targeted to the early and late stages of the replicative cycle is a new approach that presents promising perspectives. Effective viral inhibitors of both stages are presently under study, and knowledge of the molecular targets in viral proteins involved in these process will allow the rational design of specific agents. It is a valid alternative to ribavirin or ribavirin analogues and, given the encouraging results obtained in in vitro cell culture systems, priority must be given to the continuation of these studies and the implementation of in vivo efficacy assays.

ACKNOWLEDGMENTS

The studies performed in the authors' laboratory were supported by Universidad de Buenos Aires, Agencia Nacional de Promoción Científica y Tecnológica (ANPCyT) and Consejo Nacional de Investigaciones Científicas y Técnicas (CONICET), Argentina. E.B.D. is a member of the Research Center of CONICET and C.C.G. is a fellow of the same institution.

REFERENCES

1. Clegg, J. C. S.; Bowen, M. D.; Buchmeier, M. J.; Gonzalez, J. P.; Lukashevich, I. S.; Peters, C. J.; Rico-Hesse, R.; Romanowski, V. Family Arenaviridae. In *Virus Taxonomy. Seventh Report of the International Committee for the Taxonomy of Viruses*, Regenmortel, M. H. V.; van, Fauquet, C. M.; Bishop, D. H. L.; Carstens, E. B.; Estes, M. K.; Lemon, S. M.; Maniloff, J.; Mayo, M. A.; McGeoch, D. J.; Pringle, C. R.; Wickner, R. B. (eds.). Academic Press, Orlando, 2000, pp. 633–640.

2. Wulff, H.; Lange, J. V.; Webb, P. A. Interrelationships among arenaviruses measured by indirect immunofluorescence. *Intervirology* **1978**, *9*, 344–350.

3. Howard, C. R. Antigenic diversity among the arenaviruses. In *The Arenaviridae*, Salvato, M. S. (ed.). Plenum Press, New York, 1993, pp. 37–49.

4. Armstrong, C. R.; Lillie, R. D. Experimental lymphocytic choriomeningitis of monkeys and mice produced by a virus encountered in studies of the 1933 St. Louis encephalitis epidemic. *Public Health Rep. (Washington)* **1934**, *50*, 831–842.

5. Frame, J. D.; Baldwin, J. M. Jr.; Gocke, D. J.; Troup, J. M. Lassa fever, a new virus disease of man from West Africa. I. Clinical description and pathological findings. *Am. J. Trop. Med. Hyg.* **1970**, *19*, 670–676.

6. Wulff, H.; McIntosh, B. M.; Hammer, D. B.; Johnson, K. M. Isolation of an arenavirus closely related to Lassa virus from *Mastomys natalensis* in South-East Africa. *Bull. WHO* **1977**, *55*, 441–444.

7. González, J. P.; McCormick, J. B.; Saluzzo, J. F.; Herve, J. P.; Georges, A. J.; Johnson, K. M. An arenavirus isolated from wild-caught rodents (*Praomys* species) in the Central African Republic. *Intervirology* **1983**, *19*, 105–112.

8. Swanepoel, R.; Leman, P. A.; Shepherd, A. J.; Shepherd, S. P.; Kiley, M. P.; McCormick, J. B. Identification of Ippy virus as a Lassa-fever related virus. *Lancet* **1985**, *1*, 639.

9. Parodi, A. S.; Greenway, D. Y.; Rugiero, H. R.; Rivero, E.; Frigerio, M. J.; Mettler, N. E.; Garzon, F.; Boxaca, M.; Guerrero, L. B. de; Nota, N. R. Sobre la etiología del brote epidémico en Junín. *Día Med.* **1958**, *30*, 2300–2302.

10. Downs, W. G.; Anderson, C. R.; Spence, L.; Aitken, T. H. G.; Greenhall, A. H. Tacaribe virus, a new agent isolated from Artibeus bats and mosquitoes in Trinidad, West Indies. *Am. J. Trop. Med. Hyg.* **1963**, *12*, 640–642.

11. Johnson, K. M.; Kuns, M. L.; Mackenzie, R. B.; Webb, P. A.; Yunker, C. E. Isolation of Machupo virus from wild rodent *Calomys callosus*. *Am. J. Trop. Med. Hyg.* **1966**, *15*, 103–106.

12. Pinheiro, F. P.; Shope, R. E.; de Andrade, A. H. P.; Bensabath, G.; Cacios, G. V.; Casals, J. Amapari, a new virus of the Tacaribe group from rodents and mites of Amapa territory, Brazil. *Proc. Soc. Exp. Biol. Med.* **1966**, *122*, 531–535.

13. Webb, P. A.; Johnson, K. M.; Hibbs, J. B.; Kuns, M. L. Parana, a new Tacaribe complex virus from Paraguay. *Arch. Ges. Virusforsch.* **1970**, *32*, 379–388.

14. Trapido, H.; San Martín, C. Pichinde virus. A new virus of the Tacaribe group from Colombia. *Am. J. Trop. Med. Hyg.* **1971**, *20*, 631–641.

15. Webb, P. A.; Johnson, K. M.; Peters, C. J.; Justines, G. Behaviour of Machupo and Latino viruses in *Calomys callosus* from two geographic areas of Bolivia. In *Lymphocytic Choriomeningitis Virus and Other Arenaviruses*, Lehmann-Grube, F. (ed.). Springer Verlag, Berlin, 1973, pp. 313–321.

16. Pinheiro, F. P.; Woodall, J. P.; Da Rosa, A. P. A. T.; Da Rosa, J. F. T. Studies of *Arenaviruses* in Brazil. *Medicina (Buenos Aires)* **1977**, *37*(Suppl.3), 175–181.

17. Tesh, R. B.; Jarhling, P. B.; Salas, R. A.; Shope, R. E. Description of Guanarito virus (Arenaviridae: *Arenavirus*), the etiologic agent of Venezuelan hemorrhagic fever. *Am. J. Trop. Med. Hyg.* **1994**, *50*, 452–459.

18. Coimbra, T. L. M.; Nassar, E. S.; Burattini, M. N.; de Souza, L. T. M.; Ferreira, I. B.; Rocco, I. M.; Travassos da Rosa, A. P.; Vasconcelos, P. F. C.; Pinheiro, F. P.; Le Duc,

J. W.; Rico-Hesse, R.; Gonzalez, J.-P.; Jahrling, P. B.; Tesh, R. B. New arenavirus isolated in Brazil. *Lancet* **1994**, *343*, 391–392.

19. Bowen, M. D.; Peters, C. J.; Mills, J. M.; Nichol, S. T. Oliveros virus: a novel Arenavirus from Argentina. *Virology* **1966**, *217*, 362–366.

20. Fulhorst, C. F.; Bowen, M. D.; Salas, R. A.; de Manzione, N. M. C.; Duno, G.; Utrera, A.; Ksiazek, T. G.; Peters, C. J.; Nichol, S. T.; de Miller, E.; Tovar, D.; Ramos, B.; Vasquez, C.; Tesh, R. B. Isolation and characterization of Pirital virus, a newly discovered South American arenavirus. *Am. J. Trop. Med. Hyg.* **1997**, *56*, 558–553.

21. Lozano, M. E.; Posik, D. M.; Albariño, C. G.; Schujman, G.; Ghiringhelli, P. D.; Calderón, G.; Sabattini, M. S.; Romanowski, V. Characterization of arenaviruses using a family-specific primer set of RT-PCR amplification and RFLP analysis: its potential use for detection of uncharacterized arenaviruses. *Virus Res.* **1997**, *49*, 79–89.

22. Moncayo, A. C.; Hice, C. L.; Watts, D. M.; Travassos de Rosa, A. P. A.; Guzmán, H.; Russell, K. L.; Calampa, C.; Gozalo, A.; Popov, V. L.; Weaver, S. C.; Tesh, R. B. Allpahuayo virus: a newly recognized arenavirus (Arenaviridae) from arboreal rice rats (*Oecomys bicolor and Oecomys paricola*) in northeastern Peru. *Virology* **2001**, *284*, 277–286.

23. Charrel, R. N.; Feldmann, H.; Fulhorst, C. F.; Khelifa, R.; de Chesse, R.; de Lamballerie, X. Phylogeny of New World arenaviruses based on the complete coding sequences of the small genomic segment identified an evolutionary lineage produced by intrasegmental recombination. *Biochem. Biophys. Res. Commun.* **2002**, *296*, 1118–1124.

24. Jennings, W. L.; Lewis, A. L.; Sather, G. E.; Pierce, L. V.; Bond, J. O. Tamiami virus in the Tampa Bay area. *Am. J. Trop. Med. Hyg.* **1970**, *19*, 527–536.

25. Fulhorst, C. F.; Bowen, M. D.; Ksiazek, T. G.; Rollin, P. E.; Nichol, S. T.; Kosoy, M. Y.; Peters, C. J. Isolation and characterization of Whitewater Arroyo virus, a novel North American arenavirus. *Virology* **1996**, *224*, 114–120.

26. Fulhorst, C. F.; Bennett, S. G.; Milazzo, M. L.; Murray, H. L.; Webb, J. P.; Cajimat, M. N. B.; Bradley, R. B. Bear Canyon virus: an arenavirus naturally associated with the California mouse (*Peromyscus californicus*). *Emerging Infect. Dis.* **2002**, *8*, 717–721.

27. Bowen, M. D.; Peters, C. J.; Nichol, S. T. The phylogeny of New World (Tacaribe complex) arenaviruses. *Virology* **1996**, *219*, 285–290.

28. Archer, A. A.; Rico-Hesse, R. High genetic divergence and recombination in arenaviruses from the Americas. *Virology* **2002**, *304*, 274–281.

29. Clegg, J. C. S. Molecular phylogeny of the arenaviruses. *Curr. Top. Microbiol. Immunol.* **2002**, *262*, 1–24.

30. Charrel, R. N.; Lemasson, J. J.; Garbutt, M.; Khelifa, R.; De Micco, P.; Feldmann, H.; de Lamballerie, X. New insights into the evolutionary relationships between arenaviruses provided by comparative analysis of small and large segment sequences. *Virology* **2003**, *317*, 191–196.

31. Salazar-Bravo, J.; Ruedas, L. A.; Yates, T. L. Mammalian reservoirs of arenaviruses. *Curr. Top. Microbiol. Immunol.* **2002**, *262*, 26–63.

32. Rotz, L. D.; Khan, A. S.; Lillibridge, S. R.; Ostroff, S. M.; Hughes, J. M. Public health assessment of potential biological terrorism agents. *Emerging Infect. Dis.* **2002**, *8*, 225–230.

33. Compans, R. W. Arenavirus ultrastructure and morphogenesis. In *The Arenaviridae*, Salvato, M. S. (ed.). Plenum Press, New York, 1993, pp. 3–16.

34. Rowe, W. P.; Murphy, F. A.; Bergold, G. H.; Casals, J.; Hotchin, J.; Johnson, K. M.; Lehmann-Grube, F.; Mims, C. A.; Traub, E.; Webb, P. A. Arenaviruses: proposed name for a newly defined virus group. *J. Virol.* **1970**, *5*, 651–652.

35. Leung, W. C.; Rawls, W. E. Virion-associated ribosomes are not required for the replication of Pichinde virus. *Virology* **1977**, *81*, 174–176.

36. Romanowski, V.; Bishop, D. H. L. The formation of arenaviruses that are genetically diploid. *Virology* **1983**, *126*, 87–95.

37. Southern, P. J.; Singh, M. K.; Riviere, Y.; Jacoby, D. R.; Buchmeier, M. J.; Oldstone, M. B. A. Molecular characterization of the genomic S RNA segment from lymphocytic choriomeningitis virus. *Virology* **1987**, *157*, 145–155.

38. Iapalucci, S.; Cherñavsky, A.; Rossi, C.; Burgín, M. J.; Franze-Fernández, M. T. Tacaribe virus gene expression in cytopathic and non-cytopathic infections. *Virology* **1994**, *200*, 613–622.

39. Meyer, B. J.; de la Torre, J. C.; Southern, P. J. Arenaviruses: genomic RNAs, transcription and replication. *Curr. Top. Microbiol. Immunol.* **2002**, *262*, 139–157.

40. Peters, C. J. Human infections with arenaviruses in the Americas. *Curr. Top. Microbiol. Immunol.* **2002**, *262*, 65–74.

41. Manzione, R. de; Salas, R. A.; Paredes, H.; Godoy, O.; Rojas, L.; Araoz, F.; Fulhorst, C. F.; Ksiazek, T. G.; Mills, J. N.; Ellis, B. A.; Paters, C. J.; Tesh, R. B. Venezuelan hemorrhagic fever: clinical and epidemiological studies of 165 cases. *Clin. Infect. Dis.* **1998**, *26*, 308–313.

42. Barry, M.; Russi, M.; Armstrong, L.; Geller, D. L.; Tesh, R.; Dembry, L.; Gonzalez, J. P.; Khan, A.; Peters, C. J. Treatment of a laboratory-acquired Sabiá virus infection. *N. Engl. J. Med.* **1995**, *333*, 294–296.

43. McCormick, J. B.; Fisher-Hoch, S. P. Lassa fever. *Curr. Top. Microbiol. Immunol.* **2002**, *262*, 73–109.

44. Monath, T. P.; Mertens, P. E.; Patton, R.; Moser, C. R.; Baum, J. J.; Pinneo, L; Gary, G. W.; Kissling, R. E. A hospital epidemic of Lassa fever in Zorzor, Liberia, March–April 1972. *Am. J. Trop. Med. Hyg.* **1973**, *22*, 773–779.

45. Maiztegui, J. I. Clinical and epidemiological patterns of Argentine hemorrhagic fever. *Bull. WHO* **1975**, *52*, 567–575.

46. Enría, D. A.; Briggiler, A. M.; Fernández, N. J.; Levis, S. C.; Maiztegui, J. I. Importance of dose of neutralizing antibodies in treatment of Argentine hemorrhagic fever with immune plasma. *Lancet* **1984**, *8397 (ii)*, 255–256.

47. Maiztegui, J. I.; Fernández, N.; Damilano, A. J. Efficacy of immune plasma in treatment of Argentine hemorrhagic fever and association between treatment and a late neurological syndrome. *Lancet* **1979**, *8154 (ii)*, 1216–1217.

48. Enría, D. A.; Maiztegui, J. I. Antiviral treatment of Argentine hemorrhagic fever. *Antiviral Res.* **1994**, *23*, 23–31.

49. McCormick, J. B.; King, I. J.; Webb, P. A.; Scribner, C. L.; Craven, R. B.; Johnson, K. M.; Elliot, L. H.; Belmont-Williams, R. Lassa fever. Effective therapy with ribavirin. *N. Engl. J. Med.* **1986**, *314*, 20–26.

50. Streeter, D. G.; Witkowski, J. T.; Khare, G. P.; Sidwell, R. W.; Bauer, R. J.; Robins, R. K.; Simon, L. N. Mechanism of action of 1-β-D-ribofuranosyl-1,2,4-triazole-3-carboxamide (Virazole), a new broad-spectrum antiviral agent. *Proc. Natl. Acad. Sci. U.S.A.* **1973**, *70*, 1174–1178.

51. Gilbert, B. E.; Knight, V. (1986). Biochemistry and clinical application of ribavirin. *Antimicrob. Agents Chemother.* **1986**, *30*, 201–205.

52. Goswami, B. B.; Borek, E.; Sharma, O. K.; Fujitaki, J.; Smith, R. A. The broad spectrum antiviral agent ribavirin inhibits capping of mRNA. *Biochem. Biophys. Res. Commun.* **1979**, *89*, 830–836.

53. Crotty, S.; Maag, D.; Arnold, J. J.; Zhong, W.; Lau, J. Y. N.; Hong, Z.; Andino, R.; Cameron, C. E. The broad-spectrum antiviral ribonucleotide, ribavirin, is an RNA virus mutagen. *Nat. Med.* **2000**, *6*, 1375–1379.

54. Crotty, S.; Cameron, C. E.; Andino, R. RNA virus error catastrophe: direct molecular test by using ribavirin. *Proc. Natl. Acad. Sci. U.S.A.* **2001**, *98*, 6895–6900.

55. Ruiz-Jarabo, C. M.; Ly, C.; Domingo, E.; de la Torre, J. C. Lethal mutagenesis of the prototypic arenavirus lymphocytic choriomeningitis virus (LCMV). *Virology* **2003**, *308*, 37–47.

56. Tam, R. C.; Lau, J. Y. N.; Hong, Z. Mechanisms of action of ribavirin in antiviral therapies. *Antiviral Chem. Chemother.* **2002**, *12*, 261–272.

57. Wyde, P. R. Respiratory syncytial virus (RSV) disease and prospects for its control. *Antiviral Res.* **1998**, *39*, 63–79.

58. Walker, M. P.; Appleby, T. C.; Zhong, W.; Lau, J. Y. N.; Hong, Z. Hepatitis C virus therapies: current treatments, targets and future perspectives. *Antiviral Chem. Chemother.* **2003**, *14*, 1–21.

59. Jahrling P. B.; Hesse, R. A.; Eddy, G. A.; Johnson, K. M.; Callis, R. T.; Stephen, E. L. (1980). Lassa virus infection of rhesus monkeys: pathogenesis and treatment with ribavirin. *J. Infect. Dis.* **1980**, *141*, 580–589.

60. McKee, K. T.; Huggins, J. W.; Trahan, C. J.; Mahlandi, B. G. Ribavirin prophylaxis and therapy for experimental Argentine hemorrhagic fever. *Antimicrob. Agents Chemother.* **1988**, *32*, 1304–1309.

61. Kenyon, R. H.; Canonico, P. G.; Green, D. G.; Peters, C. J. Effect of ribavirin and tributylribavirin on Argentine hemorrhagic fever (Junin virus) in guinea pigs. *Antimicrob. Agents Chemother.* **1986**, *29*, 521–523.

62. Weissenbacher, M. C.; Avila, M. M.; Calello, M. A.; Merani, M. S.; McCormick, J. B.; Rodriguez, M. Effect of ribavirin and immune serum on Junin virus infected primates. *Med. Microbiol. Immunol.* **1986**, *175*, 183–186.

63. Enría, D. A.; Briggiler, A. M.; Levis, S.; Vallejos, D.; Maiztegui, J. I.; Canonico, P. G. Tolerance and antiviral effect of ribavirin in patients with Argentine hemorrhagic fever. *Antiviral Res.* **1987**, *7*, 353–359.

64. Huggins, J. W.; Robins, R. K.; Canonico, P. G. Synergistic antiviral effects of ribavirin and the C-nucleoside analogs tiazofurin and selenazofurin against togaviruses, bunyaviruses, and arenaviruses. *Antimicrob. Agents Chemother.* **1984**, *26*, 476–480.

65. Burns, N. J. III; Barnett, B. B.; Huffman, J. H.; Dawson, M. Y.; Sidwell, R. W.; De Clercq, E.; Kende, M. A newly developed immunofluorescent assay for determining the Pichinde virus-inhibitory effects of selected nucleoside analogues. *Antiviral Res.* **1988**, *10*, 89–98.

66. Smee, D. F.; Gilbert, J.; Leonhardt, J. A.; Barnett, B. B.; Huggins, J. H.; Sidwell, R. W. Treatment of lethal Pichinde virus infections in weanling LVG/Lak hamsters with ribavirin, ribamidine, selenazofurin, and ampligen. *Antiviral Res.* **1993**, *20*, 57–70.

67. Andrei, G.; De Clercq, E. Inhibitory effect of selected antiviral compounds on arenavirus replication in vitro. *Antiviral Res.* **1990**, *14*, 287–300.

68. Smee, D. F.; Morris, J. L. B.; Barnard, D. L.; Van Aerschot, A. Selective inhibition of arthropod-borne and arenaviruses by 3'-fluoro-3'-deoxyadenosine. *Antiviral Res.* **1992**, *18*, 151–162.

69. Guillerm, G.; Guillerm, D.; Vandenplas-Vitkowski, C.; Glapski, C.; De Clercq, E. Inactivation of *S*-adenosyl-L-homocysteine hydrolase with novel 5'-thioadenosine derivatives. Antiviral effects. *Bioorg. Med. Chem. Lett.* **2003**, *13*, 1649–1652.

70. Martins Alho, M. A.; Sguerra, V. L.; Talarico, L. B.; García, C. C.; Damonte, E. B.; D'Accorso, N. Unpublished results, 2004.

71. Uckun, F. M.; Petkevich, A. S.; Vassilev, A. O.; Tibbles, H. E.; Titov, L. Stampidine prevents mortality in an experimental mouse model of viral hemorrhagic fever caused by Lassa virus. *BMC Infect. Dis.* **2004**, *4*, 1–7.

72. Burns, J. W.; Buchmeier, M. J. Protein–protein interactions in lymphocytic choriomeningitis virus. *Virology* **1991**, *163*, 620–629.

73. Bruns, M.; Cihak, J.; Müller, G.; Lehmann-Grube, F. Lymphocytic choriomeningitis virus. VI. Isolation of a glycoprotein mediating neutralization. *Virology* **1983**, *130*, 247–251.

74. Parekh, B. S., Buchmeier, M. J. Proteins of lymphocytic choriomeningitis virus: antigenic topography of the viral glycoproteins. *Virology* **1986**, *153*, 168–178.

75. Borrow, P.; Oldstone, M. B. A. Characterization of lymphocytic choriomeningitis virus-binding protein (s): a candidate cellular receptor for the virus. *J. Virol.* **1992**, *66*, 7270–7281.

76. Scolaro, L. A.; Mersich, S. E.; Damonte, E. B. A mouse attenuated mutant of Junin virus with an altered envelope glycoprotein. *Arch. Virol.* **1990**, *111*, 257–262.

77. Cao, W.; Henry, M. D.; Borrow, P.; Yamada, H.; Elder, J. H.; Ravkov, E. V.; Nichol, S. T.; Compans, R. W.; Campbell, K. P.; Oldstone, M. B. A. Identification of α-dystroglycan as a receptor for lymphocytic choriomeningitis virus and Lassa fever virus. *Science* **1998**, *282*, 2079–2081.

78. Henry, M. D.; and Campbell, K. P. Dystroglycan inside and out. *Curr. Opin. Cell Biol.* **1999**, *11*, 602–607.

79. Spiropoulou, C. F.; Kunz, S.; Rollin, P. E.; Campbell, K. P.; Oldstone, M. B. A. New World arenaviruses clade C, but not clade A and B viruses, utilizes α-dystroglycan as its major receptor. *J. Virol.* **2002**, *76*, 5140–5146.

80. Raiger Iustman, L. J.; Candurra, N.; Mersich, S. E. Influencia del tratamiento enzimático sobre la interacción virus Junín-células Vero. *Rev. Arg. Microbiol.* **1995**, *27*, 28–32.

81. Schneider-Schaulies, J. Cellular receptors for viruses: links to tropism and pathogenesis. *J. Gen. Virol.* **2000**, *81*, 1413–1429.

82. Smelt, S. C.; Borrow, P.; Kunz, S.; Cao, W.; Tishon, A.; Lewicki, H.; Campbell, K. P.; Oldstone, M. B. A. Differences in affinity of binding of lymphocytic choriomeningitis virus strains to the cellular receptor α-dystroglycan correlate with viral tropism and disease kinetics. *J. Virol.* **2001**, *75*, 448–457.

83. Witvrouw, M.; Desmyter, J.; De Clercq, E. Antiviral portrait series: 4. Polysulfates as inhibitors of HIV and other enveloped viruses. *Antiviral Chem. Chemother.* **1994**, *5*, 345–359.

84. Glushakova, S. E.; Lukashevich, I. S. Early events in arenavirus replication are sensitive to lysosomotropic compounds. *Arch. Virol.* **1989**, *194*, 157–161.

85. Castilla, V.; Mersich, S. E.; Candurra, N. A.; Damonte, E. B. The entry of Junin virus into Vero cells. *Arch. Virol.* **1994**, *36*, 363–374.

86. Borrow, P.; Oldstone, M. B. A. Mechanism of lymphocytic choriomeningitis virus entry into cells. *Virology* **1994**, *198*, 1–9.

87. Castilla, V.; Palermo, L. M.; Coto, C. E. Involvement of vacuolar proton ATPase in Junin virus multiplication. *Arch. Virol.* **2001**, *146*, 251–263.

88. Di Simone, C.; Buchmeier, M. J. Kinetics and pH dependence of acid-induced structural changes in the lymphocytic choriomeningitis virus glycoprotein complex. *Virology* **1995**, *209*, 3–9.

89. Di Simone, C.; Zandonatti, M. A.; Buchmeier, M. J. Acidic pH triggers LCMV membrane fusion activity and conformational change in the glycoprotein spike. *Virology* **1994**, *198*, 455–465.

90. Castilla, V.; Mersich, S. E. Low-pH-induced fusion of Vero cells infected with Junin virus. *Arch. Virol.* **1996**, *141*, 1307–1317.

91. Glushakova, S. E.; Omelyanenko V. G.; Lukashevich, I. S.; Bogdanov, A. A.; Moshnikova, A. B.; Kozytch, A. T.; Torchilin, V. P. The fusion of artificial lipid membranes induced by the synthetic arenavirus fusion peptide. *Biochim. Biophys. Acta* **1992**, *1110*, 202–208.

92. Coto, C. E.; Calello, M. A.; Parodi, A. S. Efecto de la amantadina-HCl sobre la infectividad del virus Junín (FHA) in vitro e in vivo. *Rev. Argent. Microbiol.* **1969**, *1*, 3–8.

93. Pfau, C. J.; Trowbridge, R. S.; Welsh, R. M.; Staneck, L. D.; O'Connell, C. M. Arenaviruses: inhibition by amantadine hydrochloride. *J. Gen. Virol.* **1972**, *14*, 209–211.

94. Pfau, C. J. Arenavirus chemotherapy—retrospect and prospect. *Bull. WHO* **1975**, *52*, 737–744.

95. Candurra, N. A.; Maskin, L.; Damonte, E. B. Inhibition of arenavirus multiplication in vitro by phenotiazines. *Antiviral Res.* **1996**, *31*, 149–158.

96. Candurra, N. A.; Damonte, E. B. Acción inhibitoria de la cafeína sobre la multiplicación del virus Junín. *Rev. Argent. Microbiol.* **1999**, *31*, 135–141.

97. Wang, L. H.; Rothberg, K. G.; Anderson, R. G. Mis-assembly of clathrin lattices on endosomes reveals a regulatory switch for coated pit formation. *J. Cell Biol.* **1993**, *123*, 1107–1117.

98. Candurra, N. A.; Lago, M. J.; Maskin, L.; Damonte, E. B. Involvement of the cytoskeleton in Junin virus multiplication. *J. Gen. Virol.* **1999**, *80*, 147–156.

99. Andrei, G.; Couto, A. S.; de Lederkremer, R. M.; Coto, C. E. Purification and partial characterization of an antiviral active peptide from *Melia azedarach* L. *Antiviral Chem. Chemother.* **1994**, *5*, 105–110.

100. Castilla, V.; Barquero, A. A.; Mersich, S. E.; Coto, C. E. In vitro anti-Junin virus activity of a peptide isolated from *Melia azedarach* L. leaves. *Int. J. Antimicrob. Agents* **1998**, *10*, 67–75.

101. Andrei, G. M.; Lampuri, J. S.; Coto, C. E.; de Torres, R. A. An antiviral factor from *Melia azedarach* L. prevents Tacaribe virus encephalitis in mice. *Experientia* **1986**, *42*, 843–845.

102. Murphy, F. A.; Webb, P. A.; Johnson, K. M.; Whitfield, S. G.; Chappell, W. A. Arenaviruses in Vero cells: ultrastructural studies. *J. Virol.* **1970**, *6*, 507–518.

103. Lenz, O.; ter Meulen, J.; Feldmann, H.; Klenk, H.-D.; Garten, W. Identification of a novel consensus sequence at the cleavage site of the Lassa virus glycoprotein. *J. Virol.* **2000**, *74*, 11418–11421.

104. Lenz, O.; ter Meulen, J.; Klenk, H. D.; Seidah, N. G.; Garten, W. The Lassa virus glycoprotein precursor GPC is proteolytically processed by subtilase SKI-1/S1P. *Proc. Natl. Acad. Sci. U.S.A.* **2001**, *98*, 12701–12705.

105. Beyer, W. R.; Popplau, D.; Garten, W.; von Laer, D.; Lenz, O. Endoproteolytic processing of the lymphocytic choriomeningitis virus glycoprotein by the subtilase SKI-1/S1P. *J. Virol.* **2003**, *77*, 2866–2872.

106. Wright, K. E.; Spiro, R. C.; Burns, W.; Buchmeier, M. J. Post-translational processing of the glycoproteins of lymphocytic choriomeningitis virus. *Virology* **1990**, *177*, 175–183.

107. Candurra, N. A.; Damonte, E. B. Effect of inhibitors of the intracellular exocytic pathway on glycoprotein processing and maturation of Junin virus. *Arch. Virol.* **1997**, *142*, 2179–2193.

108. Damonte, E. B.; Mersich, S. E.; Candurra, N. A. Intracellular processing and transport of Junin virus glycoproteins influences virion infectivity. *Virus Res.* **1994**, *34*, 317–326.

109. Kunz, S.; Edelmann, K. H.; de la Torre, J. C.; Gorney, R.; Oldstone, M. B. A. Mechanisms for lymphocytic choriomeningitis virus glycoprotein cleavage, transport, and incorporation into virions. *Virology* **2003**, *314*, 168–178.

110. Silber, A. M.; Candurra, N. A.; Damonte, E. B. The effects of oligosaccharide trimming inhibitors on glycoprotein expression and infectivity of Junin virus. *FEMS Microbiol. Lett.* **1993**, *109*, 39–44.

111. Romanowski, V. Genetic organization of Junin virus, the etiological agent of Argentine hemorrhagic fever. In *The Arenaviridae*, Salvato, M. S. (ed.). Plenum Press, New York, 1993, pp. 51–84.

112. Cordo, S. M.; Candurra, N. A.; Damonte, E. B. Myristic acid analogs are inhibitors of Junin virus replication. *Microbes Infect.* **1999**, *1*, 609–614.

113. Bartolotta, S.; García, C. C.; Candurra, N. A.; Damonte, E. B. Effect of fatty acids on arenavirus replication: inhibition of virus production by lauric acid. *Arch. Virol.* **2001**, *146*, 777–790.

114. Salvato, M. S.; Shimomaye, E. M. The completed sequence of lymphocytic choriomeningitis virus reveals a unique RNA structure and a gene for a zinc finger protein. *Virology* **1989**, *173*, 1–10.

115. Iapalucci, S.; López, N.; Rey, O.; Zakin, M. M.; Cohen, G. N.; Franze-Fernandez, M. T. The 5' region of Tacaribe virus L RNA encodes a protein with a potential metal binding domain. *Virology* **1989**, *173*, 357–361.

116. Djavani, M.; Lukashevich, I. S.; Sanchez, A.; Nichol, S. T.; Salvato, M. S. Completion of the Lassa fever virus sequence and identification of a RING finger open reading frame at the L RNA 5' end. *Virology* **1997**, *235*, 414–418.

117. Gibadulinova, A.; Zelnik, V.; Reiserova, L.; Zavodska, E.; Zatovicova, M.; Ciampor, F.; Pastorekova, S.; Pastorek, J. Sequence and characterisation of the Z gene encoding ring finger protein of the lymphocytic choriomeningitis virus MX strain. *Acta Virol.* **1998**, *42*, 369–374.

118. Salvato, M. S.; Schweighofer, K. J.; Burns, J.; Shimomaye, E. M. Biochemical and immunological evidence that the 11-kDa zinc-binding protein of lymphocytic choriomeningitis virus is a structural component of the virus. *Virus Res.* **1992**, *22*, 185–198.

119. Garcin, D.; Rochat, S.; Kolakofsky, D. The Tacaribe arenavirus small zinc finger protein is required for both mRNA synthesis and genome replication. *J. Virol.* **1993**, *67*, 807–812.

120. Lee, K. J.; Novella, I. S.; Teng, M. N.; Oldstone, M. B. A.; de la Torre, J. C. NP and L proteins of lymphocytic choriomeningitis virus (LCMV) are sufficient for efficient transcription and replication of LCMV genomic RNA analogs. *J. Virol.* **2000**, *74*, 3470–3477.

121. Cornu, T. I.; de la Torre, J. C. RING finger Z protein of lymphocytic choriomeningitis virus (LCMV) inhibits transcription and RNA replication of an LCMV S-segment minigenome. *J. Virol.* **2001**, *75*, 9415–9426.

122. López, N.; Jácamo, R.; Franze-Fernández, M. T. Transcription and RNA replication of Tacaribe virus genome and antigenome analogs require N and L proteins: Z protein is an inhibitor of these processes. *J. Virol.* **2001**, *75*, 12241–12251.

123. Borden, K. L.; Campbell-Dwyer, E. J.; Salvato, M. S. The promyelocytic leukemia protein PML has a pro-apoptotic activity mediated through its RING domain. *FEBS Lett.* **1997**, *418*, 30–34.

124. Borden, K. L.; Campbell-Dwyer, E. J.; Salvato, M. S. An arenavirus RING (zinc-binding) protein binds the oncoprotein promyelocyte leukemia protein (PML) and relocates PML nuclear bodies to the cytoplasm. *J. Virol.* **1998**, *72*, 758–766.

125. Borden, K. L. B.; Campbell-Dwyer, E. J.; Carlile, G. W.; Djavani, M.; Salvato, M. S. Two RING finger proteins, the oncoprotein PML and the arenavirus Z protein, colocalize with the nuclear fraction of the ribosomal P proteins. *J. Virol.* **1998**, *72*, 3819–3826.

126. Campbell-Dwyer, E. J.; Lai, H.; MacDonald, R. C.; Salvato, M. S.; Borden, K. L. B. The lymphocytic choriomeningitis virus RING protein Z associates with eukaryotic initiation factor 4E and selectively represses translation in a RING-dependent manner. *J. Virol.* **2000**, *74*, 3293–3300.

127. Salvato, M. S. Molecular biology of the prototype arenavirus, lymphocytic choriomeningitis virus. In *The Arenaviridae*, Salvato, M. S. (ed.). Plenum Press, New York, 1993, pp. 133–156.

128. Garoff, H.; Hewson, R.; Opstelten, D. J. Virus maturation by budding. *Microbiol. Mol. Biol. Rev.* **1998**, *62*, 1171–1190.

129. Strecker, T.; Eichler, R.; ter Meulen, J.; Weissenhorn, W.; Klenk, H. D.; Garten, W.; Lenz, O. Lassa virus Z protein is a matrix protein and sufficient for the release of virus-like particles. *J. Virol.* **2003**, *77*, 10700–10705.

130. Perez, M; Craven, R. C.; de la Torre, J. C. The small RING finger protein Z drives arenavirus budding: implications for antiviral strategies. *Proc. Natl. Acad. Sci. U.S.A.* **2003**, *100*, 12978–12983.

131. Eichler, R.; Strecker, T.; Kolesnikova, L.; ter Meulen, J.; Weissenhorn, W.; Becker, S.; Klenk, H. D.; Garten, W.; Lenz, O. Characterization of the Lassa virus matrix protein: electron microscopic study of virus-like particles and interaction with the nucleoprotein (NP). *Virus Res.* **2004**, *100*, 249–255.

132. Freed, E. O. Viral late domains. *J. Virol.* **2002**, *76*, 4679–4687.

133. Cornu, T. I.; de la Torre, J. C. Characterization of the arenavirus RING finger protein regions required for Z-mediated inhibition of viral RNA synthesis. *J. Virol.* **2002**, *76*, 6678–6688.

134. García, C. C.; Candurra, N. A.; Damonte, E. B. Antiviral and virucidal activities against arenaviruses of zinc-finger active compounds. *Antiviral Chem. Chemother.* **2000**, *11*, 231–238.

135. Rice, W. G.; Turpin, J. A.; Schaeffer, C. A.; Graham, L.; Clanton, D.; Buckheit, R. W. Jr.; Zaharevitz, D.; Summers, M. F.; Wallquist, A.; Covell, D. G. Evaluation of selected chemotypes in coupled cellular and molecular target-based screens identifies novel HIV-1 zinc finger inhibitors. *J. Med. Chem.* **1996**, *39*, 3603–3616.

136. Rice, W. G.; Turpin, J. A.; Huang, M.; Clanton, D.; Buckheit, R. W. Jr.; Covell, D. G.; Wallquist, A.; McDonnell, N. B.; de Guzman, R. N.; Summers, M. F.; Zalkow, L.; Bader, J. P.; Haugwitz, R.; Sausville, E. A. Azodicarbonamide inhibits HIV-1 replication by targeting the nucleocapsid protein. *Nat. Med.* **1997**, *3*, 341–345.

137. Tummino, P. J.; Harvey, P. J.; McQuade, T.; Domagala, J.; Gogliotti, R.; Sanchez, J.; Song, Y.; Hupe, D. The human immunodeficiency virus type 1 (HIV-1) nucleocapsid protein zinc ejection activity of disulfide benzamides and benzisothiazolones: correlation with anti-HIV and virucidal activities. *Antimicrob. Agents Chemother.* **1997**, *41*, 394–400.

138. García, C. C.; Candurra, N. A.; Damonte, E. B. Mode of inactivation of arenaviruses by disulfide-based compounds. *Antiviral Res.* **2002**, *55*, 437–446.

139. García, C. C.; Candurra, N. A.; Damonte, E. B. Differential inhibitory action of two azoic compounds against arenaviruses. *Int. J. Antimicrob. Agents* **2003**, *21*, 319–324.

140. García, C. C.; Candurra, N. A.; Damonte, E. B. Arenavirus inactivation with conservation of virus surface glycoprotein and blockade in viral transcription. *Antiviral Res.* **2003**, *57*, A91.

141. García, C. C. Unpublished results, **2004**.

142. Wachsman, M. B.; López, E. M. F.; Ramírez, J. A.; Galagovsky, L. R.; Coto, C. E. Antiviral effect of brassinosteroids against herpes virus and arenaviruses. *Antiviral Chem. Chemother.* **2000**, *11*, 71–77.

143. Comin, M. J.; Maier, M. S.; Roccatagliata, A. J.; Pujol, C. A.; Damonte, E. B. Evaluation of the antiviral activity of natural sulfated polyhydroxysteroids and their synthetic derivatives and analogs. *Steroids* **1999**, *64*, 335–340.

144. García, C. C.; Rosso, M. L.; Bertoni, M. D.; Maier, M. S.; Damonte, E. B. Evaluation of the antiviral activity against Junin virus of macrocyclic trichothecenes produced by the hypocrealean epibiont of *Baccharis coridifolia*. *Planta Med.* **2002**, *68*, 209–212.

145. García, C. C.; Brousse, B. N.; Carlucci, M. J.; Moglioni, A. G.; Martins Alho, M.; Moltrassio, G. Y.; D'Accorso, N. B.; Damonte, E. B. Inhibitory effect of thiosemicar-bazone derivatives on Junin virus replication in vitro. *Antiviral Chem. Chemother.* **2003**, *14*, 99–105.

146. Albiol Matanic, V.; Castilla, V. Antiviral activity of antimicrobial cationic peptides against Junin virus and herpes simplex virus. *Int. J. Antimicrob. Agents* **2004**, *23*, 382–389.

147. Maiztegui, J. I.; McKee, K. T.; Barrera Oro, J. G.; Harrison, L. H.; Gibbs, P. H.; Feuillade, M. R.; Enria, D. A.; Briggiler, A. M.; Levis, S. C.; Ambrosio, A. M.; Halsey, N. A.; Peters, C. J.; AHF Study Group. Protective efficacy of a live attenuated vaccine against Argentine hemorrhagic fever. *J. Infect. Dis.* **1998**, *177*, 277–283.

S-Adenosylhomocysteine Hydrolase Inhibitors as a Source of Anti-Filovirus Agents

STEWART W. SCHNELLER and MINMIN YANG

Department of Chemistry and Biochemistry, Auburn University

6.1 INTRODUCTION

There is evidence that, upon infection, the filoviruses inhibit the natural production of interferon in the host cells. This effect can be reversed by the carbocyclic nucleoside 3-deazaneplanocin A and, possibly, 3-deazaaristeromycin, which are inhibitors of S-adenosylhomocysteine hydrolase. This effect is further manifested in blocking viral mRNA processing. This chapter outlines the infectious properties of the filoviruses Ebola and Marburg; the current status of therapeutic (vaccine and drug) development; the role that interferon immunotherapy can play in therapy design; the biochemical stages associated with inhibiting viral mRNA and its relationship to anti-filoviral agents; and the status of current efforts to avail significant amounts of 3-deazaneplanocin A and 3-deazaaristerocmycin for further therapeutic investigations.

6.2 FILOVIRUSES

The small lipid enveloped zoonotic RNA viruses that are responsible for viral hemorrhagic fevers (VHFs) exist in four taxonomic families: the Filoviridae (Ebola and Marburg), Arenaviridae (Junin, Lassa, Tacaribe, Machupo, Guanarito), Bunyaviridae (Hantavirus, Rift Valley fever, Crimean-Congo HF), and Flaviviridae (yellow fever, dengue).[1,2] The VHF designation is the result of the damage that occurs to the vascular system following infection.[2] This often is accompanied by

Antiviral Drug Discovery for Emerging Diseases and Bioterrorism Threats. Edited by Paul F. Torrence
Copyright © 2005 John Wiley & Sons, Inc.

hemorrhaging, which in some instances is severe and life-threatening.[2] Many of the VHFs have been identified as possible bioweapons against civilians because of (1) high morbidity and mortality, (2) person-to-person transmission, (3) low dose/high infectivity with delivery by aerosol, (4) unavailability of treatment methods, (5) pathogen availability, (6) stressful circumstances the infection would cause for health care workers, (7) capability of large-scale production, (8) environmental stability, and (9) previous research on the pathogens.[1]

In the latter regard, there are reports that the hemorrhagic fevers have been weaponized,[1,3,4] and that until 1992, the Soviet Union/Russia produced large quantities of Marburg (filo), Ebola (filo), Lassa (arena), Junin (arena), and Machupo (flavi) viruses.[1] Successful infection of nonhuman primates with aerosolized Ebola,[5] Marburg,[6] Lassa,[7] and New World arenaviruses[8] has also been documented.[1] There is also reason to believe that the filoviruses were subjected to biotechnology modifications either to enhance their pathogenicity and/or to produce agents with characteristics not typical of the virus,[3] which mousepox experiments appeared to have validated.[9] The possibility that some of the scientists who worked on these projects (as well as with smallpox) may now be in countries capable of bioterrorism activities adds to the concerns.

Interestingly, prior to 1969, yellow fever and Rift Valley fever were being developed in the U.S. offensive biological weapons program.[1,10]

Of the hemorrhagic fevers, the filoviruses Ebola (EBO) and Marburg (MBG) cause the most severe effects in humans with fever and death appearing within a few days.[11] There is a single species of Marburg. Marburg was the first filovirus discovered (1967); this occurred at a vaccinia production facility in Marburg, Germany, where workers came in contact with monkey carriers imported from Uganda. Marburg virus, however, remains confined to Africa.

Ebola virus was encountered (1976) at a missionary hospital in Zaire (now the Democratic Republic of the Congo), where it reached epidemic proportions. The filovirus genus contains four subtypes of Ebola: (1) Zaire, (2) Sudan, and (3) Ivory Coast, which infect human, and (4) Reston, which causes disease only in nonhuman primates. Ebola-Zaire (EBO-Z) causes the most virulent VHF in humans.[1]

While the natural reservoir for the filoviruses remains unknown,[12] their potency requires that they be handled in a BSL-4 containment facility.

There are, presently, no vaccines or therapeutic candidates available for combating Ebola and Marburg viruses but they are urgently needed.[13–18]

6.3 THERAPEUTIC AGENTS FOR FILOVIRUSES

Despite recent animal model advances in vaccine development to protect against the effects of filovirus infection, a number of issues must be resolved before vaccines qualify for human use. This places the need for therapeutics as a priority. Efforts in this regard have been limited,[14] until recently, because of insufficient biochemical information on filoviral replication at the molecular level. By analyzing the similarities in filoviral replication with the more thoroughly studied

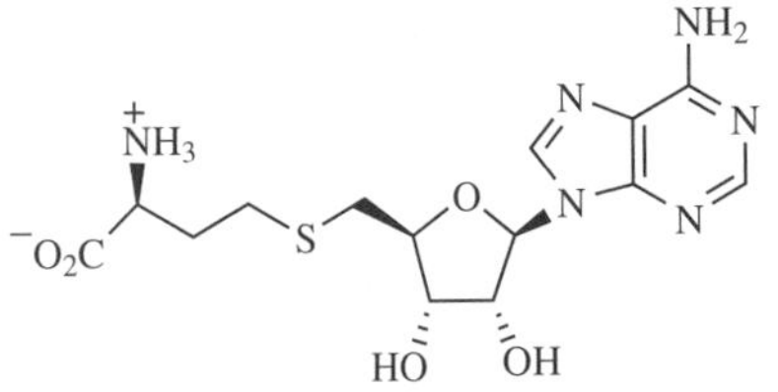

FIGURE 6.1   *S*-Adenosylhomocysteine and *S*-adenosylmethionine.

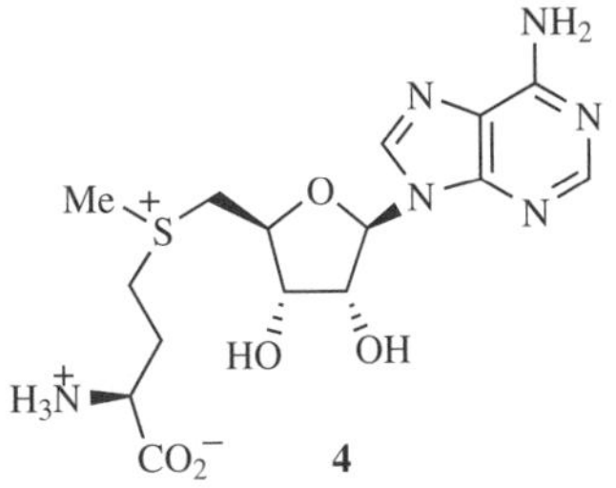

rhabdo- and paramyxoviruses,[19] it was concluded that inhibitors of *S*-adenosyl-L-homocysteine (**1**, AdoHcy, Figure 6.1) hydrolase would have an inhibitory effect on the filoviruses,[20] and that EBO and MBG share common drug targets,[14,21] suggesting an agent effective against one will have cross-efficaciousness against the other.

In 2000 Bray, Driscoll, and Huggins reported[20] that 3-deazaaristeromycin (**2**, Figure 6.2) and 3-deazaneplanocin A (c³-NpcA, **3**), well-known AdoHcy hydrolase inhibitors, showed significant activity (high therapeutic index) toward Ebola. In mice, **3** was found to have considerable activity. These results would predict that **3** was acting by inhibiting AdoHcy hydrolase that was, in turn, manifested in decreased viral mRNA methyl capping. A recent paper[22] does not refute this but provides further insight into what could be the consequence of incomplete mRNA processing.[23] In that regard, **3** is described as causing reversal of the EBO-induced suppression of the innate antiviral interferon (IFN-α)[23,24] production in infected mice. This is a very noteworthy observation in developing an immunotherapeutic approach to anti-filovirus agents. This possibility gains support from Bray and his colleagues,[20] who stated "unlike other IFN inducers (e.g., poly ICLC), which stimulate IFN-α production in both infected and uninfected cells, **3** induces massive IFN-α production only in virus-infected cells." This suggests further studies to overcome undesirable side effects of **3** (e.g., short serum and tissue half-lives[25]) should be undertaken to provide improved therapeutic candidates based on AdoHcy hydrolase inhibitors (such as **3**). This will, in turn, broaden the base of

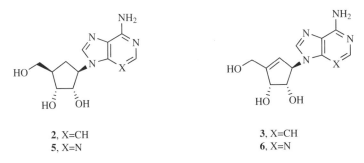

2, X=CH
5, X=N

3, X=CH
6, X=N

FIGURE 6.2   Various carbocyclic nucleosides.

understanding the relationship between AdoHcy hydrolase inhibition and IFN-α production suppression upon viral infection, which may not be limited to filo-viruses, and the role of AdoHcy hydrolase inhibitors in future drug design. This provides the foundation for the research in our laboratories at Auburn. However, before presenting the current status of that effort, some mention of the relationship between messenger RNA (mRNA) and the S-adenosylmethionine (**4**)/AdoHcy (**1**) ratio and the role that can play in antiviral drug design is in order.

6.4   VIRAL mRNA METHYLATION

In recent years, nucleoside derivatives have been one of the major areas of pursuit in seeking new antiviral agents.[26] Out of this, several adenosine analogues have been described. A common characteristic of these compounds is that they are potent product inhibitors of S-adenosyl-L-homocysteine (AdoHcy) hydrolase. AdoHcy catalyzes the reversible hydrolysis of AdoHcy to adenosine (Ado) and homocys-teine.[27] Inhibition of AdoHcy hydrolase results in accumulation of AdoHcy, which is both the product and a feedback inhibitor of essential S-adenosylmethionine (AdoMet)-dependent methylation reactions (Figure 6.3). Such methylation reac-tions are required for final processing of the 5′-capped structure of mRNA (as m⁷Gppp⁶AᵐpApᵐ...) from cellular and viral sources.[28–30] Therefore, inhibitors of AdoHcy hydrolase may be expected to inhibit maturation of viral mRNAs and, in turn, the production of the requisite proteins and enzymes for generation of progeny virus particles.[29] In fact, it has been shown that the vaccinia virus-specific AdoMet-dependant enzymes,[31] which catalyze these reactions for processing its mRNAs (i.e., guanine-7-methyltransferase, 2′-O-nucleoside methyltransferase)[32,33] are sus-ceptible to inhibition by AdoHcy.[34] It is not surprising, therefore, that potential

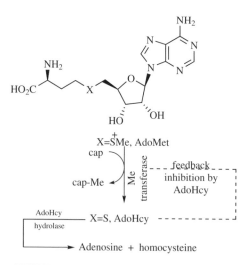

FIGURE 6.3   AdoMet/AdoHcy metabolism.

inhibitors of AdoHcy hydrolase elicit inhibitory activity toward vaccinia virus,[19,35] smallpox,[36] and Ebola.[20]

Since AdoHcy hydrolase is a cellular enzyme, it might be expected that the design of AdoHcy hydrolase inhibitors would lead to general suppression of protein synthesis and subsequent host toxicity. In considering how inhibition of AdoHcy hydrolase could succeed in the treatment of filovirus infections without intolerable associated toxicity, two possibilities exist. First, viral infection is likely to lead to increased demand for protein synthesis in virally infected cells relative to uninfected cells. This, in turn, would place a greater demand for methylation of viral mRNA in the infected cells, which would make the methyltransferase reactions more vulnerable to perturbation by increased AdoHcy levels. Borchardt and colleagues[35] have provided support for this possibility by reporting that infection of murine L-929 cells with vaccinia virus causes a large increase in the AdoHcy hydrolase activity.

Second, qualitative differences between the virally encoded methyltransferases (as is the case for orthopox virus) and those of the uninfected cells can be expected to present different binding domains for the feedback inhibitor AdoHcy and, in turn, different binding constants that could favor preferential inhibition of the viral transferases by AdoHcy over the uninfected cell. In fact, Borchardt has concluded "that there exists differences in the AdoHcy-binding sites on AdoMet-dependent methyltransferases" and he has reported differential inhibition of the transferases.[37]

Undoubtedly, prolonged inhibition of AdoHcy hydrolase will overtake general cellular protein synthesis, leading to severe toxicity. Wolfe and Borchardt have noted, however, that "a temporary and partial inhibition, while not seriously altering cell function, may allow phosphatases and ribonucleases to destroy the foreign mRNAs. After removal of the AdoHcy hydrolase inhibitor, cellular mRNA cap methylation could resume and full protein synthesis would ensue."[29]

Among the most promising antiviral agents based on inhibition of AdoHcy hydrolase are carbocyclic nucleosides,[19,38] which are nucleosides wherein the ribofuranose moiety is replaced by a cyclopentane ring [e.g., **5**, aristeromycin, which is carbocyclic adenosine, and neplanocin (**6**) (Figure 6.2).[38,39] This structural alteration renders the analogues resistant to phosphorylases, which cleave the glycosidic bond of standard nucleosides, and, consequently, improves their stability as potential medicinal agents.[39] Also, conformational changes and stereoelectronic perturbations that occur with replacing the ribofuranose unit with a cyclopentyl ring bring about the unique biological properties of carbocyclic nucleosides.[39] In addition to their antiviral properties, carbocyclic nucleosides can serve as substrates for standard nucleoside processing enzymes (e.g., kinases),[38,39] as anti-tumor,[38] anti-leishmanial,[40a] and anti-trypanosomal[40b] candidates and as probes to enlighten biochemical processes.[41]

6.5   3-DEAZAARISTEROMYCIN AND 3-DEAZANEPLANOCIN A

The unique properties of **3** in its apparent role in counteracting the attenuating effects that Ebola virus has on IFN levels in its host cells offers a unique

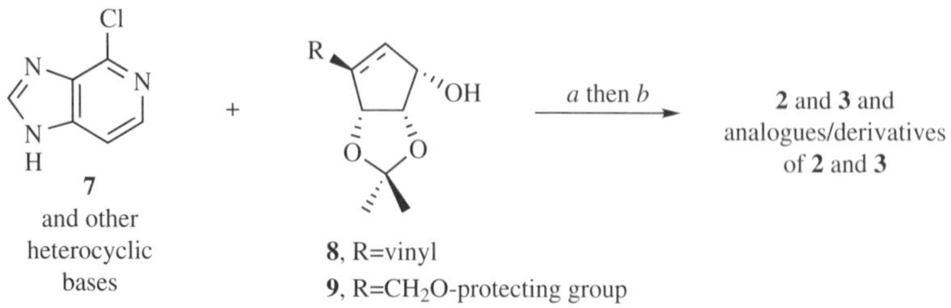

SCHEME 6.1 Synthetic plan. Reaction conditions: *a*, Mitsunobu coupling; *b*, a series of steps.

immunotherapeutic approach to drug design not heretofore reported with AdoHcy hydrolase inhibitors. We have set out to exploit this structural entity (**3** and, since it is also Ebola active, **2**) for the development of anti-filovirus drugs. To begin this study we found it necessary to overcome existing synthetic routes to **2** and **3**, which are expensive, low yielding and lacking in stereospecificity, and not easily adaptable for accessing derivatives and analogues.

Our synthetic approach was based on a Mitsunobu coupling of a heterocyclic base with an appropriately functionalized cyclopentanol as in Scheme 6.1.

To begin, 6-chloro-3-deazapurine (**7**) was the obvious heterocyclic base to use (Scheme 6.1). To date, literature procedures to **7** are few in number, low yielding, and not amenable to safe scale-up. By combining the most efficient and practical steps in existing heterocyclic chemistry literature and existing procedures to **7**, we have developed the convenient pathway to **7** as shown in Scheme 6.2.

Using a convergent synthetic approach,[42] we recently completed a convenient preparation of **2** from readily available **8**[43] (Scheme 6.3). In that direction, Mitsunobu reaction of **8** with **7** gave the coupled product **10** (Scheme 6.3). Transformation of the ethylene of **10** to the requisite hydroxymethyl group was accomplished in a two-step sequence: (1) oxidative cleavage of the double bond with osmium tetroxide/sodium periodate followed by (2) sodium borohydride

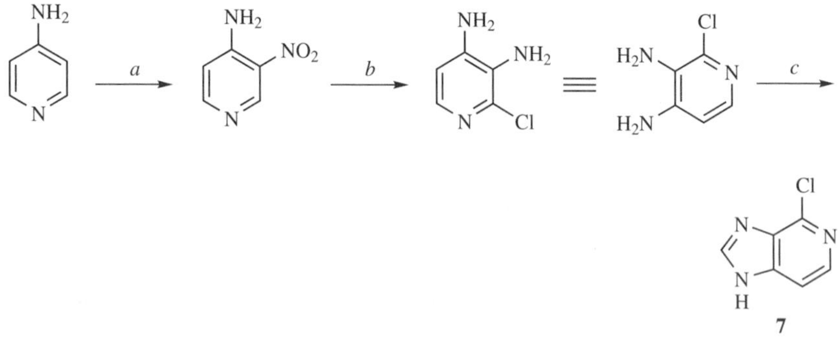

SCHEME 6.2 Synthesis of 6-chloro-3-deazapurine. Reaction conditions: *a*, HNO$_3$/H$_2$SO$_4$, 61%; *b*, SnCl$_2$•2H$_2$O, HCl, 89%; *c*, (EtO)$_3$CH, HCO$_2$H, 88%.

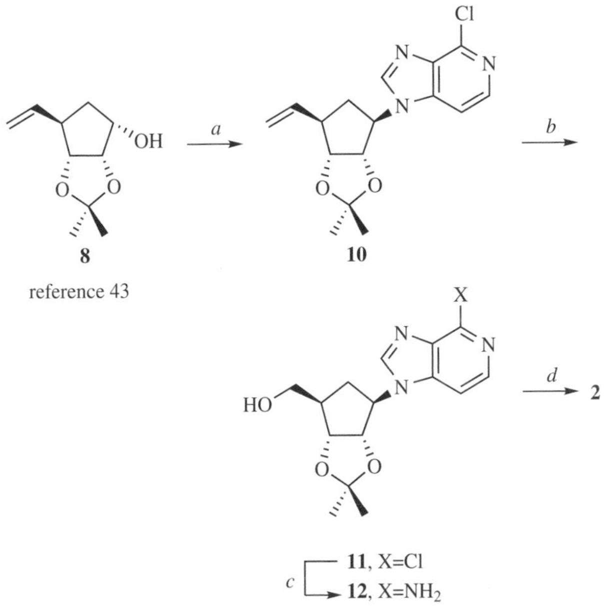

SCHEME 6.3 Synthesis of 3-deazaaristeromycin. Reaction conditions: *a*, 6-chloro-3-deazapurine (**7**), DIAD, Ph$_3$P, THF, 70%; *b*, (i) NaIO$_4$, OsO$_4$, MeOH/H$_2$O; (ii) NaBH$_4$, MeOH, 81%, 2 steps from **10**; *c*, (i) N$_2$H$_4$, MeOH; (ii) Raney Ni, 75%, 2 steps from **11**; *d*, HCl/MeOH, 95%.

reduction to provide **11**. Conversion of **11** into **12** was carried out by, first, reaction with hydrazine to displace the heterocyclic chloro substituent followed by Raney nickel reduction. Deprotection of **12** availed large quantities of **2**. Replacing **7** with other heterocyclic bases in reaction with **8** permits[44] entry into a large number of analogues of 3-deazaaristeromycin for Ebola virus investigations.

The success in obtaining **2** suggested a similar approach to **3** (i.e., Scheme 6.1 and reaction between **7** and **9**). Thus, a retrosynthetic analysis (Scheme 6.4) to **9** was designed. The novel synthesis of **9** from **13** recently reported by Lee, Cass, and Jacobson[45] was considered too lengthy for our intention to develop a convenient process to **3** for anti-filovirus studies. However, the procedure did call forth the ring closure metathesis (RCM) reaction,[47] which we later incorporated into our plan.

The oxidative rearrangement of tertiary alcohols **14** and **15** was another possible route to **9**. Johnson and co-workers reported[48] that, under oxidative rearrangement conditions, **14** failed to give the desired product. This led us to conclude that this failure was due to the concave structure of **14**, which prevented approach of the pyridinium chlorochromate (PCC) oxidizing agent to the hydroxyl on the α-face of **14**. On the other hand, we reasoned that approach of the PCC to a β-hydroxyl (as in **15**) was unlikely to encounter a similar steric effect. Thus, the plan was to proceed via the *tertiary* allylic alcohol **15** by employing a RCM reaction on the bisalkene **16**. Compound **16** was envisioned as accessible from **17**, which, in turn, was desired

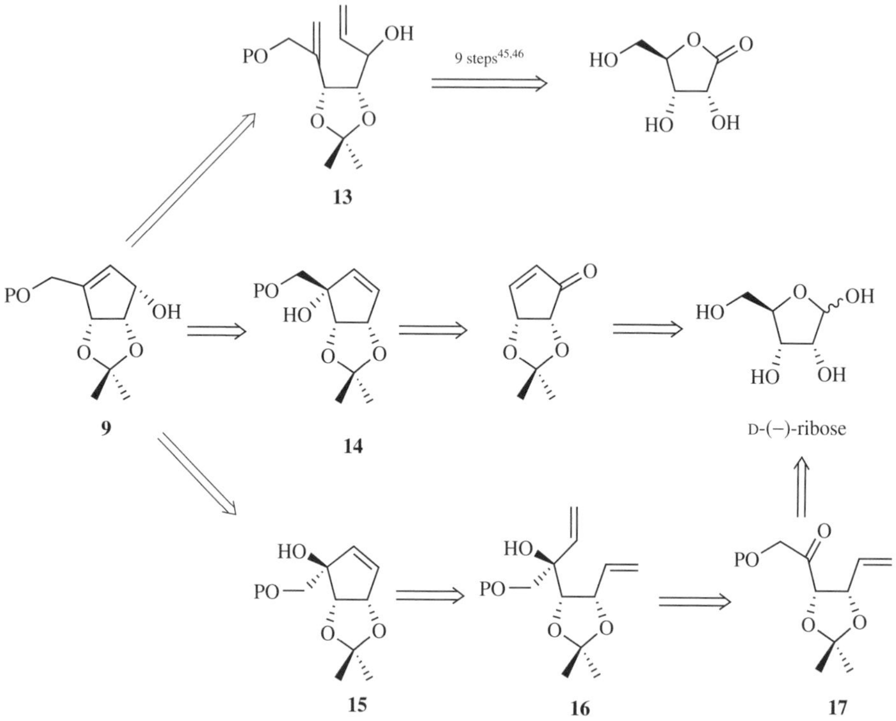

SCHEME 6.4   Retrosynthetic considerations to 3-deazaneplanocin A precursor.

(for synthetic versatility) to be obtainable from ribose. The stereochemistry of the *tertiary* carbon in **16** was predicted by the chelation transition state of the addition of vinylmagnesium bromide to **17** (Figure 6.4).

The actual synthesis was then commenced considering the TBS protecting group (for **9**) (Scheme 6.5). Subjecting **18** to a Wittig reaction with methyl triphenylphosphonium bromide afforded the desired product **19** along with its isomer **20** arising from silyl migration. These two isomers could not be separated cleanly by column

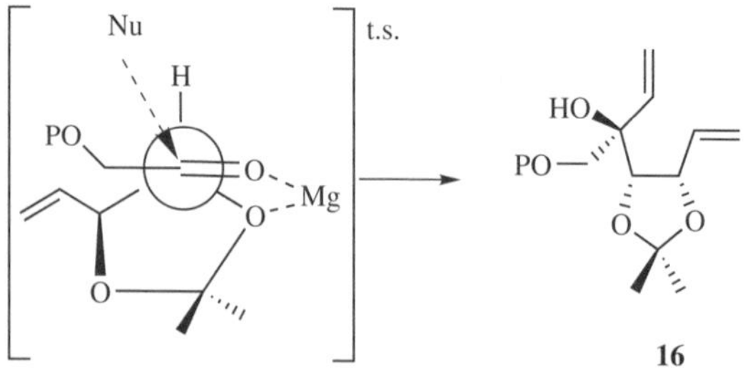

FIGURE 6.4   Transition state in nucleophilic addition.

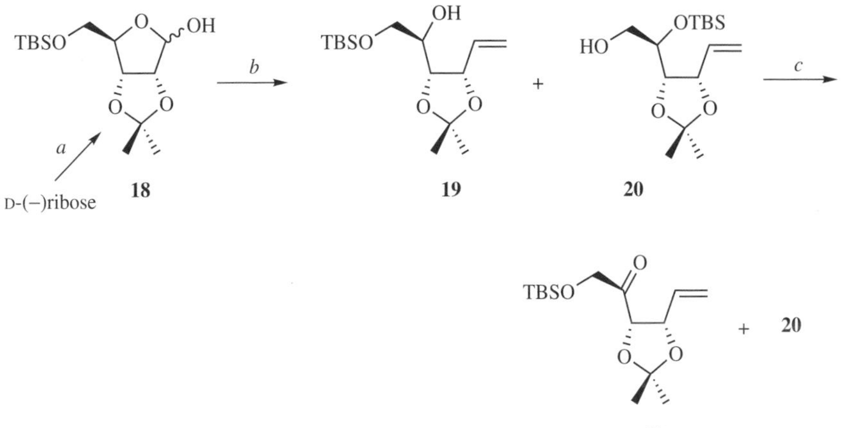

SCHEME 6.5   Preliminary evaluation of using a protected ribose precursor. Reaction conditions: *a*, (i) acetone, H_2SO_4; (ii) TBSCl, imidazole, CH_2Cl_2, 80%; *b*, Ph_3PCH_3Br, *t*-BuOK, THF, 81%, **19**:**20** = 3:1 by NMR; *c*, Dess–Martin periodinane, 91% from **19**.

chromatography. Consequently, a follow-up oxidation of this mixture with Dess–Martin periodinane (DMP) afforded the desired product ketone **21** and, surprisingly, **20** with its hydroxyl unaffected. To the best of our knowledge, this is the first example of selective oxidation of a secondary alcohol over a primary alcohol with DMP.

Due to the silyl migration of this route (Scheme 6.5), a different protecting group was sought. Reaction of **22a** with trityl chloride (to **22b**) followed by a Wittig reaction afforded high overall yield of **23** from D-ribose (Scheme 6.6). Dess–Martin periodinane oxidation of **23** cleanly furnished the desired product **24** (compare to **17** in Scheme 6.4). Grignard reaction of **24** with vinyl magnesium bromide afforded the diene **25** (compare to **16**, Scheme 6.4) in high selectivity. With **25** in hand, it was subjected to RCM reaction conditions with 1 mol% of Grubbs' first generation catalyst. This reaction produced the desired **26** (compare to **15**, Scheme 6.4). The stereochemistry of C-4$'$ in **26** was determined by a NOESY spectral analysis.

With **26** available, the oxidative rearrangement of its *tertiary* allylic alcohol was investigated. In this direction, with PCC as the oxidizing agent, enone **27** was rapidly formed but in low yield. Since PCC was known to cleave trityl groups, pyridinium dichromate (PDC), a less acidic oxidizing agent, was investigated. This reaction was found to be successful to **27** if conducted under refluxing conditions. Luche reduction of **27** afforded **28** (compare to **9**). This stereoselective reduction gave the allylic alcohol possessing the α-hydroxyl configuration because of the concave structure **27**, preventing hydride attack from the bottom face.

Conversion of **28** into **29** was carried out under Mitsunobu conditions. Compound **29** was easily transformed into **3** following the procedures of Marquez and co-workers.[49]

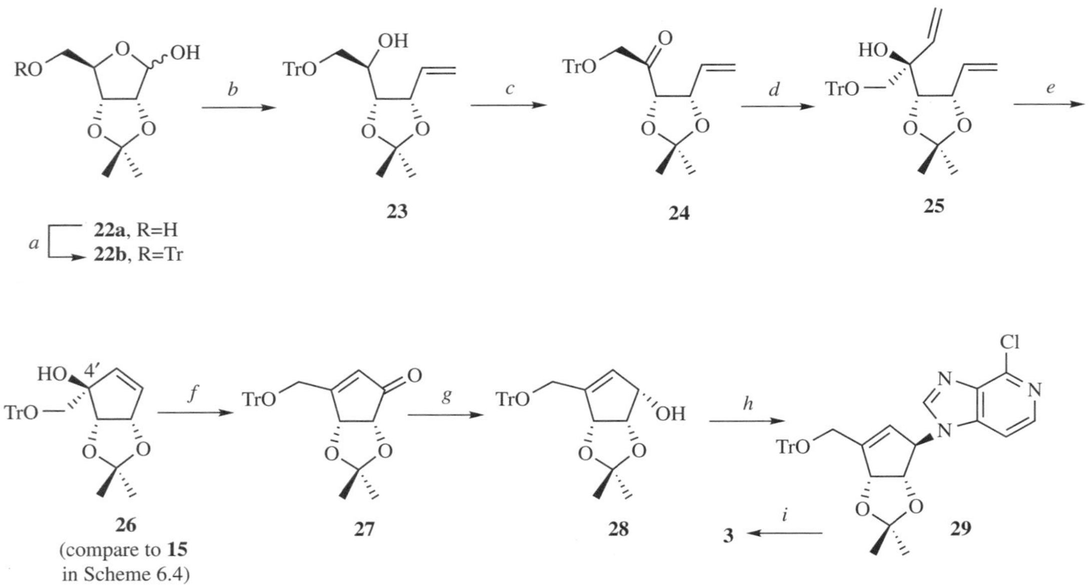

SCHEME 6.6 Synthesis of 3-deazaneplanocin. Reaction conditions: *a*, TrCl, pyridine, DMAP, CH$_2$Cl$_2$, 91%; *b*, on **22**, Ph$_3$PMeBr, *t*-BuOK, THF, 87%; *c*, Dess–Martin periodinane, CH$_2$Cl$_2$, 92%; *d*, vinylmagnesium bromide, CH$_2$Cl$_2$, 97%, *dr* = 20:1; *e*, Grubbs' catalyst, CH$_2$Cl$_2$, 95%; *f*, PDC, CH$_2$Cl$_2$, 88%; *g*, NaBH$_4$, CeCl$_3$•7 H$_2$O, MeOH, 95%; *h*, 6-chloro-3-deazapurine (**7**), DIAD, Ph$_3$P, THF, 41%; *i*, reference 49.

148

As with **8**, the cyclopentenol **28** lends itself to reaction with a variety of heterocyclic bases to avail many analogues of **3** in large amounts.

Simultaneous to our development of this route to **28**, Jeong and co-workers were considering an analogous pathway.[50]

6.6 CONCLUSION

With the report that the 3-deaza carbocyclic nucleosides, 3-deazaneplanocin A (**3**) and 3-deazaaristeromycin (**2**), which are inhibitors of *S*-adenosylhomocysteine hydrolase, show significant anti-filovirus potential by affecting interferon production in infected cells, convenient and practical syntheses of these compounds became important for more extensive investigations. In that direction, successful preparative routes to **2** and **3**, also adaptable for providing numerous analogues, are outlined beginning with readily available starting materials.

ACKNOWLEDGMENT

This research was supported by funds from the Department of Health and Human Services (AI 48495 and AI 56540), for which the authors are appreciative.

REFERENCES

1. Borio, L.; Inglesby, T.; Peters, C. J.; Schmaljohn, A. L.; Hughes, J. M.; Jahrling, P. B.; Ksiazek, T.; Johnson, K. M.; Meyerhoff, A.; O'Toole, T.; Ascher, M. S.; Bartlett, J.; Breman, J. G.; Eitzen, E. M.; Hamburg, M.; Hauer, J.; Henderson, D. A.; Johnson, R. T.; Kwik, G.; Layton, M.; Lillibridge, S.; Nabel, G. J.; Osterholm, M. T.; Perl, T. M.; Russell, P.; Tonat, K. Hemorrhagic fever viruses as biological weapons—medical and public health management. *JAMA* **2002**, *287*, 2391–2405.

2. (a) Center for Biosecurity of UPMC, Viral Hemorrhagic Fevers Fact Sheet (2003), http://www.upmc-biosecurity.org/pages/agents/vhf_facts.html (accessed April 14, 2004). (b) Centers for Disease Control and Prevention, Viral Hemorrhagic Fevers (2003), http://www.cdc.gov/ncidod/dvrd/spb/mnpages/dispages/vhf.htm (accessed April 14, 2004).

3. Alibek, K.; Handelman, S. *Biohazard: The Chilling True Story of the Largest Covert Biological Weapons Program in the World, Told from the Inside by the Man Who Ran It*, Random House, New York, 1999, p. 319.

4. Miller, J.; Engelberg, S.; Broad, W. *Germs: Biological Weapons and America's Secret War*, Simon & Schuster, New York, 2001, p. 382.

5. Johnson, E.; Jaax, N.; White, J.; Jahrling, P. Lethal experimental infections of rhesus-monkeys by aerosolized Ebola-virus. *Int. J. Exp. Pathol.* **1995**, *76*, 227–236.

6. References 16 and 19 of Reference 1.

7. Stephenson, E. H.; Larson, E. W.; Dominik, J. W. Effect of environmental factors on aerosol-induced Lassa virus infection. *J. Med. Virol.* **1984**, *14*, 295–303.

8. Kenyon, R. H.; Mckee, K. T.; Zack, P. M.; Rippy, M. K.; Vogel, A. P.; et al. Aerosol infection of rhesus macaques with Junin virus. *Intervirology* **1992**, *33*, 23–31.

9. Jackson, R. J.; Ramsay, A. J.; Christensen, C. D.; Beaton, S.; Hall, D. F.; Ramshaw, I. A. Expression of mouse interleukin-4 by recombinant ectromelia virus suppresses cytolytic lymphocyte responses and overcomes genetic resistance to mousepox. *J. Virol.* **2001**, *75*, 1205–1210.

10. Center for Nonproliferation Studies, Chemical and Biological Weapons: Possession and Programs Past and Present (2002), `http://cns.miis.edu/research/cbw/possess.htm` (accessed 14 April 2004).

11. Leroy, E. M.; Rouquet, P.; Formenty, P.; Souquiere, S.; Kilbourne, A.; Froment, J.-M.; Bermejo, M.; Smit, S.; Karesh, W.; Swanepoel, R.; Zaki, S. R.; Rollin, P. E. Multiple Ebola transmission events and rapid decline of central African wildlife. *Science* **2004**, *303*, 387–390.

12. (a) Geisbert, T. W.; Hensley, L. E.; Larsen, T.; Young, H. A.; Reed, D. S.; Geisbert, J. B.; Scott, D. P.; Kagan, E.; Jahrling, P. B.; Davis, K. J. Pathogenesis of Ebola hemorrhagic fever in cynomolgus macaques: Evidence that hemorrhage is not a direct effect of virus-induced cytolysis of endothelial cells. *Am. J. Pathol.* **2003**, *163*, 2347–2370. (b) Peterson, A. T.; Bauer, J. T.; Mills, J. N. Ecologic and geographic distribution of filovirus disease. *Emerging Infect. Dis.* **2004**, *10*, 40–47.

13. Steinberg, D. Antiterror agenda promotes Ebola vaccine and immunotherapy. *Scientist* **2002**, *16* 32–33.

14. (a) Andrei, G.; De Clercq, E. Molecular approaches for the treatment of hemorrhagic fever virus infections. *Antiviral Res.* **1993**, *22*, 45–75. (b) Bray, M.; Paragas, J. Experimental therapy of filovirus infections. *Antiviral Res.* **2002**, *54*, 1–17.

15. Nabel, G. J. Vaccine for AIDS and Ebola virus infection. *Virus Res.* **2003**, *92*, 213–217.

16. Feldmann, H.; Jones, S.; Klenk, H.-D.; Schnittler, H.-J. Ebola virus: from discovery to vaccine. *Nat. Rev. Immunol.* **2003**, *3*, 677–685.

17. Nelson, R. Novel Ebola vaccine begins first human trials. *Lancet* **2003**, *362*, 1815.

18. Barrientos, L. G.; O'Keefe, B. R.; Bray, M.; Sanchez, A.; Gronenborn, A. M.; Boyd, M. R. Cyanovirin-N binds to the viral surface glycoprotein, $GP_{1,2}$ and inhibits infectivity of Ebola virus. *Antiviral Res.* **2003**, *58*, 47–56.

19. De Clercq, E. Antiviral activity spectrum and target of action of different classes of nucleoside analogs. *Nucleosides Nucleotides* **1994**, *13*, 1271–1295.

20. Bray, M.; Driscoll, J.; Huggins, J. W. Treatment of lethal Ebola virus infection in mice with a single dose of an S-adenosyl-L-homocysteine hydrolase inhibitor. *Antiviral Res.* **2000**, *45*, 135–147.

21. Huggins, J.; Zhang, Z.-X.; Bray, M. Antiviral drug therapy of filovirus infections: S-adenosylhomocysteine hydrolase inhibitors inhibit Ebola virus *in vitro* and in a lethal mouse model. *J. Infect. Dis.* **1999**, *179* (Suppl. 1), S240–S247.

22. Bray, M.; Raymond, J. L.; Geisbert, T. W.; Baker, R. O. 3-Deazaneplanocin A induces massively increased interferon-α production in Ebola virus-infected mice. *Antiviral Res.* **2002**, *55*, 151–159.

23. Basler, C. F.; Wang, X.; Muhlberger, E.; Volchkov, V.; Paragas, J.; Klenk, H.-D; Garcia-Sastre, A.; Palese, P. The Ebola virus VP35 protein functions as a type I IFN antagonist. *Proc. Natl. Acad. Sci. U.S.A.* **2000**, *97*, 12289–12294.

24. Bray, M. The role of type 1 interferon response in the resistance of mice to filovirus infection. *J. Gen. Virol.* **2001**, *82*, 1365–1373.

25. Coulombe, R. A.; Sharma, R. P.; Huggins, J. W. Phamacokinetics of the antiviral agent 3-deazaneplanocin A. *Eur. J. Drug Metab. Pharmacokinet.* **1995**, *20*, 197–202.

26. *Recent Advances in Nucleosides: Chemistry and Chemotherapy*, Chu, C. K. (ed.). Elsevier, Amsterdam, 2002.

27. Palmer, J. L.; Abeles, R. H. The mechanism of action of *S*-adenosylhomocysteinase. *J. Biol. Chem.* **1979**, *254* 1217–1226.

28. Borchardt, R. T. *S*-Adenosyl-L-methionine-dependent macromolecule methyltransferases—potential targets for the design of chemotherapeutic agents. *J. Med. Chem.* **1980**, *23*, 347–357.

29. Wolfe, M. S.; Borchardt, R. T. *S*-Adenosyl-L-homocysteine hydrolase as a target for antiviral chemotherapy. *J. Med. Chem.* **1991**, *34*, 1521–1530.

30. Saha, N.; Shuman, S.; Schwer, B. Yeast based genetic system for functional analysis of poxvirus mRNA cap methyltransferase. *J. Virol.* **2003**, *77*, 7300–7307.

31. Gong, C.; Shuman, S. Mapping the active site of vaccinia virus RNA triphosphatase. *Virology* **2003**, *309*, 125–134.

32. (a) Barbosa, E.; Moss, B. Messenger RNA(nucleoside-2′-)-methyltransferase from vaccinia virus—purification and physical properties. *J. Biol. Chem.* **1978**, *253*, 7692–7697. (b) Barbosa, E.; Moss, B. Messenger RNA(nucleoside-2′-)-methyltransferase from vaccinia virus—characteristics and substrate-specificity. *J. Biol. Chem.* **1978**, *253*, 7698–7702.

33. Martin, S. A.; Moss, B. Modification of RNA by mRNA guanylyltransferase and mRNA(guanine-7)-methyltransferase from vaccinia virions. *J. Biol. Chem.* **1975**, *250*, 9330–9335.

34. Oxenrider, K. A.; Bu, G.; Sitz, T. O. Adenosine analogs inhibit the guanine-7-methylation of mRNA cap structures. *FEBS Lett.* **1993**, *316*, 273–277.

35. Borchardt, R. T.; Keller, B. T.; Patelthombre, U. Neplanocin-A—a potent inhibitor of *S*-adenosylhomocysteine hydrolase and of vaccinia virus multiplication in mouse L929 cells. *J. Biol. Chem.* **1984**, *259*, 4353–4358.

36. Huggins, J. W.; Schneller, S. W., unpublished results.

37. Houston, D. M.; Matuszewska, B.; Borchardt, R. T. Potential inhibitors of *S*-adenosylmethionine-dependent methyltransferases. 10. Base acid and amino acid modified analogs of *S*-aristeromycinyl-L-homocysteine. *J. Med. Chem.* **1985**, *28*, 478–482.

38. (a) Crimmins, M. T. New developments in the enantioselective synthesis of cyclopentyl carbocyclic nucleosides. *Tetrahedron* **1998**, *54*, 9229–9272. (b) Borthwick, A. D.; Biggadike, K. Synthesis of chiral carbocyclic nucleosides. *Tetrahedron* **1992**, *48*, 571–623. (c) Agrofoglio, L.; Suhas, E.; Farese, A.; Condom, R.; Challand, S. R.; et al. Synthesis of carbocyclic nucleosides. *Tetrahedron* **1994**, *50*, 10611–10670. (d) Marquez, V. E.; Lim, M. I. Carbocyclic nucleosides. *Med. Res. Rev.* **1986**, *6*, 1–40.

39. Marquez, V. E. Carbocyclic nucleosides. *Adv. Antiviral Drug Design* **1996**, *2*, 89–146.

40. (a) Da Silva, A. D.; Coimbra, E. S.; Fourrey, J. L.; Machado, A. S.; Robert-Gero, M. Expeditious enantioselective synthesis of carbocyclic nucleosides with anti-leishmanial activity. *Tetrahedron Lett.* **1993**, *34*, 6745–6748. (b) Seley, K. L.; Schneller, S. W.; Lane, S.; Rattendi, D.; Bacchi, C. J. Synthesis and anti-trypanosomal activities of a series of 7-deaza-5′-noraristeromycin derivatives with variations in the cyclopentyl ring substituents. *Antimicrob. Agents Chemother.* **1997**, *41*, 1658–1661.

41. (a) Caperelli, C. A.; Price, M. F. Carbocyclic glycinamide ribonucleotide is a substrate for glycinamide ribonucleotide transformylase. *Arch. Biochem. Biophys.* **1988**, *264*, 340–342. (b) Slama, J. T.; Simmons, A. M. Inhibition of NAD glycohydrolase and ADP-ribosyl transferases by carbocyclic analogs of oxidized nicotinamide adenine-dinucleotide. *Biochemistry* **1989**, *28*, 7688–7694. (c) Szemzo, A.; Szecsi, J.; Sagi, J.; Otvos, L. First synthesis of carbocyclic oligothymidylates. *Tetrahedron Lett.* **1990**, *31*, 1463–1466. (d) Parry, R. J.; Haridas, K. Synthesis of 1α-pyrophosphoryl-2α,3α-dihydroxy-4β-cyclopentanemethanol-5-phosphate, a carbocyclic analog of 5-phosphoribosyl-1-pyrophosphate (PRPP). *Tetrahedron Lett.* **1993**, *34*, 7013–7016.

42. Ludek, O. R.; Meier, C. New convergent synthesis of carbocyclic nucleoside analogues. *Synthesis* **2003**, 2101–2109.

43. Yang, M.; Ye, W.; Schneller, S. W. *J. Org. Chem.*, **2004**, *69*, 3993–3996.

44. Hegde, V. R.; Seley, K. L.; Schneller, S. W. Carbocyclic 5'-norcytidine (5'-norcarbodine). *J. Heterocycl. Chem.* **2000**, *37*, 1361–1362.

45. Lee, K.; Cass, C.; Jacobson, K. A. Synthesis using ring closure metathesis and effect on nucleoside transport of a (*N*)-methanocarba *S*-(4-nitrobenzyl)thioinosine derivative. *Org. Lett.* **2001**, *3*, 597–599.

46. Ohira, S.; Sawamoto, T.; Yamato, M. Synthesis of (−)-neplanocin A via C-H insertion of alkylidenecarbene. *Tetrahedron Lett.* **1995**, *36*, 1537–1538.

47. Grubbs, R. H.; Chang, S. Recent advances in olefin metathesis and its application in organic synthesis. *Tetrahedron* **1998**, *54*, 4413–4450.

48. Medich, J. R.; Kunnen, K. B.; Johnson, C. R. Synthesis of the carbocyclic nucleoside (−)-neplanocin A. *Tetrahedron Lett.* **1987**, *28*, 4131–4134.

49. Tseng, C. K. H.; Marquez, V. E.; Fuller, R. W.; Goldstein, B. M.; Haines, D. R.; McPherson, H.; Parsons, J. L.; Shannon, W. M.; Arnett, G.; Hollingshead, M.; Driscoll, J. S. Synthesis of 3-deazaneplanocin A, a powerful inhibitor of *S*-adenosylhomocysteine hydrolase with potent and selective *in vitro* and *in vivo* antiviral activities. *J. Med. Chem.* **1989**, *32*, 1442–1446.

50. Choi, W. J.; Moon, H. R.; Kim, H. O.; Yoo, B. N.; Lee, J. A.; Shin, D. H.; Jeong, L. S. Preparative and stereoselective synthesis of the versatile intermediate for carbocyclic nucleosides: effects of the bulky protecting groups to enforce facial selectivity. *J. Org. Chem.* **2004**, 69, 2634–2636.

CHAPTER 7

Antiviral Strategies for Ebola Virus

JILLIAN M. LICATA and RONALD N. HARTY

Department of Pathobiology, School of Veterinary Medicine, University of Pennsylvania

7.1 INTRODUCTION

Filoviruses have been categorized by the U.S. government as select agents, possessing the potential for biological weaponization. No effective vaccines or therapeutics are currently available; however, such reagents will be vital to combat prospective mass attacks. A complete understanding of the viral life cycle has been hindered somewhat due to limited availability of viral isolates and containment restrictions. Nonetheless, great strides have been made in understanding the processes of viral entry, replication, and budding, as well as disease pathogenesis. This information has revealed a wide array of potential targets for antiviral therapies, as well as methods by which the most effective vaccination strategies may be achieved. Indeed, a combination of some of these recently explored strategies may prove to be the best defense against a future outbreak. A comprehensive review of recent developments in the field of filovirology and antiviral research is provided in this chapter.

Ebola and Marburg viruses comprise the Filoviridae family of viruses. These filamentous, thread-like virions have a single-stranded, negative-sense RNA genome of ~19.0 kb in length. The genome encodes the envelope glycoprotein (GP), the matrix proteins VP40 and VP24, the nucleoprotein (NP), nonstructural proteins VP30 and VP35, and the viral polymerase (L) (as reviewed[1]).

The first documented reports of Ebola virus occurred in 1976 in two simultaneous outbreaks in Zaire (now the Democratic Republic of the Congo) and Sudan.[2] The Zaire and Sudan subtypes of Ebola virus have caused the majority of human outbreaks, whereas the Cote d'Ivoire subtype has only been implicated in one human case.[3] A fourth subtype, Reston, was identified in an outbreak in a primate

---

Antiviral Drug Discovery for Emerging Diseases and Bioterrorism Threats. Edited by Paul F. Torrence
Copyright © 2005 John Wiley & Sons, Inc.

colony in the United States and has not shown the potential for fatal disease in humans.[4] During outbreaks of Ebola, the virus is most commonly transmitted through intimate contact with virus-containing blood or body fluids. Aerosol transmission has also been documented during experimental infection of nonhuman primates,[5,6] and the virus appears to be relatively stable in the environment.[7]

Pathogenesis of filovirus infections may include severe hemorrhagic fever, often leading to death.[8] The initial symptoms of filovirus infection may include flu-like symptoms such as fever, chills, muscle and head aches, nausea, vomiting, loss of appetite, and malaise. The disease quickly runs its course, and more devastating symptoms, including severe bleeding, coagulation defects, maculopapular rash, exaggerated inflammatory responses, and hemorrhaging into the skin, mucous membranes, and organs ensue. As viremia overtakes the immune system, disseminated intravascular coagulopathy (DIC) occurs and the patient may go into shock or coma. Mortality rates are typically between 50% and 90% with the time to death ranging from 14 to 21 days (as reviewed[9,10]).

The U.S. Centers for Disease Control and Prevention (CDC) has classified filoviruses as "Category A" biological weapons.[11] The Working Group on Civilian Biodefense has cited some of the features of such agents as high morbidity/mortality, ease of person-to-person transmission, environmental stability, and the potential to cause public anxiety.[12] Filoviruses have allegedly been evaluated for their potential to be used as biowarfare agents by the former Soviet Union.[13]

Perhaps most daunting is the fact that, currently, there are no effective vaccines, nor therapeutics in use to prevent filovirus infection. This is mainly due to the fact that few laboratories have the proper containment facilities necessary to work with these agents, and investigators have had difficulty in obtaining samples from the limited number of confirmed human infections following the first recognition of the disease (<2000).[14] To overcome these obstacles, researchers have adapted the filoviruses to lower species, such as mice and guinea pigs, for the study of disease pathogenesis and treatment efficacies. When evaluating such studies, it should be kept in mind that viral adaptation can cause sequence changes in the virus as well as alterations to pathogenesis, and these occurrences have in fact been reported.[15–18] Researchers have also benefited from the isolation of viral cDNAs, which has enabled them to generate expression systems to study isolated viral gene products and their roles in the virus life cycle. Therefore, despite the aforementioned limitations, much progress has been made in understanding the molecular aspects of filovirus replication and pathogenesis. As a result, these efforts have brought to light a number of potential targets for antiviral therapies and methods to effectively treat infected individuals. For example, antivirals currently under investigation include those that may be used prophylactically, as well as those that may be used therapeutically. In addition, antivirals that act directly on the virus as well as those that act indirectly by changing the course of disease are also under investigation. In this chapter we highlight some of the antiviral strategies currently being pursued for Ebola virus including the development of drugs to target specific steps of the viral life cycle, agents that may alter disease pathogenesis, and effective immunization strategies to prevent infection during an outbreak.

7.2 INHIBITION OF VIRUS ENTRY

The surface glycoprotein (GP) of Ebola virus exists as a trimeric spike protruding from the viral surface and enables the virus to achieve penetration of the cell by a two-step process of receptor binding and membrane fusion. Therefore, targeting GP with antiviral drugs to block these early processes has been an active area of antiviral research.

7.2.1 Neutralizing Antibodies

The importance of neutralizing antibodies during Ebola virus infection remains unclear, as they are often present at low to insignificant titers in the serum of infected patients, and their presence is generally detected very late in the convalescent period.[1] During the 1995 Ebola virus outbreak in Kikwit, Democratic Republic of the Congo, attempts were made to transfuse convalescent-phase whole blood into infected individuals.[19,20] Further studies on antibody transfusions have demonstrated that the passive transfer of commercially available IgG from hyperimmunized horses protected guinea pigs from lethal infection with Ebola virus.[21,22] However, when transferred to primates, the horse IgG only served to reduce the viral burden, and all animals succumbed to disease by day 8 postinfection.[23] Alternatively, immune plasma from goats was protective in challenge experiments in both guinea pigs and baboons.[24] The transfer of this polyclonal immune serum to mice infected subcutaneously with Ebola virus led to the development of high anti-Ebola virus IgG titers,[25] resembling that which has been seen in human survivors.[26,27] Furthermore, it was demonstrated that administration of immune serum did not completely block viral replication.[25] This latter finding highlights the importance of defining antiviral strategies that will target additional stages of the viral life cycle.

Aside from transfer of convalescent serum to patients, attempts to use monoclonal antibodies (mAb) as a treatment for Ebola virus infection have been pursued. For example, 14 monoclonal antibodies (mAbs) targeting the GP of Ebola virus (Zaire) were created in BALB/c mice. Ten of these mAbs were able to confer protection to lethally challenged mice when administered within an acceptable human therapeutic dose up to 24 hours prior to challenge.[28] In another study, the bone marrow from convalescent donors was used to construct an antibody phage display library, which resulted in the isolation of a variety of mAbs against viral NP, GP, or sGP. These antibodies displayed neutralization activity in a plaque reduction assay, establishing the principle that antibodies elicited during a natural infection represent treatment candidates.[29] One mAb from this study, KZ52, was used in a follow-up animal study. Dose-dependent protection of lethally challenged guinea pigs was observed when KZ52 was administered up to 1 hour postchallenge. Notably, in the group of guinea pigs completely protected from infection by KZ52, all but one animal possessed low to intermediate serum titers. This finding suggests that, aside from neutralization, mAb KZ52 may also possess the ability to act against infected cells, thus controlling critical tissue damage and reducing viremia.[17] Although initial studies on protective effects of KZ52 proved successful in rodents, it was recently reported that administration of this mAb to rhesus macaques did not confer protection from disease.[30]

An important note when considering mAb treatment of patients is that few cross-neutralizing epitopes exist among various strains of Ebola virus. To overcome this deficiency, the development of cocktails of neutralizing antibodies has been proposed to ensure protective effects and select against emerging antigenic variants.[31] Another important consideration is the possibility of antibody-dependent enhancement (ADE) of infection (as reviewed[32]). Indeed, the infectivity of VSV pseudotyped with Ebola virus GP was enhanced in both human 293T cells and endothelial cells by antibodies produced in mice immunized with Ebola virus GP.[33] On the contrary, a second study failed to detect ADE in Ebola virus-infected monkeys,[18] although whether the ADE detection conditions were optimal in these experiments remains questionable. Finally, more than half of the samples of convalescent serum isolated from Ebola virus-infected patients following the 1995 outbreak enhanced infectivity of the virus in vitro.[34]

7.2.2 Receptor Binding

A variety of specific strategies aimed at blocking receptor binding mediated by GP have been investigated. For example, approaches utilizing drugs to coat the viral surface as well as those to develop competitive inhibitors of GP–receptor interactions have been pursued.

The drug cyanovirin-N (CV-N) was originally discovered in a screen of natural products as candidates for antiviral agents against HIV-1. CV-N was shown to block adsorption of HIV-1 to target cells by binding to high-mannose oligosaccharides within the HIV-1 envelope gp120.[35] Similar to gp120, Ebola GP is known to be heavily glycosylated with both N- and O-linked carbohydrates.[36] Thus, a study was undertaken to determine whether CV-N was able to interfere with the adsorption of Ebola virus to target cells. Indeed, CV-N was shown by ELISA to bind to the GP1 subunit of Ebola virus GP, block viral cytopathic effects in cell culture, and increase the mean time to death in lethally challenged mice.[37] In addition, CV-N has been shown to prevent the transduction of HeLa cells by Ebola GP- and Marburg GP-pseudotyped lentiviruses.[38] As with other drug therapies, CV-N exhibited a narrow "therapeutic index," suggesting that further study in nonhuman primate models is warranted. In addition, the development of CV-N mimetics to mask specific sugar side chains of Ebola virus GP may provide a new avenue of Ebola virus therapy.

Drugs that can competitively inhibit binding of Ebola virus GP to its cell receptor also represent viable candidates for antivirals. Folate-receptor-α (FR-α) was proposed recently to serve as a receptor for Ebola virus[39]; however, a follow-up study raised significant concerns regarding this finding.[40] Simmons et al.[40] suggest that FR-α is not a requirement for viral entry, as a variety of cell types that lack FR-α expression, but are susceptible to infection with Ebola virus, exist. A broad range of cell types are indeed susceptible to filovirus infection,[41,42] suggesting that either multiple receptors can mediate entry of Ebola virus or the receptor is widespread and highly conserved. If the latter scenario is true, receptor binding would represent an attractive target for the development of small molecule inhibitors.

While the receptor for Ebola virus remains elusive, the discovery that DC- (dendritic cell-) and L-SIGN (liver/lymph node-specific intercellular adhesion molecule 3-grabbing nonintegrin) can act as trans-receptors for Ebola virus[43,44] has provided another potential target for antiviral drugs. For HIV-1, cells expressing DC- and L-SIGN are able to bind and capture virus and subsequently disseminate infectious particles to susceptible cells. It remains to be determined whether or not a similar mechanism of dissemination of Ebola virus occurs. The advent of glyco-dendrimer technology[45] has provided a potential means of interference with Ebola virus binding to the aforementioned lectins. Glycodendrimers are carbohydrate multivalent structures designed to hinder low affinity carbohydrate interactions,[46] such as those between Ebola virus GP and DC- and/or L-SIGN.[44] Furthermore, the ability of such molecules to block viral receptors has been illustrated in other systems.[47,48] One study to date has examined the use of this technology in inhibiting Ebola virus infection.[49] In this study, the ability of Ebola-GP-pseudo-typed lentiviral vectors to infect Jurkat cells stably transduced with DC-SIGN was inhibited in the presence of the glycodendritic structure BH30sucMan.[49] Thus, evaluation of such compounds in animal models of infection represents a logical next step in the pursuit of therapies of this sort.

7.2.3 Fusion

The Ebola virus GP is proteolytically cleaved into disulfide-linked GP1 and GP2 subunits as part of its maturation process during infection.[50] The GP2 subunit was shown to contain a coiled-coil motif, which is highly conserved among viral glycoproteins, and assumed to be important for oligomerization and membrane fusion.[51,52] Notably, peptides corresponding to a similar structure within the HIV-1 gp41 protein, such as T-20, have been shown to inhibit replication of the virus in vitro and in vivo. The mechanism of inhibition appears to involve binding of the peptide to gp41, which blocks fusion of the glycoprotein with the target cell membrane.[53,54] A study by Watanabe and colleagues demonstrated that a peptide corresponding to the C-terminal helix present in Ebola virus GP2 inhibited entry of a recombinant virus expressing Ebola GP.[55] It should be noted that unlike the peptides utilized in HIV-1 studies, high concentrations of the Ebola-specific peptides were necessary to prevent fusion. The need for large amounts of Ebola-specific peptides may reflect differences in the cellular location of the fusion event—at the plasma membrane for HIV-1[56] and in the endosome for Ebola virus.[57,58] These initial results are promising, and optimization of peptide length, concentration, and composition will allow for further evaluation of these peptides as antiviral agents for Ebola virus infection.

7.2.4 Lipid Rafts

Lipid rafts are specialized membrane microdomains that are rich in cholesterol and adopt a liquid-ordered phase with reduced fluidity and mobility.[59] Restriction of molecular movement within these microdomains is thought to allow for more efficient function (e.g., signal transduction) by concentrating the molecules. Increasing evidence suggests that lipid rafts serve as platforms for entry of several viral pathogens, including HIV-1, influenza A virus, SV40, and Sindbis virus.[60] Similarly, recent findings suggest that filoviruses utilize lipid rafts (caveolae) for entry into cells.[61,62] Treatment of cells with agents known to disrupt raft formation or stability, such as filipin, nystatin, PMA, and cyclodextrin, resulted in decreased filovirus infectivity.[61,62] Although no studies to date have formally developed or tested antiviral agents that can disrupt the targeting of viral proteins to lipid rafts and/or the assembly of such platforms, the concept represents yet another potential avenue of therapeutics targeting entry of Ebola virus.

7.3 EBOLA VIRUS REPLICATION

Potential antiviral therapies for Ebola virus may also be designed to target viral replication. Replication and transcription of the negative-sense RNA genome of Ebola virus is mediated by four viral proteins: NP, VP35, L, and VP30. Briefly, the RNA-dependent RNA polymerase (L protein) transcribes a leader RNA and discrete capped and polyadenylated mRNAs encoding the individual viral proteins in a $3' \rightarrow 5'$ direction. Accumulation of NP and VP35, the polymerase cofactor, is thought to trigger a switch from transcription of mRNAs to replication of the full-length genome (as reviewed[1]). The process of replication (synthesis of genomic RNA) appears to occur independently of VP30; however, the presence of VP30 serves to enhance transcription (synthesis of viral mRNAs).[63]

7.3.1 Targeting VP30

Recent insights into a role for VP30 during transcription of the Ebola virus genome have revealed some potential new targets for antiviral drugs. For example, Weik et al.[64] found that the integrity of a secondary structure in the leader sequence of the NP gene, an experimentally predicted stem-loop, was necessary for VP30-regulated transcription to occur. Weik and colleagues propose that VP30 may bind directly, or recruit a cofactor, to the stem-loop structure, thereby inhibiting its formation and suppressing its ability to impede movement of the viral polymerase along the template RNA.[64] A complete understanding of this mechanism may allow for the generation of molecules that may block VP30 from accessing the stem-loop structure.

Another study focused on the mediation of VP30-activated transcription through phosphorylation of the viral protein. Phosphorylation of VP30 occurs at the N terminus of the protein and involves one threonine and six serine residues. The phosphorylated form of VP30 was found associated with NP inclusions and was transcriptionally inactive, whereas the nonphosphorylated form of VP30 was evenly distributed in the cytoplasm and was transcriptionally active.[65] Interestingly, treatment of Ebola virus infected cells with okadaic acid (OA), an inhibitor of PP1 and PP2A phosphatases[66] and thereby VP30 phosphorylation, caused a dose-dependent decrease in the number of infected cells.[65] Unfortunately, treatment with OA has been reported to result in severe side effects, such as induction of tumor growth and genetic instability.[67,68]

As with many other transcription factors, VP30 was shown recently to form homo-oligomers in transfected cells.[69] Moreover, supplementation of the mini-genome system with oligomerization mutants of VP30 resulted in a complete inhibition of viral transcription.[69] Interestingly, delivery of a synthetic peptide ($E30_{pep}$-wt) comprised of the 25 amino acid oligomerization domain of VP30 into Ebola virus-infected cells inhibited viral replication.[69] This represents yet another potential mechanism by which Ebola virus replication may be inhibited.

7.3.2 Adenosine Analogues

More generic approaches have also been attempted to target replication of Ebola virus in infected individuals. Traditionally, ribavirin has been used to inhibit the polymerase activity of many RNA viruses, although it has not proved effective in vitro, or in animal models of lethal Ebola virus infection.[70,71] Alternatively, drugs such as S-adenosyl-L-homocysteine (SAH) inhibitors have shown promising protective results in animal models of Ebola virus infection. These adenosine analogues, in particular, carbocyclic 3-deazaadenosine (C-c^3 Ado) and 3-deazane-planocin A (c^3-Npc A), function to indirectly limit $5'$ cap methylation of viral mRNAs,[72] and these analogues have demonstrated clear antiviral potential both in vitro and in vivo.[73,74] Both of these drugs specifically inhibit replication of Ebola virus Zaire and Sudan strains, as well as Marburg virus in vitro with low cytotoxicity.[75] Studies in both SCID and immunocompetent mice have shown that a three times daily (TID) treatment regimen was able to protect animals from lethal challenge.[75,76] In a more recent study, Bray and colleagues were able to reduce the treatment to a single inoculation and found that when administered between days 1 and 2 postinfection, the drugs were able to cure Ebola virus-infected mice.[77] Thus, adenosine analogues have promising potential in the battle against Ebola virus infection.

7.3.3 RNA Interference

A new class of potential therapeutics is based on the use of small interfering RNAs (siRNAs) to target replication of viruses such as HIV-1 and respiratory syncytial virus (RSV). RNA interference (RNAi) is based on the notion that double-stranded RNA, which is achieved when siRNAs bind to complementary target RNA sequences, directs degradation of the target mRNA in cells.[78] Encouraging results using RNAi have been obtained for HIV-1 recently. Specifically, synthetic siRNAs targeted against distinct regions of the HIV-1 genome were found to inhibit virus replication in primary cells.[79] Unfortunately, similar approaches using antisense RNA have thus far been unsuccessful when applied to Ebola virus replication.[80] While the potential use of antisense RNA and siRNA as antiviral therapies is intriguing, much work remains to be done in both identifying appropriate, accessible genomic targets of these RNAs, and in optimizing the stability and delivery[81] of these molecules to infected patients.

7.4   ANTIVIRAL RESPONSE TO INFECTION

Filoviruses initially infect cells of the monocyte lineage such as macrophages. The virus subsequently spreads in a pantropic manner to many other cell types, including endothelial cells.[82] While endothelial cells are not believed to represent an early target of viral replication, Ebola virus does appear to induce damage to these cells by indirect mechanisms, perhaps involving the secretion of host factors.[83] It is noteworthy that endothelial cells are a viral target, as they are known to play an important role in mediating the host antiviral response by appropriating expression of immunomodulatory genes.[84] Induction of the antiviral state in the host is attributed to the presence of double-stranded RNA (dsRNA) as well as other infection indicators. The presence of these indicators results in the synthesis and secretion of type 1 interferon (IFN), including variants of IFN-α and IFN-β.[85] Numerous viruses have developed strategies to evade the type 1 IFN antiviral response,[86] including Ebola virus.[87–90]

7.4.1   VP35 Protein and the IFN Response

In addition to its vital role in viral RNA synthesis and assembly, VP35 has been shown to potentiate an inhibitory effect on the cellular IFN response to Ebola virus infection. A role for VP35 as an IFN antagonist came from an initial study by Basler and colleagues, which demonstrated that VP35 was able to complement an influenza A virus lacking the NS1 protein, a well-documented IFN antagonist.[89] A preliminary mechanism of action for this suppressive effect of VP35 appears to be the ability of VP35 to inhibit phosphorylation, and therefore activation of interferon regulatory factor (IRF)-3,[91] a transcription factor. IRF-3 plays a central role in host cell IFN response to viral infection and has been shown to activate IFN-β and a subset of IFN-α genes (as reviewed[92]). Elucidation of the precise mechanism of VP35-mediated suppression of the IFN response is an active area of investigation, and a better understanding of the IFN antagonist activity associated with Ebola virus would clearly be important for future development of both antivirals and vaccines.[89]

7.4.2   Adenosine Analogues Revisited

The surprisingly robust inhibition of Ebola virus-induced death conveyed by only a single dose of adenosine analogues C-c[3] Ado and c[3]-Npc A[77] prompted two follow-up studies to explore further the mechanisms of action of these analogues. Findings from the first study indicated that the efficacy of adenosine analogue administration was diminished when coadministered with antibodies targeting both IFN-α and IFN-β in a murine model of Ebola virus infection,[93] suggesting a role for the type 1 IFN response in the effectiveness of this treatment. Results from the second study indicated that delivery of the analogue c^3-NpcA resulted in a massive production of IFN-α by virus-infected cells. IFN-α levels were not elevated in the serum of drug-treated mice that were not infected with Ebola virus.[94] However, the authors do point out that enhancement of IFN-α production was not observed in Ebola virus-infected primates treated with c^3-NpcA, suggesting that rodent and nonhuman primate models of infection differ greatly in regard to immune induction.[94]

In addition to potentially enhancing type 1 IFN responses to viral infection, adenosine homologues may affect immune response to infection in a variety of other manners. Notably, two adenosine homologues were shown to impair proper functioning of murine macrophages,[95] and C-c^3 Ado was shown to block the release of interleukin-1 from activated human monocytes.[96] Therefore, in addition to their ability to inhibit viral replication, it is intriguing to speculate that treatment with these drugs may additionally affect normal macrophage functioning, thereby rendering these cells poor hosts for supporting initial infection by Ebola virus.[77]

7.4.3 Treatment with Exogenous IFN

In response to the inhibition of type 1 IFN production by Ebola virus, a number of attempts have been made to treat patients by supplementation with exogenous IFN. For example, it has been reported that mice treated with a recombinant chimeric B/D form of human IFN-α were protected against infection with Ebola virus.[80] Similarly, treatment of guinea pigs with reaferon (IFN-α) and ridostatin (a single-stranded/dsRNA mixture) appeared to confer protection against Marburg virus and increased the time to death an average of 3 days following Ebola virus infection.[97] Contrasting results were obtained in another study, where treatment of guinea pigs with homologous IFN-α was not beneficial in a lethal-challenge model.[98] Finally, in a cynomolgus macaque model, treatment with IFN-α2b delayed viremia for several days; however, all treated animals ultimately succumbed to disease.[21]

Variations to the approach of directly administering IFN have also been investigated. CpG-oligodeoxynucleotides (ODN) have the ability to enter antigen-presenting cells and lymphocytes and stimulate the release of immunoprotective cytokines such as IFN.[99] The protective effects of CpG-ODN have been examined in a mouse model of Ebola virus infection.[100] Indeed, treatment of mice with 10–50 μg CpG-ODN completely protected the animals from 10^2–10^3 LD$_{50}$ Ebola virus challenge.[100]

7.5 VIRAL PATHOGENESIS

Ebola virus infection is associated with the rapid induction of devastating disease conditions in the host. The development of antivirals targeting pathogenesis will undoubtedly be helpful in ameliorating the disease outcome. Additionally, such drugs may serve to lengthen the window of opportunity during which therapies targeting viral replication can be effective.

7.5.1 Coagulation Defects

One of the hallmarks of infection with Ebola virus is the development of coagulation abnormalities, leading to DIC and thrombosis-related organ failure. Ebola virus replication has been shown to induce the overexpression of tissue factor in monocytes and macrophages, leading to DIC characteristic of infection.[101,102] Tissue factor is a key player in the blood coagulation cascade and, therefore, its inappropriate expression can trigger thrombotic disorders.[101] The discovery of recombinant nematode anticoagulant protein c2 (rNAPc2), a small protein previously shown to inhibit the pathway leading from tissue factor formation to thrombin,[103] has provided a new drug therapy to target the course of disease in Ebola virus-infected animals. The efficacy of rNAPc2 in the treatment of Ebola virus-infected rhesus macaques was evaluated in a study by Geisbert et al.[104] Using the highest dose deemed safe, the drug was administered daily to infected animals beginning either 10 minutes or 24 hours postinfection. Out of nine animals treated with rNAPc2, three survived with no adverse health effects up to a year after initiation of the study.[104] The remaining animals saw a significant prolongation of survival before ultimately succumbing to disease, perhaps due to the apparent ability of drug treatment to significantly reduce plasma viremia levels.[104] Coagulation defects may also result from the abundance of cytokine production, induced by inflammation associated with severe infection.[105] Interestingly, rNAPc2 treatment appeared to reduce IL-6 production in a majority of the animals, particularly those that survived disease.[104] Overall, these initial results demonstrate potential for the use of rNAPc2 in the treatment of the disease progression of Ebola virus, through prevention of coagulation abnormalities and perhaps reduction in the host inflammatory response.

7.5.2 Apoptosis

In recent years, induction of apoptosis has been shown to occur rapidly following Ebola virus infection as evidenced by detection of 41/7 nuclear matrix protein (NMP) in the plasma, DNA fragmentation in leukocytes, and in situ TUNEL positive staining of lymphocytes isolated from infected individuals.[27,106,107] Apoptosis is now believed to be a compounding factor in the dismal outcome of Ebola virus infection. Interestingly, Ebola virus replication is nonexistent in lymphocytes,[58,108] suggesting that apoptosis of lymphocytes during Ebola virus infection is the result of a bystander effect. Although no exact mechanism of viral-induced apoptosis exists to date, one speculation is that soluble factors such as TNF-α, IFN-α, nitric oxide (NO), and other reactive oxygen species are secreted by infected cells and serve to induce apoptosis of neighboring, noninfected cells.[27,106,109] In addition, it has been postulated that viral proteins, such as secreted forms of the viral GP,[110] may stimulate apoptosis, although there is no direct evidence for this mechanism.[27,106,109] Insight into the specific pathways that Ebola virus utilizes to induce apoptosis will surely help to identify novel targets for antiviral therapy.

7.6   ASSEMBLY AND BUDDING OF EBOLA VIRUS

Assembly of viral proteins at the site of release and subsequent budding of virions represent the late stages of Ebola virus replication. Recent findings regarding the mechanisms of assembly and budding of Ebola virus have revealed the potential for developing antivirals to target these late steps in replication. For example, Ebola virus VP40 and GP, as well as lipid raft microdomains, are thought to be important for efficient budding of progeny virions, and disruption of the functions of these components of budding through the use of antivirals may be feasible.

7.6.1   Late (L) Budding Domains

The VP40 matrix protein alone can associate with the plasma membrane and induce the formation and release of virus-like particles (VLPs) from mammalian cells.[111] These VLPs are morphologically similar to authentic Ebola virus particles.[112–114] Thus, VP40 possesses all of the information necessary to promote virus budding. Efficient release of VP40 VLPs is due in part to the presence of two proline-rich L-domain motifs, $_7PTAP_{10}$ and $_{10}PPxY_{13}$, present at the N terminus of VP40.[111,114,115] L-domain motifs are found in a variety of viral matrix proteins and are believed to serve as protein–protein interaction modules, which recruit cellular machinery to the site of virus budding. Indeed, L-domain mutations lead to decreased budding efficiency of both VLPs and infectious virus.[116]

One of the best characterized viral L-domains is the PTAP motif. PTAP is present in both the gag protein of HIV-1 and VP40 of Ebola virus and is known to interact with the cellular protein tsg101.[115,117–119] On the other hand, the PPxY-type L-domain present in the M protein of VSV and VP40 of Ebola virus is known to interact with the cellular ubiquitin ligase Nedd4.[111,112,119–122] In sum, host proteins that participate in endosomal sorting and multivesicular body (MVB) formation in cells are thought to play a role in facilitating virus budding (as reviewed[116]). While much has been learned regarding the molecular aspects of Ebola virus budding, the precise function of the L-domain motifs remains unclear. Nevertheless, it has been postulated that small molecule inhibitors designed to compete with host proteins for binding to viral L-domains may effectively interfere with budding of viruses such as Ebola. Subsequent reduction in virus budding and spread may allow for clearance of the virus by the host immune system. Since diverse viruses including retroviruses, filoviruses, rhabdoviruses, and arenaviruses all utilize L-domains for efficient egress, the potential for such inhibitors to have a broad-based activity is intriguing.

7.6.2 Lipid Rafts

Lipid rafts have been implicated in serving as recruiting platforms for the assembly and budding of several RNA viruses (as reviewed[123]). Recent findings suggest that Ebola virus utilizes lipid raft domains for both entry and exit.[62] Indeed, VP40 and GP of Ebola virus have been detected in lipid raft domains in Ebola virus-infected cells.[62] It has been suggested that virus–host interactions between VP40 and tsg101, for example, may contribute to recruitment of viral components to lipid rafts.[62,115,124] Since VP40 interacts with host proteins typically found on endosomal membranes, the possibility that lipid raft domains present on endosomal membranes may be important for virus budding cannot be ruled out.[125]

In addition to L-domains, other regions of VP40 involved in membrane binding and oligomerization have been identified and are clearly important for VP40 function. For example, a recent study suggests that oligomeric forms of VP40 preferentially reside in lipid raft domains, and that membrane association and oligomerization of VP40 are dependent on the C-terminal 18 amino acids, particularly proline residues at positions 283 and 286.[124] Therefore, antiviral drugs targeting membrane binding and oligomerization domains of VP40, as well as those that can disrupt lipid raft stability, may represent attractive candidates for therapeutic intervention.

7.7 VACCINATION

While the pursuit of antivirals for Ebola virus is important and necessary, the gold standard for protection against any viral disease is vaccination. The quest for a vaccine against Ebola virus is an active area of investigation by many laboratories. Some of the ongoing approaches being employed to develop an effective vaccine for Ebola virus are highlighted below.

7.7.1 Replicons

The use of viral replicons has been explored as a strategy for developing an Ebola virus vaccine. The efficacy of replicon-based vaccines seems to be dependent on dosing, viral proteins utilized, and the animal choice of study. A replicon system based on the alphavirus Venezuelan equine encephalitis (VEE) virus is one of the best characterized. An important advantage of this replicon is that most animal populations have no preexisting immunity to VEE, and sequential immunization with the replicon does not induce VEE-specific antibodies.[126] In addition, VEE replicon particles (VRPs) have been shown to target expression of genes to the lymph nodes and to antigen-presenting dendritic cells, thereby inducing high levels of mucosal and cell-mediated immunity.[127]

Most studies involving VRP vaccination have examined the ability of filovirus GP and/or NP to elicit protective immune responses. For example, a study by Hevey and colleagues demonstrated that a VRP expressing Marburg virus GP conveyed complete protection to cynomolgus monkeys infected with Marburg virus. Furthermore, enhanced levels of protection were observed when NP was also expressed.[128] When a similar VRP-vaccination strategy was employed for Ebola virus, although VRPs expressing Ebola GP and/or NP were protective in rodents lethally challenged with Ebola virus,[129] the vaccine was not protective in cynomolgus monkeys.[18] This finding suggests that pathogenesis of Marburg and Ebola virus infection differs, perhaps with regard to infection course, tropism, and/or host responses. In a separate study, a bivalent VRP vaccine composed of the viral glycoproteins of both Lassa virus and Ebola virus proved to be protective in guinea pigs lethally challenged with Ebola virus. It should be noted that the vaccinated animals that did succumb to disease had no virus in their tissues upon post mortem analysis.[130]

Additional viral proteins, such as VP24, VP40, VP30, and VP35, have been explored as possible vaccine candidates. For example, VRPs expressing VP24 proved to be the best candidate to induce protection in BALB/c mice, with VP40 and VP30 yielding protection levels between 55% and 85% depending on dose numbers. In contrast, VP35 was the only protein offering protection in C57BL/6 mice.[131] Recombinant vaccinia viruses expressing NP, VP35, VP40, or VP24 did not elicit protection in guinea pigs lethally challenged with Ebola virus.[132,133] As the development of these types of vaccination strategies proceeds, it will be important to keep in mind that primate models remain essential for evaluation of these therapies for humans.

7.7.2 DNA Vaccines

DNA vaccines represent another approach to elicit protection against Ebola virus. Plasmids encoding either Ebola virus GP, or NP, were shown to be protective in lethally challenged mice and guinea pigs.[134,135] Working to improve the efficacy of current replicon-based vaccination strategies, two groups have combined DNA vaccination with replicon administration in a prime–boost manner. Sullivan and colleagues were successful in protecting macaques from challenge by administering a GP-expressing plasmid first, followed by a boost with a GP-expressing adenoviral vector. Indeed, high antibody titers and increased cytotoxic T-lymphocyte (CTL) responses were observed in fully protected animals.[136] A safety study involving 27 volunteers is underway for an initial evaluation of DNA primer vaccines in human subjects.[137] Most recently, it was determined that immunization of nonhuman primates with only the adenoviral component (ADV-GP or ADV-NP) of this prime–boost strategy induced a more rapid antibody response in animals, albeit less immunologically potent. Nonetheless, animals were protected against lethal challenge with virus.[138] The rapidity of this vaccination strategy makes it an attractive candidate for the containment of sudden outbreaks of Ebola virus.

7.7.3 Recombinant Vaccines

Researchers have also examined the potential of heterologous live viral vectors in effectively preventing Ebola virus infection. Vesicular stomatitis virus (VSV)-based vectors are fine contenders, as VSV is known to elicit strong antibody and cellular immune responses.[139] Rose and colleagues previously demonstrated that vaccination of mice with a recombinant VSV containing the glycoprotein of HIV-1 elicited high antibody titers as well as robust long-term memory and cellular immune responses.[140,141] Based on this strategy, Feldmann and colleagues have generated a recombinant VSV vector expressing the Ebola virus GP. Protection against lethal challenge was conferred within a month and animals required only a single administration.[30]

7.7.4 Ebola Virus VLPs

There is precedent in the literature for the use of VLPs as vaccines. Indeed, VLPs have been shown to generate humoral and cell-mediated immunity toward the viral components they are engineered to express.[142–146] Because coexpression of the Ebola virus proteins GP and VP40 have been shown to induce efficient formation of Ebola virus VLPs (eVLPs), and since both of these viral proteins are known to be immunogenic in animals, the use eVLPs as a vaccine is an important new area of investigation. The eVLPs generated by VP40 and GP coexpression are the most recently examined vaccine strategy being tested by researchers. For example, a study by Warfield and co-workers demonstrated the ability of eVLPs to activate dendritic cells in vitro, induce a transient activation (days 1–5 postadministration) of B and T cells in vaccinated BALB/c mice, and elicit a dose-dependent antibody response.[147] In a lethal challenge experiment, BALB/c mice vaccinated with 10 μg of eVLPs and subsequently infected with a high dose of Ebola virus (300 pfu) were 100% protected and showed no signs of morbidity for up to 28 days postchallenge.[147] These preliminary results are promising, although examination of the protective ability of these eVLPs in primates is necessary. Notably, a VLP vaccine developed for the treatment of papillomavirus infection has recently entered Phase III human trials, suggesting precedent for the efficacy of such a vaccine strategy.[137] This vaccine approach may be improved upon by incorporating other viral proteins, such as NP, into the delivered VLP to enhance CTL responses, or by incorporating viral genes from various strains of Ebola virus to generate a more comprehensive vaccine.

7.7.5 Cell-Mediated Immunity

For some time, development of a vaccine for Ebola virus had focused on the use of immune serum and elicitation of humoral responses as a defense. Because these therapies never proved to be completely successful in disease prevention, the need for robust cellular immune mechanisms was likely critical for efficient protection. Thus, several investigations into the role of cell-mediated immunity for protection against Ebola virus infections have been initiated. For example, adoptive transfer of CTLs from mice vaccinated with a VEE replicon encoding viral NP into naïve mice protected the recipients from lethal challenge with Ebola virus.[148] These findings provided definitive proof for a role of cell-mediated immunity in combating Ebola virus infection. With this knowledge, improvements to the aforementioned vaccine strategies have been attempted, focusing on induction of cellular immune responses. For example, immunization of mice with irradiated Ebola virus in liposomes (L) containing lipid A elicited CTL responses toward GP peptides.[149] Liposomes serve as vehicles for the transfer of viral antigens, and, upon delivery, these peptides enter the major histocompatibility complex (MHC) I pathway, thereby eliciting CTL responses.[150] Vaccination of mice with L-encapsidated irradiated Ebola virus protected mice from a 300-LD_{50} Ebola virus challenge, prevented the development of viremia, and generated CTLs to two GP peptides. Elicitation of GP CTLs appears to be due to the presence of the liposome, as immunization with unencapsidated virus did not generate CTLs.[151]

7.8 CONCLUSION

Numerous advances have been made in recent years concerning the development of effective antiviral drugs and vaccination strategies to protect against Ebola virus infection. The requirements for such strategies are multifaceted; while antivirals designed to treat the disease are clearly important, those that can prevent the establishment of disease will be more highly beneficial. Many of the preliminary studies to evaluate the efficacies of the treatments outlined here yielded promising results; however, more comprehensive studies in relevant animal models, while difficult, will be necessary before widespread use of these antivirals is realized. Ultimately, oral methods of administration may be essential for the effective treatment of large populations in the instance of a mass attack. Clearly, combination therapies capable of both targeting particular stages of the virus life cycle, thereby blocking replication, and altering disease pathogenesis to reduce symptoms remain our greatest hope in combating future filovirus outbreaks.

ACKNOWLEDGMENTS

The authors would like to thank Dr. Jason Paragas and Dr. Michael Bray for their critical evaluation of this chapter.

REFERENCES

1. Sanchez, A.; Khan, A. S.; Zaki, S. R.; Nabel, G. J.; Ksiazek, T. G.; et al. Filoviridae. In *Fields Virology*, Lippincott, Williams, & Wilkins, Philadelphia, 2001, pp. 1279–1304.

2. Johnson, K. M.; Lange, J. V.; Webb, P. A.; Murphy, F. A. Isolation and partial characterisation of a new virus causing acute haemorrhagic fever in Zaire. *Lancet* **1977**, *i*, 569–571.

3. Peters, C. J.; Khan, A. S. Filovirus diseases. *Curr. Top. Microbiol. Immunol.* **1999**, *235*, 85–95.

4. Jahrling, P. B.; Geisbert, T. W.; Dalgard, D. W.; Johnson, E. D.; Ksiazek, T. G.; et al. Preliminary report: isolation of Ebola virus from monkeys imported to USA. *Lancet* **1990**, *335*, 502–505.

5. Johnson, E.; Jaax, N.; White, J.; Jahrling, P. Lethal experimental infections of rhesus monkeys by aerosolized Ebola virus. *Int. J. Exp. Pathol.* **1995**, *76*, 227–236.

6. Jaax, N.; Jahrling, P.; Geisbert, T.; Geisbert, J.; Steele, K.; et al. Transmission of Ebola virus (Zaire strain) to uninfected control monkeys in a biocontainment laboratory [see comments]. *Lancet* **1995**, *346*, 1669–1671.

7. Belanov, E. F.; Muntianov, V. P.; Kriuk, V. D.; Sokolov, A. V.; Bormotov, N. I.; et al. Survival of Marburg virus infectivity on contaminated surfaces and in aerosols. *Vopr. Virusol.* **1996**, *41*, 32–34.

8. Feldmann, H.; Klenk, H.-D. Marburg and Ebola viruses. *Adv. Virus Res.* **1996**, *47*, 1–52.

9. Bray, M. Filoviridae. In *Clinical Virology*, 2nd ed., ASM Press, Washington, DC, 2002, pp. 875–890.

10. Colebunders, R.; Borchert, M. Ebola haemorrhagic fever—a review. *J. Infect.* **2000**, *40*, 16–20.

11. Rotz, L.; Khan, A.; Lillibridge, S.; Ostroff, S.; Hughes, J. Public health assessment of potential biological terrorism agents. *Emerging Infect. Dis.* **2002**, *8*, 225–229.

12. Borio, L.; Inglesby, T.; Peters, C. J.; et al. Hemorrhagic fever viruses as biological weapons—medical and public health management. *JAMA* **2002**, *287*, 2391–2405.

13. Alibek, J.; Handelman, S. *Biohazard*, Random House, New York, 1999.

14. Bray, M. Defense against filoviruses used as biological weapons. *Antiviral Res.* **2003**, *57*, 53–60.

15. Volchkov, V. E.; Chepurnov, A. A.; Volchkova, V. A.; Ternovoi, V. A.; Klenk, H.-D. Molecular characterisation of guinea pig-adapted variants of Ebola virus. *Virology* **2000**, *277*, 147–155.

16. Hart, M. K. Vaccine research efforts for filoviruses. *Int. J. Parasitol.* **2003**, *33*, 583–595.

17. Parren, P. W. H. I.; Geisbert, T. W.; Maruyama, T.; Jahrling, P. B.; Burton, D. R. Pre- and postexposure prophylaxis of Ebola virus infection in an animal model by passive transfer of a neutralizing human antibody. *J. Virol.* **2002**, *76*, 6408–6412.

18. Geisbert, T. W.; Pushko, P.; Anderson, K.; Smith, J.; Davis, K. J.; et al. Evaluation in nonhuman primates of vaccines against Ebola virus. *Emerging Infect. Dis.* **2002**, *8*, 503–507.

19. Mupapa, K.; Massamba, M.; Kibadi, K.; Kuvula, K.; Bwaka, A.; et al. Treatment of Ebola hemorrhagic fever with blood transfusions from convalescent patients. International Scientific and Technical committee. *J. Infect. Dis.* **1999**, *179* (Suppl. 1), 18–23.

20. Sadek, R. F.; Khan, A. S.; Stevens, G.; Peters, C. J. Ebola hemorrhagic fever, Democratic Republic of Congo, 1995: determinants of survival. *J. Infect. Dis.* **1999**, *179* (Suppl. 1), S24–27.

21. Jahrling, P. B.; Geisbert, T. W.; Geisbert, J. B.; Swearengen, J. R.; Bray, M.; et al. Evaluation of immune globulin and recombinant interferon-alpha2b for treatment of experimental Ebola virus infections. *J. Infect. Dis.* **1999**, *179* (Suppl. 1), S224–234.

22. Hevey, M.; Negley, D.; Geisbert, J.; Jahrling, P. B.; Schmaljohn, A. Antigenicity and vaccine potential of Marburg virus glycoprotein expressed by baculovirus recombinants. *Virology* **1997**, *239*, 206–216.

23. Jahrling, P. B.; Geisbert, J.; Swearengen, J. R.; Jaax, G. P.; Lewis, T.; et al. Passive immunization of Ebola virus-infected cynomolgus monkeys with immunoglobulin from hyperimmune horses. *Arch. Virol. Suppl.* **1996**, *11*, 135–140.

24. Kudoyarova-Zubavichene, N. M.; Sergeyev, N. N.; Chepurnov, A. A.; Netesov, S. V. Preparation and use of hyperimmune serum for prophylaxis and therapy of Ebola virus infections. *J. Infect. Dis.* **1999**, *179* (Suppl. 1), S218–223.

25. Gupta, M.; Mahanty, S.; Bray, M.; Ahmed, R.; Rollin, P. E. Passive transfer of antibodies protects immunocompetent and immunodeficient mice against lethal Ebola virus infection without complete inhibition of viral replication. *J. Virol.* **2001**, *75*, 4649–4654.

26. Ksiazek, T. G.; Rollin, P. E.; Williams, A. J.; Bressler, D. S.; Martin, M. L.; et al. Clinical virology of Ebola hemorrhagic fever (EHF): virus, virus antigen, and IgG and IgM antibody findings among EHF patients in Kikwit, Democratic Republic of the Congo, 1995. *J. Infect. Dis.* **1999**, *179* (Suppl. 1), S177–198.

27. Baize, S.; Leroy, E. M.; Georges-Courbot, M. C.; Capron, M.; Lansoud-Soukate, J.; et al. Defective humoral responses and extensive intravascular apoptosis are associated with fatal outcome in Ebola virus-infected patients. *Nat. Med.* **1999**, *5*, 423–426.

28. Wilson, J. A.; Hevey, M.; Bakken, R.; Guest, S.; Bray, M.; et al. Epitopes involved in antibody-mediated protection from Ebola virus. *Science* **2000**, *287*, 1664–1666.

29. Maruyama, T.; Rodriguez, L. L.; Jahrling, P. B.; Sanchez, A.; Khan, A. S.; et al. Ebola virus can be effectively neutralized by antibody produced in natural human infection. *J. Virol.* **1999**, *73*, 6024–6030.

30. Enserink, M. New vaccine and treatment excite Ebola researchers. *Science* **2003**, *302*, 1141–1142.

31. Takada, A.; Kawaoka, Y. The pathogenesis of Ebola hemorrhagic fever. *Trends Microbiol.* **2001**, *9*, 506–511.

32. Porterfield, J. S. Antibody-dependent enhancement of viral infectivity. *Adv. Virus Res.* **1986**, *31*, 335–355.

33. Takada, A.; Watanabe, S.; Okazaki, K.; Kida, H.; Kawaoka, Y. Infectivity-enhancing antibodies to Ebola virus glycoprotein. *J. Virol.* **2001**, *75*, 2324–2330.

34. Takada, A.; Kawaoka, Y. Antibody-dependent enhancement of viral infection: molecular mechanisms and *in vivo* implications. *Rev. Med. Virol.* **2003**, *13*, 387–398.

35. Boyd, M. R.; Gustafson, K. R.; McMahon, J. B.; Shoemaker, R. H.; O'Keefe, B. R.; et al. Discovery of cyanovirin-N, a novel human immunodeficiency virus-inactivating protein that binds viral surface envelope glycoprotein gp120: potential applications to microbicide development. *Antimicrob. Agents Chemother.* **1997**, *41*, 1521–1530.

36. Feldmann, H.; Volchkov, V. E.; Volchkova, V. A.; Klenk, H.-D. The glycoproteins of Marburg and Ebola virus and their potential roles in pathogenesis. *Arch. Virol. Suppl.* **1999**, *15*, 159–169.

37. Barrientos, L. G.; O'Keefe, B. R.; Bray, M.; Sanchez, A.; Gronenborn, A. M.; et al. Cyanovirin-N binds to the viral surface glycoprotein, $GP_{1,2}$ and inhibits infectivity of Ebola virus. *Antiviral Res.* **2003**, *58*, 47–56.

38. Barrientos, L. G.; Lasala, F.; Otero, J. R.; Sanchez, A.; Delgado, R. In vitro evaluation of cyanovirin-N antiviral activity, by use of lentiviral vectors pseudotyped with filovirus envelope glycoproteins. *J. Infect. Dis.* **2004**, *189*, 1440–1443.

39. Chan, S. Y.; Empig, C. J.; Welte, F. J.; Speck, R. F.; Schmaljohn, A.; et al. Folate receptor-alpha is a cofactor for cellular entry by Marburg and Ebola viruses. *Cell* **2001**, *106*, 117–126.

40. Simmons, G.; Rennekamp, A. J.; Chai, N.; Vandenberghe, L. H.; Riley, J. L.; et al. Folate receptor alpha and caveolae are not required for Ebola virus glycoprotein-mediated viral infection. *J. Virol.* **2003**, *77*, 13433–13438.

41. Ryabchikova, A. I.; Kolesnikova, L. V.; Netesov, S. V. Animal pathology of filoviral infections. *Curr. Top. Microbiol. Immunol.* **1999**, *235*, 145–173.

42. Takada, A.; Watanabe, S.; Ito, H.; Okazaki, K.; Kida, H.; et al. Downregulation of beta-1 integrins by Ebola virus glycoprotein: implication for virus entry. *Virology* **2000**, *278*, 20–26.

43. Alvarez, C. P.; Lasala, F.; Carrillo, J.; Muniz, O.; Corbi, A. L.; et al. C-type lectins DC-SIGN and L-SIGN mediate cellular entry by Ebola virus in *cis* and in *trans*. *J. Virol.* **2002**, *76*, 6841–6844.

44. Simmons, G.; Reeves, J. D.; Grogan, C. C.; Vandenberghe, L. H.; Baribaud, F.; et al. DC-SIGN and DC-SIGNR bind Ebola glycoproteins and enhance infection of macrophages and endothelial cells. *Virology* **2003**, *305*, 115–123.

45. Bezouska, K. Design, functional evaluation and biomedical application of carbohydrate dendrimers (glycodendrimers). *J. Biotechnol.* **2002**, *90*, 269–290.

46. Arce, E.; Nieto, P. M.; Diaz, V.; Garcia-Castro, R.; Bernad, A.; et al. Glycodendritic structures based on Boltorn hyperbranched polymers and their interactions with Lens culinaris lectin. *Bioconjug. Chem.* **2003**, *14*, 817–823.

47. Reuter, J. D.; Myc, A.; Hayes, M. M.; Gan, Z.; Roy, R.; et al. Inhibition of viral adhesion and infection by sialic acid-conjugated dendritic polymers. *Bioconjug. Chem.* **1999**, *10*, 271–278.

48. Landers, J. J.; Cao, Z.; Lee, I.; Piehler, L. T.; Myc, P. P.; et al. Prevention of influenza pneumonitis by sialic acid-conjugated dendritic polymers. *J. Infect. Dis.* **2002**, *186*, 1222–1230.

49. Lasala, F.; Arce, E.; Otero, J. R.; Rojo, J.; Delgado, R. Mannosyl glycodendritic structure inhibits DC-SIGN-mediated Ebola virus infection in *cis* and in *trans*. *Antimicrob. Agents Chemother.* **2003**, *47*, 3970–3972.

50. Volchkov, V. E.; Feldmann, H.; Volchkova, V. A.; Klenk, H.-D. Processing of the Ebola virus glycoprotein by the proprotein convertase furin. *Proc. Natl. Acad. Sci. U.S.A.* **1998**, *95*, 5762–5767.

51. Malashkevich, V. N.; Schneider, B. J.; McNally, M. L.; Milhollen, M. A.; Pang, J. X.; et al. Core structure of the envelope glycoprotein GP2 from Ebola virus at 1.9-angstrom resolution. *Proc. Natl. Acad. Sci. U.S.A.* **1999**, *96*, 2662–2667.

52. Weissenhorn, W.; Carfi, A.; Lee, K.-H.; Skehel, J.; Wiley, D. C. Crystal structure of the Ebola virus membrane fusion subunit, GP2, from the envelope glycoprotein ectodomain. *Mol. Cell* **1998**, *2*, 605–616.

53. Kilby, J. M.; Hopkins, S.; Venetta, T. M.; DiMassimo, B.; Cloud, G. A.; et al. Potent suppression of HIV-1 replication in humans by T-20, a peptide inhibitor of gp41-mediated virus entry. *Nat. Med.* **1998**, *4*, 1302–1307.

54. Chan, D. C.; Chutkowski, C. T.; Kim, P. S. Evidence that a prominent cavity in the coiled coil of HIV type 1 gp41 is an attractive drug target. *Proc. Natl. Acad. Sci. U.S.A.* **1998**, *95*, 15613–15617.

55. Watanabe, S.; Takada, A.; Watanabe, T.; Ito, H.; Kida, H.; et al. Functional importance of the coiled-coil of the Ebola virus glycoprotein. *J. Virol.* **2000**, *74*, 10194–10201.

56. Chan, D. C.; Kim, P. S. HIV entry and its inhibition. *Cell* **1998**, *93*, 681–684.

57. Takada, A.; Robison, C.; Goto, H.; Sanchez, A.; Murti, K. G.; et al. A system for functional analysis of Ebola virus glycoprotein. *Proc. Natl. Acad. Sci. U.S.A.* **1997**, *94*, 14764–14769.

58. Wool-Lewis, R. J.; Bates, P. Characterization of Ebola virus entry by using pseudo-typed viruses: identification of receptor-deficient cell lines. *J. Virol.* **1998**, *72*, 3155–3160.

59. Simons, K.; Toomre, D. Lipid rafts and signal transduction. *Nat. Rev. Immunol.* **2000**, *1*, 31–39.

60. Campbell, S. M.; Crowe, S. M.; Mak, J. Lipid rafts and HIV-1: from viral assembly to assembly of progeny virions. *J. Clin. Virol.* **2001**, *22*, 217–227.

61. Empig, C. J.; Goldsmith, M. A. Association of the caveola vesicular system with cellular entry by filoviruses. *J. Virol.* **2002**, *76*, 5266–5270.

62. Bavari, S.; Bosio, C. M.; Wiegand, E.; Ruthel, G.; Will, A. B.; et al. Lipid raft microdomains: a gateway for compartmentalized trafficking of Ebola and Marburg viruses. *J. Exp. Med.* **2002**, *195*, 593–602.

63. Muhlberger, E.; Weik, M.; Volchkov, V.; Klenk, H.-D.; Becker, S. Comparison of transcription and replication strategies of Marburg and Ebola virus by using artificial replication systems. *J. Virol.* **1999**, *73*, 2333–2342.

64. Weik, M.; Modrof, J.; Klenk, H.-D.; Becker, S.; Muhlberger, E. Ebola virus VP30-mediated transcription is regulated by RNA secondary structure formation. *J. Virol.* **2002**, *76*, 8532–8539.

65. Modrof, J.; Muhlberger, E.; Klenk, H.-D.; Becker, S. Phosphorylation of VP30 impairs Ebola virus transcription. *J. Biol. Chem.* **2002**, *277*, 33099–33104.

66. Bialojin, C.; Takai, A. Inhibitory effect of a marine-sponge toxin, okadaic acid, on protein phosphatases. Specificity and kinetics. *Biochem. J.* **1988**, *256*, 283–290.

67. Nagao, M.; Shima, H.; Nakayasu, M.; Sugimura, T. Protein serine/threonine phosphatases as binding proteins for okadaic acid. *Mutat. Res.* **1995**, *333*, 173–179.

68. Suganuma, M.; Fujiki, H.; Suguri, H.; Yoshizawa, S.; Hirota, M.; et al. Okadaic acid: an additional non-phorbol-12-tetradecanoate-13-acetate-type tumor promoter. *Proc. Natl. Acad. Sci. U.S.A.* **1988**, *85*, 1768–1771.

69. Hartlieb, B.; Modroft, J.; Muhlberger, C.; Klenk, H.-D.; Becker, S. Oligomerization of Ebola virus VP30 is essential for viral transcription and can be inhibited by a synthetic peptide. *J. Biol. Chem.* **2003**, *278*, 41830–41836.

70. Huggins, J. W. Prospects for treatment of viral hemorrhagic fevers with ribavirin, a broad-spectrum antiviral drug. *Rev. Infect. Dis.* **1989**, *11* (Suppl 4), S750–761.

71. Ignatyev, G.; Steinkasserer, A.; Streltsova, M.; Atrasheuskaya, A.; Agafonov, A.; et al. Experimental study on the possibility of treatment of some hemorrhagic fevers. *J. Biotechnol.* **2000**, *83*, 67–76.

72. Wolfe, M.; Borchardt, R. *S*-adenosyl-L-homocysteine hydrolase as a target for antiviral chemotherapy. *Med. Chem.* **1991**, *34*, 1523–1530.

73. De Clercq, E. Molecular targets for antiviral agents. *J. Pharmacol. Exp. Ther.* **2001**, *297*, 1–10.

74. Tseng, C. K. H.; Marquez, V. E.; Fuller, R. W.; Goldstein, B. M.; Haines, D. R.; et al. Synthesis of 3 deazaneplanocin a powerful inhibitor of *S*-adenosylhomocysteine hydrolase with potent and selective in-vitro and in-vivo antiviral activities. *J. Med. Chem.* **1989**, *32*, 1442–1446.

75. Huggins, J. W.; Zhang, Z.; Monath, T. I. Inhibition of Ebola virus replication in vitro and in a SCID mouse model by *S*-adenosylhomocysteine hydrolase inhibitors. *Antiviral Res. Suppl.* **1995**, *1*, 122.

76. Huggins, J.; Zhang, Z. X.; Bray, M. Antiviral drug therapy of filovirus infections: *S*-adenosylhomocysteine hydrolase inhibitors inhibit Ebola virus in vitro and in a lethal mouse model. J. Infect. Dis. **1999**, *179* (Suppl. 1), S240–247.

77. Bray, M.; Driscoll, J.; Huggins, J. W. Treatment of lethal Ebola virus infection in mice with a single dose of an *S*-adenosyl-L-homocysteine hydrolase inhibitor. *Antiviral Res.* **2000**, *45*, 135–147.

78. Elbashir, S. M. Duplexes of 21-nucleotide RNAs mediate RNA interference in cultured mammalian cells. *Nature* **2001**, *411*, 494–498.

79. Jacque, J.-M.; Triques, K.; Stevenson, M. Modulation of HIV-1 replication by RNA interference. *Nature* **2002**, *418*, 435–438.

80. Bray, M.; Paragas, J. Experimental therapy of filovirus infections. *Antiviral Res.* **2002**, *54*, 1–17.

81. Boden, D.; Pusch, O.; Silbermann, R.; Lee, F.; Tucker, L.; et al. Enhanced gene silencing of HIV-1 specific siRNA using microRNA designed hairpins. *Nucleic Acids Res.* **2004**, *32*, 1154–1158.

82. Zaki, S. R.; Goldsmith, M. A. Pathologic features of filovirus infections in humans. *Curr. Top. Microbiol. Immunol.* **1998**, *235*, 97–116.

83. Geisbert, T. W.; Young, H. A.; Jahrling, P. B.; Davis, K. J.; Larsen, T.; et al. Pathogenesis of Ebola hemorrhagic fever in primate models: evidence that hemorrhage is not a direct effect of virus-induced cytolysis of endothelial cells. *Am. J. Pathol.* **2003**, *163*, 2371–2382.

84. Ruszczak, Z.; Schwartz, R. A. Vascular endothelium in the regulation of immune response. *Res. Commun. Mol. Pathol. Pharmacol.* **1996**, *94*, 3–21.

85. Sen, G. C. Viruses and interferons. *Annu. Rev. Microbiol.*. **2001**, *55*, 255–281.

86. Katze, H. The war against the interferon-induced dsRNA-activated protein kinase: can viruses win? *J. Interferon Res.* **1992**, *12*, 241–248.

87. Harcourt, B. H.; Sanchez, A.; Offermann, M. K. Ebola virus inhibits induction of genes by double-stranded RNA in endothelial cells. *Virology* **1998**, *252*, 179–188.

88. Harcourt, B. H.; Sanchez, A.; Offermann, M. K. Ebola virus selectively inhibits responses to interferons but not to interleukin-1B, in endothelial cells. *J. Virol.* **1999**, *73*, 3491–3496.

89. Basler, C. F.; Wang, X.; Muhlberger, E.; Volchkov, V.; Paragas, J.; et al. The Ebola virus VP35 protein functions as a type I IFN antagonist. *Proc. Natl. Acad. Sci. U.S.A.* **2000**, *97*, 12289–12294.

90. Basler, C. F.; Palese, P. Modulation of innate immunity by filoviruses. In *Ebola and Marburg Viruses: Molecular and Cellular Biology*, Horizon Bioscience, Norwich, UK, 2004.

91. Basler, C. F.; Mikulasova, A.; Martinez-Sobrido, L.; Paragas, J.; Muhlberger, E.; et al. The Ebola virus VP35 protein inhibits activation of interferon regulatory factor 3. *J. Virol.* **2003**, *77*, 7945–7956.

92. Barnes, B.; Lubyova, B.; Pitha, P. M. On the role of IRF in host defense. *J. Interferon Cytokine Res.* **2002**, *22*, 59–71.

93. Bray, M. The role of the type I interferon response in the resistance of mice to filovirus infection. *J. Gen. Virol.* **2001**, *82*, 1365–1373.

94. Bray, M.; Raymond, J. L.; Geisbert, T.; Baker, R. O. 3-Deazaneplanocin A induces massively increased interferon-alpha production in Ebola virus-infected mice. *Antiviral Res.* **2002**, *55*, 151–159.

95. Lambert, L.; Frondorf, K.; Berling, J.; Wolos, J. Effects of an *S*-adenosyl-L-homocysteine hydrolase inhibitor on murine macrophage activation and function. *Immunopharmacology* **1995**, *29*, x–x.

96. Schmidt, J.; Bomford, R.; Gao, X.; Rhodes, J. 3-Deazaadenosine—an inhibitor of interleukin 1 production by human peripheral blood monocytes. *Int. J. Immunopharmacol.* **1990**, *12*, 89–97.

97. Sergeev, A. N.; Ryzhikov, A. B.; Bulychev, L. E.; Evtin, N. K.; P'iankov, O. V.; et al. [Study of the treatment-prophylactic effect of immunomodulators in experimental infections, caused by Marburg, Ebola, and Venezuelan equine encephalitis viruses]. *Vopr. Virusol.* **1997**, *42*, 226–229.

98. Ignat'ev, G. M.; Strel'tsova, M. A.; Agafonov, A. P.; Kashentseva, E. A.; Prozorovskii, N. S. [Experimental study of possible treatment of Marburg hemorrhagic fever with desferal, ribavirin, and homologous interferon]. *Vopr. Virusol.* **1996**, *41*, 206–209.

99. Nichani, A. K.; Kaushik, R. S.; Mena, A.; Popowych, Y.; Dent, D.; et al. CpG oligodeoxynucleotide induction of antiviral effector molecules in sheep. *Cell. Immunol.* **2004**, *227*, 24–37.

100. Klinman, D. M.; Verthelyi, D.; Takeshita, F.; Ishii, K. J. Immune recognition of foreign DNA: a cure for bioterrorism? *Immunity* **1999**, *11*, 123–129.

101. Arai, A.; Hirano, H.; Ueta, Y.; Hamada, T.; Mita, T.; et al. Detection of mononuclear cells as the source of the increased tissue factor mRNA in the liver from lipopolysaccharide-treated rats. *Thromb. Res.* **2000**, *97*, 153–162.

102. Geisbert, T. W.; Young, H. A.; Jahrling, P. B.; Davis, K. J.; Kagan, E.; et al. Mechanism underlying coagulation abnormalities in Ebola hemorrhagic fever: overexpression of tissue factor in primate monocytes/macrophages. *J. Infect. Dis.* **2003**, *188*, 1618–1629.

103. Vlasuk, G. P.; Rote, W. E. Inhibition of factor VIIa/tissue factor with nematode anticoagulant protein c2: from unique mechanism to a promising new clinical anticoagulant. *Trends Cardiovasc. Med.* **2002**, *12*, 325–331.

104. Geisbert, T. W.; Hensley, L. E.; Jahrling, P. B.; Larsen, T.; Geisbert, J. B.; et al. Treatment of Ebola virus infection with a recombinant inhibitor of factor VIIa/tissue factor: a study in rhesus monkeys. *Lancet* **2003**, *362*, 1953–1958.

105. de Jonge, E.; Friederich, P. W.; Vlasuk, G. P.; Rote, W. E.; Vroom, M. B.; et al. Activation of coagulation by administration of recombinant factor VIIa elicits interleukin 6 (IL-6) and IL-8 release in healthy human subjects. *Clin. Diagn. Lab. Immunol.* **2003**, *10*, 495–497.

106. Geisbert, T. W.; Hensley, L. E.; Gibb, T. R.; Steele, K. E.; Jaax, N. K.; et al. Apoptosis induced in vitro and in vivo during infection by Ebola and Marburg viruses. *Lab. Invest.* **2000**, *80*, 171–186.

107. Geisbert, T. W.; Hensley, L. E.; Larsen, T.; Young, H. A.; Reed, D. S.; et al. Pathogenesis of Ebola hemorrhagic fever in cynomolgus macaques. *Am. J. Pathol.* **2003**, *163*, 2347–2370.

108. Connolly, B. M.; Steele, K. E.; Davis, K. J.; Geisbert, T. W.; Kell, W. M.; et al. Pathogenesis of experimental Ebola virus infection in guinea pigs. *J. Infect. Dis.* **1999**, *179* (Suppl. 1), S203–217.

109. Hensley, L. E.; Young, H. A.; Jahrling, P. B.; Geisbert, T. W. Proinflammatory response during Ebola virus infection of primate models: possible involvement of the tumor necrosis factor receptor superfamily. *Immunol. Lett.* **2002**, *80*, 169–179.

110. Volchkov, V. E. Processing of the Ebola virus glycoprotein. *Curr. Top. Microbiol. Immunol.* **1999**, *235*, 35–47.

111. Harty, R. N.; Brown, M. E.; Wang, G.; Huibregtse, J.; Hayes, F. P. A PPxY motif within the VP40 protein of Ebola virus interacts physically and functionally with a ubiquitin ligase: implications for filovirus budding. *Proc. Natl. Acad. Sci. U.S.A.* **2000**, *97*, 13871–13876.

112. Timmins, J.; Scianimanico, S.; Schoehn, G.; Weissenhorn, W. Vesicular release of Ebola virus matrix protein VP40. *Virology* **2001**, *283*, 1–6.

113. Noda, T.; Sagara, H.; Suzuki, E.; Takada, A.; Kida, H.; et al. Ebola virus VP40 drives the formation of virus-like filamentous particles along with GP. *J. Virol.* **2002**, *76*, 4855–4865.

114. Jasenosky, L. D.; Neumann, G.; Lukashevich, I.; Kawaoka, Y. Ebola virus VP40-induced particle formation and association with the lipid bilayer. *J. Virol.* **2001**, *75*, 5205–5214.

115. Licata, J. M.; Simpson-Holley, M.; Wright, N. T.; Han, Z.; Paragas, J.; et al. Overlapping motifs (PTAP and PPEY) within the Ebola virus VP40 protein function independently as late budding domains: involvement of host proteins tsg101 and vps-4. *J. Virol.* **2003**, *77*, 1812–1819.

116. Freed, E. O. Viral late domains. *J. Virol.* **2002**, *76*, 4679–4687.

117. Garrus, J. E.; von Schwedler, U. K.; Pornillos, O. W.; Morham, S. G.; Zavitz, K. H.; et al. Tsg101 and the vacuolar protein sorting pathway are essential for HIV-1 budding. *Cell* **2001**, *107*, 55–65.

118. Martin-Serrano, J.; Zang, T.; Bieniasz, P. D. HIV-1 and Ebola virus encode small peptide motifs that recruit tsg101 to sites of particle assembly to facilitate egress. *Nat. Med.* **2001**, *7*, 1313–1319.

119. Timmins, J.; Schoehn, G.; Ricard-Blum, S.; Scianimanico, S.; Vernet, T.; et al. Ebola virus matrix protein VP40 interaction with human cellular factors tsg101 and nedd4. *J. Mol. Biol.* **2003**, *326*, 493–502.

120. Harty, R. N.; Paragas, J.; Sudol, M.; Palese, P. A proline-rich motif within the matrix protein of vesicular stomatitis virus and rabies virus interacts with WW domains of cellular proteins: implications for viral budding. *J. Virol.* **1999**, *73*, 2921–2929.

121. Kikonyogo, A.; Bouamr, F.; Vana, M. L.; Xiang, Y.; Aiyar, A.; et al. Proteins related to the Nedd4 family of ubiquitin protein ligases interact with the L domain of Rous sarcoma virus and are required for gag budding from cells. *Proc. Natl. Acad. Sci. U.S.A.* **2001**, *98*, 11199–11204.

122. Yasuda, J.; Nakao, M.; Kawaoka, Y.; Shida, H. Nedd4 regulates egress of Ebola virus-like particles from host cells. *J. Virol.* **2003**, *77*, 9987–9992.

123. Briggs, J. A. G.; Wilk, T.; Fuller, S. D. Do lipid rafts mediate virus assembly and pseudotyping? *J. Gen. Virol.* **2003**, *84*, 757–768.

124. Panchal, R. G.; Ruthel, G.; Kenny, T. A.; Kallstrom, G. H.; Lane, D.; et al. *In vivo* oligomerization and raft localization of Ebola virus protein VP40 during vesicular budding. *Proc. Natl. Acad. Sci. U.S.A.* **2003**, *100*, 15936–15941.

125. Kolesnikova, L.; Bugany, H.; Klenk, H.-D.; Becker, S. VP40, the matrix protein of Marburg virus is associated with membranes of the late endosomal compartment. *J. Virol.* **2002**, *76*, 1825–1838.

126. Pushko, P.; Parker, M.; Ludwig, G. V.; Davis, N. L.; Johnston, R. E.; et al. Replicon-helper systems from attenuated Venezuelan equine encephalitis virus: expression of heterologous genes in vitro and immunization against heterologous pathogens in vivo. *Vaccine* **1997**, *239*, 389–401.

127. MacDonald, G. H.; Johnston, R. E. Role of dendritic cell targeting in Venezuelan equine encephalitis virus. *J. Virol.* **2000**, *74*, 914–922.

128. Hevey, M.; Negley, D.; Pushko, P.; Smith, J.; Schmaljohn, A. Marburg virus vaccines based upon alphavirus replicons protect guinea pigs and nonhuman primates. *Virology* **1998**, *251*, 28–37.

129. Pushko, P.; Bray, M.; Ludwig, G. V.; Parker, M.; Schmaljohn, A.; et al. Recombinant RNA replicons derived from attenuated Venezuelan equine encephalitis virus protect guinea pigs and mice from Ebola hemorrhagic fever virus. *Vaccine* **2000**, *19*, 142–153.

130. Pushko, P.; Geisbert, J.; Parker, M.; Jahrling, P.; Smith, J. Individual and bivalent vaccines based on alphavirus replicons protect guinea pigs against infection with Lassa and Ebola viruses. *J. Virol.* **2001**, *75*, 11677–11685.

131. Wilson, J. A.; Bray, M.; Bakken, R.; Hart, M. K. Vaccine potential of Ebola virus VP24, VP30, VP35, and VP40 proteins. *Virology* **2001**, *286*, 384–390.

132. Gilligan, K. J.; Geisbert, J. B.; Jahrling, P. B.; Anderson, K. A. Assessment of protective immunity conferred by recombinant vaccinia viruses to guinea pigs challenged with Ebola virus. In *Vaccines 97*, Cold Spring Harbor Laboratory Press, Cold Spring Harbor, NY, 1997, pp. 87–92.

133. Chepurnov, A. A.; Ternovoi, V. A.; Dadaeva, A. A.; Dmitriev, I. P.; Sizikova, L. P.; et al. Immunobiological properties of VP24 protein of Ebola virus expressed by recombinant vaccinia virus. *Vopr. Virusol.* **1997**, *3*, 115–120.

134. Vanderzanden, L.; Bray, M.; Fuller, D.; Roberts, T.; Custer, D.; et al. DNA vaccines expressing either the GP or NP genes of Ebola virus protect mice from lethal challenge. *Virology* **1998**, *246*, 134–144.

135. Xu, L.; Sanchez, A.; Yang, Z.; Zaki, S. R.; Nabel, E. G.; et al. Immunization for Ebola virus infection. *Nat. Med.* **1998**, *4*, 16–17.

136. Sullivan, N.; Sanchez, A.; Rollin, P. E.; Yang, Z.; Nabel, G. J. Development of a preventive vaccine for Ebola virus infection in primates. *Nature* **2000**, *408*, 605–609.

137. Vastag, B. Ebola vaccines tested in humans, monkeys. *JAMA* **2004**, *291*, 549–550.

138. Sullivan, N. J.; Geisbert, T. W.; Geisbert, J. B.; Xu, L.; Yang, Z.; et al. Accelerated vaccination for Ebola virus haemorrhagic fever in non-human primates. *Nature* **2003**, *424*, 681–684.

139. Roberts, A.; Buonocore, L.; Price, R.; Forman, J.; Rose, J. K. Attenuated vesicular stomatitis viruses as vaccine vectors. *J. Virol.* **1999**, *73*, 3723–3732.

140. Haglund, K.; Leiner, I.; Kerksiek, K.; Buonocore, L.; Pamer, E.; et al. Robust recall and long-term memory T-cell responses induced by prime-boost regimens with heterologous live viral vectors expressing human immunodeficiency virus type 1 Gag and Env proteins. *J. Virol.* **2002**, *76*, 7506–7517.

141. Rose, N. F.; Roberts, A.; Buonocore, L.; Rose, J. K. Glycoprotein exchange vectors based on vesicular stomatitis virus allow effective boosting and generation of neutralizing antibodies to a primary isolate of human immunodeficiency virus type 1. *J. Virol.* **2000**, *74*, 10903–10910.

142. Palker, T. J.; Monteiro, J. M.; Martin, M. M.; Kakareka, C.; Smith, J. F.; et al. Antibody, cytokine, and cytotoxic T lymphocyte responses in chimpanzees immunized with human papillomavirus virus-like particles. *Vaccine* **2001**, *19*, 3733–3743.

143. Touze, A.; Dupuy, C.; Chabaud, M.; LeCann, P.; Coursaget, P. Production of human papillomavirus type 45 virus-like particles in insect cells using a recombinant baculovirus. *FEMS Microbiol. Lett.* **1996**, *141*, 111–116.

144. Buonaguro, L.; Buonaguro, F. M.; Tornesello, M. L.; Mantas, D.; Beth-Giraldo, E.; et al. High efficient production of Pr55(gag) virus-like particles expressing multiple HIV-1 epitopes, including a gp120 protein derived from an Ugandan HIV-1 isolate of subtype A. *Antiviral Res.* **2001**, *49*, 35–47.

145. Casal, J. I.; Rueda, P.; Hurtado, A. Parvovirus-like particles as vaccine vectors. *Methods* **1999**, *19*, 174–186.

146. Conner, M. E.; Zarley, C. D.; Hu, B.; Parsons, S.; Drabinski, D.; et al. Virus-like particles as a rotavirus subunit vaccine. *J. Infect. Dis.* **1996**, *174* (Suppl. 1), S88–92.

147. Warfield, K. L.; Bosio, C. M.; Welcher, B. C.; Deal, E. M.; Mohamadzadeh, M.; et al. Ebola virus-like particles protect from lethal Ebola virus infection. *Proc. Natl. Acad. Sci. U.S.A.* **2003**, *100*, 15889–15894.

148. Wilson, J. A.; Hart, M. K. Protection from Ebola virus mediated by cytotoxic T lymphocytes specific for the viral nucleoprotein. *J. Virol.* **2001**, *75*, 2660–2664.

149. Rao, M.; Matyas, G. R.; Grieder, F.; Anderson, K.; Jahrling, P. B.; et al. Cytotoxic T lymphocytes to Ebola Zaire virus are induced in mice by immunization with liposomes containing lipid A. *Vaccine* **1999**, *17*, 2991–2998.

150. Alving, C. R.; Koulchin, V.; Glenn, G. M.; Rao, M. Liposomes as carriers of peptide antigens: induction of antibodies and cytotoxic T lymphocytes to conjugated and unconjugated peptides. *Immunol. Rev.* **1995**, *145*, 5–31.

151. Rao, M.; Bray, M.; Alving, C. R.; Jahrling, P.; Matyas, G. R. Induction of immune responses in mice and monkeys to Ebola virus after immunization with liposome-encapsulated irradiated Ebola virus: protection in mice requires $CD4^+T$ cells. *J. Virol.* **2002**, *76*, 9176–9185.

EMERGING

EID
Online

INFECTIOUS DISEASES

A Peer-Reviewed Journal Tracking and Analyzing Disease Trends   Vol.8, No.5, May 2002

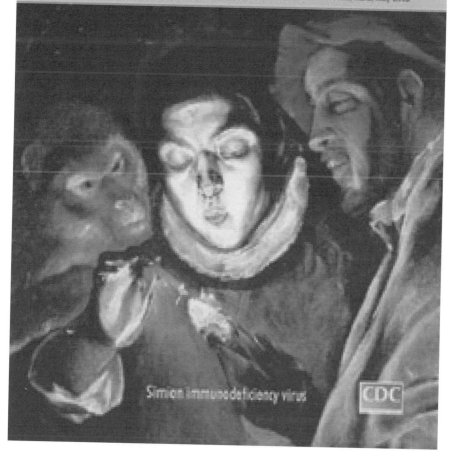

Simian immunodeficiency virus

CDC

CHAPTER 8

IMPDH Inhibitors: Discovery of Antiviral Agents Against Emerging Diseases

VASU NAIR

Department of Pharmaceutical and Biomedical Sciences and The Center for Drug Discovery, The University of Georgia

8.1 INTRODUCTION

While the discovery and development of various vaccines have provided successful therapeutic approaches to eradicate some serious viral pathogens such as smallpox, polio, measles, mumps, and rubella, there are many existing and emerging viruses that cause serious infectious diseases for which there are no vaccines or therapeutically effective antiviral agents. This is particularly so for some of the RNA viruses that are etiological agents for hemorrhagic fevers. In addition, some viruses, both existing and well-known and others that are emerging, may represent potential weapons of bioterrorism. This chapter presents a brief overview of these viruses and discusses the approach from our laboratory involving rational design, synthesis, and enzymology for the discovery of potential antiviral compounds directed at these viruses.

8.2 SELECTED VIRUSES

The genus *Orthopoxvirus* of the Poxviridae family of viruses includes variola, cowpox, vaccinia, and monkeypox viruses, all of which can cause human infections.[1-5] The etiologic agent of smallpox is the variola virus. Smallpox has killed tens of millions of people worldwide and, in addition, has disfigured innumerable millions.[1] Of the potential biological weapons of bioterrorism, smallpox poses one of the greatest threats,[6-8] because in the period between 1977 and 1979, it was

Antiviral Drug Discovery for Emerging Diseases and Bioterrorism Threats. Edited by Paul F. Torrence
Copyright © 2005 John Wiley & Sons, Inc.

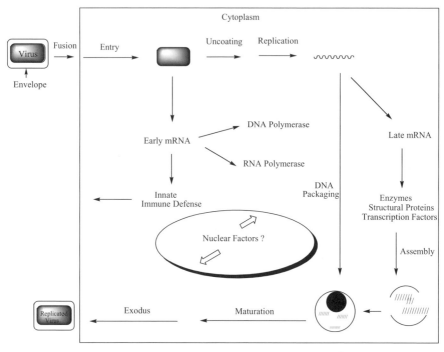

FIGURE 8.1 Replication cycle of the poxvirus.[1]

concluded that smallpox had been eradicated worldwide and vaccination programs were discontinued.[9] For this reason, a majority of the U.S. population and the world (estimated to be 80%) are vulnerable to smallpox.[8]

The genome of orthopoxviruses consists of linear, covalently closed, double-stranded DNA of approximately 200 kbp packaged in a large virion.[10] Viral DNA and RNA replication occurs in the cytoplasm (Figure 8.1).[1] Numerous proteins are present in virions, including a DNA-dependent DNA polymerase, a DNA-dependent RNA polymerase, mRNA guanine 7-methyltransferase, mRNA 2'-O-methyltransferase, and DNA topoisomerase. Other poxvirus-encoded enzymes include thymidine kinase and ribonucleotide reductase. The viral mRNAs are capped, polyadenylated at their 3' termini, and not spliced. Poxviruses are more complex in their replication than other DNA viruses and encode more viral enzymes for their replication. DNA replication, which is not fully understood, is directed mainly by viral enzymes and apparently involves a self-priming, strand displacement mechanism in which replicative intermediates serve as templates for the synthesis of genomic DNA.[10]

Of particular significance in the replication of poxviruses is that the DNA of poxviruses encode DNA-dependent RNA polymerases for the synthesis of mRNAs, which subsequently undergo processing called mRNA capping, and then are involved in the synthesis of the many viral proteins of these viruses.[10] This viral mRNA processing or capping is essential for viral replication (Figure 8.2).

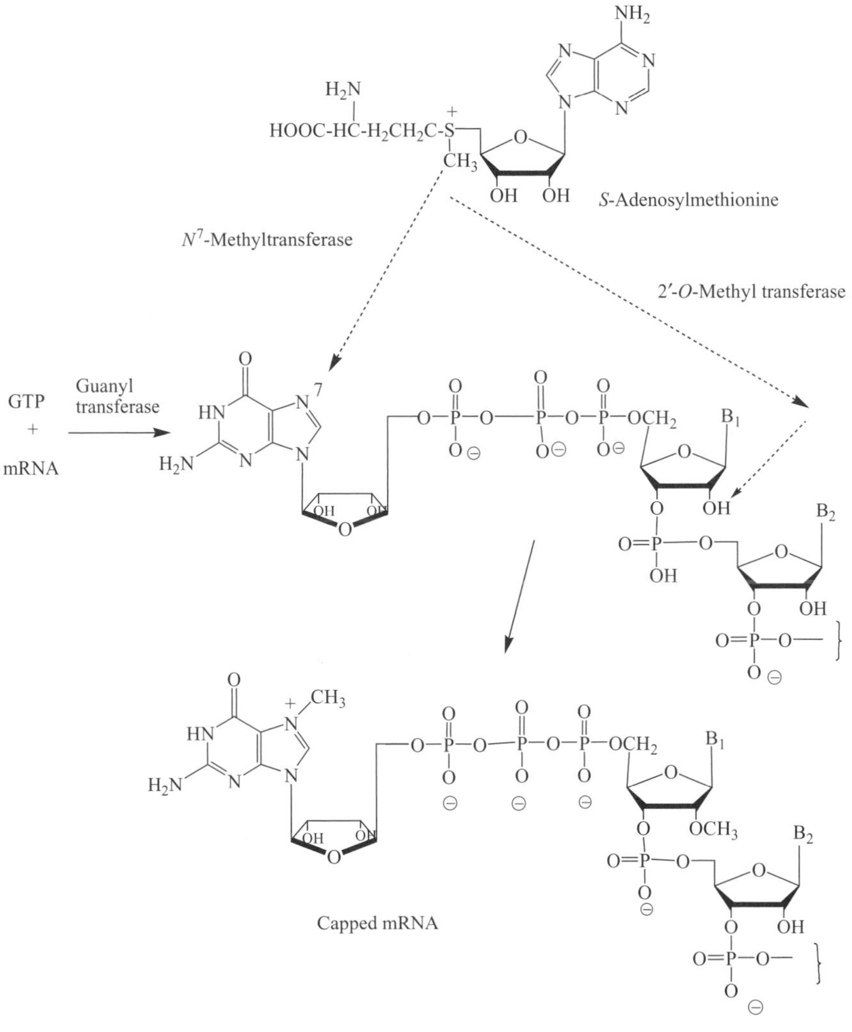

FIGURE 8.2 Chemistry of the capping of viral mRNA.

The family Filoviridae appears to have a single genus, *Filovirus*, and has two known species, Ebola and Marburg. They cause severe hemorrhagic fever with accompanying high rates of mortality.[11,12]

The Marburg virus was first recognized in 1967 and the Ebola virus in 1976. Although filoviruses are viewed with much fear and concern in Africa where they have been uncovered, they appear to be largely nonexistent in other parts of the world. However, the potential use of these viruses in warfare or bioterrorism is of very serious concern. There are no drugs available that provide significant therapeutic activity against the Marburg or Ebola virus.[13]

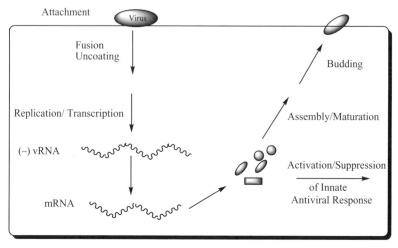

FIGURE 8.3 Replication of filoviruses.[12]

Filoviruses possess a single-stranded, negative-sense RNA genome that is approximately 19 kb.[12] The seven viral genes are arranged in a linear mode and the arrangement resembles that of paramyxoviruses. The replication of filoviruses (Figure 8.3) has a number of steps that can be targeted by antiviral agents and include, among others, attachment to receptor, fusion, transcription of viral genes, and viral mRNA methylation.[12] Two of the steps in the replication cycle of filoviruses, viral RNA-dependent RNA polymerase and viral RNA methylation, represent two potential biochemical points of attack in the rationale design of anti-filovirus agents. Inhibitors of IMPDH may also provide a possible mechanism for inhibition of filovirus replication (see Section 8.4 for a discussion of inhibitors of IMPDH).

In addition to the filoviruses, some other RNA viruses that cause viral hemorrhagic fevers include the flaviviruses (dengue and yellow fever), arenaviruses (Junin and Lassa), and bunyaviruses (Rift Valley fever and Hantavirus).[14] Infectious diseases caused by these viruses result in high mortality because of the lack of availability of therapeutic agents or vaccines. Because many of these viruses are stable and can be delivered by aerosol methods, they may also be considered as potential weapons of bioterrorism.

8.3 INOSINE MONOPHOSPHATE DEHYDROGENASE (IMPDH)

The enzyme inosine monophosphate dehydrogenase [IMPDH (EC 1.1.1.205)] catalyzes the conversion of IMP to XMP at the metabolic branch point in the de novo purine nucleotide synthetic pathway (Figure 8.4).[15–18] NAD$^+$ is the coenzyme for this conversion and is reduced to NADH. The enzymatic reaction and its inhibition can be observed by UV spectroscopy through monitoring of the

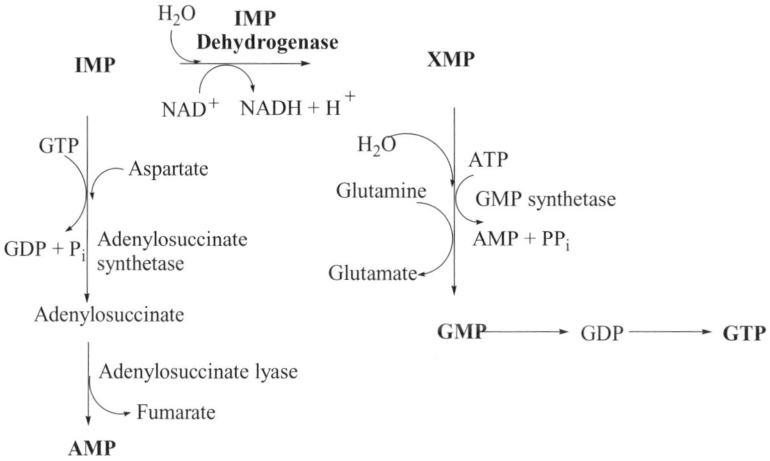

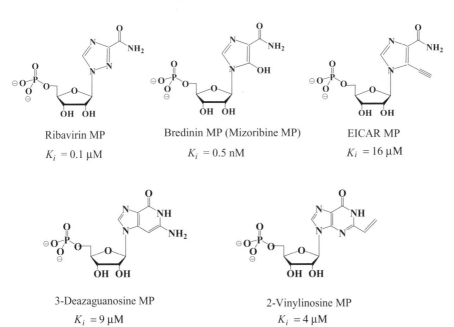

FIGURE 8.4 Conversion of IMP to GTP showing the role of IMPDH in GTP biosynthesis.

formation of NADH, which absorbs at 340 nm (discussed in Section 8.4.5 with the example of fluorovinylinosine). IMPDH has received considerable interest in recent years as an important target enzyme for cancer and antiviral therapies.[19–32] In support of this is the observation that compounds that are potent inhibitors of IMPDH as their monophosphates (Figure 8.5), such as ribavirin, tiazofurin,

Ribavirin MP

$K_i = 0.1\ \mu M$

Bredinin MP (Mizoribine MP)

$K_i = 0.5\ nM$

EICAR MP

$K_i = 16\ \mu M$

3-Deazaguanosine MP

$K_i = 9\ \mu M$

2-Vinylinosine MP

$K_i = 4\ \mu M$

FIGURE 8.5 Examples of some inhibitors of IMPDH (K_i values cited in Refs. 15,36,37, and 39).

3-deazaguanosine, bredinin (mizoribine), and 2-vinylinosine, have all shown broad-spectrum antiviral activity against a number of viruses including the vaccinia virus.[24,31,33-39] Inhibitors of IMPDH may also be of interest as antiviral agents for filoviruses and other viruses that cause hemorrhagic fevers.

Other support for using the IMPDH approach to drug discovery particularly against highly pathogenic RNA viruses comes from the suggestion that a common trait of many RNA viruses is a high frequency of mutation and a susceptibility to the phenomenon of error catastrophe.[40-43] Indeed, it has been suggested that animal RNA viruses maintain themselves on the borderline of error catastrophe.[40] Thus, it is of interest that the IMPDH inhibitor, ribavirin, produced positive responses when used in combination with interferon-α against chronic hepatitis C when patients did not respond to interferon alone.[44-46] It has also been suggested that in the case of the poliovirus and perhaps other RNA viruses, ribavirin may have a lethal mutagenic effect following its incorporation (via its triphosphate) into the viral genome catalyzed by the viral RNA-dependent RNA polymerase[41,42]. The result is to force the RNA viruses into a lethal accumulation of errors, which are augmented by reduction of GTP pools caused by the inhibition of IMPDH by ribavirin monophosphate.[47] The reason for this is that the decrease in the cellular GTP pools is likely to increase the frequency of incorporation of ribavirin triphosphate incorporation as a mutagenic GTP analogue.

The mechanism of the biochemical conversion of IMP to XMP catalyzed by IMPDH[15-18] involves interaction of the enzyme (Cys 331) and coenzyme (NAD$^+$) at the 2-position of IMP (Figure 8.6). It appears that the enzyme actually binds covalently at the 2-position of IMP through the sulfhydryl group of Cys 331. This is

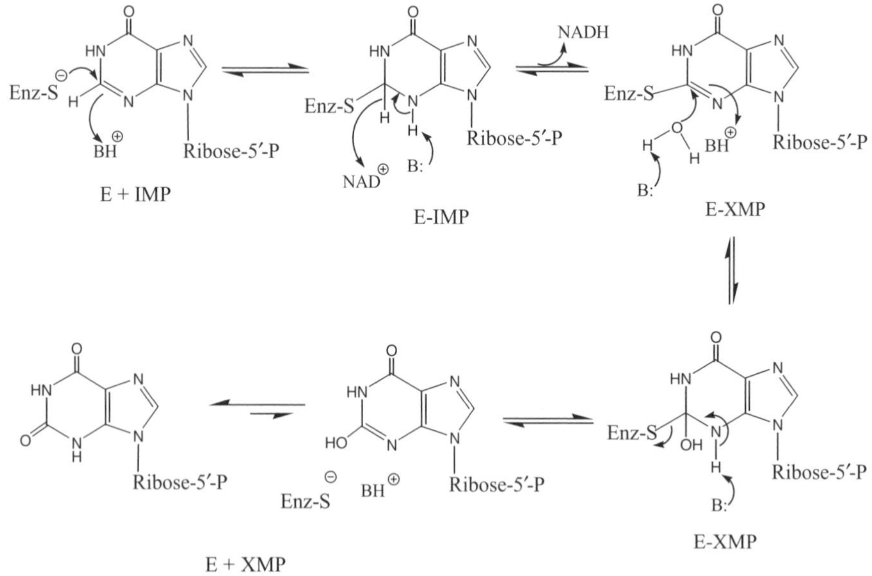

FIGURE 8.6 Mechanism of the reaction catalyzed by IMPDH.[15]

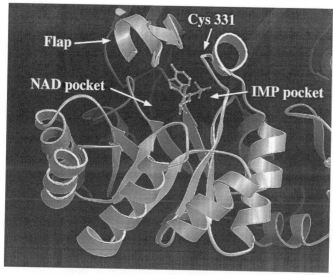

FIGURE 8.7 Ribbon diagram of IMPDH II with bound IMP.[53] (Adapted with permission from *Journal of Applied Crystallography.*)

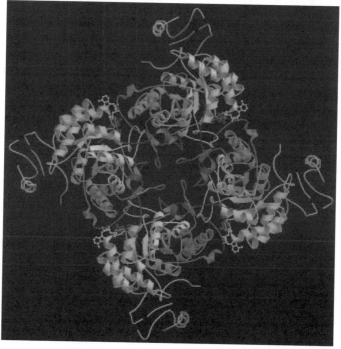

FIGURE 8.8 X-ray structure of the ternary complex of the human Type II IMPDH with 6-chloropurine riboside 5'-monophosphate and nicontinamide adenine dinucleotide.[56] (Reproduced with permission from the *Protein Data Bank.*) (See insert for color representation.)

followed by an oxidation step (hydride abstraction) at the 2-position involving NAD^+ followed by hydration at this position and ejection of the enzyme. All of the chemistry taking place at the 2-position is of significance in the design of inhibitors of IMPDH and this has has been the focus of some of our work in this area. The human enzyme exists in two isoforms, Type I (expressed in normal cells) and Type II (predominates in neoplastic and fast replicating cells).[48,49] Human Type I and II enzymes have been cloned and expressed in *Escherichia coli*.[50] There has been much renewed interest in this enzyme in the last few years (e.g. see Refs. 29, 36, 38, 39, 51, and 52). Several recent crystal structures of IMPDH have been determined (Figures 8.7 and 8.8).[53–56] In our laboratory, we have isolated and studied bacterial IMPDH (from *E. coli* B3 strain) and human recombinant IMPDH II.[39]

8.4 INHIBITORS OF IMPDH WITH ACTIVITY AGAINST VIRUSES OF EMERGING DISEASES AND BIOTERRORISM THREATS

Of the potential weapons of bioterrorism, smallpox poses one of the greatest threats. There are a number of compounds that are known to be inhibitors of orthopoxviruses and some of their biochemical mechanisms of action are as follows: inhibition of inosine monophosphate dehydrogenase (IMPDH) [e.g., ribavirin, ethynylimidazolecarboxamide riboside (EICAR), fluoroimidazole-carboxamide riboside (FICAR), tiazofurin and selenazole, 2-vinylinosine], S-adenosylhomocysteine hydrolase (SAHase) inhibitors (e.g., neplanocin and its analogues, 5′-noraristeromycin and its analogues), thymidylate synthase inhibitors [e.g., (E)-5-(2-bromovinyl)deoxyuridine (BVDU)], and viral DNA synthesis inhibitors [e.g., cidofovir (HPMPC)].[31,34,57–61] A few of these compounds are inhibitors of orthopox virus replication by more than one mechanism of action. Representative examples are discussed below.

8.4.1 Ribavirin

1

The modified ribonucleoside ribavirin (1-β-D-ribofuranosyl-1,2,4-triazole-3-carboxamide, **1**) can be viewed as a structural analogue of guanosine.[33] Ribavirin can be synthesized enzymatically by coupling of 3-carbamoyl-1,2,4-triazole

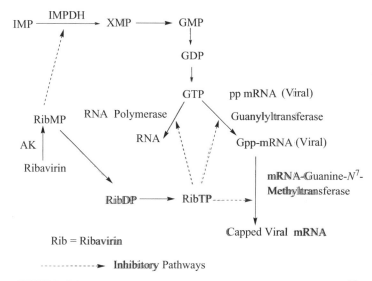

FIGURE 8.9   Proposed mechanism of antiviral activity of ribavirin.[36]

through a transferase reaction catalyzed by purine nucleoside phosphorylases.[62] Chemical methods for synthesis are also available.[62] Ribavirin 5′-monophosphate is an inhibitor of IMPDH with a K_i of 4.1 μM.[15,33,36] Ribavirin exhibits broad-spectrum antiviral activity[31,33,34] against a number of viruses including some toga-, bunya-, and arenaviruses. Adenoviruses are also inhibited by ribavirin. This very interesting nucleoside is also active against the vaccinia virus (4–20 μg/mL).[31] The mechanism of antiviral action of ribavirin[33,35,36] follows several pathways (Figure 8.9). Its monophosphate is an inhibitor of IMPDH, which results in depletion of cellular guanosine triphosphate (GTP) pools. Ribavirin, in its several phosphory-lated forms, can inhibit transcription by RNA polymerases. Of interest also is that ribavirin 5′-triphosphate has been shown to inhibit vaccinia virus mRNA guanylyl-transferase, thus blocking the "capping" of viral mRNA.[33,35,36]

Ribavirin is in clinical use as an antiviral drug for hepatitis C, respiratory syncytial virus, and Lassa virus infections.[44–46] Its mechanism of action as an antiviral agent may be interpreted in another light. It has been suggested that in the case of the poliovirus and perhaps other RNA viruses, ribavirin may have a lethal mutagenic effect following its incorporation into the viral genome catalyzed by the viral RNA-dependent RNA polymerase.[41] Incorporation into the viral genome may force the RNA viruses into a lethal accumulation of errors, which are augmented by reduction of GTP pools caused by the inhibition of IMPDH by ribavirin mono-phosphate.[47] Decrease in the cellular GTP pools is likely to increase the frequency of incorporation of ribavirin triphosphate incorporation as a mutagenic GTP analogue.

8.4.2   1-(4-Carboxamido-5-ethynylimidazole)-β-D-ribofuranoside or Ethynylimidazole Carboxamide Riboside (EICAR)

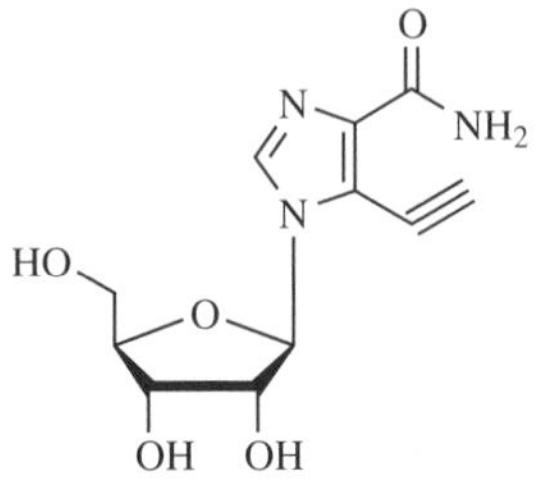

2

The compound referred to as EICAR (**2**) can be synthesized from protected 5-aminoimidazole-carboxamide riboside, AICAR (**3**) (Scheme 8.1) by conversion of the 5-amino functionality to the 5-iodo group (**4**) by a radical deamination/halogenation methodology previously developed by Nair et al.[63–65] followed by the Stille palladium-catalyzed cross-coupling reaction[66,67] with trimethyl[(tributylstannyl)ethynyl] silane to give the 5-ethynyl intermediate, which can be deprotected to give EICAR (**2**).[68]

EICAR is a congener of ribavirin but apparently exhibits more potency. The activity includes both DNA and RNA viruses.[31] Among the existing and emerging RNA viruses are picorna-, toga-, flavi-, bunya-, arena-, reo-, rhabdo-, ortho-, and paramyxoviruses. The mechanism of action of this compound appears to be

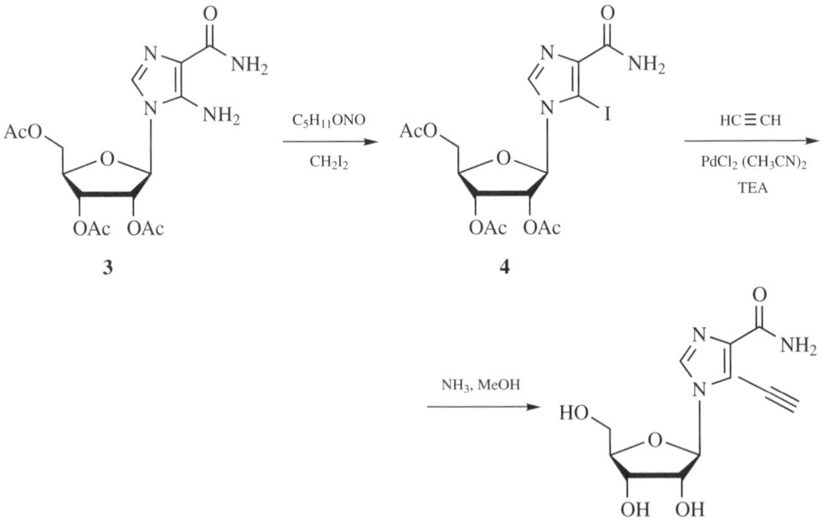

SCHEME 8.1   Synthesis of EICAR from AICAR triacetate.

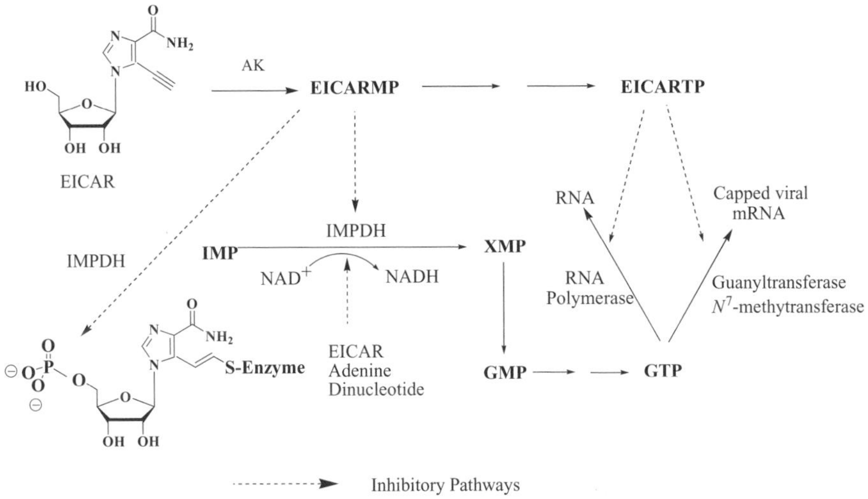

FIGURE 8.10 Proposed mechanism for inhibition of viral replication by EICAR.[38]

multipronged and may include inhibition of IMPDH through its $5'$-monophosphate, inhibition of IMPDH through an NAD^+ analogue (EICAR adenine dinucleotide), inhibition of viral RNA polymerase through EICAR triphosphate, and inhibition of viral mRNA capping (Figure 8.10).

8.4.3 Tiazofurin and Selenazofurin

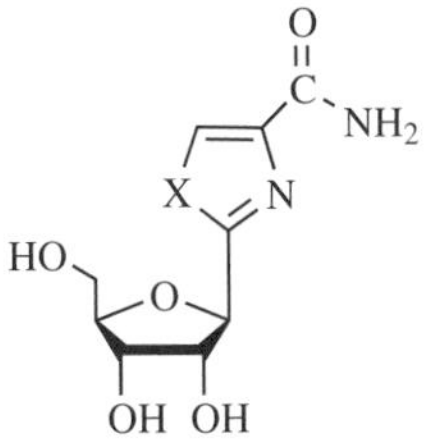

5 X = S, Tiazofurin
6 X = Se, Selenazofurin

Tiazofurin [2-(β-D-ribofuranosyl)thiazole-4-carboxamide] (**5**) was first synthesized in 1977 by Robins and co-workers (59). It is a C-nucleoside and can be viewed as a structural analogue of ribavirin. This compound was found to have antiproliferative activity and antiviral activity.[31,36,38,59] It is converted cellularly to an anabolite, thiazole-4-carboxamide adenine dinucleotide, TAD^+ (**7**), which is a structural analogue of the coenzyme, nicotinamide adenine dinucleotide (NAD^+). Tiazofurin is phosphorylated in cells to its monophosphate (TiazMP), which is the precursor of

TAD$^+$. TAD$^+$ is a noncompetitive inhibitor of IMPDH with respect to NAD$^+$ and the K_i for this inhibition is 0.2 μM.[36,60]

7 X = S, TAD$^+$
8 X = Se, SAD$^+$

The selenium analogue of tiazofurin referred to as selenazofurin (**6**) was also synthesized by Robins and co-workers.[69] Like tiazofurin, selenazofurin exhibits both in vitro and in vivo antitumor activity.[70,71] It is also an inhibitor of IMPDH ($K_i = 0.05$ μM)[70] apparently through its dinucleotide, SAD$^+$ (Figure 8.11), which is also a structural analogue of NAD$^+$. X-ray crystallographic data[54] suggest that TAD$^+$ binds to the NAD$^+$ site on IMPDH.

Selenazofurin was found to have in vitro activity against both DNA and RNA viruses. For example, selenazofurin shows in vitro antiviral activity against the vaccinia virus (3 μg/mL).[31]

8.4.4 Bredinin

9

The natural product bredinin (**9**) or mizoribine (4-carbamoyl-1-β-D-ribofuranosylimidazolium-5-olate) is a derivative of AICAR.[62] X-ray analysis of this compound confirmed its chemical structure and its zwitterionic nature. It can be synthesized by standard Vorbruggen coupling methods.[72] Bredinin can be synthesized also by enzymatic coupling of 4-carbamoylimidazolium-5-olate through a transferase reaction catalyzed by purine nucleoside phoshporylases.[62] Bredinin 5'-monophosphate is a potent inhibitor of IMPDH ($K_i = 0.5$ nM).[15]

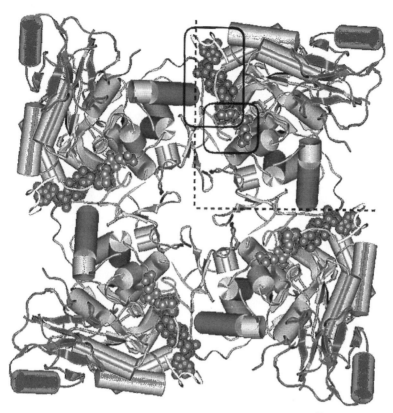

FIGURE 8.11   Human type II IMPDH: crystal structure of tetramer.[54] (Reproduced with permission of *Proceedings of the National Academy of Sciences of the United States of America*.) (See insert for color representation.)

Bredinin exhibits potent immunosuppressive activity. It also exhibits broad-spectrum antiviral activity including activity against three strains of RSV, one strain each of the influenza virus (FluV) types A and B, parainfluenza virus (PFluV) types 2 and 3, mumps virus (MPSV), and measles virus (MLSV).[73] It has also been reported to be active against the vaccinia virus.[74] The mechanism of viral inhibition appears to be associated with the inhibition of IMPDH by the monophosphate of this compound. As in the case of ribavirin, other mechanisms may also be possible.

8.4.5   2-[2(Z)-Fluorovinyl]inosine

2-Fluorovinylinosine (2-FVIMP, **10**), an analogue of the broad-spectrum antiviral compound 2-vinylinosine (discussed is Section 8.4.6) has been synthesized recently by us[75] through a multistep route, which is described in detail in Scheme 8.2.

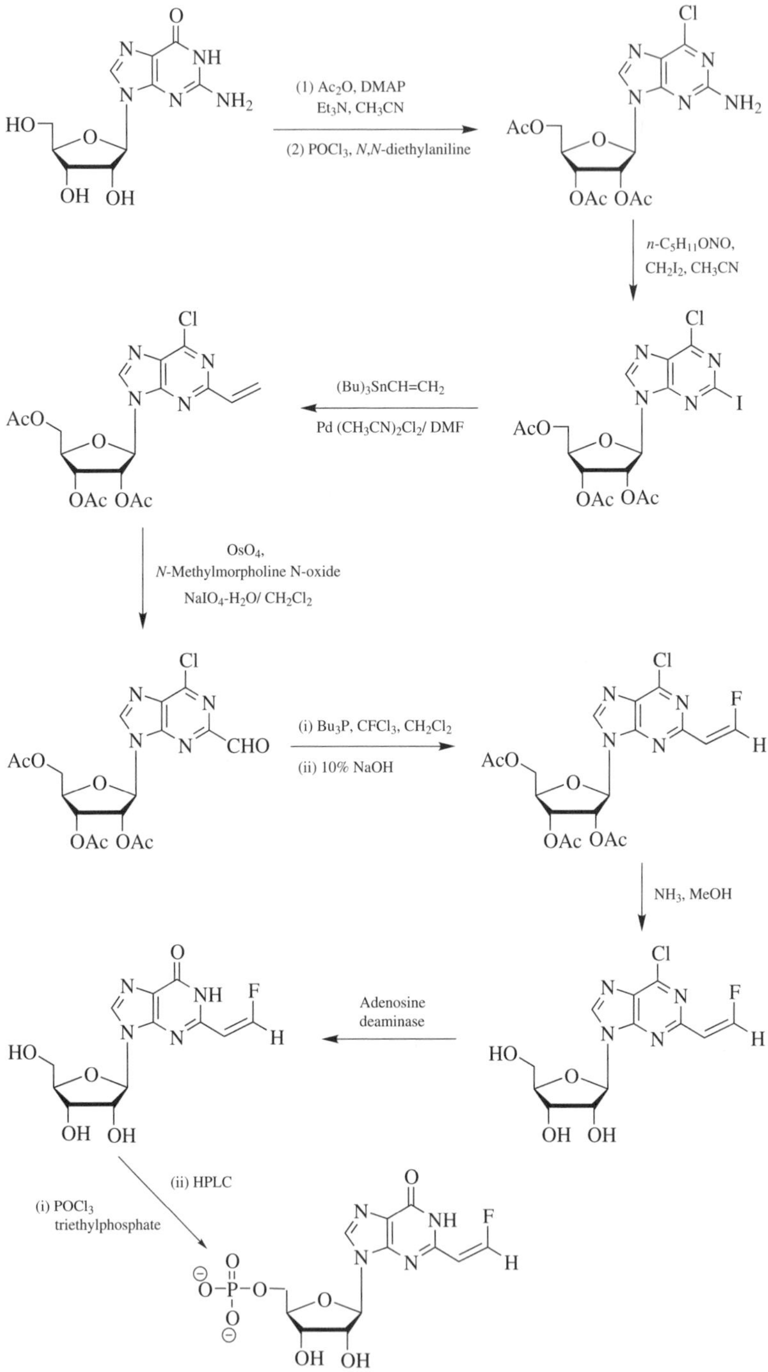

SCHEME 8.2   Synthesis of 2-fluorovinylinosine and its 5′-monophosphate.

10

We have carried out detailed studies of the inhibition of bacterial IMPDH by 2-fluorovinylinosine 5′-monophosphate.[76] The inhibition reaction was monitored by following the increase in absorbance at 340 nm due to the formation of NADH. The data were fitted into the following equation [1]:

$$\ln(V_t/V_0) = -k_{obs}t \qquad [1]$$

where V_t is the activity at time t and V_0 is the activity at time t = 0. The k_{obs} values obtained for inactivation of IMPDH were then fitted into the equation [2]:

$$k_{obs} = k_{inact}[I]/(K_i + [I]) \qquad [2]$$

where k_{inact} is the inactivation rate constant, K_i is the apparent dissociation constant, and [I] is the inhibitor (2-FVIMP) concentration. Incubation of IMPDH with 2-FVIMP exhibited a time-dependent decrease in V_t/V_0 as shown in Figure 8.12. This is an indication that 2-FVIMP inactivates the enzyme.

For further understanding of the mechanism of inhibition, the k_{obs} values obtained by using equation [1] were plotted against inhibitor concentration. The hyperbolic relationship observed between k_{obs} and 2-FVIMP concentration (Figure 8.13) suggests that 2-FVIMP interacts with IMPDH through a two-step mechanism as follows:

$$E + I \underset{k_{-1}}{\overset{k_1}{\rightleftharpoons}} E.I \xrightarrow{K_{inact}} E - I$$

where $K_i = k_1/k_{-1}$, E is IMPDH, E.I is the reversibly bound enzyme–inhibitor complex, and E–I is the irreversibly inactivated enzyme. Thus, it appears that the mechanism of inactivation of IMPDH by 2-FVIMP involves the initial reversible formation of an E.I complex followed by the inactivation step. The values of k_{inact} and K_i were determined using equation [2] by plotting the reciprocal of k_{obs} versus the reciprocal of inhibitor concentration. The values of k_{inact} and K_i were 0.0269 s^{-1} and 1.11 μM, respectively, whereas the well-known IMPDH inhibitor 6-chloropurine ribonucleoside monophosphate in these studies

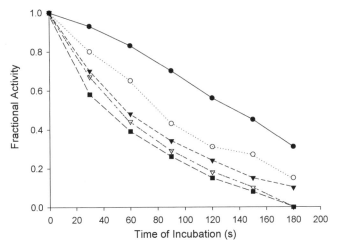

FIGURE 8.12 Inhibition of *E. coli* IMPDH by 2-FVIMP with respect to time.[76] (●, 0.25 μM; ○, 0.50 μM; ◄, 0.75 μM; △, 1.0 μM; ■, 1.5 μM.)

gave values of 0.076 min^{-1} and 62.0 μM. The type of inactivation of IMPDH shown by 2-FVIMP is related to that exhibited by ethynylimidazole carbox-amide riboside monophosphate (EICARMP).[37] Antiviral screening of **10** against the vaccinia and cowpox viruses (HFF cell line) showed moderate acti-vity (T.I.~4).[77] The mechanism of this antiviral activity is likely associated with the ability of the cellularly produced monophosphate to be an inhibitor of IMPDH.

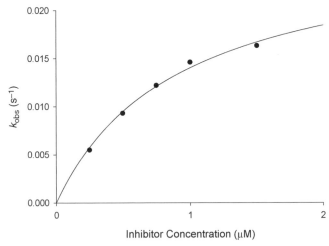

FIGURE 8.13 Relationship of k_{obs} with inhibitor (2-FVIMP) concentration.[76]

8.4.6 2-Vinylinosine

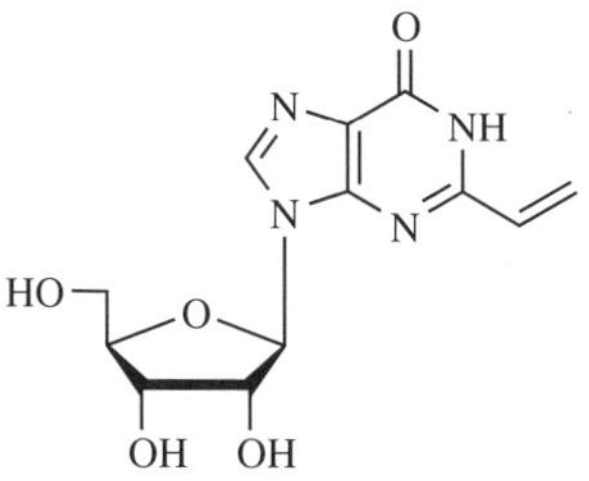

11

2-Vinylinosine (**11**) was first synthesized in our laboratory.[66,67] Since the original synthesis, we have improved the methodology for the preparation of this interesting compound.[75] Our current chemoenzymatic synthetic approach is summarized in Scheme 8.3.

2-Vinylinosine 5′-monophosphate can be synthesized by either chemical or enzymatic phosphorylation of 2-vinylinosine. 2-Vinylinosine is a poor substrate for adenosine kinase. However, even the low substrate activity is sufficient for the small-scale enzymatic synthesis of the 5′-monophosphate of this compound. We have also shown that 2-vinylinosine monophosphate may be formed, at least in part in cells, through cleavage of 2-vinylinosine by purine nucleoside phosphorylase and subsequent phosphoribosylation with HGPRT and PRPP. 2-Vinylinosine 5′-monophosphate is a strong inhibitor of IMPDH with a K_i of 4 μM.[39] IMPDH is inactivated by this compound.

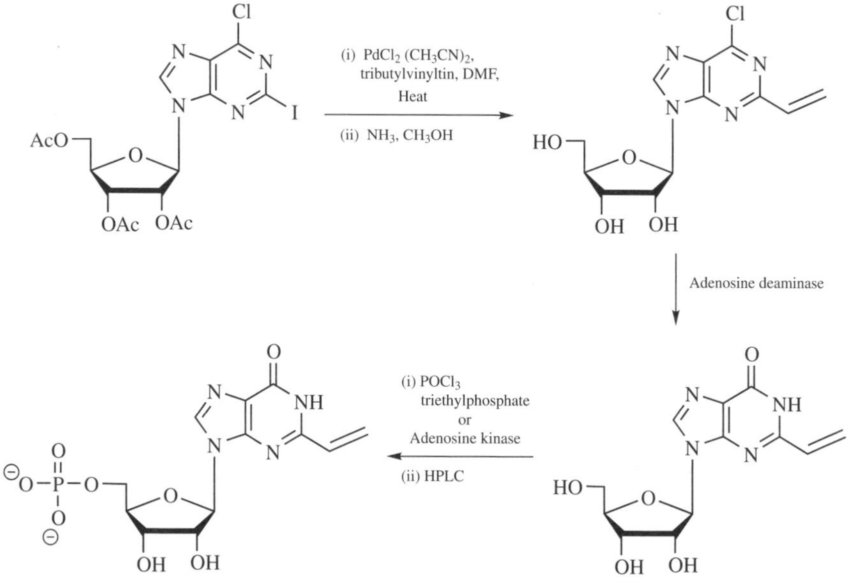

SCHEME 8.3 Chemoenzymatic synthesis of 2-vinylinosine.

Of interest to the focus of this book is the observation that 2-vinylinosine shows broad-spectrum in vitro antiviral activity against a number of viruses (IC_{50} in Vero cells except for AD2, which was in Hep2 cells): VV, vaccinia virus (poxvirus, 13.0 μg/mL); JEV, Japanese encephallitis virus (flavivirus, 3.2 μg/mL); PIC, Pichinde (arenavirus, 2.5 μg/mL); PT, Punta Toro (phlebovirus, 2.7 μg/mL); RVF, Rift Valley fever (phlebovirus, 24 μg/mL); VEE, Venezuelan equine encephalo-myelitis (alphavirus, 7.7 μg/mL); and YF, yellow fever (flavivirus, 7.7 μg/mL); and AD2, adenovirus type 2 (adenovirus, 12.6 μg/mL).[61,75,77]

8.4.7   6-Chloro-2-ethynylpurine-β-ᴅ-ribofuranoside

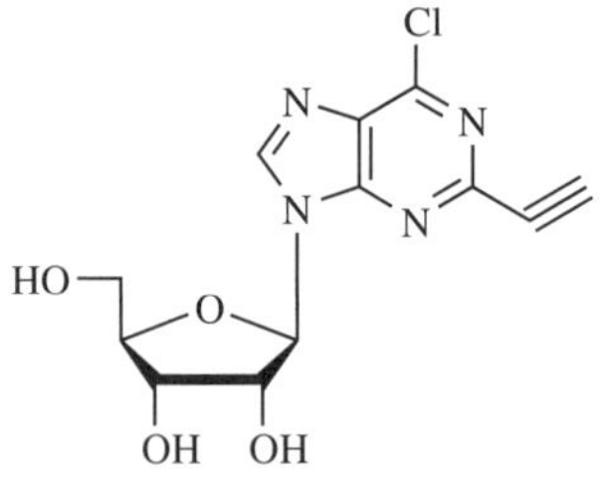

12

The 2,6-disubstituted nucleoside, **12**, can be synthesized by a methodology similar to that described for the synthesis of 2-vinylinosine (**11**).[75] The 5′-monophosphate of **12** is an inhibitor of IMPDH (k_{inact} and K_i were 0.03 s^{-1} and 4.2 μM, respectively).[39,76,77] 6-Chloro-2-ethynylpurine ribonucleoside (**12**) showed potent in vitro activity against the vaccinia virus (HFF cells): $IC_{50} > 0.8$ μg/mL and the cowpox virus (HFF cells): $IC_{50} > 0.8$ μg/mL. However, this compound was also toxic to HFF cells.[77,78].

8.4.8   2-Acetonylinosine

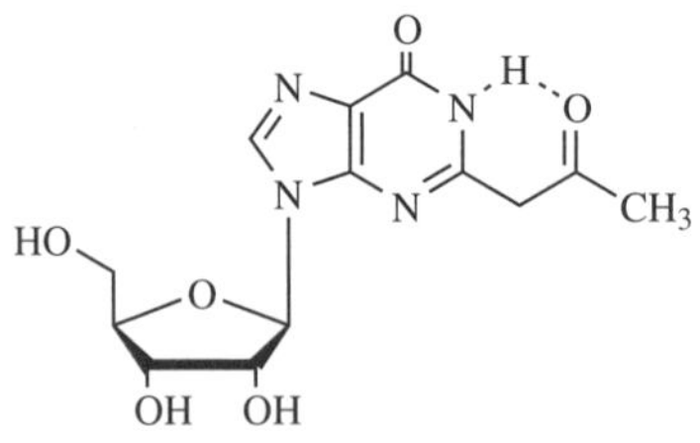

13

Another example of a 2-substituted purine nucleoside with antiviral activity against emerging viruses is 2-acetonylinosine (**13**). This compound was synthesized in our laboratory[66,67,78] through a chemoenzymatic approach as shown in Scheme 8.4. While 2-acetonylinosine (**13**) does not exhibit the broad-spectrum activity shown

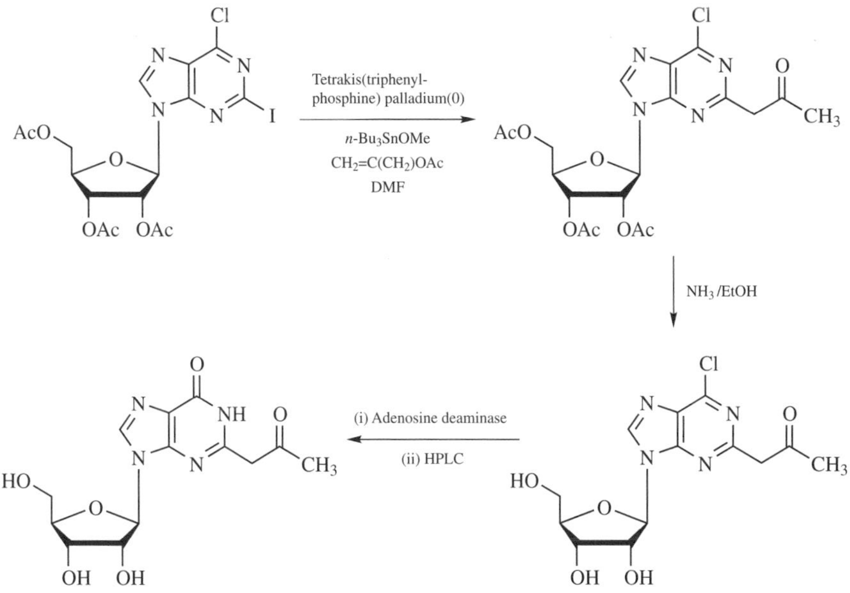

SCHEME 8.4 Chemoenzymatic synthesis of 2-acetonylinosine.

by 2-vinylinosine (**11**), it shows potent and selective antiviral activity against the sandfly fever virus (SFV)[61] with a therapeutic index of >1000! The Sandfly fever virus is a phlebovirus of the genus Bunyavirus,[14] and these viruses have single-stranded, segmented RNA genomes.[79] The mechanism of the antiviral activity of **11** is not understood. Compound **11** is not a substrate for adenosine kinase and its cellular monophosphorylation may be through the PNP/HGPRT pathway. The mechanism of inhibition may not be through IMPDH inhibition because the monophosphate of **13** is not an inhibitor of IMPDH. It is possible that the triphosphate of **13** is an inhibitor of the SFV viral RNA polymerase. The low in vitro cellular toxicity of this compound implies that it is very selective.

ACKNOWLEDGMENT

The research work from our laboratory described in this chapter was supported by grants from the National Institutes of Health (NIAID). Its contents are solely the responsibility of the author and do not necessarily represent the official views of the NIH.

REFERENCES

1. Fenner, F. Poxviruses, in *Fields Virology*, Fields, B. N., Knipe, D. M., Howley, P. M. (eds.). Lippincott-Raven, Philadelphia, 1996, pp. 2673–2702.

2. LeDuc, J. W.; Damon, I.; Meegan, J. M.; Relman, D. A.; Huggins, J.; Jahrling, P. B. Smallpox research activities: U.S. interagency collaboration, 2001. *Emerging Infect. Dis.* **2002**, *8*, 743–745.

3. Heymann, D. L.; Szczeniowski, M.; Esteves, K. Re-emergence of monkeypox in Africa: a review of the past six years. *Br. Med. Bull.* **1998**, *54*, 693–702.

4. Jezek, Z.; Szczeniowski, M.; Paluku, K. M.; Mutombo, M. Human monkeypox: clinical features of 282 patients. *J. Infect. Dis.* **1987**, *156*, 293–298.

5. Hooper, J. W.; Thompson, E.; Wilhelmsen, C.; Zimmerman, M.; Ichou, M. Ait; Steffen, S. E.; Schmaljohn, C. S.; Schmaljohn, A. L.; Jahrling, P. B. Smallpox DNA vaccine protects nonhuman primates against lethal monkeypox. *J. Virol.* **2004**, *78*, 4433–4443.

6. Bremen, J.; Henderson, D. A. Poxvirus dilemmas—monkeypox, smallpox and biological terrorism. *N. Engl. J. Med.* **1998**, *339*, 556–559.

7. Henderson, D. A. Bioterrorism as a public health threat. *Emerging Infect. Dis.* **1998**, *4*, 488–492.

8. Henderson, D. A. The looming threat of bioterrorism. *Science* **1999**, *283*, 1279–1282, and references therein.

9. Fenner, F.; Henderson, D. A.; Arita, I.; Jezek, Z.; Ladnyi, I. D. *Smallpox and Its Eradication*, World Health Organization, Geneva, 1988.

10. Moss, B. Poxviridae: the viruses and their replication, in *Fields Virology*, B. N. Fields, D. M. Knipe, and P. M. Howley (eds.). Lippincott-Raven, Philadelphia, 1996, pp. 2637– 2671.

11. Bray, M. Filoviridae, in *Clinical Virology*, Richman, D. R., Whitley, R. J., Hayden, F. G. (eds.). ASM Press, Washington, Dc, 2002, pp. 875–890.

12. Sanchez, A., Peter, C. J., Rollin, P., Ksiazek, T. G., Murphy, F. A. Filoviridae: Marburg and Ebola viruses, in *Fields Virology*, Fields, B. N., Knipe, D. M., Howley, P. M. (eds.). Lippincott-Raven, Philadelphia, 2001, pp. 1161–1176.

13. Bray, M.; Paragas, J. Experimental therapy of filovirus infections. *Antiviral Res.* **2002**, *54*, 1–17.

14. Hay, J.; Bartkoski, M. J. Jr. Pathogenesis of viral Infections, in *Chemotherapy of Viral Infections*, Came, P. E., Caliguiri, L. A. (eds.). Springer-Verlag, Berlin, 1982, pp. 1–91.

15. Kerr, K. M.; Hedstrom, L. The roles of conserved carboxylate residues in IMP dehydrogenase and identification of a transition state analog. *Biochemistry* **1997**, *36*, 13365–13373.

16. Wang, W.; Hedstrom, L. Kinetic mechanism of human inosine 5′-monophosphate dehydrogenase type II: random addition of substrates and ordered release of products. *Biochemistry* **1997**, *36*, 8479–8483.

17. Hedstrom, L. IMP dehydrogenase: mechanism of action and inhibition. *Curr. Med. Chem.* **1999**, *6*, 545–560.

18. Kerr, K. M.; Digits, J. A.; Kuperwasser, N.; Hedstrom, L. Asp338 controls hydride transfer in *E. coli* IMP dehydrogenase. *Biochemistry* **2000**, *39*, 9804–9810.

19. Zimmermann, A. G.; Gu, J.-J.; Laliberte, J.; Mitchell, B. S. Inosine-5′-monophosphate dehydrogenase: regulation of expression and role in cellular proliferation and T lymphocyte activation. *Prog. Nucleic Acid Res. Mol. Biol.* **1998**, *61*, 181–209.

20. St. Georgiev, V. Enzymes of the purine metabolism: inhibition and therapeutic potential. In *Annals of New York Academy of Sciences, Volume 685*, St. Georgiev, V.; Yamaguchi, H. (eds.). New York Academy of Sciences, New York, 1993, pp. 207–216.

21. Pankiewicz, K. W. Inhibitors of inosine monophosphate dehydrogenase as potential chemotherapeutic agents. *Exp. Opin. Ther. Patents* **1999**, *9*, 55–65.

22. Natsumeda, Y.; Carr, S. F. Human type I and II IMP dehydrogenases as drug targets. In *Annals of New York Academy of Sciences, Volume 696*, Allison, A. C.; Lafferty, K. J.; Fliri, H. (eds.). New York Academy of Sciences, New York, 1993, pp. 88–93.

23. Pani, A.; Marongiu, M. E.; Pinna, E.; Scintu, F.; Perra, G.; De Montis, A.; Manfredini, S.; La Colla, P. *In vitro* and *in vivo* antiproliferative activity of IPCAP, a new pyrazole nucleoside analog. *Anticancer Res.* **1998**, *18*, 2623–2630.

24. Kosugi, Y.; Saito, Y.; Mori, S.; Watanabe, J.; Baba, M.; Shigeta, S. Antiviral activities of mizoribine and other inosine monophosphate dehydrogenase inhibitors against several ortho and paramyxoviruses. *Antiviral Chem. Chemother.* **1994**, *5*, 366–371.

25. Franchetti, P.; Cappellacci, L.; Grifantini, M.; Barzi, A.; Nocentini, G.; Yang, H.; O'Connor, A.; Jayaram, H. N.; Carrell, C.; Goldstein, B. M. Furanfurin and thiophenfurin: two novel tiazofurin analogues. Synthesis, structure, antitumor activity, and interactions with inosine monophosphate dehydrogenase. *J. Med. Chem.* **1995**, *38*, 3829–3837.

26. Xiang, B.; Taylor, J. C.; Markham, G. D. Monovalent cation activation and kinetic mechanism of inosine 5'-phosphate dehydrogenase. *J. Biol. Chem.* **1996**, *271*, 1435–1440.

27. Antonino, L. C.; Wu, J. C. Human IMP dehydrogenase catalyzes the dehalogenation of 2-fluoro- and 2-chloroinosine 5'-monophosphate in the absence of NAD. *Biochemistry* **1994**, *33*, 1753–1759.

28. Zhang, H.-Z.; Rao, K.; Carr, S. F.; Papp, E.; Straub, K.; Wu, J. C.; Fried, J. Rationally designed inhibitors of inosine monophosphate dehydrogenase. *J. Med. Chem.* **1997**, *40*, 4–8.

29. Franchetti, P.; Grifantini, M. Nucleoside and non-nucleoside IMP dehydrogenase inhibitors as antitumor and antiviral agents. *Curr. Med. Chem.* **1999**, *6*, 599–614.

30. Goldstein, B. M.; Colby, T. D. IMP dehydrogenase: structural aspects of inhibitor binding. *Curr. Med. Chem.* **1999**, *6*, 519–536.

31. De Clercq, E. Vaccinia virus inhibitors as a paradigm for the chemotherapy of poxvirus infections. *Clin. Microbiol. Rev.* **2001**, *14*, 382–397.

32. De Clerq, E. Strategics in the design of antiviral drugs. *Nat. Rev. Drug Disc.* **2002**, *11*, 13–25.

33. Smith, R. A.; Kirkpatrick, W. (eds.). *Ribavirin. A Broad Spectrum Antiviral Agent*, Academic Press, New York, 1980.

34. Smee, D. F.; Huggins, J. W. Potential of the IMP dehydrogenase inhibitors for antiviral therapies of poxvirus infections. *Antiviral Res.* **1998**, A89.

35. Goswami, B. B.; Borek, E.; Sharma, O. K.; Fujitaki, J.; Smith, R. A. The broad-spectrum antiviral agent ribavirin inhibits capping of mRNA. *Biochem. Biophys. Res. Commun.* **1979**, *89*, 830–836.

36. Franchetti, P.; Cappellacci, L.; Grifantini, M. IMP dehydrogenase as a target of antitumor and antiviral chemotherapy. *Il Farmaco* **1996**, *51*, 457–469.

37. Wang, W.; Papov, V. V.; Minakawa, N.; Matsuda, A.; Biemann, K.; Hedstrom, L. Inactivation of inosine 5'-monophosphate dehydrogenase by the antiviral agent 5-ethynyl-1-β-D-ribofuranosylimidazole-4-carboxamide 5'-monophosphate. *Biochemistry* **1996**, *35*, 95–101.

38. Minakawa, N.; Matsuda, A. Design of inosine 5'-monophosphate dehydrogenase inhibitors: synthesis and biological activities of 5-ethynyl-1-β-D-ribofuranosylimidazole-4-carboxamide (EICAR) and its derivatives. *Curr. Med. Chem.* **1999**, *6*, 615–628.

39. Pal, S.; Bera, B.; Nair, V. Inhibition of inosine monophosphate dehydrogenase (IMPDH) by the antiviral compound, 2-vinylinosine. *Bioorg. Med. Chem.* **2002**, *10*, 3615–3618.

40. Holland, J. J.; Domingo, E.; de la Torre, J. C.; Steinhauer, D. A. Mutation frequencies at defined single codon sites in vesicular stomatitis virus and poliovirus can be increased only slightly by chemical mutagenesis. *J. Virol.* **1990**, *64*, 3960–3962.

41. Lee, C. H.; Gilbertson, D. L.; Novella, I. S.; Huerta, R.; Domingo, E.; Holland, J. J. Negative effects of chemical mutagenesis on the adaptive behavior of vesicular stomatitis virus. *J. Virol.* **1997**, *71*, 3636–3664.

42. Crotty S; Maag, D.; Arnold, J. J.; Zhong, W.; Lau, J. Y.; Hong, Z.; Andino, R.; Cameron, C. E. The broad-spectrum antiviral ribonucleoside ribavirin is an RNA virus mutagen. *Nat. Med.* **2000**, *6*, 1375–1379.

43. Sierra, S; Davila M.; Lowenstein, P. R.; Domingo, E. Response of foot-and-mouth disease virus to increased mutagenesis: influence of viral load and fitness in loss of infectivity. *J. Virol.* **2000**, *74*, 8316–8323.

44. Davis, G. L.; Esteban-Mur, R.; Rustgi, V.; Hoefs, J.; Gordon, S. C.; Trepo, C.; Shiffman, M. L.; Zeuzem, S.; Craxi, A.; Ling, M. H.; Albrecht, J. Interferon α-2b alone or in combination with ribavirin for the treatment of relapse of chronic hepatitis C. International Hepatitis Interventional Therapy Group. *N. Engl. J. Med.* **1998**, *339*, 1493–1499.

45. McHutchison, J. G.; Gordon, S. C.; Schiff, E. R.; Shiffman, M. L.; Lee, W. M.; Rustgi, V. K.; Goodman, Z. D.; Ling, M. H.; Cort, S.; Albrecht, J. K. Interferon α-2b alone or in combination with ribavirin as initial treatment for chronic hepatitis C. International Hepatitis Interventional Therapy Group. *N. Engl. J. Med.* **1998**, *339*, 1485–1492.

46. Wyde, P. R. Respiratory syncytial virus (RSV) disease and prospects for its control. *Antiviral Res.* **1998**, *39*, 63–79.

47. Crotty, S.; Cameron, C. E.; Andino, R. RNA virus error catastrophe: direct molecular test by using ribavirin. *Proc. Natl Acad. Sci. U.S.A.* **2001**, *98*, 6895–6900.

48. Konno, Y.; Natsumeda, Y.; Nagai, M.; Yamaji, Y.; Ohno, S.; Suzuki, K.; Weber, G. Expression of human IMP dehydrogenase types I and II in *Escherichia coli* and distribution in human normal lymphocytes and leukemic cell lines. *J. Biol. Chem.* **1991**, *266*, 506–509.

49. Carr, S. F.; Papp, E.; Wu, J. C.; Natsumeda, Y. Characterization of human type I and type II IMP dehydrogenases. *J. Biol. Chem.* **1993**, *268*, 27286–27290.

50. Hager, P. W.; Collart, F. R.; Huberman, E.; Mitchell, B. S. Recombinant human inosine monophosphate dehydrogenase type I and type II proteins: purification and characterization of inhibitor binding. *Biochem. Pharmacol.* **1995**, *49*, 1323–1329.

51. Schalk-Hihi, C.; Zhang, Y.-Z.; Markham, G. D. The conformation of NADH bound to inosine 5'-monophosphate dehydrogenase determined by transferred nuclear Overhauser effect spectroscopy. *Biochemistry* **1998**, *37*, 7608–7616.

52. Miyamoto, T.; Matsuno, K.; Imamura, M.; Kim, S.-I.; Honjon, K.; Hatano, S. Purification and some properties of IMP dehydrogenase of *Bacillus cereus*. *Microbiol. Res.* **1998**, *153*, 23–27.

53. Carson, M. Ribbons 2.0, IMPDH. *J. Appl. Crystallogr.* **1991**, *24*, 958–961.

54. Colby, T. D.; Vanderveen, K.; Strickler, M. D.; Markham, G. D.; Goldstein, B. M. Crystal structure of human type II inosine monophosphate dehydrogenase: implications for ligand binding and drug design. *Proc. Natl. Acad. Sci. U.S.A.* **1999**, *96*, 3531–3536.

55. Zhang, R.-G.; Evans, G.; Rotella, F. J.; Westbrook, E. M.; Beno, D.; Huberman, E.; Joachimiak, A.; Collart, F. R. Characteristics and crystal structure of bacterial inosine-5'-monophosphate dehydrogenase. *Biochemistry* **1999**, *38*, 4691–4700.

56. Risal, D.; Strickler, M. D.; Goldstein, B. M. The ternary complex of the human type II inosine monophosphate dehydrogenase with 6-Cl IMP and NAD. *Protein Data Bank* **2004** in press.

57. Naesens, L.; Snoeck, R.; Andrei, G.; Balzarini, J.; Neyts, J.; De Clercq, E. HPMPC (cidofovir), PMEA (adefovir) and related acyclic nucleoside phosphonate analogues: a review of their pharmacology and clinical potential in the treatment of viral infections. *Antivir. Chem. Chemother.* **1997**, *8*, 1–23.

58. Huggins, J. W.; Martinez, M. J.; Hartmann, C. J.; Hensley, L. E.; Jackson, D. L.; Kefauver, D. F.; Kulesh, D. A.; Larsen, T.; Miller, D. M.; Mucker, E. M.; Shamblin, J. D.; Tate, M. K.; Whitehouse, C. A.; Zwiers, S. H.; Jahrling, P. B. Successful cidofovir treatment of smallpox-like disease in *Variola* and monkeypox primate models. *Antiviral Res.* **2004**, *62*, A57.

59. Srivastava, P. D.; Pickering, M. U.; Allen, O. B.; Streeter, D. G.; Campbell, M. T.; Witkowski, J. T.; Sidwell, R. W.; Robins, R. K. Synthesis and antiviral activity of certain thiazole C-nucleosides. *J. Med. Chem.* **1977**, *20*, 256–262.

60. Cooney, D. A.; Jayaram, H. N.; Gebeyehu, G.; Betts, C. R.; Kelley, J. A.; Marquez, V. E.; Johns, D. G. The conversion of 2-β-D-ribofuranosylthiazole-4-carboxamide to an analog of NAD with potent IMP dehydrogenase-inhibitory properties. *Biochem. Pharmacol.* **1982**, *31*, 2133–2136.

61. Nair, V.; Ussery. M. A. New hypoxanthine nucleosides with RNA antiviral activity. *Antiviral Res.* **1992**, *19*, 173–178.

62. Preobrazhenskaya, M. N.; Korbukh, I. A. xxx. In *Chemistry of Nucleosides and Nucleotides*, *Vol. 3*, Townsend, L.B. (ed.). Plenum Press, New York, 1994, pp. 1–105, and references therein.

63. Nair, V.; Richardson, S. G. Modification of nucleic acid bases via radical intermediates: synthesis of dihalogenated purine nucleosides. *Synthesis* **1982**, 670–672.

64. Nair, V.; Richardson, S. G. The utility of purinyl radicals in the synthesis of base-modified nucleosides and alkyl purines: 6-amino group replacement by H, Cl, Br, and I. *J. Org. Chem.* **1980**, *45*, 3969–3974.

65. Nair, V.; Young, D. A.; DeSilvia, R. G. 2-Halogenated purine nucleosides: synthesis and reactivity. *J. Org. Chem.* **1987**, *52*, 1344–1347.

66. Nair, V.; Turner, G. A.; Buenger, G. S.; Chamberlain, S. D. New methodologies for the synthesis of C-2 functionalized hypoxanthine nucleosides. *J. Org. Chem.* **1988**, *53*, 3051–3057.

67. Nair, V.; Turner, G. A.; Chamberlain, S. D. Novel approaches to functionalized nucleosides via palladium-catalyzed cross-coupling with organostannanes. *J. Am Chem. Soc.* **1987**, *109*, 7223–7224.

68. Minakawa, N.; Takeda, T.; Sasaki, T.; Matsuda, A.; Veda, T. Nucleosides and nucleotides. 96. Synthesis and antitumor activity of 5-ethynyl-1-beta-D-ribofuranosyl-imidazole-4-carboxamide (EICAR) and its derivatives. *J. Med. Chem.* **1991**, *34*, 778–786.

69. Srivastava, P. C.; Robins, R. K. Synthesis and antitumor activity of 2-beta-D-ribofuranosylselenazole-4-carboxamide and related derivatives. *J. Med. Chem.* **1983**, *26*, 445–448.

70. Jayaram, H. N.; Ahluwalia, G. S.; Dion, R. L.; Gebeyehu, G.; Marquez, V. E.; Kelley, J. A.; Robins, R. K.; Cooney, D. A.; Cooney, D. A.; Johns, D. G. Conversion of 2-beta-D-ribofuranosylselenazole-4-carboxamide to an analogue of NAD with potent IMP dehydrogenase-inhibitory properties. *Biochem. Pharmacol.* **1983**, *32*, 2633–2636.

71. Streeter, D. R.; Robins, R. K. Comparative in vitro studies of tiazofurin and a selenazole analog. *Biochem. Biophys. Res. Commun.* **1983**, *115*, 544.

72. Tarumi, Y.; Takebayaski, Y.; Atsumi, T. Studies on imidazole derivatives and related compounds. 4. Synthesis of *O*-glycosides of 4-carbamoylimidazolium-5-olate. *J. Heterocycl. Chem.* **1984**, *21*, 849–854.

73. Kosugi, Y.; Saito, Y.; Mori, S.; Watanabe, J.; Baba, M.; Shigeta, S. Antiviral activities of mizoribine and other inosine monophosphate dehydrogenase inhibitors against ortho- and paramyxoviruses. *Antiviral Chem. Chemother.* **1994**, *5*, 366–371.

74. Suhadolnik, R. J. *Nucleosides as Biological Probes*, Wiley, New York, 1979, pp. 149–154.

75. Nair, V.; Bera, B.; Kern, E. R. Synthesis and antiviral activities of 2-functionalized purine ribonucleosides. *Nucleosides Nucleotides Nucleic Acids* **2003**, *22*, 115–127.

76. Nair, V.; Kamboj, R. C. Inhibition of inosine monophosphate dehydrogenase (IMPDH) by 2-[2-(Z)-fluorovinyl] inosine 5′-monophosphate. *Bioorg. Med. Chem. Lett.* **2003**, *13*, 645–647.

77. Nair, V.; Kern, E. R.; Bera, B. Antiviral ribonucleosides: inhibitors of inosine monophosphate dehydrogenase. *Antiviral Res.* **2002**, *53*, A63.

78. Nair, V.; Story, S.; Gupta, M.; Bonsu, E. Antiviral ribonucleosides: inhibitors of inosine monophosphate dehydrogenase. *Antiviral Res.* **2004**, *62*, A72.

79. Bishop, D. H. Virion polymerases. In *Comprehensive Virology, Vol. 10*, Plenum Press, New York, 1977, pp. 117–253.

CHAPTER 9

Lethal Mutagenesis: Exploiting Error-Prone Replication of Riboviruses for Antiviral Therapy

JASON D. GRACI and CRAIG E. CAMERON

Department of Biochemistry and Molecular Biology, Pennsylvania State University

9.1 INTRODUCTION

Riboviruses, whose genetic information is encoded in RNA rather than DNA, are the causative agents of numerous emerging diseases. SARS-associated coronavirus, Hantavirus, and West Nile virus are just a few of the many viruses responsible for recent public health challenges. Even well-characterized RNA viruses, such as influenza virus, continue to pose a significant public health threat. Riboviruses are also prominent among the potential agents of bioterrorism and biowarfare. The CDC has classified probable biowarfare agents into three categories (A, B, and C) according to factors including ease of acquisition, potential for dissemination, and potential impact on public health and safety.[1] RNA viruses have been included in each category. Category A contains the hemorrhagic fever viruses, including members of the Filoviridae, Flaviviridae, and Arenaviridae families. Included in Category B are agents of viral encephalitis, including alphaviruses such as Venezuelan equine encephalitis virus, eastern equine encephalitis virus, and western equine encephalitis virus. Finally, a number of emerging diseases have been classified as Category C agents, including Hantaviruses and Nipah virus.

Despite extensive research into the replication and pathogenesis of these viruses, few clinically useful therapeutics have resulted for treatment of RNA virus infections. Although a handful of compounds inhibitory to specific virus families have been developed, little success has been achieved in developing broad-spectrum antivirals. The only broad-spectrum antiviral in clinical use is the nucleoside analogue ribavirin.[2] Due to the potentially devastating consequences

Antiviral Drug Discovery for Emerging Diseases and Bioterrorism Threats. Edited by Paul F. Torrence
Copyright © 2005 John Wiley & Sons, Inc.

of an outbreak of a clinically uncontrollable virus infection, it is imperative to develop new and effective antiviral therapies.

An important and unique property of RNA viruses is that replication of their genomes is inherently error-prone, leading to at least one mutation per genome per replication cycle. Over the past decade, the concept of lethal mutagenesis has arisen. This is based on the idea that an increase in mutation frequency beyond an error threshold will lead to the rapid loss of essential genetic information, resulting in substantial decreases in viability.

Over the past few years, renewed interest in lethal mutagenesis has led to a number of important discoveries. Significant advances have given promise for the translation of lethal mutagenesis into use as a clinical antiviral strategy. In this chapter, we summarize our current knowledge of lethal mutagenesis and expound upon its utility in developing suitable clinical therapeutics for treatment of RNA virus infections.

9.2 ERROR-PRONE NATURE OF RIBOVIRUS REPLICATION AND THE CONCEPT OF LETHAL MUTAGENESIS

Although the precise determination of mutation frequency in naturally evolving virus populations is complex, numerous studies have estimated the mutation frequency of RNA virus replication to be orders of magnitude higher than for DNA replication.[3] It has been postulated that viral RNA-dependent RNA polymerases (RdRPs), the virus-encoded enzymes responsible for replication of genomic RNA, are inherently less faithful in regard to nucleotide selection and incorporation. However, recent dissection of the mechanism of the poliovirus RdRP suggests that this is not the case.[4a] A more plausible explanation is that the apparent lack of a $3' \rightarrow 5'$ exonuclease ("proofreading") activity of RdRPs, in addition to the absence of any postincorporation error repair mechanism, limits the fidelity of RNA replication.[4b]

The ultimate result of this "error-prone" process is the generation of approximately one mutation per RNA genome per round of replication.[5] Therefore, RNA virus populations are envisioned as a diverse and heterogeneous distribution of genomes termed a quasispecies. The concept of quasispecies was first developed by Eigen.[6] A quasispecies hovers around a "most fit" consensus sequence, but most, if not all, individual genomes in the population will contain variations from this consensus. Existence as a quasispecies is presumably advantageous in that the presence of abundant genetic variants allows for the rapid adaptation of the population in response to changing environmental conditions, for example, adaptation to a new host range, evasion of host immune defenses, or resistance to clinical therapy. In this sense, existence as a quasispecies aids in the continued survival of the species.

However, the extremely small genomes of RNA viruses necessitate that the genetic information be as compact as possible. RNA viruses have evolved a number of mechanisms to maximize the efficiency of their limited genomes, which would otherwise present constraints to their evolution.[7] These strategies include the use of multiple, overlapping reading frames for translation and the use of the same sequence space for multiple purposes, such as utilizing structural elements of RNA in addition to the protein-coding sequence. This highly compact nature of RNA genomes implies that they will be extremely sensitive to mutation, and that adaptive mutations are subject to fitness trade-offs.

The deleterious effects of higher mutation frequency (and concomitant lowered genetic stability) are presumably offset by the adaptive advantage provided by the quasispecies in maximizing the chances for population survival. The large population sizes and rapid replication times exhibited by riboviruses also assist in dealing with the limitations of quasispecies. Quasispecies theory has been described extensively elsewhere.[3,8]

A corollary to quasispecies theory postulates the existence of an error threshold, an error frequency beyond which insufficient genetic information is retained to allow continued propagation of the population. Beyond the error threshold, genetic information essentially loses meaning as it is driven toward randomness. If obtaining maximal diversity is important for RNA virus survival, it is likely that these viruses have evolved to exist at the edge of error catastrophe, the point of maximal adaptability.

Evidence that riboviruses exist at or near the error threshold was first provided by Holland and colleagues.[9] This work showed that mutations at single sites, as measured by a defined phenotype in vesicular stomatitis virus and poliovirus, could only be increased by less than threefold when using the mutagen 5-fluorouracil. The mutation frequency was not increased beyond these levels even when virus viability was decreased significantly. Hence, only small increases in mutation frequency can be tolerated by RNA genomes. This observation suggests that RNA viruses exist at the edge of error catastrophe, and that significant reductions in viability can result from relatively minor decreases in the fidelity of replication.

Later, work by Crotty and colleagues suggested that poliovirus exists at the error threshold.[10] Capsid-coding regions of poliovirus were sequenced after growth of the virus in a mutagen. Untreated poliovirus contained approximately 1.5 mutations per genome. An increase in mutation beyond this level resulted in surprisingly significant effects on virus viability. Importantly, relatively minor increases in mutation frequency were sufficient to cause extreme decreases in specific infectivity (Figure 9.1). When mutations per genome increased from 1.5 to 2, a 50% reduction in specific infectivity was observed. An approximately fourfold increase in mutation frequency caused a 95% reduction in specific infectivity of poliovirus RNA.

Loeb and colleagues examined the effects of mutagens on HIV-1.[11] Viability was dramatically decreased in the presence of only mild mutagens. Additionally, a mutagen that increased the mutation frequency only threefold was sufficient to cause extinction of the virus population during serial passage. From these experiments the term "lethal mutagenesis" was coined.

The strategy of lethal mutagenesis is based on increasing the viral mutation frequency in order to drive the population beyond the error threshold. All

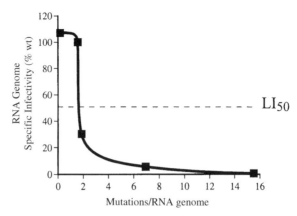

FIGURE 9.1   Poliovirus exists near the edge of error catastrophe. Poliovirus was produced in HeLa cells treated with varying levels of ribavirin, and specific infectivity was determined by transfection of isolated viral RNA. Genomic equivalents of capsid-coding regions were sequenced to determine the average number of mutations per genome. Untreated poliovirus was found to have approximately 1.5 mutations/genome. The LI_{50} (50% loss of specific infectivity) is the point at which 50% of the genomes are lethally mutated. (Reproduced with permission from *Proceedings of the National Academy of Science of the United States of America.*)[10]

indications are that only a small increase in mutagenesis is necessary for dramatic effects on RNA virus viability. Hence, an extremely effective mutagen (i.e., one that induces a very high level of mutation) is probably not required to develop an effective antiviral agent.

9.3   EVIDENCE FOR LETHAL MUTAGENESIS IN VITRO

Ribavirin was previously mentioned as the only broad-spectrum antiviral compound in clinical use. Ribavirin is a synthetic nucleoside analogue first described by Sidwell and co-workers over 30 years ago.[2] It has demonstrated antiviral activity against a wide range of viruses in vitro and is clinically approved for the treatment of a number of different viral infections, most notably in combination with interferon-α as therapy for hepatitis C virus (HCV) infection.[12,13] Research toward understanding the antiviral mechanism of ribavirin has a complicated and contentious history, with a number of distinct mechanisms being proposed. It seems most likely that this nucleoside analogue has multiple methods of action depending on the context in which it is employed. This controversy has been reviewed elsewhere.[14,15] One important property of ribavirin is the compelling evidence that has recently accumulated pointing to the ability of ribavirin to act as a lethal mutagen.

Early in the investigation of ribavirin, the observation was made that ribavirin could be phosphorylated by cellular nucleoside and nucleotide kinases. More importantly, the triphosphorylated form of ribavirin was found to accumulate within treated cells and was the most abundant metabolite.[16,17] This discovery immediately raised the question as to whether ribavirin triphosphate (RTP) could be incorporated into nascent RNA as a ribonucleotide analogue during replication or transcription. Unfortunately, early experiments were unable to detect incorporation of radioisotope-labeled ribavirin into viral RNA.

The first demonstration of ribavirin incorporation by a viral RdRP was performed by Crotty and co-workers utilizing poliovirus.[18] Using an in vitro primer-extension assay, it was shown that the poliovirus RdRP could incorporate ribavirin at approximately the rate of an incorrect nucleotide. Importantly, ribavirin was incorporated with approximately equal efficiency when either cytidine or uridine was the templating nucleotide. The reverse was also true: a template containing ribavirin was able to direct incorporation of either cytidine or uridine with equal efficiency. Hence, ribavirin could act as an ambiguous purine analogue. This property is likely mediated by rotation of the carboxamide moiety of the pseudo-base, allowing for two distinct hydrogen bonding configurations (Figure 9.2). Incorporation of ribavirin into nascent genomes did not affect the further elongation of the polynucleotide chain; hence, ribavirin was not a chain terminator. Experiments utilizing a poliovirus subgenomic replicon indicated that ribavirin had only minimal effects on the processes of translation and RNA synthesis. Hence, ribavirin does not primarily act by inhibiting or slowing these processes during virus replication.

Incorporation of an ambiguously pairing base into a genome should lead to an increase in mutation frequency. Ribavirin, as a general purine analogue, should therefore induce A-to-G and U-to-C transitions into poliovirus genomic RNA depending on the polarity of the RNA strand into which it is incorporated. Using a phenotypic screen, Crotty and colleagues observed that treatment of poliovirus did indeed result in an increase in transition mutations.[18] Together, the data obtained in these experiments provided strong evidence that lethal mutagenesis was responsible, at least in part, for the antiviral activity of ribavirin against poliovirus in vitro.

Similar results have been obtained with other viruses. Lanford and co-workers demonstrated ribavirin-induced mutagenesis of GB virus B, a surrogate model for HCV.[19] In this case, a significant reduction in viral RNA and a severe decrease in

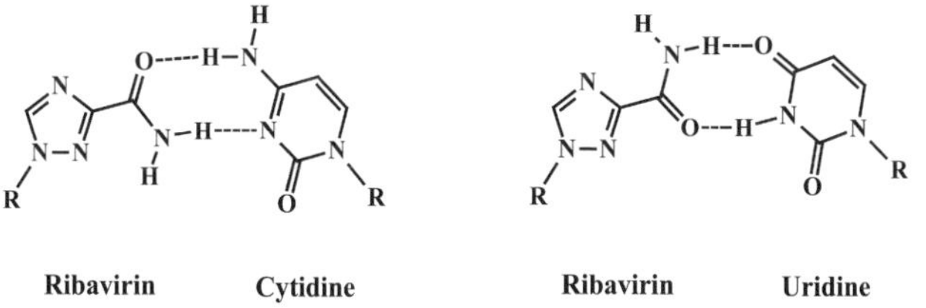

FIGURE 9.2 The nucleoside analogue ribavirin exhibits ambiguous base pairing. Rotation of the carboxamide moiety of the pseudobase of ribavirin can allow base pairing with either cytosine or uracil at approximately equal efficiency.

specific infectivity was seen after GB virus B infection of ribavirin-treated tamarin hepatocytes. After one passage in culture, viral RNA was undetectable and no resistant variants emerged. Ribavirin triphosphate has also been shown to be an ambiguously base pairing substrate for the HCV RdRP.[20] Further evidence suggesting error catastrophe as the mechanism of action of ribavirin against HCV has been obtained using a binary T7 polymerase/HCV cDNA replication system[21] and in a subgenomic replicon system,[22] although both of these are surrogate models for HCV replication. Unfortunately, authentic cell culture or small-animal models for HCV do not exist to further verify these results. The effects of mutagenesis on HIV was summarized in the preceding section, and lethal mutagenesis has also been observed for foot-and-mouth disease virus[23,24] and the arenavirus lymphocytic choriomeningitis virus.[25]

Severson and colleagues investigated the effect of ribavirin treatment on Hantaan virus.[26] Sequencing of S-segment coding regions derived from ribavirin-exposed virus showed that the mutation frequency was increased more than eightfold relative to untreated virus (about 4 substitutions per 1289 base pair S-segment). An observed decrease in viral mRNA and protein production was attributed to mutagenesis during transcription, leading to nonfunctional or unstable mRNAs. Levels of all nucleotide substitutions (both transitions and transversions) were increased. Additionally, a high number of insertions (approximately 8 per S-segment) were found. The inserted nucleotide was always identical to the preceding nucleotide in the sequence. The authors interpreted these results to indicate that ribavirin acts as a mutagen to Hantaan virus, and that the antiviral effect is mediated by transition into error catastrophe.

One factor that is clearly of importance for the efficacy of a lethal mutagen is the frequency of incorporation of the nucleoside. The fidelity of the particular polymerase in question will impact the ability of a nucleoside to be effectively incorporated. It is apparent that polymerases vary in respect to the incorporation of non-natural nucleosides. This can affect the efficiency of incorporation, as well as the templating specificity. However, another consideration is the susceptibility of a particular genomic sequence to mutation. That is, do RNA genomes themselves differ in their inherent susceptibility to lethal mutagenesis?

Research in the authors' laboratory has shown that coxsackievirus B3 (CVB3) is much more susceptible to ribavirin treatment in cell culture than the closely related poliovirus (PV) (Figure 9.3). Interestingly, ribavirin is incorporated less efficiently by the CVB3 polymerase in vitro (J. D. Graci, C. Castro, and C. E. Cameron, unpublished data). One potential explanation for this apparent discrepancy is that mutations in the CVB3 genome are more deleterious than the same level of mutation in the PV genome. In other words, the CVB3 genome is less "flexible" in regard to the sequence space that it can occupy.

One measure of the apparent flexibility of a genome is the rate of nonsynonymous mutation (d_N) in relation to the rate of synonymous mutation(d_S).[27,28] The ratio d_N/d_S can be interpreted as a measure of the selective constraints imposed on a virus population. This value has been determined for a number of different RNA viruses, and the d_N/d_S ratio has been shown to vary widely between viruses.[29] It is

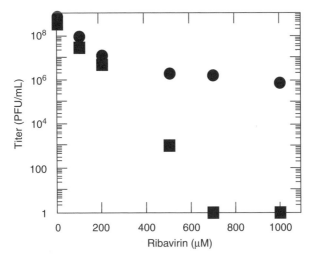

FIGURE 9.3 Coxsackievirus is more susceptible to ribavirin than poliovirus. HeLa cells (1×10^5) were pretreated with ribavirin for 18 hours and then infected with 2000 PFU PV ($\bullet$) or CVB3/0($\blacksquare$). Infected cells were incubated in the presence of compound until cell death. Virus was harvested by freeze–thaw and titer was determined. No viable CVB3/0 could be detected when ribavirin was present at a concentration of 750 μM or greater.

likely that a virus with a more diverse host range, either in terms of multiple organisms or just multiple sites of infection in the same host, may be more severely constrained in terms of variability. Even differences between cells of a single host can have severe effects on virus viability and pathogenicity. For instance, a minimal number of mutations in the poliovirus IRES results in attenuation due to a failure to replicate in neuronal cells.[30] This specificity is affected by the constraints to RNA evolution mentioned above, particularly the coevolution of multiple functions for a particular genome segment. Because RNA viruses have evolved to maximize the use of their limited genome sizes, a single nucleotide change may impact a number of separate functions. The degree to which this is true will limit the ability of the genome to tolerate additional mutations.

The extensive investigations summarized above have given credence to the notion of lethal mutagenesis as an antiviral strategy. It is apparent that small increases in mutation frequency can have significant effects on virus viability. It is also apparent from the range of viruses examined thus far that this strategy holds promise as a broad-spectrum approach for treatment of general RNA virus infection.

9.4 RESISTANCE TO LETHAL MUTAGENS

An important consideration in the investigation of new antiviral strategies is the possibility of resistance and what the impact of resistance will be on disease progression and transmission. Presumably, general viral resistance to lethal mutagens would arise primarily through an increase in polymerase fidelity, although drug-specific mechanisms may be possible. In the case of lethal mutagens, a number of recent studies have shed light on this issue.

Pfeiffer and Kirkegaard were successful in isolating a ribavirin-resistant variant of poliovirus through serial passage in the presence of the drug.[31] A single transition mutation in the RdRP, a glycine to serine substitution at position 64 of the fingers subdomain, was sufficient to confer resistance, albeit modest, to ribavirin in cell culture. This resistant virus had a threefold reduction in error frequency measured by using a phenotypic screen. Cross-resistance was demonstrated to another mutagen, 5-azacytidine. The authors hypothesized that decreased susceptibility to ribavirin was due to a reduction in mutation frequency (and consequently a lower susceptibility to mutagenesis) mediated by a higher-fidelity polymerase. This fidelity could potentially lead to resistance by either decreasing the frequency of incorporation of non-natural nucleosides or by increasing the overall fidelity of replication, thereby distancing the population from the error threshold. This circumstance would allow the genome to limit genetic damage induced by mutagens. Biochemical analysis of this polymerase variant indicated that the fidelity of this enzyme was indeed increased relative to the wild-type polymerase.[60]

Another important observation made in the Kirkegaard study was that resistant poliovirus variants were only selected when initially passaged at a low concentration of ribavirin. Higher concentrations led to apparent virus extinction after continuous passage. This observation explains the failure of other laboratories to detect ribavirin-resistant variants because limitations in experimental design may have prevented the emergence of resistance. This finding also has important implications for the clinical use of lethal mutagens in that administration of mutagens at a dosage insufficient for strong virus inhibition may increase the possibility of resistant populations emerging. There is clinical evidence that high-dose treatment with ribavirin is superior for patients who were resistant to normal therapy.[32]

Young and co-workers investigated the effect of ribavirin on HCV derived from clinical samples.[33] Sequencing of HCV-coding regions from patients receiving ribavirin monotherapy revealed a modest increase in mutation frequency, particularly in A-to-G and U-to-A substitutions. More importantly, a particular mutation in the RdRP of genotype 1a HCV emerged in all patients treated with ribavirin. This variant, containing a phenylalanine to tyrosine substitution at position 415 of the polymerase thumb subdomain, was replaced by the parental strain in some patients upon cessation of ribavirin therapy. The effect of this tyrosine substitution was investigated in cell culture using an HCV subgenomic replicon. HCV replicons containing phenylanine at this position were susceptible to ribavirin treatment while replicons with tyrosine at the same position exhibited resistance. The detailed biochemical mechanism of this resistance mutation has not yet been investigated, but these data implicate the RdRP as the target of ribavirin in vivo.

The precise effect that increased replication fidelity would have in a biological context, as opposed to cell culture, is unknown. It has been hypothesized that RNA viruses have evolved to exist on the edge of error catastrophe due to the advantages conferred by increased adaptability in a complex biological environment. The reduction in the quasispecies nature of the virus population that would be conferred by increased fidelity could impact the ability of the virus to adapt to the immune response or clinical treatment and even hinder transmission across species barriers. Thus, even though resistance may arise, its ultimate effect may be to reduce pathogenicity through attenuation or the inability to replicate efficiently in vivo.

9.5 LETHAL MUTAGENESIS AS AN ANTIVIRAL STRATEGY

Lethal mutagenesis has not firmly been established as an effective clinical antiviral therapy. This situation is partially due to the fact that the majority of known mutagenic nucleosides exhibit pronounced cellular toxicity, and the corresponding nucleotides would need to be present at high enough intracellular levels to be incorporated at a significant frequency during RNA genome replication. Thus, ribavirin is the only antiviral in clinical use which has been hypothesized to possibly exert its effects via lethal mutagenesis.

Ribavirin is effective against a broad range of both RNA and DNA viruses in vitro. It is approved for clinical treatment of HCV infection when administered in combination with interferon-α. It is also approved for use against respiratory syncitial virus infection in children, in which case it is administered as an aerosol, and as a treatment for Lassa virus infection. Ribavirin has shown some activity both in vivo and in vitro against hemorrhagic fever viruses, particularly members of the Arenaviridae and Bunyaviridae families,[34,35] but ribavirin has no apparent clinical efficacy against viral hemorrhagic fever induced by filoviruses or flaviviruses. Ribavirin has also been used to treat infection by Nipah virus,[36] Hantavirus,[37] and other emerging diseases.

Little data exist to strongly support any mechanism of action of ribavirin in clinical cases, and the actual effect of ribavirin on infections in human patients is still under debate. A number of factors have complicated the efforts to detect lethal mutagenesis in clinical samples, including the transient nature of lethally mutated RNA genomes, limitations in detection technology and sample collection, and the possibility of clinical virus populations rapidly acquiring resistance. Monitoring antiviral therapy by reverse transcription-polymerase chain reaction adds the complication that this technology cannot distinguish lethally mutated, unviable genomes from infectious, viable genomes. Thus, conclusions drawn from this data can be misleading. Additionally, current drug delivery methods may not allow sufficient accumulation of lethal mutagens at sites of infection. Clinical doses required to duplicate drug concentrations used in cell culture studies may be toxic or otherwise unattainable. It has been suggested that ribavirin may not accumulate to high enough clinical levels to cause substantial mutagenesis in vivo.[23]

In many cases, antiviral activity attributed to lethal mutagenesis in vitro or in cell culture has not been duplicated in animal models or in clinical investigations. Although ribavirin presumably acts via lethal mutagenesis when employed against

GB virus B infection in cultured tamarin hepatocytes, no significant antiviral effect was seen in infected tamarins fed ribavirin at high doses.[19]

However, the recent work by Young and colleagues has provided support for lethal mutagenesis as at least contributing to the effect seen when ribavirin is administered to patients infected with hepatitis C virus.[33] A modest mutagenic effect was noted in hepatitis C samples isolated from ribavirin-treated patients. More importantly, the discovery of a specific mutation in the polymerase of virus isolated from patients treated with ribavirin strongly suggests that the RdRP is the ultimate target of ribavirin therapy in clinical practice. Interestingly, HCV genotype 1a contain a phenylalanine at this position that can be mutated to tyrosine to give resistance, but all other HCV genotypes already contain a consensus tyrosine in this position. Therefore, other genotypes may already be less susceptible to ribavirin treatment.

An important consideration in development of mutagenic antivirals as a clinical treatment is the effect on the host. Nucleoside analogues can have considerable toxicity in vivo due to the numerous vital functions nucleosides play in the cell. Nucleotide metabolism is a strictly regulated process, and introduction of an analogue that can inhibit enzymes of these pathways can have quite dramatic effects on cellular viability. Many known nucleoside analogues do in fact act as strong inhibitors of these enzymes.[38] Furthermore, conversion of a mutagenic ribonucleoside analogue to the corresponding deoxynucleoside has the potential to cause heritable genetic damage. Ribavirin is not thought to be converted to the deoxynucleoside in any substantial quantities,[17] but the structural characteristics responsible for this property are unknown. Ribavirin is a teratogen and interferes with sperm development. It has been suggested that this may be due to incorporation via a cellular RdRP utilized in the cellular RNA interference (RNAi) process.[15] All of these possible side effects will need to be considered in the development of lethal mutagens.

Recent experiments with SARS-associated coronavirus infection of Vero 76 cells have suggested that ribavirin is ineffective against this virus.[39] However, previous work with West Nile virus has shown differences in the efficacy of ribavirin in cell culture depending on the cell line employed.[40] This is likely due to a 13-fold reduction in the accumulation of ribavirin monophosphate in Vero cells.[41] Similar results have been obtained in the authors' laboratory with poliovirus (J. D. Graci and C. E. Cameron, unpublished data). Ribavirin had only a minimal effect on poliovirus infection of Vero 76 cells as compared to HeLa cells (Figure 9.4). The differences observed between cell types argue that cell culture-based approaches may be insufficient in determining the potential clinical value of a compound of interest. At the least, results obtained with cultured cells should be viewed with caution unless results can be verified with well-characterized cell lines as controls. Importantly, this underscores the fact that the effectiveness of a particular nucleoside analogue is highly dependent on the characteristics of the target cell.

Another important discovery has generated significant interest in lethal mutagenesis: the realization that cells may have evolved mutagenic activity as an innate

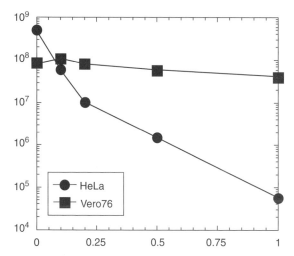

FIGURE 9.4   Ribavirin has minimal effect on poliovirus in Vero 76 cells. HeLa cells (•) or Vero 76 cells (■) (1×10^5) were pretreated with ribavirin for 18 hours, then infected with 2000 PFU PV. Infected cells were incubated in the presence of compound until cell death. Virus was harvested by freeze–thaw and titer was determined.

antiviral defense mechanism. Recently, the enzyme APOBEC3G has been showned to be responsible for the reduced infectivity of Δvif HIV in "nonpermissive" cells.[42] This enzyme is a DNA-specific cytidine deaminase, and its expression causes an increase in dC-to-dU mutations in E. coli.[43] Currently, it is believed that APOBEC3G is included in virions and, upon entry of HIV into a new host cell, deaminates the first retroviral negative strand during replication, causing dC-to-dU transitions.[44] The resultant increase in mutation frequency should have a deleterious effect on genome stability and fidelity of replication. This antiviral activity was found to be absent in the presence of Vif.

Recent investigations into this property of Vif have suggested that Vif can induce ubiquitination and subsequent degradation of APOBEC3G via cellular proteasomal pathways, therefore preventing its incorporation into virions.[45–49] It has also been reported that APOBEC3G expression leads to enhanced degradation of Vif via ubiquitination, suggesting a reciprocal relationship in which both proteins may be degraded in a single complex.[49] APOBEC3G is active against other retroviruses[44,50] and has also been shown to inhibit hepatitis B virus of the family Hepadnaviridae, although mutagenesis was not detected in this particular study.[51]

This discovery of a cellular mutagenic antiviral activity raises many important questions. Do cells possess other antiviral activities that can induce mutagenesis of foreign genomes? Is such a strategy utilized against other DNA- or RNA-based viruses? Clearly, HIV Vif has evolved to suppress this cellular response. But have other viruses acquired similar countermeasures, and can these be exploited for therapeutic approaches? Further understanding of this innate antiviral defense mechanism may help in developing lethal mutagenesis as a clinical strategy.

The ADAR (adenosine deaminase that acts on RNA) family of enzymes has provocative characteristics that may suggest it can target viral RNA genomes for mutation. The enzymes bind to RNA that is highly doubled-stranded and catalyze the conversion of adenosine to inosine, which is generally recognized as guanosine by most enzymes.[52] Human ADAR1-L is highly active in the cytoplasm [53] and expressed as part of the interferon response. Whether this enzyme acts as part of an innate antiviral defense mechanism has yet to be thoroughly investigated.

9.6   DIRECTIONS FOR FUTURE RESEARCH

Recent research has demonstrated the promise of lethal mutagenesis as an antiviral strategy. Exploitation of this strategy to produce broad-spectrum antiviral mutagens has become an exciting possibility. Unfortunately, many of the hurdles to be overcome in translating these discoveries into clinical use are not well understood. In this final section of the chapter, we provide a brief overview of some challenges to overcome in order to develop lethal mutagenesis into a clinically useful antiviral strategy.

Investigation of Known Mutagens as Antivirals and Development of New Nucleoside Analogues. An extensive compendium of information has accumulated on synthetic nucleoside chemistry, and numerous nucleoside analogues have already been synthesized and characterized. In light of recent results with lethal mutagenesis, it may be worthwhile to reevaluate known mutagenic analogues for antiviral activity. In addition, novel nucleoside analogues should be developed in the search for more effective lethal mutagens. Work in this area has already begun.[54–56] The goal should be not only to develop mutagenic analogues but also to work toward understanding the molecular charactersitics and structure–function relationships underlying incorporation and fidelity characteristics of nucleoside analogues in the context of viral RdRPs. In addition, further elucidation of the properties required for effective cellular import and phosphorylation, essential for in vitro utilization of mutagenic nucleosides, is required (reviewed previously).[14]

Understanding the Effect of Lethal Mutagenesis on Different Viruses. As mentioned earlier, coxsackievirus B3 was found to be more susceptible to ribavirin-induced mutagenesis than poliovirus. Thus, even closely related viruses may have widely varying responses to an increase in error frequency. This differential susceptibility may be due either to differences in the fidelity of the virus polymerases or to increased susceptibility of the genome itself to mutation. However, the biological basis for this is not understood. One possibility is that viruses which must replicate in a variety of different host cells (or in different organisms, as in the vectorborne viruses) may be more constrained in the breadth of sequences that can be tolerated. Understanding the relationship between polymerase fidelity, constraints on sequence variability, and the effect of mutagenesis on pathology and spread of different viruses should lead to insight into the development of effective antivirals.

Understanding and Controlling Host Cytotoxicity. The majority of known biologically active nucleoside analogues have some degree of cytostatic and/or cytotoxic effects. This problem could be caused by a number of factors, most importantly mutagenesis of host cell DNA and gross aberrations of cellular nucleotide pools and metabolism. Developing a greater understanding of cellular nucleotide metabolism may allow development of analogues that exhibit minimal cellular toxicity, yet remain highly mutagenic to viral RNA genomes. Recent work with 2′-substituted nucleosides has been promising in relieving cellular toxicity.[57,58] Also of great importance is understanding what, if any, structural characteristics can prevent ribonucleoside analogues from being converted to deoxyribonucleoside analogues in order to prevent incorporation by host DNA polymerases.

Understanding the Impact of Resistance. It has become quite clear that resistance to mutagens can occur in virus populations. This observation has brought a number of new questions to the forefront. Most importantly, what effect will the development of resistance have on the pathology and transmission of a particular virus? It can be inferred that the ribavirin-resistant phenotypes of HCV and PV are of significant lower fitness than "wild-type" virus populations due to the fact that the resistance phenotype quickly gives way to wild-type virus upon cessation of ribavirin exposure. Presumably, resistance is due to enhanced fidelity of the RdRP, but it is unknown what the effect of this "reduction" of quasispecies character will have on the virus population. Because these populations are thought to have evolved to exist on the edge of error catastrophe, low-fidelity replication must be beneficial. It is likely the reduction in variability of the population would affect the ability of a virus to evade the immune defenses of the host, or diminish the ability of the virus to develop further resistance to unrelated antivirals. Further investigation of enhanced-fidelity riboviruses (such as the ribavirin-resistant variant of poliovirus) in their natural biological context should provide insight into these issues. Lethal mutagens may therefore be a logical addition to drug "cocktails," such as those used currently in the treatment of HIV. In fact, Mansky reported an apparent increase in virus mutation frequency during potent antiretroviral therapy (ART).[59] Additionally, a high-fidelity virus may be less likely to infect a new host or even be prevented from replicating throughtout its entire host range.

9.7 CONCLUSION

Successful antimicrobial strategies have been based on exploiting differences in the biology of host and pathogen. In this chapter, we have explored the strategy of lethal mutagenesis, which targets two important properties of riboviruses: the use of RNA rather than DNA as the genetic material and the error-prone replication of the viral genome. Because these characteristics exist in all known RNA viruses, lethal mutagens have potential as broad-spectrum antiviral agents.

Recent work with lethal mutagens has resulted in promising advances in understanding the mechanism of lethal mutagenesis as an antiviral strategy. However, there is still much to learn, particularly regarding the effect of mutagenic nucleoside analogues on host processes. Continued study of lethal mutagens and lethal mutagenesis holds great promise for the development of strategies to treat emerging and established RNA virus diseases.

ACKNOWLEDGMENTS

The authors thank Dr. Nora Chapman and Dr. Steven Tracy (University of Nebraska Medical Center) for providing CVB3/0 cDNA. Data for incorporation of ribavirin by the CVB3/0 polymerase was obtained by Dr. Christian Castro (Pennsylvania State University). Evaluation of ribavirin in Vero 76 cells was performed by Joshua Kucharski (Pennsylvania State University). Research on lethal mutagenesis performed in the Cameron laboratory is funded by grants from the American Heart Association (0340028N) and the National Institutes of Health (AI054776).

REFERENCES

1. Rotz, L. D.; Khan, A. S.; Lillibridge, S. R.; Ostroff, S. M.; Hughes, J. M. Public health assessment of potential biological terrorism agents. *Emerging Infect. Dis.* **2002**, *8*, 225–230.

2. Sidwell, R. W.; Huffman, J. H.; Khare, G. P.; Allen, L. B.; Witkowski, J. T.; et al. Broad-spectrum antiviral activity of Virazole: 1-beta-D-ribofuranosyl-1,2,4-triazole-3-carboxamide. *Science* **1972**, *177*, 705–706.

3. Domingo, E.; Escarmis, C.; Sevilla, N.; Moya, A.; Elena, S. F.; et al. Basic concepts in RNA virus evolution. The quasispecies (extremely heterogeneous) nature of viral RNA genome populations: biological relevance—a review. *FASEB J.* **1996**, *10*, 859–864.

4. (a) Steinhauer, D. A.; Domingo, E.; Holland, J. J. Lack of evidence for proofreading mechanisms associated with an RNA virus polymerase. *Gene* **1992**, *122*, 281–288. (b) Arnold, J. J.; Cameron, C. E. Poliovirus RNA-dependent RNA polymerase (3D^{pol}): Presteady-state kinetic analysis of ribonucleotide incorporation in the presence of Mg^{2+}. *Biochemistry* **2004**, *43*, 5126–5137.

5. Drake, J. W.; Holland, J. J. Mutation rates among RNA viruses. *Proc. Natl. Acad. Sci. U.S.A.* **1999**, *96*, 13910–13913.

6. Eigen, M. Selforganization of matter and the evolution of biological macromolecules. *Naturwissenschaften* **1971**, *58*, 465–523.

7. Holmes, E. C. Error thresholds and the constraints to RNA virus evolution. *Trends Microbiol.* **2003**, *11*, 543–546.

8. Domingo, E.; Holland, J. J.; Escarmis, C.; Sevilla, N.; Moya, A.; et al. RNA virus mutations and fitness for survival. Basic concepts in RNA virus evolution. *Annu. Rev. Microbiol.* **1997**, *51*, 151–178.

9. Holland, J. J.; Domingo, E.; de la Torre, J. C.; Steinhauer, D. A. Mutation frequencies at defined single codon sites in vesicular stomatitis virus and poliovirus can be increased only slightly by chemical mutagenesis. *J. Virol.* **1990**, *64*, 3960–3962.

10. Crotty, S.; Cameron, C. E.; Andino, R. RNA virus error catastrophe: direct molecular test by using ribavirin. *Proc. Natl. Acad. Sci. U.S.A.* **2001**, *98*, 6895–6900.

11. Loeb, L. A.; Essigmann, J. M.; Kazazi, F.; Zhang, J.; Rose, K. D.; et al. Lethal mutagenesis of HIV with mutagenic nucleoside analogs. *Proc. Natl. Acad. Sci. U.S.A.* **1999**, *96*, 1492–1497.

12. Cummings, K. J.; Lee, S. M.; West, E. S.; Cid-Ruzafa, J.; Fein, S. G.; et al. Interferon and ribavirin vs interferon alone in the re-treatment of chronic hepatitis C previously nonresponsive to interferon: a meta-analysis of randomized trials. *JAMA* **2001**, *285*, 193–199.

13. Davis, G. L.; Esteban-Mur, R.; Rustgi, V.; Hoefs, J.; Gordon, S. C.; et al. Interferon α-2b alone or in combination with ribavirin for the treatment of relapse of chronic hepatitis C. International Hepatitis Interventional Therapy Group. *N. Engl. J. Med.* **1998**, *339*, 1493–1499.

14. Graci, J. D.; Cameron, C. E. Challenges for the development of ribonucleoside analogues as inducers of error catastrophe. *Antiviral Chem. Chemother.* **2004**, *15*, 1–13.

15. Cameron, C. E.; Castro, C. The mechanism of action of ribavirin: lethal mutagenesis of RNA virus genomes mediated by the viral RNA-dependent RNA polymerase. *Curr. Opin. Infect. Dis.* **2001**, *14*, 757–764.

16. Page, T.; Connor, J. D. The metabolism of ribavirin in erythrocytes and nucleated cells. *Int. J. Biochem.* **1990**, *22*, 379–383.

17. Miller, J. P.; Kigwana, L. J.; Streeter, D. G.; Robins, R. K.; Simon, L. N.; et al. The relationship between the metabolism of ribavirin and its proposed mechanism of action. *Ann. N.Y. Acad. Sci.* **1977**, *284*, 211–229.

18. Crotty, S.; Maag, D.; Arnold, J. J.; Zhong, W.; Lau, J. Y.; et al. The broad-spectrum antiviral ribonucleoside ribavirin is an RNA virus mutagen. *Nat. Med.* **2000**, *6*, 375–1379.

19. Lanford, R. E.; Chavez, D.; Guerra, B.; Lau, J. Y.; Hong, Z.; et al. Ribavirin induces error-prone replication of GB virus B in primary tamarin hepatocytes. *J. Virol.* **2001**, *75*, 8074–8081.

20. Maag, D.; Castro, C.; Hong, Z.; Cameron, C. E. Hepatitis C virus RNA-dependent RNA polymerase (NS5B) as a mediator of the antiviral activity of ribavirin. *J. Biol. Chem.* **2001**, *276*, 46094–46098.

21. Contreras, A. M.; Hiasa, Y.; He, W.; Terella, A.; Schmidt, E. V.; et al. Viral RNA mutations are region specific and increased by ribavirin in a full-length hepatitis C virus replication system. *J. Virol.* **2002**, *76*, 8505–8517.

22. Zhou, S.; Liu, R.; Baroudy, B. M.; Malcolm, B. A.; Reyes, G. R. The effect of ribavirin and IMPDH inhibitors on hepatitis C virus subgenomic replicon RNA. *Virology* **2003**, *310*, 333–342.

23. Airaksinen, A.; Pariente, N.; Menendez-Arias, L.; Domingo, E. Curing of foot-and-mouth disease virus from persistently infected cells by ribavirin involves enhanced mutagenesis. *Virology* **2003**, *311*, 339–349.

24. Pariente, N.; Sierra, S.; Lowenstein, P. R.; Domingo, E. Efficient virus extinction by combinations of a mutagen and antiviral inhibitors. *J. Virol.* **2001**, *75*, 9723–9730.

25. Ruiz-Jarabo, C. M.; Ly, C.; Domingo, E.; de la Torre, J. C. Lethal mutagenesis of the prototypic arenavirus lymphocytic choriomeningitis virus (LCMV). *Virology* **2003**, *308*, 37–47.

26. Severson, W. E.; Schmaljohn, C. S.; Javadian, A.; Jonsson, C. B. Ribavirin causes error catastrophe during Hantaan virus replication. *J. Virol.* **2003**, *77*, 481–488.

27. Yang, Z.; Nielsen, R.; Goldman, N.; Pedersen, A. M. Codon-substitution models for heterogeneous selection pressure at amino acid sites. *Genetics* **2000**, *155*, 431–449.

28. Miyata, T.; Yasunaga, T. Molecular evolution of mRNA: a method for estimating evolutionary rates of synonymous and amino acid substitutions from homologous nucleotide sequences and its application. *J. Mol. Evol.* **1980**, *16*, 23–36.

29. Woelk, C. H.; Holmes, E. C. Reduced positive selection in vector-borne RNA viruses. *Mol. Biol. Evol.* **2002**, *19*, 2333–2336.

30. Kawamura, N.; Kohara, M.; Abe, S.; Komatsu, T.; Tago, K.; et al. Determinants in the 5′ noncoding region of poliovirus Sabin 1 RNA that influence the attenuation phenotype. *J. Virol.* **1989**, *63*, 1302–1309.

31. Pfeiffer, J. K.; Kirkegaard, K. A single mutation in poliovirus RNA-dependent RNA polymerase confers resistance to mutagenic nucleotide analogs via increased fidelity. *Proc. Natl. Acad. Sci. U.S.A.* **2003**, *100*, 7289–7294.

32. da Silva, L. C.; Bassit, L.; Ono-Nita, S. K.; Pinho, J. R.; Nishiya, A.; et al. High rate of sustained response to consensus interferon plus ribavirin in chronic hepatitis C patients resistant to alpha-interferon and ribavirin: a pilot study. *J. Gastroenterol* **2002**, *37*, 732–736.

33. Young, K. C.; Lindsay, K. L.; Lee, K. J.; Liu, W. C.; He, J. W.; et al. Identification of a ribavirin-resistant NS5B mutation of hepatitis C virus during ribavirin monotherapy. *Hepatology* **2003**, *38*, 869–878.

34. Mardani, M.; Jahromi, M. K.; Naieni, K. H.; Zeinali, M. The efficacy of oral ribavirin in the treatment of Crimean-Congo hemorrhagic fever in Iran. *Clin. Infect. Dis.* **2003**, *36*, 1613–1618. Epub 2003 Jun 1614.

35. Huggins, J. W. Prospects for treatment of viral hemorrhagic fevers with ribavirin, a broad-spectrum antiviral drug. *Rev. Infect. Dis.* **1989**, *11*, S750–761.

36. Chong, H. T.; Kamarulzaman, A.; Tan, C. T.; Goh, K. J.; Thayaparan, T.; et al. Treatment of acute Nipah encephalitis with ribavirin. *Ann. Neurol.* **2001**, *49*, 810–813.

37. Huggins, J. W.; Hsiang, C. M.; Cosgriff, T. M.; Guang, M. Y.; Smith, J. I.; et al. Prospective, double-blind, concurrent, placebo-controlled clinical trial of intravenous ribavirin therapy of hemorrhagic fever with renal syndrome. *J. Infect. Dis.* **1991**, *164*, 1119–1127.

38. De Clercq, E. Antiviral agents: characteristic activity spectrum depending on the molecular target with which they interact. *Adv. Virus. Res.* **1993**, *42*, 1–55.

39. Cinatl, J.; Morgenstern, B.; Bauer, G.; Chandra, P.; Rabenau, H.; et al. Glycyrrhizin, an active component of liquorice roots, and replication of SARS-associated coronavirus. *Lancet* **2003**, *361*, 2045–2046.

40. Morrey, J. D.; Smee, D. F.; Sidwell, R. W.; Tseng, C. Identification of active antiviral compounds against a New York isolate of West Nile virus. *Antiviral Res.* **2002**, *55*, 107–116.

41. Smee, D. F.; Bray, M.; Huggins, J. W. Antiviral activity and mode of action studies of ribavirin and mycophenolic acid against orthopoxviruses in vitro. *Antiviral Chem. Chemother.* **2001**, *12*, 327–335.

42. Sheehy, A. M.; Gaddis, N. C.; Choi, J. D.; Malim, M. H. Isolation of a human gene that inhibits HIV-1 infection and is suppressed by the viral Vif protein. *Nature* **2002**, *418*, 646–650.

43. Harris, R. S.; Petersen-Mahrt, S. K.; Neuberger, M. S. RNA editing enzyme APOBEC1 and some of its homologs can act as DNA mutators. *Mol. Cell.* **2002**, *10*, 1247–1253.

44. Harris, R. S.; Bishop, K. N.; Sheehy, A. M.; Craig, H. M.; Petersen-Mahrt, S. K.; et al. DNA deamination mediates innate immunity to retroviral infection. *Cell* **2003**, *113*, 803–809.

45. Yu, X.; Yu, Y.; Liu, B.; Luo, K.; Kong, W.; et al. Induction of APOBEC3G ubiquitination and degradation by an HIV-1 Vif-Cul5-SCF complex. *Science* **2003**, *302*, 1056–1060. Epub 2003 Oct 1016.

46. Stopak, K.; de Noronha, C.; Yonemoto, W.; Greene, W. C. HIV-1 Vif blocks the antiviral activity of APOBEC3G by impairing both its translation and intracellular stability. *Mol. Cell.* **2003**, *12*, 591–601.

47. Marin, M.; Rose, K. M.; Kozak, S. L.; Kabat, D. HIV-1 Vif protein binds the editing enzyme APOBEC3G and induces its degradation. *Nat. Med.* **2003**, *9*, 1398–1403. Epub 2003 Oct 1395.

48. Sheehy, A. M.; Gaddis, N. C.; Malim, M. H. The antiretroviral enzyme APOBEC3G is degraded by the proteasome in response to HIV-1 Vif. *Nat. Med.* **2003**, *9*, 1404–1407. Epub 2003 Oct 1405.

49. Mehle, A.; Strack, B.; Ancuta, P.; Zhang, C.; McPike, M.; et al. Vif overcomes the innate antiviral activity of APOBEC3G by promoting its degradation in the ubiquitin-proteasome pathway. *J. Biol. Chem.* **2004**, *279*, 7792–7798. Epub 2003 Dec 7713.

50. Mangeat, B.; Turelli, P.; Caron, G.; Friedli, M.; Perrin, L.; et al. Broad antiretroviral defence by human APOBEC3G through lethal editing of nascent reverse transcripts. *Nature* **2003**, *424*, 99–103.

51. Turelli, P.; Mangeat, B.; Jost, S.; Vianin, S.; Trono, D. Inhibition of hepatitis B virus replication by APOBEC3G. *Science* **2004**, *303*, 1829.

52. Bass, B. L. RNA editing by adenosine deaminases that act on RNA. *Annu. Rev. Biochem.* **2002**, *71*, 817–846.

53. Wong, S. K.; Sato, S.; Lazinski, D. W. Elevated activity of the large form of ADAR1 in vivo: very efficient RNA editing occurs in the cytoplasm. *RNA* **2003**, *9*, 586–598.

54. Moriyama, K.; Otsuka, C.; Loakes, D.; Negishi, K. Highly efficient random mutagenesis in transcription–reverse-transcription cycles by a hydrogen bond ambivalent nucleoside 5′-triphosphate analogue: potential candidates for a selective anti-retroviral therapy. *Nucleosides Nucleotides Nucleic Acids* **2001**, *20*, 1473–1483.

55. Moriyama, K.; Negishi, K.; Briggs, M. S.; Smith, C. L.; Hill, F.; et al. Synthesis and RNA polymerase incorporation of the degenerate ribonucleotide analogue rPTP. *Nucleic Acids Res.* **1998**, *26*, 2105–2111.

56. Harki, D. A.; Graci, J. D.; Korneeva, V. S.; Ghosh, S. K.; Hong, Z.; et al. Synthesis and antiviral evaluation of a mutagenic and non-hydrogen bonding ribonucleoside analogue: 1-beta-D-Ribofuranosyl-3-nitropyrrole. *Biochemistry* **2002**, *41*, 9026–9033.

57. Carroll, S. S.; Tomassini, J. E.; Bosserman, M.; Getty, K.; Stahlhut, M. W.; et al. Inhibition of hepatitis C virus RNA replication by 2′-modified nucleoside analogs. *J. Biol. Chem.* **2003**, *278*, 11979–11984.

58. Migliaccio, G.; Tomassini, J. E.; Carroll, S. S.; Tomei, L.; Altamura, S.; et al. Characterization of resistance to non-obligate chain terminating ribonucleoside analogs which inhibit HCV replication in vitro. *J. Biol. Chem.* **2003**, *8*, 8.

59. Mansky, L. M. Mutagenic outcome of combined antiviral drug treatment during human immunodeficiency virus type 1 replication. *Virology* **2003**, *307*, 116–121.

60. Arnold, J. J.; Vignozzi, M.; Stone, J. K.; Andino, R; Cameron, C. E. Remote-site control of an active site fidelity checkpoint in a viral RNA-dependent RNA polymerase. *J. Biol. Chem.* **2005**, May 5. (epublication).

EMERGING
INFECTIOUS DISEASES

A Peer-Reviewed Journal Tracking and Analyzing Disease Trends   Vol. 9, No. 7, July 2003

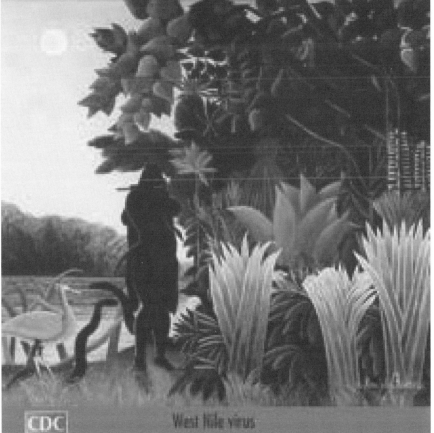

West Nile virus

CDC

CHAPTER 10

Structural Biology of Flaviviral Replication and Opportunities for Drug Design

KRISHNA MURTHY

Center for Biophysical Sciences and Engineering, University of Alabama at Birmingham

10.1 INTRODUCTION

Flaviviral diseases are widespread in tropical regions and are caused by infections due to viruses such as dengue, yellow fever, Japanese encephalitis, and West Nile. Information that has been obtained from genetic, molecular biological, biochemical, and structural studies has elucidated the key processes involved in the life cycle of flaviviruses and identified several therapeutic targets. These include viral structural proteins such as the envelope protein and nonstructural proteins such as the viral protease, helicase, RNA polymerase, and methyl transferase. This chapter summarizes the information that is currently available on each of these proteins and the work that is being done to target them using suitable inhibitory compounds.

10.2 FLAVIVIRAL DISEASES

The *Flavivirus* genus of Flaviviridae numbers approximately seventy identified members and includes many potent human pathogens.[1] These include yellow fever, dengue, Japanese encephalitis, and West Nile viruses, among others. Flaviviruses are arboviruses transmitted by ticks or mosquitoes. Although successful eradication of flaviviral vectors have banished infections from North America, flaviviruses pervade many of the tropical regions of the world, causing death, disease, and

Antiviral Drug Discovery for Emerging Diseases and Bioterrorism Threats. Edited by Paul F. Torrence
Copyright © 2005 John Wiley & Sons, Inc.

enormous economic damage. For a comprehensive series of reviews on flaviviral structure, replication, evolution, pathogenesis, immunity, epidemiology, detection, diagnosis, and vaccine development, the reader is referred to recent volumes of *Advances in Virus Research.*[2] Some reviews on potential drug design strategies against flaviviral diseases are also available.[3–5] Only brief background sketches of some of these topics that are relevant to a discussion of potential pharmacological targets will be presented here.

Currently, dengue viruses (Den) are by far the most widespread and most virulent and pose the largest public health thereat. Quiescent mosquito reservoirs of the four serotypes of dengue (Den 1–4) in almost all tropical regions result in eruptions of frequent epidemics among the resident human population. It has been estimated that approximately 2.5 billion people, 40% of the world's population, live in areas that are endemic to dengue viruses and are at risk for infection.[6] Estimated annual dengue infections number 100 million, with 500,000 cases of dengue hemorrhagic fever, resulting in an average of 25,000 deaths.[7] Japanese encephalitis (JE), St. Louis encephalitis (SLE), and tickborne encephalitis (TBE) are also prevalent in many tropical regions, although they affect smaller proportions of the human population.[8–11] West Nile virus (WNV), also present in many tropical regions, has been recently reintroduced into North America and has rapidly spread into many temperate regions.[12–14] Other members that have recently infected human populations include Kyasanur Forest disease (KFD) virus, Omsk hemorrhagic fever (OHF) virus, and the Alkhurma virus.[15–17] Besides being significant public health threats, Den, KFD, and OHF are thought to have bioterrorism potential.[18] Vaccines are available to provide immunity against some of the flaviviruses. The highly efficacious YF17D vaccine currently provides immunity against the eponymous yellow fever virus, once the most widespread of flaviviruses.[19] Vaccines are also either available or in the advanced clinical trial stages for TBE, JE, and WNV.[20–25] Progress on development of vaccines for KFD is also being made.[26,27] The four serotypes of dengue appear to present a harder problem for vaccine design, because dengue infections are subject to antibody-dependent enhancement (ADE). Infection of any of the four serotypes results in the usually survivable dengue fever. However, a subsequent infection by a different serotype causes the more frequently fatal dengue hemorrhagic fever/dengue shock syndrome; apparently due to non-neutralizing cross-reaction of antibodies from the first infection with the heterotypic virus followed by efficient uptake of the antibody-bound virus via Fcγ and complement receptors. Thus, although tetravalent dengue vaccines are under clinical trials, their efficacy is yet to be demonstrated.[21,28–32]

10.3 MECHANISMS OF VIRAL ENTRY

Flaviviruses normally enter host cells by initial binding to virus-specific, cell-surface receptors, aided by glycosaminoglycan (GAG) coreceptors, followed by endocytosis. Using virus overlay blot techniques, existence of specific cell surface receptor molecules have been demonstrated for Den1,[33] Den2,[34–37] Den4,[38–41] TBE,[42] and WNV.[43] In addition, CD209, a receptor required for entry of all dengue serotypes,[44,45] has also been identified. Isolation of a Den4 receptor protein has recently[46] been accomplished. Potential utilization of GAG receptors has been demonstrated for some dengue serotypes.[33,47,48] In addition to normal entry, some flaviviruses also gain entry through receptors other than specific flaviviral receptors via ADE. This phenomenon has been particularly well documented for dengue viruses. Fcγ receptors are utilized by IgG-bound but non-neutralized viruses, while complement receptors are similarly exploited by IgM-bound viruses.[31]

10.4 FLAVIVIRAL REPLICATION

Flaviviruses are positive-stranded RNA viruses with an approximately 11 kb genome size. The RNA is terminated at the 5' end by a type I cap structure that consists of a $m^7GpppAmpN_2$.[49] A single coding frame in the genome is flanked by an approximately 100 nucleotide 5' noncoding region and a 400–700 nucleotide 5' noncoding region. Mutational and biochemical studies carried out on Den4 and WNV indicate that the noncoding regions interact with host-specific proteins during replication and modulate translation of the viral RNA.[50–56] The coding region of the RNA specifies a long viral polyprotein, which is cleaved by a combination of host and viral proteases into at least 10 polypeptides. Three of these (C, PrM, E) are structural proteins, and at least seven (NS1, NS2A, NS2B, NS3, NS4A, NS4B, NS5) are nonstructural proteins.[57] Cleavage of the viral polyprotein into its component polypeptides is one of the best characterized steps in flaviviral replication and occurs in the endoplasmic reticulum both cotranslationally and posttranslationally. Figure 10.1 summarizes the cleavages and the proteases that mediate this process. Four of the cleavages, those between C–PrM, PrM–E, E–NS1, and NS4A–NS4B, are carried out by a host signalase.[58–62] Studies on dengue, YFV, JEV, and WNV have established that a viral serine protease is responsible for

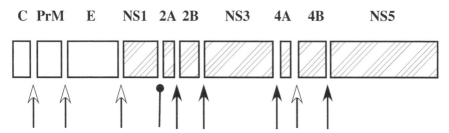

FIGURE 10.1 Flaviviral polyprotein and its cleavage. Each protein product is represented by a rectangular box roughly proportional to the molecular mass of the protein. Nonstructural protein boxes are stippled. The proteins are labeled at the top. Solid arrows indicate cleavage by the viral serine protease. Open-headed arrows indicate cleavage by a host signalase. Line terminated by a round head indicates cleavage by a currently unknown protease.

cleavages between NS2A–NS2B, NS2B–NS3, and NS3–NS4A.[63–65] Identity of the protease that processes the NS1–NS2A junction is currently unknown.[66] The viral NS2B/NS3 protease, originally detected through sequence comparisons,[67,68] recognizes a dibasic amino acid side chain motif and is an essential part of the viral replication machinery, as shown by mutational analyses.[69–75] The RNA replicase of flaviviruses is localized on host cytoplasmic membranes and is a complex assembly of its nonstructural proteins along with several host factors. However, there is currently incomplete information about the topological disposition of the components or about the temporal sequence and involvement of individual components.[76] It is nevertheless known that replication proceeds through the initial formation of a negative RNA strand, which is used as a template repeatedly for synthesis of many positive strands.[49,77,78] From studies on Den2, it is thought that priming of positive-strand synthesis on templates occurs through a "copy-back" mechanism similar to that suggested for HCV replication.[79] Although it is known that 5′ cap formation occurs through the combined involvement of the RNA triphosphatase activity of NS3 and the methyltransferase activity of NS5, the exact mechanisms are still obscure.[80]

10.5 POTENTIAL PHARMACOLOGICAL TARGETS

Studies on the molecular details of viral entry, replication, and assembly suggest that flaviviruses are vulnerable to attack at several stages during their life cycle. Both structural and enzymatically active viral proteins, which play critical roles in the viral lifecycle, are plausible targets.

10.5.1 Nonstructural Proteins

Flaviviruses express four enzymatic activities in host cells: a serine protease that is required for cleavages at four of the polyprotein junctions, an RNA helicase and an RNA polymerase required for replication, and a methyltransferase needed for 5′ cap synthesis. These four activities are carried out by two viral proteins; NS3, which has both serine protease and RNA helicase activities, and NS5, which possesses RNA-dependent RNA polymerase (RdRP) and methyltransferase functions.

10.5.2 Serine Protease/RNA Helicase/NTPase (NS3)

The NS3 protein of flaviviruses is multifunctional, possessing serine protease, RNA helicase, NTPase, and RNA 5′-triphosphatase activities. The nucleic acid processing activities are located in the carboxyl terminal two-thirds of the protein, which has sequence similarity to the DEXH family of RNA helicases.[81–83] The N-terminal trypsin-like serine protease domain of NS3 (NS3-pro) and NS2B are required for cleavages at the NS2A–NS2B, NS2B–NS3, NS3–NS4A, and NS4B–NS5 polyprotein junctions (Figure 10.1) in mammalian cells as well as in vitro for Den, YF, and WNV.[61,69,70,84–86] In a manner similar to that of several other two-component

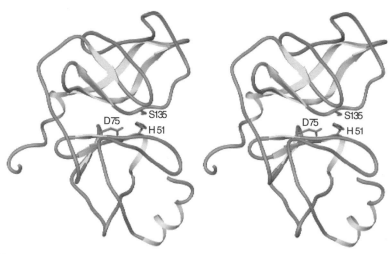

FIGURE 10.2   Stereo view of unliganded dengue 2 NS3-pro with catalytic triad shown as sticks and labeled. (See insert for color representation.)

viral proteases,[87,88] NS2B functions as an activator of NS3-pro.[61,64,73,74,89,90] The activation of NS3-pro by NS2B, a predominantly hydrophobic protein that is 130 residues in length, can be duplicated by a 40 residue hydrophilic domain [NS2B(H)] derived from it.[72,75,91,92] All the NS2B/NS3 cleavage sites share an invariant Arg or Lys residue at P1 (nomenclature of Schechter and Berger[93]), with a second basic residue occupying P2 at most cleavage sites. An amino acid with a short side chain (Ala, Gly, or Ser) frequents the P1' position. Mutations that inactivate the NS3 protease are lethal for viral replication, underscoring an indispensable role for the protease in the viral life cycle.

The structure of NS3-pro (Figure 10.2) has shown it to be a prototypical serine protease,[94] with an orientation of the catalytic triad similar to many other serine proteases.[95] The structure also closely resembles that of the hepatitis C virus (HCV) NS4A/NS3 protease,[96–98] with which the Den2 NS3-pro shares significant sequence similarity. Similarities in sequence among NS3-pro domains of flaviviruses[99] suggest that their structures are likely to be similar to that of Den2. For example, a similar structure for WNV protease can readily be constructed through homology modeling (V. K. Ganesh, unpublished data). The structure of the 2:1 complex of NS3-pro[100] with the mung bean Bowman–Birk Inhibitor (MbBBI) showed that the enzyme was inhibited by classical serine protease inhibitors by the standard mechanism (Figure 10.3); the main chains of the two inhibitory heads form a short β sheet with the enzyme, the C–O bond of the scissile carbonyl for each P1 residue is stretched to near single bond length (1.42 Å) and nestles in the oxy-anion holes formed by enzyme residues G133, S135, and G151; the carbon atoms possess near tetrahedral geometry and the oxygen atoms make sub van der Waals contacts (2.3 Å and 2.2 Å) with Oγ of the catalytic S135. Distinct differences were observed however, between binding of a P1 Lys residue compared with a P1

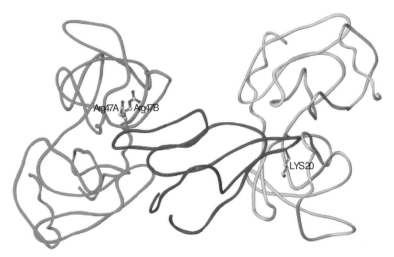

FIGURE 10.3 A ribbon drawing of the 2:1 Den2-NS3-pro:mung bean Bowman–Birk inhibitor (MbBBI) complex. Two different conformations of Arg 47 at one P1 position, and Lys 20 at the other P1 position, of MbBBI are shown as balls and sticks. (See insert for color representation.)

Arg in MbBBI by dengue NS3-pro. While the Lys side chain made hydrogen bonding interactions with Y150 and S163 in the enzyme S1 site, the Arg at P1 on the second "head" of MbBBI exhibited a disordered binding mode with one conformation (A) making electrostatic interactions with the aromatic cloud of Y150 and the second (B) salt bridge with D129[100]; the Arg interaction is shown in Figure 10.4. The structure of the MbBBI complex is also conceptually consistent with

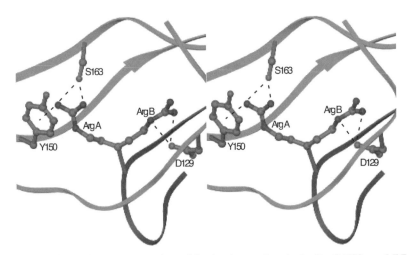

FIGURE 10.4 A close-up stereo view of the Arg interactions in the Den2 NS3-pro:MbBBI complex. Residues that make electrostatic interactions with the P1 Arg side chain are shown as balls and sticks. (See insert for color representation.)

mutational studies that have shown that mutating both Asp129 and Tyr150 to Ala is necessary to inactivate the protease.[101] However, neither of these structures contains either NS2B or NS2B(H), making it difficult to determine the mechanism of activation and the conformation of the fully activated protease. The strongly hydrophilic nature of NS2B(H) indicates that NS2B/NS3-pro interaction is likely to be dominated by hydrophilic contacts, some evidence for which has been obtained from mutagenesis studies on the YFV protease.[102] Using the NS2B(H)/NS3-pro mimic of the dengue protease, and NS3-pro domain alone, it has been demonstrated[103] that NS3-pro can hydrolyze the chromogenic substrate, Arg-*p*-nitrophenylanilide, efficiently but was essentially inactive on fluorogenic tripeptide substrate, Boc-Gly-Arg-Arg-AMC (7-amido-4-methylcoumarin). Furthermore, NS2B(H) activates NS3-pro by approximately four orders of magnitude in hydrolysis of tripeptide substrates, while it has little effect on hydrolysis of substrates that possess only a P1 side chain, suggesting that interactions between the P1 residue and the enzyme are not strongly dependent on NS2B. These kinetic results were used to suggest two plausible hypothetical mechanisms for activation of Den2 NS3-pro by NS2B. The first posits conformational changes induced in NS3-pro by interaction with NS2B, which induces greater structural complementarity of the binding pockets in the former for the side chains of the substrate. The second mechanism postulates a direct interaction of NS2B with substrate side chains, resulting in greater stabilization of the enzyme–activator–substrate ternary complex.[103] Both mechanisms have parallels in functioning of other two-component proteases.[87,98] Although a modeling study[104] has proposed structural details for NS2B–NS3-pro interaction, in the absence of supportive experimental data, the molecular mechanism of activation of NS3-pro by NS2B is currently obscure. Despite reservations about the eventual significance of the MbBBI complex in flaviviral polyprotein processing, the two structures Den2–NS3-pro[94] and its complex with MbBBI[100] are the only two flaviviral protease structures that are currently available for use in structure-assisted design of inhibitors.

Proteases are ubiquitous in biological processes and have been considered to be attractive targets for therapy of a variety of viral and nonviral diseases.[105] However, because all proteases of a given class share common mechanistic features and differ only in their choice of substrates, making strongly selective or specific inhibitors for a given protease is a challenging task. One generally adopted strategy in a search for specific inhibitors is to modify a specific substrate, commonly a short peptide, through substituting the peptide bond by a nonhydrolyzable analogue. Several α-keto amide analogues of peptide substrate-derived sequences at polyprotein cleavage sites have been reported,[106] tested against a covalently linked NS2B-3 construct of Den2. The hexapeptide analogue based on the NS3/4A site had the best K_i of 47 μM. The same study also reported an irreversible inhibition by an aldehyde analogue with a K_i of 16 μM.[106] Although there are no structural data at present, these inhibitors are expected to bind and behave as nonhydrolyzable substrates. Appropriate three-dimensional structures of inhibited complexes generally provide useful data for design of inhibitors using methods of structure-assisted methods.[107] Although it is tempting, in structural terms, to use the bifurcated Arg conformation in the MbBBI complex[100] in designing selective inhibitors, the uncertain physiological relevance of this structure suggests caution. There is no other structural platform that can currently be used in structure-assisted design of flaviviral serine protease inhibitors. However, with the increasing interest in flaviviral enzymes, a suitable template structure might soon become available.

Among alternative strategies that have been suggested for inhibiting flaviviral proteases is the possibility of disrupting the interaction between NS3-pro and NS2B.[101] Such an approach has also been suggested in the case of HCV protease.[98] This strategy may be more effective for flaviviral proteases than for HCV because of the greater enhancement of the activity of the former by NS2B compared to that of HCV NS3 protease by NS4A. While the activity of HCV NS3 protease is enhanced by a factor of 3–100 by NS4A, depending on the cleavage site,[108] Den2 NS3-pro is activated by 4–5 orders of magnitude by NS2B[103] and the WNV enzyme by a similar magnitude (R. Padmanabhan, personal communication). Thus, the flaviviral proteases might be more critically dependent on their activation factors for attaining physiologically meaningful levels of activity. Evidence obtained from measuring the change in activation levels of Den2 NS2B/NS3-pro, as a function of NaCl concentration,[103] and the strongly hydrophilic nature of the sequence of NS2B(H)[70,75,91] indicate that electrostatic forces might make a significant contribution to NS3-pro–NS2B interaction in flaviviruses. In addition, mutational studies on YFV[102] and Den2 (B. Falgout, personal communication) have suggested that not all residues of NH2B(H) are equally important for interaction with NS3-pro. While this and other information could potentially be used in exploring peptides that might antagonize the NS2B(H)–NS3-pro interaction, no published data appears to be currently available. Clues to nonpeptide molecular entities that could disrupt this interaction must await a structure that incorporates NS2B or NS2B(H).

The RNA helicase activity of NS3 is encoded in the carboxyl terminal two-thirds of the protein and this region has significant sequence similarity to the DEXd/H superfamily of RNA helicases.[109,110] A prerequisite for helicase activity is an RNA-stimulated ATPase activity that provides the energy for helix unwinding. NS3 proteins from JEV,[111,112] YFV,[113] WNV,[83] and Den2[82] have been shown to express this activity. Mutational disruption of helicase activity has been used to demonstrate the essential nature of this enzyme in flaviviral replication.[114] The C-terminal regions of flaviviral NS3 proteins also express an RNA triphosphatase (RTPase) activity, which might be important for 5' cap addition.[80] Both the NTPase and the RTPase activities are sensitive to Mg^{2+}, ionic strength, and nonhydrolyzable ATP analogues, as demonstrated for the WNV[80] and Den2[115] enzymes. In addition, work on Den2 NS3[115] has established that mutation of Lys199, part of the presumed nucleotide binding site, abolishes both NTPase and RTPase activities. No three-dimensional structure has been reported for this part of a flaviviral protein, but structures of the closely related hepatitis C virus NS3 helicase, as well as its complexes with nucleic acids, are available.[98,116,117] The structure of the entire NS3 protein of the hepatitis C virus protein has also been reported.[118] Viral helicases, due to their mandatory involvement in one of the central events in viral

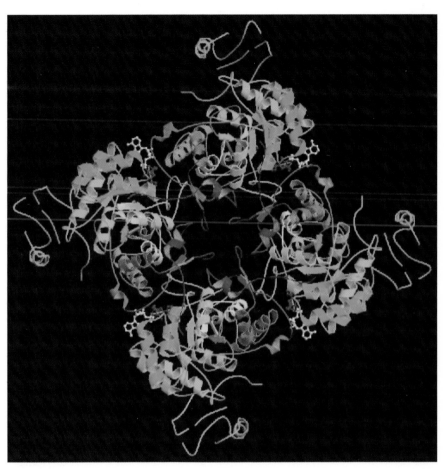

FIGURE 8.8 X-ray structure of the ternary complex of the human Type II IMPDH with 6-chloropurine riboside 5′-monophosphate and nicontinamide adenine dinucleotide.[56] (Reproduced with permission from the *Protein Data Bank*.)

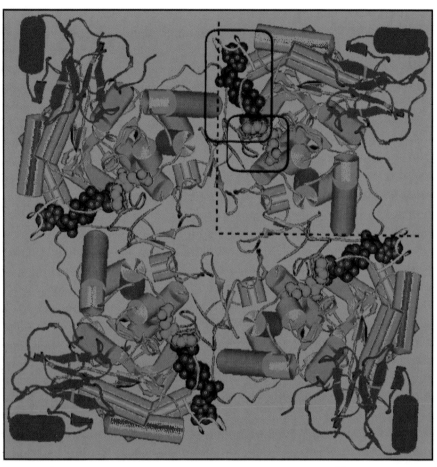

FIGURE 8.11 Human type II IMPDH: crystal structure of tetramer.[54] (Reproduced with permission of *Proceedings of the National Academy of Sciences of the United States of America*.)

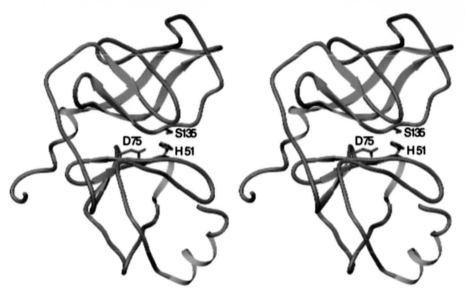

FIGURE 10.2 Stereo view of unliganded dengue 2 NS3-pro with catalytic triad shown as sticks and labeled.

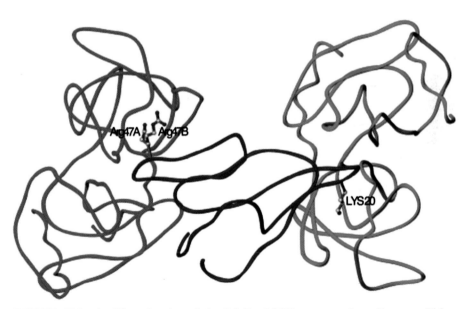

FIGURE 10.3 A ribbon drawing of the 2:1 Den2-NS3-pro:mung bean Bowman–Birk inhibitor (MbBBI) complex. Two different conformations of Arg 47 at one P1 position, and Lys 20 at the other P1 position, of MbBBI are shown as balls and sticks.

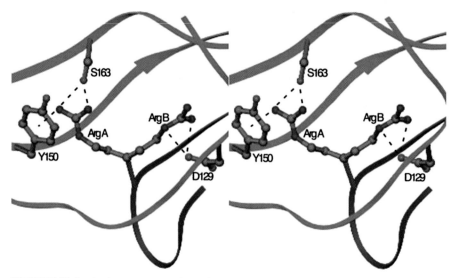

FIGURE 10.4 A close-up stereo view of the Arg interactions in the Den2 NS3-pro:MbBBI complex. Residues that make electrostatic interactions with the P1 Arg side chain are shown as balls and sticks.

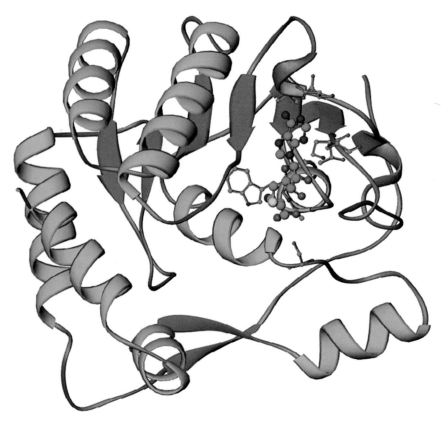

FIGURE 10.5 Crystal structure of the Den2 NS5 methyltransferase domain. The S-adenosylhomocysteine molecule is shown as balls and sticks.

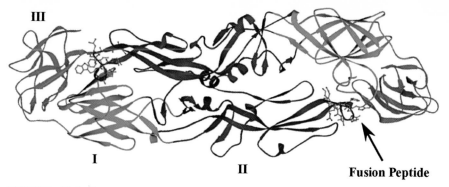

FIGURE 10.6 Structure of the E protein dimer. Beta strands in each monomer are represented by ribbons. Carbohydrate attached to the glycosylation site is not shown.

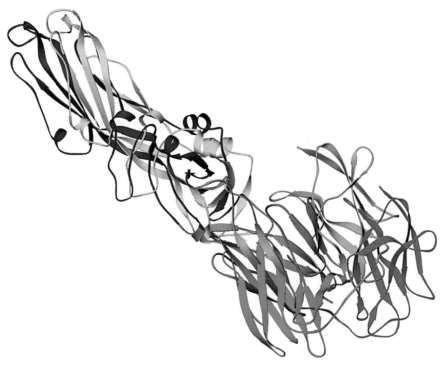

FIGURE 10.7 Comparison of the structure of dengue 2 E protein monomer between pre- and postfusion conformations.

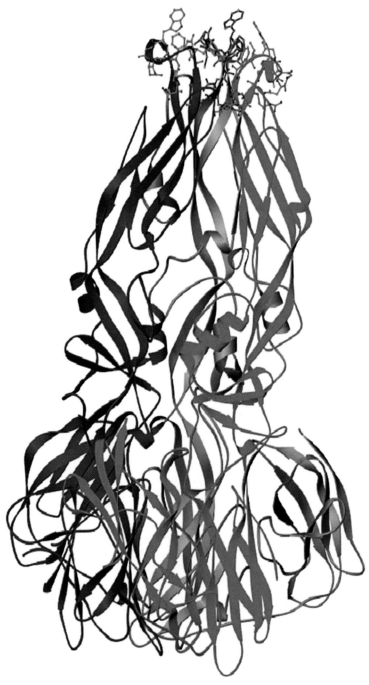

FIGURE 10.8 Dengue 2 E protein trimers formed after fusion at low pH.

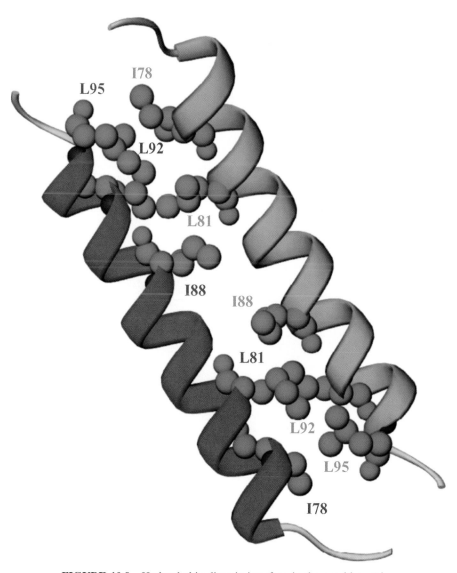

FIGURE 10.9 Hydrophobic dimeric interface in the capsid protein.

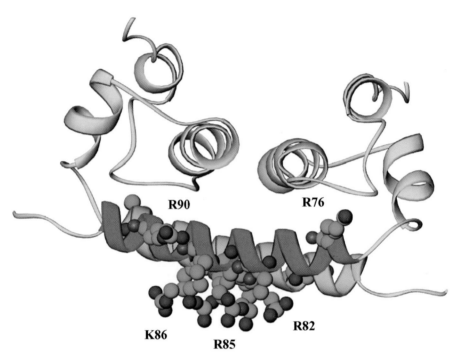

FIGURE 10.10 Positive charge cluster in the capsid protein. Only the residues in one monomer are numbered.

replication, are attractive targets for drug design.[119,120] Several nucleoside and nucleotide analogues have been investigated for inhibitory activity toward WNV and JEV helicases.[121–123]

10.5.3 RNA Polymerase/Methyltransferase (NS5)

The NS5 polypeptide carries two enzymatic activities—a carboxyl terminal RNA-dependent RNA polymerase (RdRP), and an amino terminal methyltransferase activity—both of which are critical for RNA replication. NS5 is an approximately 105 kDa protein that is post-translationally phosphorylated by a Ser/Thr kinase. Differential phosphorylation of NS5 has been suggested to be responsible for its association with NS3 in replication complexes in vivo, and potential modulation of its activity during replication.[124–126] Experiments carried out on the Den1 NS5 have shown that association of NS5 with NS3 stimulates the latter's NTPase activity, and that NS5 associates with the helicase domain of NS3, through a short stretch of residues between the polymerase and methyltransferase domains.[127,128] Sequence analysis of the C-terminal portion of NS5 has shown the presence of motifs that are found in other viral RdRPs.[57,129] Enzymological studies on several flaviviral RdRPs have been carried out and demonstrated that the Kunjin enzyme is highly processive,[130] and the Den2 enzyme exhibits an RNA initiation step that is temperature sensitive, although subsequent chain elongation is less sensitive.[131] Earlier studies on the Den1 enzyme had established that the enzyme synthesized template-sized, double-stranded, product RNA,[132] and deletion mutagenesis of active site residues of the KUN enzyme abolished polymerase activity and viral replication.[133] Comparison of sequences of available NS5 proteins from flaviviruses (V. K. Ganesh, unpublished data) indicates an average identity of 43%, with an additional 17–27% of residues that are similar, resulting in approximately 60% sequence similarity among flaviviral NS5 proteins of known sequence. Although there are three-dimensional structures available for similar viral RdRPs, such as the poliovirus 3D polymerase,[134] their sequence similarity with flaviviral RdRPs appears not to be great enough for three-dimensional model building (V. K. Ganesh et al., unpublished data). Because of the central importance of nucleic acid synthesis in viral replication, viral polymerases are important targets for chemotherapy of viral diseases.[5,135,136] There is currently no three-dimensional structure of a flaviviral polymerase that can be used in structure-assisted inhibitor design. Although compounds that have shown promise against other polymerases have been screened against WNV RdRP,[137,138] there are no clinically effective inhibitors of flaviviral polymerases.

A methyltransferase activity resides within the amino terminal third of the NS5 protein that is important for RNA capping at the 5′ terminus. The first 130 residues of flaviviral NS5 proteins have significant sequence similarity to S-adenosylmethionine (SAM)-dependent methyltransferases,[129] and SAM-dependent transferase activity has been demonstrated for Den2 NS5.[139] Deletion mutagenesis of putative SAM binding regions of KUN have shown that this activity is necessary for replication.[133] The crystal structure[139] of the methyltransferase domain (residues

1–267), in a ternary complex with *S*-adenosylhomocysteine (SAH) and β,γ-methylene GTP (GDPMP), showed that the core of the enzyme responsible for this activity is an α-β protein, with a seven-stranded β sheet flanked by four α helices (Figure 10.5). The structure is topologically similar to other SAM-dependent methyltransferases and most closely resembles the structures of *E.coli* FTsJ[140] and vaccinia VP39.[141] SAH is bound through a multitude of hydrogen bonds and van der Waals contacts. The adenine is nestled within a hydrophobic pocket, while the ribose is stabilized mainly through electrostatic interactions with protein side chains, water molecules, and sulfate ions. The GDPMP binding pocket appears to be designed specifically for guanine and the interactions with the protein side chains possible for a guanine would not be possible for an adenine moiety. In addition, the binding motif used to stabilize GDPMP appears to be unique to this enzyme, which makes exploration of specific inhibitors of this interaction an attractive proposition.[139]

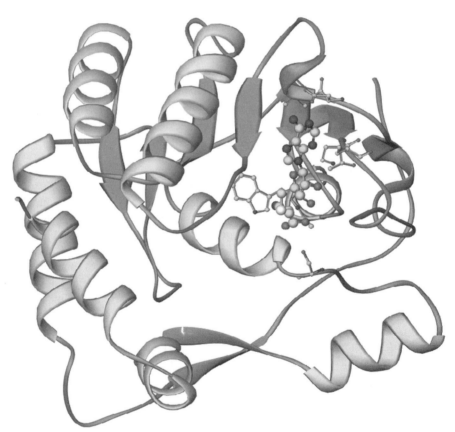

FIGURE 10.5 Crystal structure of the Den2 NS5 methyltransferase domain. The *S*-adenosylhomocysteine molecule is shown as balls and sticks. (See insert for color representation.)

10.5.4 Envelope Protein (E)

The E protein of flavivirus is the major glycosylated structural protein (495 amino acid residues (~60 kDa for Den2) exposed on the surface of the virion. The E protein mediates receptor binding on the host cell surface, and at least for initial binding, cell-surface haparan sulfate proteoglycan seems important.[47] Binding is followed by internalization of the virus via specific receptor-mediated endocytosis, inducing fusion of the virion envelope with the host cell membrane, and virus entry. The E protein is a major target of the host cell response, containing hemagglutination and neutralizing antigenic epitopes conferring protective immunity, as well as non-neutralizing antigenic epitopes responsible for ADE.[31,142–150] The E protein is therefore important for vaccine development as well as for diagnostic strategies. The E protein together with prM are on the surface of the virion, while the lipid bilayer and the viral capsid protein C tightly associated with viral RNA genome form the inner core of the virion.[144,151–157] During virion morphogenesis, prM undergoes cleavage, mediated by furin-like protease, in a late trans-Golgi compartment, resulting in mature M protein, with a concomitant loss of the ectodomain of prM. The resultant mature particle is competent in fusion with the cell membrane.[60,62,86,89,158–162] The presence of a flavivirus receptor binding site on the envelope E was revealed by a clustering of mutations that affect virulence and analyses using monoclonal antibodies.[38,42,143,150,163–165] The E protein of flavivirus resembles the alphavirus E1 protein in possessing a class II viral fusion peptide. Structures of the dengue and TBE E proteins strongly suggest that flaviviral E proteins are likely to have similar three-dimensional structures. The dengue E protein (Figure 10.6) is a dimer, arranged in three distinct domains, each of which forms a β barrel and is oriented parallel to the membrane. The central domain, I, consists of predominantly type-specific non-neutralizing epitopes and is the molecular hinge region involved in low pH-induced conformational changes. The dimerization domain, II, makes contact with a copy of itself in the homodimer and is involved in virus-mediated membrane fusion. It contains many of the

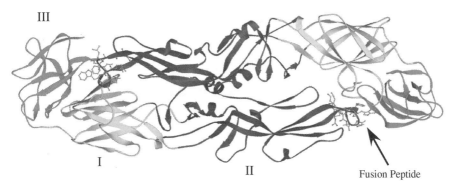

FIGURE 10.6 Structure of the E protein dimer. Beta strands in each monomer are represented by ribbons. Carbohydrate attached to the glycosylation site is not shown. (See insert for color representation.)

cross-reactive epitopes recognized by neutralizing and non-neutralizing Mabs. Domain III has an immunoglobulin-like structure, containing the most distal projecting loops from the virion surface. This domain contains multiple type- and subtype-specific epitopes, eliciting virus-neutralizing antibody response, and is thought to contain virus receptor binding site as well as being involved in tissue tropism. Several lines of evidence suggest that this overall structure of the E protein is conserved across Flaviviridae.[144,148,151,152,166] After the virus binds to cell-surface receptors and is internalized into the endosome, the flaviviral E homodimers are converted to a more stable homotrimeric form, as recently shown for both dengue and Semliki Forest viruses.[149,167] The lower endosomal pH causes structural changes, which result in relative movements of domains I and III with respect to domain II (Figure 10.7) and bring the C terminus nearly 40 Å closer to the fusion loop, while exposing the loop.[149] The fusion loop inserts into the host cell membrane, and the trimer is formed, initially through stabilizing interactions between the three fusion loops, propagating toward the base (Figure 10.8). This is followed by injection of viral RNA and replication.[149] The structure of the Den virion also shows that the surface has an icosahedral symmetrical network of E homodimers.[155]

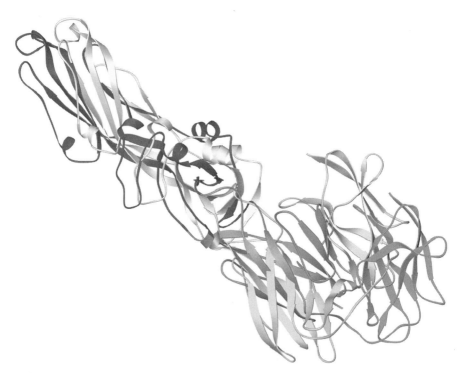

FIGURE 10.7 Comparison of the structure of dengue 2 E protein monomer between pre- and postfusion conformations. (See insert for color representation.)

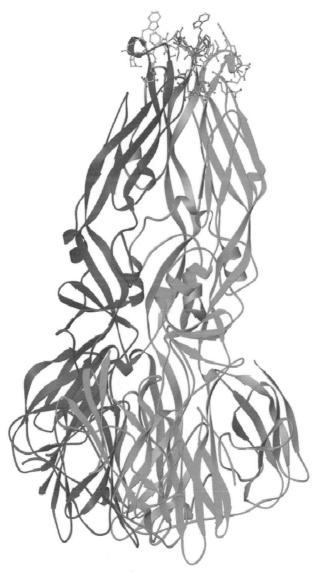

FIGURE 10.8 Dengue 2 E protein trimers formed after fusion at low pH. (See insert for color representation.)

A hydrophobic ligand binding pocket, which is defined by the kl loop in the dimeric dengue E protein, is occupied by a molecule of β-octyl glucoside in the crystal structure. Changes in this loop are pivotal for the dimer-to-trimer conformational change that accompanies insertion into host cell membrane. Thus, a strategy for inhibition of viral entry has been suggested, which would be dependent on use of synthetic compounds that bind in this pocket and prevent this obligatory conformational change.[148] Analysis of the trimer structure has also been used to suggest development of peptides, derived from the stem sequences (Figure 10.8), that would interact with domain II and prevent the stabilization of the rotated domain III, and hence formation of stable trimers.[149]

10.5.5 Capsid (C) Protein

The capsid protein has a molecular mass of about 11 kDa and, as expected, is highly basic.[57] Sequence analysis of the KUN and Den2 proteins shows the charged residues near the amino and carboxyl termini, with a hydrophobic domain that mediates membrane association.[168,169] The C protein is indispensable for specific packaging of the viral RNA and the dimeric structure of the Den2 protein has recently been determined by NMR.[170] The structure displays a new fold and a dimerization surface formed from two pairs of helices, one of which is shown in Figure 10.9. The structure shows an asymmetric charge structure with the basic

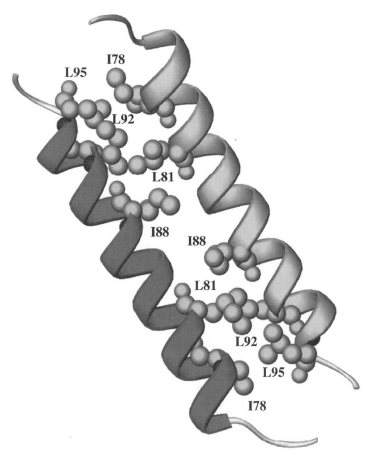

FIGURE 10.9 Hydrophobic dimeric interface in the capsid protein. (See insert for color representation.)

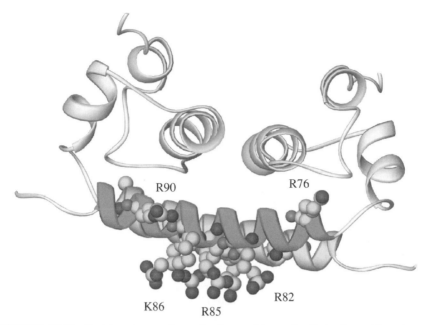

FIGURE 10.10   Positive charge cluster in the capsid protein. Only the residues in one monomer are numbered. (See insert for color representation.)

residues lining one side (Figure 10.10) and the hydrophobic residues on the opposite site. This charge distribution, coupled with those of hydrophobic residues, has been used to suggest a model for capsid–RNA interaction and membrane association.[170]

10.5.6   Other Nonstructural Proteins (NS1, NS2A, NS4A, and NS4B)

The function of NS1 is unknown in detail, although it appears to be important for viral RNA replication.[171] This 46 kDa glycoprotein is cleaved from the polyprotein by a host peptidase and occurs in both secreted and cell-surface associated forms.[66,172–175] It dimerizes after synthesis, and the cell surface association probably occurs through a glycosyl-phosphatidylinositol anchor.[176] Glycosylation is important for its participation in RNA replication, since mutation of either *N*-glycosylation site in YFV NS1 led to decreases in synthesized RNA.[177]

A small, hydrophobic, probably membrane resident protein of 22 kDa, NS2A is thought to be involved in the shift between RNA replication and RNA packaging, during flaviviral replication, as indicated by studies on KUN.[178] Its two ends are cleaved from the polyprotein by a currently unknown host enzyme and by the viral serine protease, respectively.[66] Recent studies in YFV have demonstrated that mutations in NS2A prevent production of infectious viral particles.[179]

Both NS4A and NS4B are hydrophobic proteins, with molecular masses of 16 and 27 kDa, respectively. Studies on YFV suggest involvement of NS4A in RNA replication.[180] Their functions are otherwise currently unclear.

ACKNOWLEDGMENTS

I would like thank Dr. V. K. Ganesh and Dr. M. Suresh Kumar for creating the figures. Work in my laboratory on structural and functional studies of flaviviral proteins is supported by grants from NIH and from the Johnson and Johnson Corporate Office of Science and Technology.

REFERENCES

1. Kuno, G.; Gwong-Jen, J.; Chang, K.; Tsuchiya, K. R.; et al. Phylogeny of the genus *Flavivirus. J. Virol.* **1998**, *72*, 73–83.

2. Chambers, T. J.; Monath, T. P. (eds.) *Advances in Virus Research*, Elsevier/Academic Press, Boston, 2003.

3. Andrei, G.; De Clercq, E. Molecular approaches for the treatment of hemorrhagic fever virus infections. *Antiviral Res.* **1993**, *22*, 45–75.

4. Leyssen, P.; De Clercq, E.; Neyts, J. Perspectives for the treatment of infections with Flaviviridae. *Clin. Microbiol. Rev.* **2000**, *13*, 67–82.

5. Leyssen, P.; Charlier, N.; Paeshuyse, J.; De Clercq, E.; Neyts, J. Prospects for antiviral therapy. *Adv. Virus Res.* **2003**, *61*, 511–553.

6. Gubler, D. J.; Clark, G. G. Dengue/dengue hemorrhagic fever: the emergence of a global health problem. *Emerging Infect. Dis.* **1995**, *1*, 55–57.

7. Gubler, D. J. Dengue and dengue hemorrhagic fever. *Clin. Microbiol. Rev.* **1998**, *11*, 480–496.

8. Gritsun, T. S.; Lashkevich, V. A.; Gould, E. A. Tick-borne encephalitis. *Antiviral Res.* **2003**, *57*, 129–146.

9. Gubler, D. J. The global emergence/resurgence of arboviral diseases as public health problems. *Arch. Med. Res.* **2002**, *33*, 330–342.

10. Tsai, T. F. Arboviral infections in the United States. *Infect. Dis. Clin. North Am.* **1991**, *5*, 73–102.

11. Monath, T. P.; Tsai, T. F. St. Louis encephalitis: lessons from the last decade. *Am. J. Trop. Med. Hyg.* **1987**, *37*, 40S–59S.

12. Marfin, A. A.; Peterson, C. R.; Edison, M.; Miller, J.; et al. Widespread West Nile virus activity, eastern United States, 2000. *Emering Infect. Dis.* **2001**, *7*, 730–735.

13. Petersen, L. R.; Roehrig, J. T. West Nile virus: a reemerging global pathogen. *Emerging Infect. Dis.* **2001**, *7*, 611–614.

14. Roehrig, J. T.; Layton, M.; Smith, P.; Campbell, G. C.; et al. The emergence of West Nile virus in North America: ecology, epidemiology, and surveillance. *Curr. Top. Microbiol. Immunol.* **2002**, *267*, 223–240.

15. Charrel, R. N.; de Lamballerie, X. [The Alkhurma virus (family Flaviviridae, genus *Flavivirus*): an emerging pathogen responsible for hemorrhage fever in the Middle East]. *Med. Trop. (Mars)* **2003**, *63*, 296–299.

16. Banerjee, K. Emerging viral infections with special reference to India. *Indian J. Med. Res.* **1996**, *103*, 177–200.

17. Solomon, T.; Mallewa, M. Dengue and other emerging flaviviruses. *J. Infect.* **2001**, *42*, 104–115.

18. Borio, L.; Inglesby, T.; Peters, C. J.; Schmalijohn, A. L.; et al. For the Working Group on Civilian Biodefense: hemorrhagic fever viruses as biological weapons. *JAMA* **2002**, *287*, 2391–2405.

19. Barrett, A. D. Current status of flavivirus vaccines. *Ann. N.Y. Acad. Sci.* **2001**, *951*, 262–271.

20. Baize, S.; Marianneau, P.; Georges-Courbot, M. C.; Deubel, V. Recent advances in vaccines against hemorrhagic fevers. *Curr. Opin. Infect. Dis.* **2001**, *14*, 513–518.

21. Chang, G. J.; Davis, B. S.; Hunt, A. R.; Holms, D. A.; Kuno, G. Flavivirus DNA vaccines: current status and potential. *Ann. N.Y. Acad. Sci.* **2001**, *951*, 272–285.

22. Lai, C. J.; Monath, T. P. Chimeric flaviviruses: novel vaccines against dengue fever, tick-borne encephalitis, and Japanese encephalitis. *Adv. Virus Res.* **2003**, *61*, 469–509.

23. Monath, T. P. Prospects for development of a vaccine against the West Nile virus. *Ann. N.Y. Acad. Sci.* **2001**, *951*, 1–12.

24. Pletnev, A. G.; Putnak, R.; Speicher, J.; Wanger, E. J.; et al. Molecularly engineered live-attenuated chimeric West Nile/dengue virus vaccines protect rhesus monkeys from West Nile virus. *Virology* **2003**, *314*, 190–195.

25. Tsai, G. F.; Chang, T. A.; Yu, Y. X. Japanese encephalitis vaccines. In *Vaccines*, Orenstein, W. A. (ed.). Saunders, Philadelphia, 1999, pp. 672–710.

26. Dandawate, C. N.; Desai, G. B.; Achar, T. R.; Banerjee, K. Field evaluation of formalin inactivated Kyasanur Forest disease virus tissue culture vaccine in three districts of Karnataka state. *Indian J. Med. Res.* **1994**, *99*, 152–158.

27. Thind, I. S. Attenuated Langat E5 virus as a live virus vaccine against Kyasanur Forest disease virus. *Indian J. Med. Res.* **1981**, *73*, 141–149.

28. Halstead, S. B.; Deen, J. The future of dengue vaccines. *Lancet* **2002**, *360*, 1243–1245.

29. Jacobs, M.; Young, P. Dengue vaccines: preparing to roll back dengue. *Curr. Opin. Invest. Drugs* **2003**, *4*, 168–171.

30. Putnak, R.; Porter, K.; Schmaljohn, C. DNA vaccines for flaviviruses. *Adv. Virus Res.* **2003**, *61*, 445–468.

31. Halstead, S. B. Neutralization and antibody-dependent enhancement of dengue viruses. *Adv. Virus Res.* **2003**, *60*, 421–467.

32. Cardosa, M. J. Dengue vaccine design: issues and challenges. *Br. Med. Bull.* **1998**, *54*, 395–405.

33. Hilgard, P.; Stockert, R. Heparan sulfate proteoglycans initiate dengue virus infection of hepatocytes. *Hepatology* **2000**, *32*, 1069–1077.

34. Rothwell, S. W.; Putnak, R.; La Russa, V. F. Dengue-2 virus infection of human bone marrow: characterization of dengue-2 antigen-positive stromal cells. *Am. J. Trop. Med. Hyg.* **1996**, *54*, 503–510.

35. Ramos-Castaneda, J.; Imbert, J. L.; Barron, B. L.; Ramos, C. A 65-kDa trypsin-sensible membrane cell protein as a possible receptor for dengue virus in cultured neuroblastoma cells. *J. Neurovirol.* **1997**, *3*, 435–440.

36. Bielefeldt-Ohmann, H.; Meyer, M.; Fitzpatrick, D. R.; Mackenzie, J. S. Dengue virus binding to human leukocyte cell lines: receptor usage differs between cell types and virus strains. *Virus Res.* **2001**, *73*, 81–89.

37. Munoz, M. L.; Cisneros, A.; Cruz, J.; Das, P.; et al. Putative dengue virus receptors from mosquito cells. *FEMS Microbiol. Lett.* **1998**, *168*, 251–258.

38. Martinez-Barragon, J. J.; Angel, R. M. Identification of a putative coreceptor on Vero cells that participates in dengue 4 virus infection. *J. Virol.* **2001**, *75*, 7818–7827.

39. Salas-Benito, J. S.; del Angel, R. M. Identification of two surface proteins from C6/36 cells that bind dengue type 4 virus. *J. Virol.* **1997**, *71*, 7246–7252.

40. Yazi Mendoza, M.; Salas-Benito, J. S.; Lanz-Mendoza, H.; Hernandez-Martinez, S.; del Angel, R. M. A putative receptor for dengue virus in mosquito tissues: localization of a 45-kDa glycoprotein. *Am. J. Trop. Med. Hyg.* **2002**, *67*, 76–84.

41. Yocupicio-Monroy, R. M.; Medina, F.; Reyes-del Valle, J.; del Angel, R. M. Cellular proteins from human monocytes bind to dengue 4 virus minus-strand 3′ untranslated region RNA. *J. Virol.* **2003**, *77*, 3067–3076.

42. Kopecky, J.; Grubhoffer, L.; Kovar, V.; Jindrak, L.; Vokurkova, D. A putative host cell receptor for tick-borne encephalitis virus identified by anti-idiotypic antibodies and virus affinoblotting. *Intervirology* **1999**, *42*, 9–16.

43. Chu, J. J.; Ng, M. L. Characterization of a 105-kDa plasma membrane associated glycoprotein that is involved in West Nile virus binding and infection. *Virology* **2003**, *312*, 458–469.

44. Navarro-Sanchez, E.; Altmeyer, R.; Amara, A.; Schwartz, O.; et al. Dendritic-cell-specific ICAM3-grabbing non-integrin is essential for the productive infection of human dendritic cells by mosquito-cell-derived dengue viruses. *EMBO Rep.* **2003**, *4*, 723–728.

45. Tassaneetrithep, B.; Burgess, T-H.; Granelli-Piperno, A.; Trumpsheller, C.; et al. DC-SIGN (CD209) mediates dengue virus infection of human dendritic cells. *J. Exp. Med.* **2003**, *197*, 823–829.

46. Reyes-del Valle, J.; del Angel, R. M. Isolation of putative dengue virus receptor molecules by affinity chromatography using a recombinant E protein ligand. *J. Virol. Methods* **2004**, *116*, 95–102.

47. Chen, Y.; Maguire, T.; Marks, R. M. Dengue virus infectivity depends on envelope protein binding to target cell heparan sulfate. *Nat. Med.* **1997**, *3*, 8765–8772.

48. Marks, R. M.; Lu, H.; Sunderesan, R.; Toida, T.; et al. Probing the interaction of dengue virus envelope protein with heparin: assessment of glycosaminoglycan-derived inhibitors. *J. Med. Chem.* **2001**, *44*, 2178–2187.

49. Wengler, G.; Gross, H. J. Studies on virus-specific nucleic acids synthesized in vertebrate and mosquito cells infected with flaviviruses. *Virology* **1978**, *89*, 423–437.

50. Brinton, M. A.; Dispoto, J. H. Sequence and secondary structure analysis of the 5′-terminal region of flavivirus genome RNA. *Virology* **1988**, *162*, 290–299.

51. Cahour, A.; Pletnev, A.; Vazielle-Falcoz, M.; Rosen, L.; Lai, C. J. Growth-restricted dengue virus mutants containing deletions in the 5′ noncoding region of the RNA genome. *Virology* **1995**, *207*, 68–76.

52. Li, W.; Li, Y.; Kedersha, N.; Anderson, P.; et al. Cell proteins TIA-1 and TIAR interact with the 3′ stem-loop of the West Nile virus complementary minus-strand RNA and facilitate virus replication. *J. Virol.* **2002**, *76*, 11989–12000.

53. Shi, P. Y.; Li, W.; Brinton, M. A. Cell proteins bind specifically to West Nile virus minus-strand 3′ stem-loop RNA. *J. Virol.* **1996**, *70*, 6278–6287.

54. Hahn, C. S.; Hahn, Y. S.; Rice, C. M.; Lee, E.; et al. Conserved elements in the 3′ untranslated region of flavivirus RNAs and potential cyclization sequences. *J. Mol. Biol.* **1987**, *198*, 33–41.

55. Brinton, M. A.; Fernandez, A. V.; Dispoto, J. H. The 3′-nucleotides of flavivirus genomic RNA form a conserved secondary structure. *Virology* **1986**, *153*, 113–121.

56. Zeng, L.; Falgout, B.; Markoff, L. Identification of specific nucleotide sequences within the conserved 3′-SL in the dengue type 2 virus genome required for replication. *J. Virol.* **1998**, *72*, 7510–7522.

57. Rice, C. M.; Lenches, E. M.; Eddy, S. R.; Shin, S. J.; et al. Nucleotide sequence of yellow fever virus: implications for flavivirus gene expression and evolution. *Science* **1985**, *229*, 726–733.

58. Svitkin, Y. V.; Lyapustin, V. N.; Lashkevich, V. A.; Agol, V. I. Differences between translation products of tick-borne encephalitis virus RNA in cell-free systems from Krebs-2 cells and rabbit reticulocytes: involvement of membranes in the processing of nascent precursors of flavivirus structural proteins. *Virology* **1984**, *135*, 536–541.

59. Markoff, L. In vitro processing of dengue virus structural proteins: cleavage of the pre-membrane protein. *J. Virol.* **1989**, *63*, 3345–3352.

60. Nowak, T.; Farber, P. M.; Wengler, G.; Wengler, G. Analyses of the terminal sequences of West Nile virus structural proteins and of the in vitro translation of these proteins allow the proposal of a complete scheme of the proteolytic cleavages involved in their synthesis. *Virology* **1989**, *169*, 365–376.

61. Cahour, A.; Falgout, B.; Lai, C.-J. Cleavage of the dengue virus polyprotein at the NS3/NS4A and NS4B/NS5 junctions is mediated by viral protease NS2B-NS3, whereas NS4A/NS4B may be processed by a cellular protease. *J. Virol.* **1992**, *66*, 1535–1542.

62. Ruiz-Linares, A.; Cahour, A.; Despres, P.; Girard, M.; Bouloy, M. Processing of yellow fever virus polyprotein: role of cellular proteases in maturation of the structural proteins. *J. Virol.* **1989**, *63*, 4199–4209.

63. Chambers, T. J.; Nestorowicz, A.; Amberg, S. M.; Rice, C. M. Mutagenesis of the yellow fever virus NS2B protein: effects on proteolytic processing, NS2B-NS3 complex formation, and viral replication. *J. Virol.* **1993**, *67*, 6797–6807.

64. Arias, C. F.; Preugschat, F.; Strauss, J. H. Dengue 2 virus NS2B and NS3 form a stable complex that can cleave NS3 within the helicase domain. *Virology* **1993**, *193*, 888–899.

65. Jan, L. R.; Yang, C. S.; Trent, D. W.; Falgout, B.; Lai, C. J. Processing of Japanese encephalitis virus non-structural proteins: NS2B-NS3 complex and heterologous proteases. *J. Gen. Virol.* **1995**, *76*(Pt 3), 573–580.

66. Falgout, B.; Markoff, L. Evidence that flavivirus NS1-NS2A cleavage is mediated by a membrane-bound host protease in the endoplasmic reticulum. *J. Virol.* **1995**, *69*, 7232–7243.

67. Bazan, J. F.; Fletterick, R. J. Detection of a trypsin-like serine protease domain in flaviviruses and pestiviruses. *Virology* **1989**, *171*, 637–639.

68. Gorbalenya, A. E.; Donchenko, A. P.; Koonin, E. V.; Blinov, V. M. N-terminal domains of putative helicases of flavi- and pestiviruses may be serine proteases. *Nucleic Acid Res.* **1989**, *17*, 3889–3897.

69. Chambers, T. J.; et al. Evidence that the N-terminal domain of nonstructural protein NS3 from yellow fever virus is a serine protease responsible for site-specific cleavages in the viral polyprotein. *Proc. Natl. Acad. Sci. U.S.A.* **1990**, *87*, 8898–8902.

70. Zhang, L.; Mohan, P. M.; Padmanabhan, R. Processing and localization of dengue virus type 2 polyprotein precursor NS3-NS4A-NS4B-NS5. *J. Virol.* **1992**, *66*, 7549–7554.

71. Preugschat, F.; Lenches, E. M.; Strauss, J. H. Flavivirus enzyme–substrate interactions studied with chimeric proteinases: identification of an intragenic locus important for substrate recognition. *J. Virol.* **1991**, *65*, 4749–4758.

72. Preugschat, F.; Yao, C. W.; Strauss, J. H. In vitro processing of dengue virus type 2 nonstructural proteins NS2A, NS2B, and NS3. *J. Virol.* **1990**, *64*, 4364–4374.

73. Falgout, B.; Pethel, M.; Zhang, Y. M.; Lai, C. J. Both nonstructural proteins NS2B and NS3 are required for the proteolytic processing of dengue virus nonstructural proteins. *J. Virol.* **1991**, *65*, 2467–2475.

74. Chambers, T. J.; Grakoui, A.; Rice, C. M. Processing of the yellow fever virus nonstructural polyprotein: a catalytically active NS3 proteinase domain and NS2B are required for cleavages at dibasic sites. *J. Virol.* **1991**, *65*, 6042–6050.

75. Falgout, B.; Miller, R. H.; Lai, C.-J. Deletion analysis of dengue virus type 4 nonstructural protein NS2B: identification of a domain required for NS2B-NS3 protease activity. *J. Virol.* **1993**, *67*, 2034–2042.

76. Lindenbach, B. D.; Rice, C. M. Molecular biology of flaviviruses. *Adv. Virus Res.* **2003**, *59*, 23–61.

77. Cleaves, G. R.; Ryan, T. E.; Schlesinger, R. W. Identification and characterization of type 2 dengue virus replicative intermediate and replicative form RNAs. *Virology* **1981**, *111*, 73–83.

78. Muylaert, I. R.; Chambers, T. J.; Galler, R.; Rice, C. M. Mutagenesis of the N-linked glycosylation sites of the yellow fever virus NS1 protein: effects on virus replication and mouse neurovirulence. *Virology* **1996**, *222*, 159–168.

79. You, S.; Padmanabhan, R. A novel in vitro replication system for dengue virus. Initiation of RNA synthesis at the 3′-end of exogenous viral RNA templates requires 5′- and 3′-terminal complementary sequence motifs of the viral RNA. *J. Biol. Chem.* **1999**, *274*, 33714–33722.

80. Wengler, G.; Wengler, G. The NS3 non-structural protein of flaviviruses contains a RNA triphosphatase activity. *Virology* **1993**, *197*, 265–273.

81. Gorbalenya, A. E.; Donchenko, A. P.; Koonin, E. V.; Blinov, V. M. N-terminal domains of putative helicases of flavi- and pestiviruses may be serine proteases. *Nucleic Acids Res.* **1989**, *17*, 3889–3897.

82. Li, H.; Clum, S.; You, S.; Ebner, K. E.; Padmanabhan, R. The serine protease and RNA stimulated NTPase/RNA helicase functional domains of dengue virus type 2 NS3 converge within a region of 20 amino acids. *J. Virol.* **1999**, *64*, 4364–4374.

83. Wengler, G.; Wengler, G. The carboxy-terminal part of the NS 3 protein of the West Nile flavivirus can be isolated as a soluble protein after proteolytic cleavage and represents an RNA-stimulated NTPase. *Virology* **1991**, *184*, 707–715.

84. Wengler, G.; Czaya, G.; Farber, P. M.; Hegemann, J. H. In vitro synthesis of West Nile virus proteins indicates that the amino-terminal segment of the NS3 protein contains the active centre of the protease which cleaves the viral polyprotein after multiple basic amino acids. *J. Gen. Virol.* **1991**, *72*, 851–858.

85. Yamshchikov, V. F.; Compans, R. W. Processing of the intracellular form of the West Nile virus capsid protein by the viral NS2B-NS3 protease: an in vitro study. *J. Virol.* **1994**, *68*, 5765–5771.

86. Zhang, L.; Padmanabhan, R. Role of protein conformation in the processing of dengue virus type 2 nonstructural polyprotein precursor. *Gene* **1993**, *129*, 197–205.

87. Ding, J.; McGrath, W. J.; Sweet, R. M.; Mangel, W. F. Crystal structure of the human adenovirus proteinase with its 11 amino acid cofactor. *EMBO J.* **1996**, *15*, 1778–1783.

88. Steinkuhler, C.; Urbani, A.; Tomei, L.; Biasiol, G.; et al. Activity of purified hepatitis C virus protease NS3 on peptide substrates. *J. Virol.* **1996**, *70*, 6694–6700.

89. Amberg, S. M.; Nestorowicz, A.; McCourt, D. W.; Rice, C. M. NS2B-3 proteinase-mediated processing in the yellow fever virus structural region: in vitro and in vivo studies. *J. Virol.* **1994**, *68*, 3794–3802.

90. Chambers, T. J.; Nestorowicz, A.; Rice, C. M. Mutagenesis of the yellow fever virus NS2B/3 cleavage site: determinants of cleavage site specificity and effects on polyprotein processing and viral replication. *J. Virol.* **1995**, *69*, 1600–1605.

91. Chambers, T. J.; Nestorowicz, A.; Amberg, S. M.; Rice, C. M. Mutagenesis of the yellow fever virus NS2B protein: effects on proteolytic processing, NS2B-NS3 complex formation, and viral replication. *J. Virol.* **1993**, *67*, 6797–6807.

92. Clum, S.; Ebner, K. E.; Padmanabhan, R. Cotranslational membrane insertion of dengue virus type 2 NS2B/NS3 serine proteinase precursor is required for efficient processing in vitro. *J. Biol. Chem.* **1997**, *272*, 30715–30723.

93. Schechter, I.; Berger, A. On the size of the active site in proteases. I. Papain. *Biochem. Biophys. Res. Commun.* **1967**, *27*, 157–162.

94. Krishna Murthy, H. M.; Clum, S.; Padmanabhan, R. Dengue virus NS3 serine protease: crystal structure and insights into interaction of the active site with substrates by molecular modeling and structural analysis of mutational effects. *J. Biol. Chem.* **1999**, *274*, 5573–5580.

95. Kraut, J. Serine proteases: structure and mechanism of catalysis. *Annu. Rev. Biochem.* **1977**, *46*, 331–358.

96. Yan, Y.; Li, Y.; Munshi, S.; Sardana, M.; et al. Complex of NS3 protease and NS4A peptide of BK strain hepatitis C virus: a 2.2 Å resolution structure in a hexagonal crystal form. *Protein Sci.* **1998**, *7*, 837–847.

97. Love, R. A.; Parge, H. E.; Wickersham, J. A.; Hostomsky, Z.; et al. The crystal structure of hepatitis C virus NS3 proteinase reveals a trypsin-like fold and a structural zinc binding site. *Cell* **1996**, *87*, 331–342.

98. Kim, J. L.; Morgenstern, K. A.; Lin, C.; Fox, T.; et al. Crystal structure of the hepatitis C virus NS3 protease domain complexed with a synthetic NS4A cofactor peptide. *Cell* **1996**, *87*, 343–355.

99. Ryan, M. D.; Monaghan, S.; Flint, M. Virus-encoded proteinases of Flaviviridae. *J. Gen. Virol.* **1998**, *79*, 947–959.

100. Krishna Murthy, H. M.; Judge, K.; DeLucas, L.; Padmanabhan, R. Crystal structure of dengue virus NS3 protease in complex with a Bowman–Birk inhibitor: implication for flaviviral polyproteain processing and drug design. *J. Mol. Biol.* **2000**, *301*, 759–767.

101. Valle, R. P.; Falgout, B. Mutagenesis of the NS3 protease of dengue virus type 2. *J. Virol.* **1998**, *72*, 624–632.

102. Droll, D. A.; Krishna Murthy, H. M.; Chambers, T. J. Yellow fever virus NS2B-NS3 protease: charged to alanine mutagenesis and deletion analysis define regions important for protease complex formation and function. *Virology* **2000**, *75*, 335–347.

103. Yusof, R.; Clum, S.; Wetzel, M.; Krishna Murthy, H. M.; Padmanabhan, R. Purified NS2B/NS3 serine protease of dengue virus type 2 exhibits cofactor NS2B dependence for cleavage of substrates with dibasic amino acids *in vitro. J. Biol. Chem.* **2000**, *275*, 9963–9969.

104. Brinkworth, R. I.; Fairlie, D. P.; Leung, D.; Young, P. R. Homology model of the dengue 2 virus NS3 protease: putative interactions with both substrate and NS2B cofactor. *J. Gen. Virol.* **1999**, *80*, 1167–1177.

105. Docherty, A. J.; Crabbe, T.; O'Connell, J. P.; Groom, C. R. Proteases as drug targets. *Biochem. Soc. Symp.* **2003**, 147–161.

106. Leung, D.; Schroder, K.; White, H.; Fang, N-H.; et al. Activity of recombinant dengue 2 virus NS3 protease in the presence of a truncated NS2B cofactor, small peptide substrates and inhibitors. *J. Biol. Chem.* **2001**, *276*, 45762–45771.

107. Kuntz, I. D. Structure-based strategies for drug design and discovery. *Science* **1992**, *257*, 1078–1082.

108. Steinkuhler, C.; Tomei, L.; De Francesco, R. In vitro activity of hepatitis C virus protease NS3 purified from recombinant *Baculovirus*-infected Sf9 cells. *J. Biol. Chem.* **1996**, *271*, 6367–6373.

109. Gorbalenya, A. E.; Koonin, E. V.; Donchenko, A. P.; Blinov, V. M. Two related superfamilies of putative helicases involved in replication, recombination, repair and expression of DNA and RNA genomes. *Nucleic Acids Res.* **1989**, *17*, 4713–4730.

110. Gallivan, J. P.; McGarvey, M. J. The importance of the Q motif in the ATPase activity of a viral helicase. *FEBS Lett.* **2003**, *554*, 485–488.

111. Kuo, M. D.; Chin, C.; Hsu, S. L.; Shiao, J. Y.; et al. Characterization of the NTPase activity of Japanese encephalitis virus NS3 protein. *J. Gen. Virol.* **1996**, *77*(Pt. 9), 2077–2084.

112. Takegami, T.; Sakamuro, D.; Furukawa, T. Japanese encephalitis virus nonstructural protein NS3 has RNA binding and ATPase activities. *Virus Genes* **1995**, *9*, 105–112.

113. Warrener, P.; Tamura, J. K.; Collett, M. S. RNA-stimulated NTPase activity associated with yellow fever virus NS3 protein expressed in bacteria. *J. Virol.* **1993**, *67*, 989–996.

114. Matusan, A. E.; Pryor, M. J.; Davidson, A. D.; Wright, P. J. Mutagenesis of dengue virus type 2 NS3 protein within and outside helicase motifs: effects on enzyme activity and virus replication. *J. Virol.* **2001**, *75*, 9633–9643.

115. Bartelma, G.; Padmanabhan, R. Expression, purification, and characterization of the RNA 5'-triphosphatase activity of dengue virus type 2 nonstructural protein 3. *Virology* **2002**, *299*, 122–132.

116. Cho, H. S.; Ha, N. C.; Kang, L. W.; Chung, K. M.; et al. Crystal structure of RNA helicase from genotype 1b hepatitis C virus. A feasible mechanism of unwinding duplex RNA. *J. Biol. Chem.* **1998**, *273*, 15045–15052.

117. Yao, N.; Hesson, T.; Cable, M.; Hong, Z.; et al. Structure of the hepatitis C virus RNA helicase domain. *Nat. Struct. Biol.* **1997**, *4*, 463–467.

118. Yao, N.; Reichert, P.; Taremi, S. S.; Prosise, W. W.; Weber, P. C. Molecular views of viral polyprotein processing revealed by the crystal structure of the hepatitis C virus bifunctional protease-helicase. *Structure Fold Des.* **1999**, *7*, 1353–1363.

119. Frick, D. N. Helicases as antiviral drug targets. *Drug News Perspect.* **2003**, *16*, 355–362.

120. Yao, N.; Weber, P. C. Helicase, a target for novel inhibitors of hepatitis C virus. *Antiviral Ther.* **1998**, *3*, 93–97.

121. Zhang, N.; Chen, H. M.; Koch, V.; Schmitz, H.; et al. Ring-expanded ("fat") nucleoside and nucleotide analogues exhibit potent in vitro activity against Flaviviridae NTPases/ helicases, including those of the West Nile virus, hepatitis C virus, and Japanese encephalitis virus. *J. Med. Chem.* **2003**, *46*, 4149–4164.

122. Zhang, N.; Chen, H. M.; Koch, V.; Schmitz, H.; et al. Potent inhibition of NTPase/ helicase of the West Nile virus by ring-expanded ("fat") nucleoside analogues. *J. Med. Chem.* **2003**, *46*, 4776–4789.

123. Borowski, P.; Niebuhr, A.; Schmitz, H.; Hosmane, R. S.; et al. NTPase/helicase of Flaviviridae: inhibitors and inhibition of the enzyme. *Acta Biochim. Pol.* **2002**, *49*, 597–614.

124. Kapoor, M.; Zhang, L; Ramachandra, M.; Kusukawa, J.; et al. Association between NS3 and NS5 proteins of dengue virus type 2 in the putative RNA replicase is linked to differential phosphorylation of NS5. *J. Biol. Chem.* **1995**, *270*, 19100–19106.

125. Morozova, O. V.; Tsekhanovskaya, N. A.; Maksimova, T. G.; Bachvalova, V. N.; et al. Phosphorylation of tick-borne encephalitis virus NS5 protein. *Virus Res.* **1997**, *49*, 9–15.

126. Reed, K. E.; Gorbalenya, A. E.; Rice, C. M. The NS5A/NS5 proteins of viruses from three genera of the family Flaviviridae are phosphorylated by associated serine/threonine kinases. *J. Virol.* **1998**, *72*, 6199–6206.

127. Johansson, M.; Brooks, A. J.; Jans, D. A.; Vasudevan, S. G. A small region of the dengue virus-encoded RNA-dependent RNA polymerase, NS5, confers interaction with both the nuclear transport receptor importin-beta and the viral helicase, NS3. *J. Gen. Virol.* **2001**, *82*, 735–745.

128. Brooks, A. J.; Johansson, M.; John, A. V.; Xu, Y.; et al. The interdomain region of dengue NS5 protein that binds to the viral helicase NS3 contains independently functional importin beta 1 and importin alpha/beta-recognized nuclear localization signals. *J. Biol. Chem.* **2002**, *277*, 36399–36407.

129. Koonin, E. V. Computer-assisted identification of a putative methyltransferase domain in NS5 protein of flaviviruses and lambda 2 protein of reovirus. *J. Gen. Virol.* **1993**, *74*, 733–740.

130. Guyatt, K. J.; Westaway, E. G.; Khromykh, A. A. Expression and purification of enzymatically active recombinant RNA-dependent RNA polymerase (NS5) of the flavivirus Kunjin. *J. Virol. Methods* **2001**, *92*, 37–44.

131. Ackermann, M.; Padmanabhan, R. De novo synthesis of RNA by the dengue virus RNA-dependent RNA polymerase exhibits temperature dependence at the initiation but not elongation phase. *J. Biol. Chem.* **2001**, *276*, 39926–39937.

132. Tan, B. H.; Fu, J.; Sugrue, R. J.; Yap, E. H.; et al. Recombinant dengue type 1 virus NS5 protein expressed in *Escherichia coli* exhibits RNA-dependent RNA polymerase activity. *Virology* **1996**, *216*, 317–325.

133. Khromykh, A. A.; Kenney, M. T.; Westaway, E. G. trans-Complementation of flavivirus RNA polymerase gene NS5 by using Kunjin virus replicon-expressing BHK cells. *J. Virol.* **1998**, *72*, 7270–7279.

134. Hansen, J. L.; Long, A. M.; Schultz, S. C. Structure of the RNA-dependent RNA polymerase of poliovirus. *Structure* **1997**, *5*, 1109–1122.

135. De Clercq, E. Strategies in the design of antiviral drugs. *Nat. Rev. Drug Discov.* **2002**, *1*, 13–25.

136. Shi, P. Y. Strategies for the identification of inhibitors of West Nile virus and other flaviviruses. *Curr. Opin. Invest. Drugs* **2002**, *3*, 1567–1573.

137. Anderson, J. F.; Rahal, J. J. Efficacy of interferon alpha-2b and ribavirin against West Nile virus in vitro. *Emerging Infect. Dis.* **2002**, *8*, 107–108.

138. Morrey, J. D.; Smee, D. F.; Sidwell, R. W.; Tseng, C. Identification of active antiviral compounds against a New York isolate of West Nile virus. *Antiviral Res.* **2002**, *55*, 107–116.

139. Egloff, M. P.; Benarroch, D.; Selisko, B.; Romette, J. L.; Canard, B. An RNA cap (nucleoside-2'-*O*-)-methyltransferase in the flavivirus RNA polymerase NS5: crystal structure and functional characterization. *EMBO J.* **2002**, *21*, 2757–2768.

140. Bugl, H.; Fauman, E. B.; Staker, B. L.; Zheng, F.; et al. RNA methylation under heat shock control. *Mol. Cell* **2000**, *6*, 349–360.

141. Hodel, A. E.; Gershon, P. D.; Shi, X.; Quiocho, F. A. The 1.85 Å structure of vaccinia protein VP39: a bifunctional enzyme that participates in the modification of both mRNA ends. *Cell* **1996**, *85*, 247–256.

142. Chambers, T. J.; Diamond, M. S. Pathogenesis of flavivirus encephalitis. *Adv. Virus Res.* **2003**, *60*, 273–342.

143. Crill, W. D.; Roehrig, J. T. Monoclonal antibodies that bind to domain III of dengue virus E glycoprotein are the most efficient blockers of virus adsorption to Vero cells. *J. Virol.* **2001**, *75*, 7769–7773.

144. Heinz, F. X.; Allison, S. L. Flavivirus structure and membrane fusion. *Adv. Virus Res.* **2003**, *59*, 63–97.

145. Henchal, E. A.; Gentry, M. K.; McCown, J. M.; Brandt, W. E. Dengue virus-specific and flavivirus group determinants identified with monoclonal antibodies by indirect immunofluorescence. *Am. J. Trop. Med. Hyg.* **1982**, *31*, 830–836.

146. Henchal, E. A.; McCown, J. M.; Burke, D. S.; Seguin, M. C.; Brandt, W. E. Epitopic analysis of antigenic determinants on the surface of dengue-2 virions using monoclonal antibodies. *Am. J. Trop. Med. Hyg.* **1985**, *34*, 162–169.

147. Megret, F.; Hugnot, J-P.; Falconar, A.; Gentry, M. K.; et al. Use of recombinant fusion proteins and monoclonal antibodies to define linear and discontinuous antigenic sites on the dengue virus envelope glycoprotein. *Virology* **1992**, *187*, 480–491.

148. Modis, Y.; Ogata, S.; Clements, D.; Harrison, S. C. A ligand-binding pocket in the dengue virus envelope glycoprotein. *Proc. Natl. Acad. Sci. U.S.A.* **2003**, *100*, 6986–6991.

149. Modis, Y.; Ogata, S.; Clements, D.; Harrison, S. C. Structure of the dengue virus envelope protein after membrane fusion. *Nature* **2004**, *427*, 313–319.

150. Roehrig, J. T. Antigenic structure of flavivirus proteins. *Adv. Virus Res.* **2003**, *59*, 141–175.

151. Rey, F. A.; Heinz, F. X.; Mandl, C.; Kunz, C.; Harrison, S. C. The envelope glycoprotein from tick-borne encephalitis virus at 2 Å resolution. *Nature* **1995**, *375*, 291–298.

152. Allison, S. L.; Schalich, J.; Stiasny, K.; Mandl, C. W.; et al. Oligomeric rearrangement of tick-borne encephalitis virus envelope proteins induced by an acidic pH. *J. Virol.* **1995**, *69*, 695–700.

153. Heinz, F. X.; Allison, S. L. The machinery for flavivirus fusion with host cell membranes. *Curr. Opin. Microbiol.* **2001**, *4*, 450–455.

154. Mukhopadhyay, S.; Kim, B. S.; Chipman, P. R.; Rossmann, M. G.; Kuhn, R. J. Structure of West Nile virus. *Science* **2003**, *302*, 248.

155. Kuhn, R. J.; Zhang, W.; Rossman, M. G.; Pletnev, S. V.; et al. Structure of dengue virus: implications for flavivirus organization, maturation, and fusion. *Cell* **2002**, *108*, 717–725.

156. Zhang, W.; Chipman, P. R.; Corver, J.; Johnson, P. R.; et al. Visualization of membrane protein domains by cryo-electron microscopy of dengue virus. *Nat. Struct. Biol.* **2003**, *10*, 907–912.

157. Zhang, Y.; Corver, J.; Chipman, P. R.; Zhang, W.; et al. Structures of immature flavivirus particles. *EMBO J.* **2003**, *22*, 2604–2613.

158. Falconar, A. K. Identification of an epitope on the dengue virus membrane (M) protein defined by cross-protective monoclonal antibodies: design of an improved epitope sequence based on common determinants present in both envelope (E and M) proteins. *Arch. Virol.* **1999**, *144*, 2313–2330.

159. Monath, T. P.; Arroyo, J.; Levenbook, I.; Zhang, Z. X.; et al. Single mutation in the flavivirus envelope protein hinge region increases neurovirulence for mice and monkeys but decreases viscerotropism for monkeys: relevance to development and safety testing of live, attenuated vaccines. *J. Virol.* **2002**, *76*, 1932–1943.

160. Yamshchikov, V. F.; Trent, D. W.; Compans, R. W. Upregulation of signalase processing and induction of prM-E secretion by the flavivirus NS2B-NS3 protease: roles of protease components. *J. Virol.* **1997**, *71*, 4364–4371.

161. Wengler, G. Cell-associated West Nile flavivirus is covered with E+pre-M protein heterodimers which are destroyed and reorganized by proteolytic cleavage during virus release. *J. Virol.* **1989**, *63*, 2521–2526.

162. Anderson, R. Manipulation of cell surface macromolecules by flaviviruses. *Adv. Virus Res.* **2003**, *59*, 229–274.

163. Roehrig, J. T.; Bolin, R. A.; Kelly, R. G. Monoclonal antibody mapping of the envelope glycoprotein of the dengue 2 virus, Jamaica. *Virology* **1998**, *246*, 317–328.

164. Roehrig, J. T.; Johnson, A. J.; Hunt, A. R.; Bolin, R. A.; Chu, M. C. Antibodies to dengue 2 virus E-glycoprotein synthetic peptides identify antigenic conformation. *Virology* **1990**, *177*, 668–675.

165. Kimura-Kuroda, J.; Yasui, K. Protection of mice against Japanese encephalitis virus by passive administration with monoclonal antibodies. *J. Immunol.* **1988**, *141*, 3606–3610.

166. Bressanelli, S.; Stiasny, K.; Allison S. L.; Stura, E. A.; et al. Structure of a flavivirus envelope glycoprotein in its low-pH-induced membrane fusion conformation. *EMBO J.* **2004**, *23*(4), 728–735.

167. Gibbons, D. L.; Vaney, M. C.; Roussel, A.; Vigouroux, A.; et al. Conformational change and protein–protein interactions of the fusion protein of Semliki Forest virus. *Nature* **2004**, *427*, 320–325.

168. Khromykh, A. A.; Westaway, E. G. RNA binding properties of core protein of the flavivirus Kunjin. *Arch. Virol.* **1996**, *141*, 685–699.

169. Markoff, L.; Falgout, B.; Chang, A. A conserved internal hydrophobic domain mediates the stable membrane integration of the dengue virus capsid protein. *Virology* **1997**, *233*, 105–117.

170. Ma, L.; Jones, C. T.; Groesch, T. D.; Kuhn, R. J.; Post, C. B. Solution structure of dengue virus capsid protein reveals another fold. *Proc. Natl. Acad. Sci. U.S.A.* **2004**, *101*, 3414–3419.

171. Westaway, E. G.; Mackenzie, J. M.; Kenney, M. T.; Jones, M. K.; Khromykh, A. A. Ultrastructure of Kunjin virus-infected cells: colocalization of NS1 and NS3 with double-stranded RNA, and of NS2B with NS3, in virus-induced membrane structures. *J. Virol.* **1997**, *71*, 6650–6661.

172. Chambers, T. J.; McCourt, D. W.; Rice, C. M. Production of yellow fever virus proteins in infected cells: identification of discrete polyprotein species and analysis of cleavage kinetics using region-specific polyclonal antisera. *Virology* **1990**, *177*, 159–174.

173. Mason, P. W. Maturation of Japanese encephalitis virus glycoproteins produced by infected mammalian and mosquito cells. *Virology* **1989**, *169*, 354–364.

174. Post, P. R.; Carvalho, R.; Galler, R. Glycosylation and secretion of yellow fever virus nonstructural protein NS1. *Virus Res.* **1991**, *18*, 291–302.

175. Winkler, G.; Randolph, V. B.; Cleaves, G. R.; Ryan, T. E.; Stollar, V. Evidence that the mature form of the flavivirus nonstructural protein NS1 is a dimer. *Virology* **1988**, *162*, 187–196.

176. Winkler, G.; Maxwell, S. E.; Ruemmler, C.; Stollar, V. Newly synthesized dengue-2 virus nonstructural protein NS1 is a soluble protein but becomes partially hydrophobic and membrane-associated after dimerization. *Virology* **1989**, *171*, 302–305.

177. Muylaert, I. R.; Galler, R.; Rice, C. M. Genetic analysis of the yellow fever virus NS1 protein: identification of a temperature-sensitive mutation which blocks RNA accumulation. *J. Virol.* **1997**, *71*, 291–298.

178. Khromykh, A. A.; Varnavski, A. N.; Sedlak, P. L.; Westaway, E. G. Coupling between replication and packaging of flavivirus RNA: evidence derived from the use of DNA-based full-length cDNA clones of Kunjin virus. *J. Virol.* **2001**, *75*, 4633–4640.

179. Kummerer, B. M.; Rice, C. M. Mutations in the yellow fever virus nonstructural protein NS2A selectively block production of infectious particles. *J. Virol.* **2002**, *76*, 4773–4784.

180. Lindenbach, B. D.; Rice, C. M. Genetic interaction of flavivirus nonstructural proteins NS1 and NS4A as a determinant of replicase function. *J. Virol.* **1999**, *73*, 4611–4621.

CHAPTER 11

Confronting New and Old Antiviral Threats: Broad Spectrum Potential of Prenylation Inhibitors

MENASHE ELAZAR

Division of Gastroenterology and Hepatology, Stanford University School of Medicine

JEFFREY S. GLENN

Division of Gastroenterology and Hepatology, Stanford University School of Medicine, and Veterans Administration Medical Center

11.1 INTRODUCTION

Although a wide selection of antibiotics exists for treating bacterial infections, our arsenal of effective antiviral agents is more limited. This is a challenge for treating many acute and chronic viral infections of traditional medical importance. The challenge is even greater when considering viral bioterror threats. Vaccines have been the classic bulwarks against viral diseases, but such an approach has a variety of important limitations when planning for biodefense against a viral agent employed as a weapon. For one, vaccines traditionally take several years to develop and test. Thus, they may not be available to counter an immediate threat. Second, they require an a priori knowledge of the specific viral agent to be targeted— information that may not be forthcoming. Finally, with current technology and distributed knowledge base it may be relatively easy for an individual to purposely engineer a virus capable of eluding the epitopes targeted by a given vaccine.

To address these gaps in our biodefense strategy, ideally, one would like to have a drug—preferably orally available and with low side effects—with potential for broad-spectrum antiviral activity. This might allow its administration even before a precise identification of the specific threat is made in the field. Perhaps most critical for confronting viral bioweapons in the near-term, however, is that such a drug be

Antiviral Drug Discovery for Emerging Diseases and Bioterrorism Threats. Edited by Paul F. Torrence
Copyright © 2005 John Wiley & Sons, Inc.

available *now*. Prenylation inhibitors are a new class of antiviral agents, which may actually be able to satisfy most of the above criteria. After a brief review of prenylation, this chapter focuses on the experience to date using prenylation inhibitors against a prototype viral target, hepatitis delta virus (HDV). We then highlight the potential broad-spectrum activity of prenylation inhibitors as well as some of their features, which combine to make them particularly attractive for confronting a collection of viruses of both medical and bioterror importance.

11.2   PROTEIN PRENYLATION: A POST-TRANSLATIONAL MODIFICATION

Prenylation is a post-translational lipid modification of proteins that involves the covalent addition of an isoprene, or prenyl, group to a cysteine residue located within a specific amino acid sequence at the carboxyl terminus of the protein to be modified.[1,2] Two types of prenyl groups participate in these modification reactions: farnesyl (a 15 carbon prenyl group) and geranylgeranyl (a 20 carbon prenyl group). These isoprenoids are intermediate products that are synthesized from mevalonate as part of the biosynthesis of cholesterol.[1,2] The fully synthesized farnesyl or geranylgeranyl groups are attached to their target polypeptides by the cellular enzymes farnesyltransferase (FTase) and geranylgeranyltransferase (GGTase), respectively. The substrate recognition motif for FTase and GGTase type I is the "CXXX box" motif (where C is a cysteine and X is one of the last three amino acids at the extreme carboxyl terminus of the protein). In most cases, the addition of the prenyl group is followed by proteolytic cleavage of the three "—XXX" amino acids and carboxylmethylation of the now terminal prenylated cysteine. A second class of prenylating enzymes is the GGTase type II whose substrate recognition motif is more complex and adds geranylgeranyl groups to proteins that end with —CC or —CXC.[1,2] Examples of farnesylated proteins are the yeast mating hormone a-factor,[3] human lamin B,[4] and the family of Ras proteins,[5] while the γ-subunit of G proteins[6] and Rab proteins[7] are geranylgeranylated. One functional consequence of prenylation is to increase the hydrophobicity of the modified protein, which helps promote the protein's association with cellular membranes.[8] Another role for the lipid moiety is its ability to function as a ligand capable of binding to a protein receptor.[8,9] Prenylation mediates a collection of host cell signaling and membrane trafficking events.[8] As detailed below, a variety of viruses appear to exploit this post-translational modification as well (for a more extensive review of prenylation see Zhang and Casey[1] and Clarke[2]).

11.3   HEPATITIS DELTA VIRUS: VIRUS ASSEMBLY AND PRENYLATION

Hepatitis delta virus (HDV) is a small RNA virus that is associated with hepatitis B virus (HBV). HBV infection alone causes acute and chronic liver disease; HDV coinfection can dramatically increase both the severity and rate of progression of the liver disease.[10] HDV affects ~15 million of HBV-infected individuals worldwide[11] and in the United States the prevalence of HDV has been estimated to be around 70,000 individuals.[12] To date, effective medical therapy has been lacking.

HDV is a single-stranded RNA virus with a 1.7 kb circular genome. The viral genome codes for only two proteins known as small and large delta antigens (SHDAg and LHDAg, respectively). These proteins are identical except that the large delta antigen contains an extra 19 amino acids at its carboxyl terminus. This extension is the result of a specific RNA editing event that occurs during replication of the genome.[13]

The complete HDV viral particle consists of a complex of the viral genome, both delta antigen isoforms, all encapsulated by a lipid envelope. The lipid envelope is embedded with HBV surface antigen (HBsAg) proteins, which are provided by a coinfecting HBV.[14] The HBV proteins present in the lipid envelope provide the means for HDV particle exit and entry into the cell. This dependence on HBV for a source of envelope proteins provides the molecular explanation for why HDV infection is always accompanied by HBV coinfection.

Although identical over most of their length, SHDAg and LHDAg differ in their function in a variety of ways. For example, while SHDAg is crucial for RNA replication the LHDAg can trans-dominantly inhibit this process.[15,16] Large delta antigen can also trans activate a variety of different genes.[17] Perhaps the most dramatic difference between the delta antigen isoforms is observed during virus assembly. Although both isoforms are found in HDV particles, only the large delta antigen can promote virus assembly in conjunction with HBsAg. An important clue as to what feature of large delta antigen is required for its role in particle assembly was revealed by a closer examination of the 19 amino acids unique to the larger isoform. In particular, it was noted that the last four amino acids of LHDAg, Cys-Arg-Pro-Gln-COOH, constitute a "CXXX box" motif that is highly conserved in all HDV isolates. This observation suggested that LHDAg is subject to prenylation and indeed this was shown to be the case.[18] Subsequent studies demonstrated that the specific type of prenyl lipid added to delta antigen is farnesyl.[19]

That large delta antigen prenylation is required for HDV particle assembly was shown by mutation of the large delta antigen CXXX box.[18] Mutation of cysteine to serine abolished both prenylation and assembly of HDV virus-like particles (VLPs) (Figure 11.1). This was the first demonstration that viral proteins can undergo prenylation and exploit this modification to mediate a critical aspect of the corresponding virus' life cycle. For HDV, the apparent crucial role of prenylation in virus assembly may be to target the thus lipid-modified large delta antigen to the membranes that contain the HBsAg envelope proteins. Alternatively, the attached farnesyl moiety could act as a ligand specifically recognized by a receptor in those membranes, such as HBsAg, somewhat analogous to the interaction of the geranylgeranylated Rab3 with GDI.[7] In either case, these results suggested the hypothesis that inhibition of LHDAg prenylation by *pharmacologic* means might similarly prevent virus particle formation and thereby represent the basis for

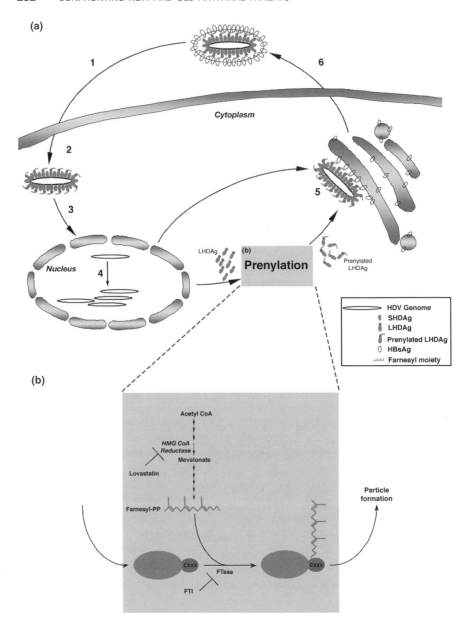

FIGURE 11.1 The hepatitis delta virus (HDV) life cycle and the role of prenylation. (a) The HDV life cycle begins with infection of a human hepatocyte (1). Upon entry, the viral particle is uncoated (2) and the genome with associated core-like delta antigens is transported to the nucleus (3), where replication (4) is mediated by small delta antigen (SHDAg). An RNA editing event that occurs during replication gives rise to the production of large delta antigen (LHDAg). LHDAg undergoes prenylation [detailed in part (b) of the figure]. The latter is necessary for assembly (5) and release (6) of new progeny viral particles in

a practical antiviral therapy. As detailed below, this hypothesis has now been successfully tested first using the VLP model system, then with complete infectious virions in a cell culture model, and finally most recently in an animal model of HDV infection.

11.4   PRENYLATION INHIBITORS AS ANTIVIRAL AGENTS

The discovery that the oncogene Ras is farnesylated and that this prenylation enables both Ras localization to the plasma membrane and Ras-mediated tranformation[20] has opened up a flourishing field of research on prenyltransferase inhibitors. For example, BZA-5B was developed as a specific inhibitor of farnesyltransferase.[21] BZA-5B was shown to inhibit prenylation of the oncoprotein H-Ras[V12] and abrogate its prenylation-mediated transformation of Rat-1 cells.[21,22]. BZA-5B was thus a logical choice for evaluating the effect of pharmacologically inhibiting prenylation of another farnesylated protein—namely, large delta antigen. Treatment of HDV VLP-producing cells with BZA-5B showed a substantial inhibition of VLP formation at $10 \, \mu M$ concentration of drug and a complete inhibition at $50 \, \mu M$.[23] Surprisingly, minimal cytotoxic effects were observed at any of these concentrations. Indeed, cells can be grown for several generations in BZA-5B without significant effects.[23]

These results demonstrated that prenylation inhibitors (PIs) are valid candidates for preventing HDV particle production. It was important to show, however, that the same effect can be exerted by other types of PIs (i.e., the observed antiviral effect was truly a result of farnesyltransferase inhibition and not related to some other feature of BZA-5B) and to extend this strategy to the inhibition of complete, genome-containing, infectious HDV particles. For these purposes a cell culture system that is capable of producing such infectious particles was utilized and treated with FTI-277,[24] a farnesyltransferase inhibitor that is structurally very different from BZA-5B. Dose-dependent inhibition of HDV infectious particle formation at micromolar concentrations of FTI-277 was observed[25] (Figure 11.2a). Furthermore, similar efficacies were achieved against another HDV genotype that is associated with particularly severe clinical disease.[25]

---

conjugation with the viral envelope proteins (HBsAg). (b) Synthesis of the isoprenoid farnesyl begins with the conversion of acetyl-CoA through several biochemical reactions to mevalonate. Mevalonate production by the action of HMG-CoA reductase is the committed step in cholesterol and prenyl lipid synthesis. Further processing reactions lead to the formation of the prenyl lipid farnesyl. Farnesyltransferase (FTase) catalyzes the final step in prenylation of LHDAg by covalently attaching the farnesyl prenyl group to a cysteine residue contained within a specific amino acid sequence known as the CXXX box motif (where C = cysteine and X = one of three amino acids at the carboxyl terminus of the protein substrate). Once prenylated, LHDAg can promote the final stage in the HDV life cycle, namely, particle formation. See text for details.

In an effort to further translate these results into a practical clinical therapy, the efficacy of prenylation inhibition-based antiviral therapy was evaluated in an in vivo animal model of HDV. This animal model combines an HBV transgenic mouse model[26] with hydrodynamic transfection[27] of the HDV genome into the tail vein of the mice. The HBV transgene helps supply a source of HBV HBsAg that is necessary for HDV particle formation, while the genome injection establishes high-efficiency HDV replication in the mouse hepatocytes.[28] This combination enables the production of infectious HDV particles in the mouse liver and their secretion into the blood. Single daily doses of two different farnesyltransferase inhibitors at 50 mg/kg/day were administered to such mice. These compounds were well tolerated, as there were no differences in measures of toxicity as compared to vehicle control. A dramatic effect on HDV viremia, however, was observed with both inhibitors achieving complete clearance of detectable viremia within one

(a)

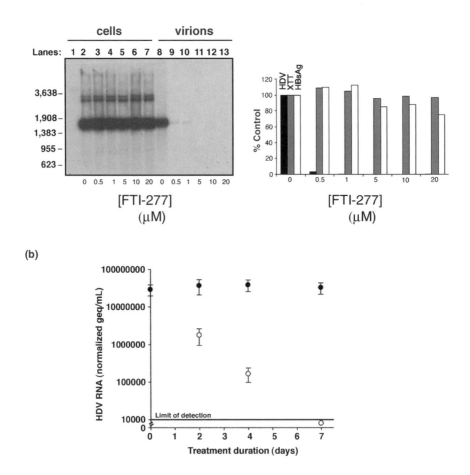

(b)

week[29] (Figure 11.2b). These results combined with the recent development of orally administered PIs that are surprisingly well tolerated in human Phase I/II clinical trials have now set the stage for the first clinical trials of this novel approach to antiviral therapy in a cohort of HDV-infected patients. Moreover, as detailed below, HDV is best considered as just the first prototype target for this novel approach to antiviral therapy.

11.5 PRENYLATION INHIBITORS: DRUGS WITH BROAD-SPECTRUM ANTIVIRAL POTENTIAL

As might be expected, exploitation of prenylation by viruses does not appear to be a phenomenon restricted only to HDV. For example, a variety of other medically important viruses encode proteins that possess potential prenylation sites (Table 11.1). These viruses represent a diverse group of viruses including double-stranded DNA viruses, single positive-stranded RNA viruses, and single negative-stranded RNA viruses. The potentially prenylated proteins in these viruses have been implicated in a diverse spectrum of functions ranging from viral assembly to viral replication as well as to date unknown functions (see Table 11.1).

←——————————

FIGURE 11.2   Prenylation inhibitors block hepatitis D virus (HDV) particle formation (a) The prenylation inhibitor FTI-277 inhibits production of HDV genome-containing particles. Huh7 cells were cotransfected with HDV and hepatitis B virus (HBV) genome-encoding constructs, which results in the formation of infectious HDV particles.[41] The cells were maintained in a daily changed medium containing carrier alone (0.2% DMSO and 400 μM DTT) (lanes 2 and 8) or carrier plus FTI-277 at the following concentrations: 0.5 μM (lanes 3 and 9), 1 μM (lanes 4 and 10), 5 μM (lanes 5 and 11), 10 μM (lanes 6 and 12), or 20 μM (lanes 7 and 13). On day 10 after transfection, cells (lanes 1 to 7) and supernatants (lanes 8 to 13) were processed for northern analysis of HDV RNA. Lane 1 corresponds to total RNA extracted from nontransfected cells subjected to carrier-containing medium (left panel). The amount of HDV RNA in the culture medium of cells treated with the indicated amount of FTI-277 was quantitated using a phosphorimager and plotted as percentage of the untreated control (0 μM) (black bars—right panel). To assess for nonspecific effects of the inhibitor, prior to total RNA extraction, XTT assays were performed to monitor cell metabolism (grey bars—right panel) and supernatant HBV surface antigen (HBsAg) levels were determined to monitor for general protein expression and secretion (empty bars—right panel). [Part (a) reproduced with permission from the *Journal Virology.*[25]] (b) In vivo treatment of HDV viremia with the prenylation inhibitor FTI-2153. HBV transgenic mice were hydrodynamically transfected with an HDV genome-encoding construct to establish HDV viremia.[29] Following transfection, the mice were treated with carrier alone (solid circles) or carrier plus FTI-2153 (open circles) for the indicated number of days prior to sacrifice. Serum HDV RNA was quantitated by RT PCR and normalized for transfection efficiency by quantitation of total HDV liver RNA. See text for details. [Part (b) reproduced with permission from *Journal of Clinical Investigation.*[29]]

TABLE 11.1 Selected Examples of CXXX Box Motif-Containing Viral Proteins

Family	Virus	Protein	CXXX-Box Motif
Deltavirus	HDV	Large δ Ag	C T P Q
Bunyaviridae	Oropouche	Nonstructural	C R D T
Herpesviridae	HSV	UL32	C T Y V
	CMV	TRL9	C R I Q
Picornaviridae	HAV	Polymerase	C D L S
	FMDV	Polymerase	C G D A
Poxiviridae	Vaccinia	A47L	C V T V
	Variola	Serpin 1	C Y P Q

The range of activities associated with these CXXX box motif-containing proteins suggests that prenylation may be important for stages in the respective viral life cycles beyond the assembly and release exemplified by HDV's LHDAg prenylation. For example, the hepatitis A virus (HAV) and foot-and-mouth disease virus (FMDV) predicted prenylation site is located in the polymerase protein of these two viruses. Like other positive-strand RNA viruses, HAV and FMDV RNA replication is believed to occur in tight association with intracellular membranes, although the mechanism of how the replication complex is assembled and maintained on these membranes is not yet known.[30] Since one consequence of prenylation is to increase the hydrophobicity of the modified protein in order to promote its membrane association,[1,8,31] a lipophilic modification may be critical for the membrane association of these polymerase proteins. Alternatively, because of protein prenylation's potential to participate in protein–protein interactions,[9] prenylation of the polymerase protein may help mediate a critical interaction with other replication complex proteins or host cell membrane anchors. In either case, one can readily envisage that abrogating this viral prenylation may prove to be detrimental for the virus. Prenylation targets are also found in both cytomegalovirus (CMV) and herpes simplex virus (HSV). Although the role of their prenylation status in the respective viral life cycles has not yet been determined, application of FTI to HSV-infected cells inhibited viral replication.[32] Finally, in addition to requiring prenylation of some of their own proteins, viruses may also depend on the prenylation of selected host cell proteins, as has been suggested for respiratory syncytial virus (RSV)[33] and hepatitis C virus (HCV).[34] Of course, inhibition of viral or host protein targets is not mutually exclusive and both mechanisms may be operative, depending on the specific virus. Taken together, the above suggests that PIs have the exciting potential to act as broad-spectrum antiviral drugs.

11.6 PRENYLATION INHIBITORS AND BIODEFENSE

Although the originally considered viral targets of PIs have been those of traditional medical importance, it is obvious that this class of drugs may also be suitable for a collection of viruses whose threat has emerged with increasing concerns about bioterrorism. The list of viruses contained in the NIAID Categories A and B Priority Pathogens encompasses a variety of viruses that might now only be encountered as a purposeful bioweapon (such as smallpox) and viruses that might be weaponized but are also of medical concern in their own right (such as HAV and bunyaviruses). As shown in Table 11.1, several of these viral agents possess proteins with conserved CXXX box motifs, suggesting they may be ideal candidates for PI-based antiviral therapy. Moreover, as mentioned above, even viruses without CXXX box-containing proteins may be susceptible to PIs. Finally, PIs may also have utility in treating some of the serious side effects associated with vaccination against certain biothreats. Indeed, one impediment to widescale anti-smallpox vaccination with vaccinia virus is the occasional severe disease caused by the latter.[35] The presence of several CXXX box-containing proteins in vaccinia virus suggests these complications may be amenable to treatment with PIs.

In addition to their potential broad-spectrum activity, PIs have another compelling feature for their inclusion in our biodefense arsenal—they are available for use right now. This is a fortunate, albeit fortuitous, situation and stems from the fact that the oncogene Ras was noted several years ago to be modified by prenylation. As a result, a tremendous effort has been mounted to develop PIs as anticancer agents. Among the products of these efforts is one of the few examples of successful rational drug design. Indeed, farnesyltransferase inhibitors like FTI-277 were designed to mimic the CXXX box peptide as found in the oncogene Ras.[24] Other classes of compounds have also been developed to inhibit prenyltransferases. These include drugs developed using benzodiazapene[21] and tricyclic scaffolds.[36] The results of these efforts is that a substantial number of PIs have been developed and the leaders of the pack have been successfully put through Phase I/II trials in humans. Although the latter have to date been exclusively for nonviral indications, much of the human pharmacokinetic and toxicity data can be used directly to support human trials of PIs as antiviral agents. Moreover, as detailed further below, such prenylation inhibition-based antiviral therapy has several additional desirable features.

11.7 PRENYLATION INHIBITORS: ATTRACTIVE FEATURES AS ANTIVIRAL DRUGS

At first glance, a strategy of treating viral infections with PIs might be expected to cause intolerable side effects because of effects on host cell pathways dependent on prenylation. Surprisingly, this does not seem to be the case, as farnesyltransferase inhibitors are tolerated by host cells in vitro[37] and more importantly in vivo by treated cancer patients.[38] This may be a reflection of the fact that most cellular proteins are geranylgeranylated rather then farnesylated,[39] that the existence of a family of prenyltransferase enzymes enables prenylation of key proteins by isoforms not targeted by an individual drug, or that the function of a given host prenylated protein may be partially restored by "cross-prenylation" with a different prenyl group. Such back-up mechanisms may not, however, be readily available to a targeted virus, especially where the prenyl group serves a ligand function and cannot be substituted by another type of prenyl group.

Where toxicities are observed, they do not appear to be the same for different types of farnesyltransferase inhibitors. This suggests such side effects are likely to be more compound-specific rather than the result of a common mechanism such as prenylation inhibition.

The strategy of prenyltransferase inhibition for antiviral therapy is different from the more classical approaches for treating viral diseases. This is because rather than targeting a specific viral protein domain, which can readily be mutated by the virus, prenylation inhibition-based antiviral therapy seeks to deprive the virus access to a *host* function, namely, prenylation. Because the locus of the targeted enzyme is not under genetic control of the virus, but rather is contained in the host cell genome, it may be a much more difficult process for viruses to easily develop resistance to this strategy. It is also important to note the fact that several PIs have been developed as oral formulations. This may help further facilitate their widespread use. Finally, it is also possible that PIs will have synergistic activity with other drugs. For example, as depicted in Figure 11.1a, farnesyl and geranylgeranyl are synthesized from the precursor mevalonate in the biosynthesis pathway of cholesterol. Mevalonate production, the committed step in prenyl group synthesis, is catalyzed by HMG-CoA reductase and several inhibitors of this enzyme are in widespread use in hypercholesterolemic patients.[40] Although HMG-CoA reductase inhibitors alone can inhibit protein prenylation in vitro, the doses required are too cytotoxic for use in humans.[40] It can, however, be contemplated that HMG-CoA reductase inhibitors in combination with PIs may have a synergistic effect on protein prenylation. Evaluation of this hypothesis may soon be forthcoming using the HDV models described herein.[23,25,29]

In summary, a growing number of viruses appear to exploit protein prenylation to mediate various aspects of their respective life cycles. This critical post-translational modification can be pharmacologically disrupted by specific prenylation inhibitors. Where tested, the latter exhibit potent antiviral effects. Prenylation inhibitors thus represent a novel class of antiviral agents with the potential for broad-spectrum activity against viruses that are of both traditional medical importance as well as potential agents of bioterrorism.

ACKNOWLEDGMENTS

This work was supported in part by the Burroughs Wellcome Fund, the Veterans Administration, the Goldman Philanthropic Partnerships and Oxnard Foundation and 1 R43 AI056641-01.

REFERENCES

1. Zhang, F. L.; Casey, P. J. Protein prenylation: molecular mechanisms and functional consequences. *Annu. Rev. Biochem.* **1996**, *65*, 241–269.

2. Clarke, S. Protein isoprenylation and methylation at carboxyl-terminal cysteine residues. *Annu. Rev. Biochem.* **1992**, *61*, 355–386.

3. Anderegg, R. J.; Betz, R.; Carr, S. A.; Crabb, J. W.; Duntze, W. Structure of *Saccharomyces cerevisiae* mating hormone a-factor. *J. Biol. Chem.* **1988**, *263*, 18236–18240.

4. Farnsworth, C. C.; Wolda, S. L.; Gelb, M. H.; Glomset, J. A. Human lamin B contains a farnesylated cysteine residue. *J. Biol. Chem.* **1989**, *264*, 20422–20429.

5. Hancock, J. F.; Magee, A. I.; Childs, J. E.; Marshall, C. J. All ras proteins are polyisoprenylated but only some are palmitoylated. *Cell* **1989**, *57*, 1167–1177.

6. Yamane, H. K.; Farnsworth, C. C.; Xie, H.; Howald, W.; Fung, B. K.-K.; et al. Brain G protein γ subunits contain an all-trans-geranylgeranyl-cysteine methyl ester at their carboxyl termini. *Proc. Natl. Acad. Sci. U.S.A.* **1990**, *87*, 5868–5872.

7. Novick, P.; Brennwald, P. Friends and family: the role of the Rab GTPases in vesicular traffic. *Cell* **1993**, *75*, 597–601.

8. Casey, P. J. Protein lipidation in cell signaling. *Science* **1995**, *268*, 221–225.

9. Hoffman, G. R.; Nassar, N.; Cerione, R. A. Structure of the Rho family GTP-binding protein Cdc42 in complex with the multifunctional regulator RhoGDI. *Cell* **2000**, *100*, 345–356.

10. Casey, J. L. Hepatitis delta virus: molecular biology, pathogenesis and immunology. *Antiviral Ther.* **1998**, *3*, 37–42.

11. Rizzetto, M.; Ponzetto, A.; Forzani, I. Epidemiology of hepatitis delta virus: Overview. In *The Hepatitis Delta Virus*, Wiley-Liss, New York, 1991, pp. 1–20.

12. Alter, M. J.; Hadler, S. C. Delta hepatitis and infection in North America. In *Hepatitis Delta Virus: Molecular Biology, Pathogenesis, and Clinical Aspects*, Wiley-Liss, New York, 1993, pp. 243–250.

13. Taylor, J. M. The structure and replication of hepatitis delta virus. *Annu. Rev. Microbiol.* **1992**, *46*, 253–276.

14. Bonino, F.; Heermann, K. H.; Rizzetto, M.; Gerlich, W. H. Hepatitis delta virus: protein composition of delta antigen and its hepatitis B virus-derived envelope. *J. Virol.* **1986**, *58*, 945–950.

15. Glenn, J. S.; White, J. M. Trans-dominant inhibition of human hepatitis delta virus genome replication. *J. Virol.* **1991**, *65*, 2357–2361.

16. Chao, M.; Hsieh, S.-Y.; Taylor, J. Role of two forms of hepatitis delta virus antigen: evidence for a mechanism of self-limiting genome replication. *J. Virol.* **1990**, *64*, 5066–5069.

17. Wei, Y.; Ganem, D. Activation of heterologous gene expression by the large isoform of hepatitis delta antigen. *J. Virol.* **1998**, *72*, 2089–2096.

18. Glenn, J. S.; Watson, J. A.; Havel, C. M.; White, J. M. Identification of a prenylation site in delta virus large antigen. *Science* **1992**, *256*, 1331–1333.

19. Otto, J. C.; Casey, P. J. The hepatitis delta virus large antigen is farnesylated both in vitro and in animal cells. *J. Biol. Chem.* **1996**, *271*, 4569–4572.

20. Willumsen, B. M.; Christensen, A.; Hubbert, N. L.; Papageorge, A. G.; Lowy, D. R. The p21 ras C-terminus is required for transformation and membrane association. *Nature* **1984**, *310*, 583–586.

21. Marsters, J. C. Jr.; McDowell, R. S.; Reynolds, M. E.; Oare, D. A.; Somers, T. C.; et al. Benzodiazepine peptidomimetic inhibitors of farnesyltransferase. *Bioorg. Med. Chem.* **1994**, *2*, 949–957.

22. James, G. L.; Goldstein, J. L.; Brown, M. S.; Rawson, T. E.; Somers, T. C.; et al. Benzodiazepine peptidomimetics: potent inhibitors of Ras farnesylation in animal cells. *Science* **1993**, *260*, 1937–1942.

23. Glenn, J. S.; Marsters, J. C. Jr.; Greenberg, H. B. Use of a prenylation inhibitor as a novel antiviral agent. *J. Virol.* **1998**, *72*, 9303–9306.

24. Lerner, E. C.; Qian, Y.; Blaskovich, M. A.; Fossum, R. D.; Vogt, A.; et al. Ras CAAX peptidomimetic FTI-277 selectively blocks oncogenic Ras signaling by inducing cytoplasmic accumulation of inactive Ras–Raf complexes. *J. Biol. Chem.* **1995**, *270*, 26802–26806.

25. Bordier, B. B.; Marion, P. L.; Ohashi, K.; Kay, M. A.; Greenberg, H. B.; et al. A prenylation inhibitor prevents production of infectious hepatitis delta virus particles. *J. Virol.* **2002**, *76*, 10465–10472.

26. Marion, P. L.; Salazar, F. H.; Liittschwager, K.; Bordier, B. B.; Seeger, C.; et al. *A Transgenic Mouse Lineage Useful for Testing Antivirals Targeting Hepatitis B Virus*, Elsevier Science, New York, 2002, pp.197–209.

27. Liu, F.; Song, Y.; Liu, D. Hydrodynamics-based transfection in animals by systemic administration of plasmid DNA. *Gene Therapy* **1999**, *6*, 1258–1266.

28. Chang, J.; Sigal, L. J.; Lerro, A.; Taylor, J. Replication of the human hepatitis delta virus genome is initiated in mouse hepatocytes following intravenous injection of naked DNA or RNA sequences. *J. Virol.* **2001**, *75*, 3469–3473.

29. Bordier, B. B.; Ohkanda, J.; Liu, P.; Lee, S. Y.; Salazar, F. H.; et al. In vivo antiviral efficacy of prenylation inhibitors against hepatitis delta virus. *J. Clin. Invest.* **2003**, *112*, 407–414.

30. Rice, C. M. Flaviviridae: the viruses and their replication. In *Fields Virology*, Lippincott-Raven Publications, Philadelphia, 1996, pp.931–959.

31. Glenn, J. S. Prenylation and virion morphogenesis. In *The Unique Hepatitis Delta Virus*, R.C. Landes Publishing, Austin, 1995, pp.83–93.

32. Farassati, F.; Yang, A. D.; Lee, P. W. Oncogenes in Ras signalling pathway dictate host-cell permissiveness to herpes simplex virus 1. *Nat. Cell Biol.* **2001**, *3*, 745–750.

33. Gower, T. L.; Graham, B. S. Antiviral activity of lovastatin against respiratory syncytial virus in vivo and in vitro. *Antimicrob. Agents Chemother.* **2001**, *45*, 1231–1237.

34. Ye, J.; Wang, C.; Sumpter, R. Jr.; Brown, M. S.; Goldstein, J. L.; et al. Disruption of hepatitis C virus RNA replication through inhibition of host protein geranylgeranylation. *Proc. Natl. Acad. Sci. U.S.A.* **2003**, *100*, 15865–15870.

35. Bray, M. Pathogenesis and potential antiviral therapy of complications of smallpox vaccination. *Antiviral Res.* **2003**, *58*, 101–114.

36. Njoroge, F. G.; Doll, R. J.; Vibulbhan, B.; Alvarez, C. S.; Bishop, W. R.; et al. Discovery of novel nonpeptide tricyclic inhibitors of Ras farnesyl protein transferase. *Bioorg. Med. Chem.* **1997**, *5*, 101–113.

37. Dalton, M. B.; Fantle, K. S.; Bechtold, H. A.; DeMaio, L.; Evans, R. M.; et al. The farnesyl protein transferase inhibitor BZA-5B blocks farnesylation of nuclear lamins and p21ras but does not affect their function or localization. *Cancer Res.* **1995**, *55*, 3295–3304.

38. Sharma, S.; Kemeny, N.; Kelsen, D. P.; Ilson, D.; O'Reilly, E.; et al. A Phase II trial of farnesyl protein transferase inhibitor SCH 66336, given by twice-daily oral

administration, in patients with metastatic colorectal cancer refractory to 5-fluorouracil and irinotecan. *Ann. Oncol.* **2002**, *13*, 1067–1071.

39. Farnsworth, C. C.; Gelb, M. H.; Glomset, J. A. Identification of geranylgeranyl-modified proteins in HeLa cells. *Science* **1990**, *247*, 320–322.

40. Sinensky, M.; Beck, L. A.; Leonard, S.; Evans, R. Differential inhibitory effects of lovastatin on protein isoprenylation and sterol synthesis. *J. Biol. Chem.* **1990**, *265*, 19937–19941.

41. Chang, F.-L.; Chen, P.-J.; Tu, S.-J.; Wang, C.-J.; Chen, D.-S. The large form of hepatitis δ antigen is crucial for assembly of hepatitis δ virus. *Proc. Natl. Acad. Sci. U.S.A.* **1991**, *88*, 8490–8494.

CHAPTER 12

West Nile Virus: New Targets for Potential Antivirals

MATTHIAS KALITZKY and HOLGER ROHDE

University Hospital Hamburg-Eppendorf, Institute for Infectious Diseases

PETER BOROWSKI

Bernhard-Nocht-Institute for Tropical Medicine, Department of Virology

12.1   INTRODUCTION

West Nile virus (WNV) is mainly an avian virus that is spread by mosquitoes. Since the WNV epidemic in New York City in 1999 the virus is gaining attention worldwide. There are currently no drugs or vaccines available to treat or prevent the disease. Although there are several potential targets for antiviral therapy, like blockade of viral entry, capping, or protein synthesis, the most promising approach appears to be the inhibition of viral enzymes directly involved in virus replication. In WNV, the replication complex consists of two main nonstructural (NS) proteins, NS3 and NS5. NS3 exerts nucleoside triphosphatase (NTPase)/helicase and protease activities, whereas NS5 acts as RNA-dependent RNA polymerase (RdRp).

This chapter summarizes our knowledge about the potential targets of anti-WNV therapy, updates the spectrum of inhibitors (blockers) of these targets, and describes the putative mechanisms by which the compounds might act. Some of the compounds presented here exhibited very low cytotoxicity combined with an unambiguous anti-WNV effect when tested in cell culture. Such compounds could show potential utility as a basis for the development of antiviral agents against WNV.

12.2   THE WEST NILE VIRUS

The West Nile virus was isolated in 1937 from the blood of a febrile woman from Uganda's West Nile province and was subsequently found in many regions of the

Antiviral Drug Discovery for Emerging Diseases and Bioterrorism Threats. Edited by Paul F. Torrence
Copyright © 2005 John Wiley & Sons, Inc.

world including Africa, the Middle East, Europe, India, and Indonesia. Epidemics with West Nile virus were first observed in the Nile Delta during the 1950s.[1] Still the virus did not infect humans in the United States until the summer of 1999, when it caused 61 human cases and seven deaths during an epidemic in New York City.[2] Since its appearance in the United States the virus has spread from the Northeast to the Eastern seaboard, to the Midwest and to the Deep South where it caused significant human, equine, and avian disease.

Birds are the principal hosts and reservoir of West Nile virus. They are also responsible for the intercontinental spread of WNV and can support replication of WNV to high levels of long-term viremia that is sufficient to infect mosquitoes.[3] The virus could be isolated from a variety of *Culex, Aedes,* and *Anopheles* species. Bird-feeding mosquito species are the principal transmission vectors of WNV.

In humans, infection with WNV usually results in an influenza-like syndrome with a duration of 3 to 5 days. Elderly people or patients with compromised immune systems are at greater risk of developing fatal neurologic complications like meningoencephalitis or poliomyelitis.[4]

Recently, the National Institutes of Health prioritized WNV together with three other flaviviruses as potential bioterrorism pathogens, which further stresses the need to develop antiviral therapeutics and vaccines for flavivirus infections.

12.3 GENOMIC REPLICATION

WNV virions are spherical in shape with a diameter of 40 to 60 nm. The viral genome is a single-stranded RNA of positive polarity and approximately 11,000 bases in length. The genomic RNA contains one single open reading frame. Both termini of the genomic RNA contain sequences that do not encode viral proteins, which are known as the 5' and 3' untranslated regions (5'-UTR and 3'-UTR).

Genomic replication proceeds similarly in all members of the family of the Flaviviridae (flaviviruses, hepaciviruses, and pestiviruses) and the replication cycle offers numerous targets for antiviral chemotherapy. After binding to a specific receptor of the target cell (that has not yet been identified for WNV), the virion is included in a lysosome by receptor-mediated endocytosis. Inside the vesicle, acid-catalyzed membrane fusion releases the nucleocapsid into the cytoplasm, a process known as "uncoating."

In hepaciviruses (such as HCV) and pestiviruses, translation is initiated by binding of the free viral RNA to an internal ribosomal entry site (IRES), which has been studied as a target for antivirals (Figure 12.1).

12.4 THE VIRAL PROTEINS

The flavivirus genome is translated as a large polypeptide that is processed co- and post-translationally by cellular and viral proteases into ten discrete products, the

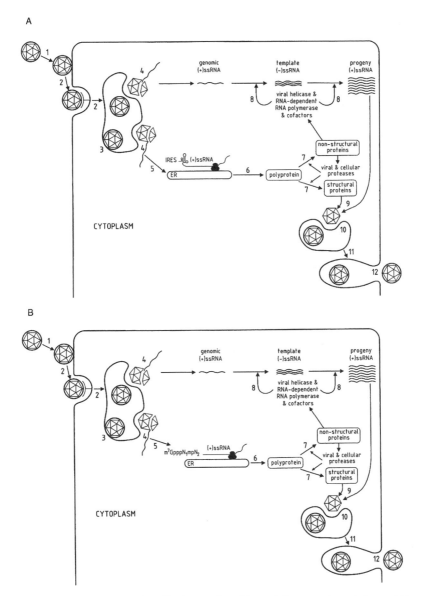

FIGURE 12.1   The presumed replicative cycles of hepaciviruses and pestiviruses (A) and of the flaviviruses (B). 1, Adsorption; 2, receptor-mediated endocytosis; 3, low-pH fusion in lysosomes; 4, uncoating; 5, IRES-mediated initiation of translation (A) or cap-mediated initiation of translation (B); 6, translation of the viral RNA into viral precursor polyprotein; 7, co- and post-translational proteolytic processing of the viral polyprotein by cellular and viral proteases; 8, membrane-associated synthesis of templated minus-strand RNA and progeny plus-strand RNA; 9, assembly of the nucleocapsid; 10, budding of virions in the endoplasmic reticulum (ER); 11, transport and maturation of virions in the ER and the Golgi complex; 12, vesicle fusion and release of mature virions. (Reproduced with permission from American Society for Microbiology[43]).

three structural and seven nonstructural proteins: NH2-C-prM-E-NS1-NS2A-NS2B-NS3-NS4A-NS4B-NS5-COOH (Figure 12.2).

Translation in WNV is associated with the rough endoplasmic reticulum. Cellular peptidase in the lumen of the ER cleaves the polypeptide to generate the N termini of prM, E, NS1, and NS4B. The cellular enzyme furin cleaves prM to form the structural protein M and the N-terminal pr-segment. The remaining cleavages of the polypeptide are mediated by the NS2B + NS3 protease complex (NS2B–3-protease) and generate the N termini of NS2B, NS3, NS4A, and NS5.

Besides the structural proteins (C-protein, E-protein, and the glycosylated progenitor protein prM), the nonstructural proteins play an important role in viral assembly and genomic replication. Although the nonstructural proteins are not part of the virion, it has been shown that their integrity is essential for virus replication. Therefore, the inhibition of the functions mediated by the nonstructural proteins seems to be a possible approach for inhibition of virus replication.

NS1 together with NS4A are required for RNA replication.[5] The hydrophobic protein NS2A has a function in the assembly and release of infectious flavivirus particles.[6] NS5 functions as the viral RNA-dependent RNA polymerase.[7] The function of the membrane-associated NS4A and NS4B peptides has not yet been identified.

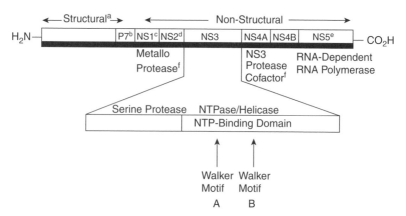

FIGURE 12.2 Simplified representation of the flaviviruses and hepaciviruses polyprotein with the expanded NS3 region. The arrows indicate the position of the Walker motifs A and B within the NTPase/helicase molecule. (a) The NH2-terminal part of the polyprotein of the members of the *Flavivirus* genus is processed into three structural proteins: a nucleocapsid protein (C), precursor membrane protein (prM), and one envelope protein (E). (b) Peptide p7 of unknown function is encoded exclusively by hepaciviruses. (c) NS1 is encoded exclusively by flaviviruses. (d) NS2 of flaviviruses is processed into two proteins: NS2A and NS2B. (e) The RNA polymerase activity of hepaciviruses is associated with the NS5B protein. (f) The functions are attributed to hepaciviruses.

Among the nonstructural proteins, NS3 appears to be the most promising target for antiviral agents because of the multiple enzymatic activities associated with this protein: NS3 exhibits serine protease activity (associated with the NH_2 terminus of the protein), nucleoside triphosphatase and RNA-helicase activities located on the COOH terminus. NS2B serves as a required cofactor for the serine protease function of NS3. It is assumed that NTPase/helicase together with NS5-associated RNA polymerase is an essential component of the viral replicase complex.

12.5 INHIBITION OF VIRAL ENTRY

Recently, Chu and Ng reported that antibodies against a 105 kDa glycoprotein on the plasma membrane of Vero and murine neuroblastoma cells with complex N-linked sugars could block virus entry efficiently[8]. Pretreatment of the cells with proteases and glycosidases strongly inhibited entry of WNV. The authors assume that this protease-sensitive 105 kDa glycoprotein could be the putative receptor for West Nile virus. Still, further understanding of the mechanisms involved in binding and entry of WNV to its target cell is needed until candidate substances can be developed.

12.6 INHIBITION OF CAPPING

In flaviviruses like WNV, translation is being initiated by a process called capping. The cap is a unique structure found at the $5'$ end of viral and cellular eukaryotic mRNA, which is important for mRNA stability and binding to the ribosome during translation. mRNA capping is a cotranscriptional modification resulting from three chemical reactions: First, $5'$-triphosphate of the mRNA is converted to diphosphate by an RNA triphosphatase. In WNV, RNA triphosphatase activity has been mapped with the C terminus of the NS3 protein. The second reaction is the transfer of guanosine monophosphate (GMP) from GTP to the $5'$-diphosphate RNA. This reaction is mediated by a guanylyltransferase, which has not yet been identified in WNV. In a third reaction the transferred guanosine moiety is methylated at the N7 position. A second methylation on the first nucleotide $3'$ to the triphosphate bridge yields $^{7Me}G\ ^{5'}\text{–ppp}\ ^{5'}\text{-}N_{Me}$. Sequence analysis revealed the presence of the characteristic motif of S-adenosyl-L-methionine-dependent methyltransferases within the N-terminal domain of the NS5 protein of flaviviruses.[9]

12.7 NTPase/HELICASES AND THEIR INHIBITION

NTPases/helicases are in general nucleotide phosphate-dependent ubiquitous proteins, capable of enzymatically unwinding double-stranded DNA or RNA structures by disrupting the hydrogen bonds that keep the two strands together.

Approximately 80% of all known plus-strand RNA viruses encode at least one potential helicase.

Structural analyses have shown that the closely related NTPase/helicase of HCV consists of three approximately equally sized domains, separated from another by deep "clefts."[10] In HCV, domain 1 and 2 of the NTPase/helicase contain seven conserved amino acid sequences (motifs I–VII). Motifs I and II are also called Walker motifs A and B.

NTPases/helicases of RNA viruses are divided into three superfamilies (SFI–III) on the basis of the amino acid sequences of the Walker motif A. Superfamily I carries the sequence GXGKS/T; the superfamilies II and III carry variations of the sequence AXXGXGKS/T and GXGXGKS, respectively.[11] The HCV enzyme is placed in superfamily II.

Superfamily II is subdivided in four groups on the basis of the amino acid sequence following the conserved DE-residue of Walker motif B. NTPase/helicase of HCV contains the motif DECH and is therefore placed in the DEXH-box subgroup.[12]

The Walker motifs A and B are not only located on all NTPases/helicases, but also in a variety of NTP binding and utilizing proteins. The function of these motifs has been described as an NTP binding pocket: Walker motif A binds to the terminal phosphate group of the NTP. Walker motif B builds a chelate complex with the Mg^{2+} ion of the Mg^{2+} – NTP complex.[13] The NTP hydrolyzing activity of NTP binding proteins could be eliminated by exchanges of the amino acid sequence of the Walker motifs.[14]

In the absence of substrate, the residues of the Walker motifs bind to one another and to the residues of the conserved T-A-T sequence on motif III. This motif is part of a flexible "switch sequence" combining domains 1 and 2.[12] The conformational changes induced by NTP hydrolysis are mediated by this "switch sequence."[12, 15]

The role of the highly conserved arginine-rich motif VI, which is located on the surface of domain 2, is surrounded by controversy. On the basis of crystallographic analysis, it can be assumed that motif VI is important for RNA binding.[12] Yet, direct involvement of its arginine residues in ATP binding is also possible.[10]

On the basis of structural and biochemical analysis, two mechanisms of helicase reaction are taken into consideration:

1. A passive mechanism in which the NTPase/helicase molecule binds to single-stranded regions of the substrate and does not participate actively in the separation of double-stranded DNA or RNA structures.[11,12,15] Consequently, the energy resulting from NTP hydrolysis would not necessarily be used for the unwinding reaction of the HCV NTPase/helicase. Consistent with the hypothesis of this "passive" mechanism is the description of an unwinding activity of HCV NTPase/helicase in the absence of ATP. Other proteins are known to be able to unwind double stranded DNA structures by an NTP-independent manner.[16]

2. The second postulated mechanism predicts the existence of two nucleic acid binding sites and an ATP-dependent unwinding reaction. Conformational changes induced by NTP binding facilitate the binding of DNA or RNA substrate to specific binding sites.[12,15]

Although the helicase activity depends on the energy resulting from NTP hydrolysis, it has been shown that the number of NTP hydrolysis events per unwinding cycle is not a constant value. It seems that the two activities of the NS3 protein are not necessarily coupled to one another. Thus, specific inhibitors of WNV NTPase/helicase could act by the following mechanisms:

1. Inhibition of the NTPase Activity by Interference with NTP Binding. If NTP hydrolysis supplies the energy for the unwinding reaction, the reduction of the accessibility of the NTP binding site for NTP may therefore lead to a reduction of the unwinding rate. When competitive inhibitors of the WNV NTPase/helicase like ADP,[17] AMP, or ATP-γ-S were tested, inhibition of the ATPase activity was measured with IC_{50} values in the low micromolar range. Surprisingly, if at all, only moderate inhibition was observed, when these compounds were tested as inhibitors of the helicase activity. Considering the low specificity of the flavivirus NTPases/ helicases toward nucleosides and nucleotides,[18] partial hydrolysis of these compounds to less potent derivatives had to be verified. Consistent with this finding is the observation that the none hydrolyzable compound α,β-CH_2-ADP not only inhibited the ATPase activity but also inhibited the helicase activity of the HCV and the WNV NTPase/helicase. However, ADP-β-S even stimulated the helicase activity of both enzymes, suggesting that the helicase and NTPase activities are not necessarily coupled to one another. In the case of α,β-CH_2-ADP, the inhibition mediated by this compound could not be explained by a simple competition with ATP for the catalytic center of the enzyme.[19]

A series of ring-expanded (so-called "fat") nucleoside and nucleotide analogues (RENs) containing the imidazo[4,5-*e*][1,3]diazepine and imidazo[4,5,-*e*][1,2,4]tria-zepine ring system has been synthesized and tested as inhibitors of the NTPases/ helicases of the Flaviviridae (Figure 12.3).

A number of RENs inhibited the viral helicase activity with IC_{50} values in the micromolar range and exhibited differential selectivity between the human enzyme Suv3 and the viral enzyme.[20,21] The mechanism of action of RENs might involve

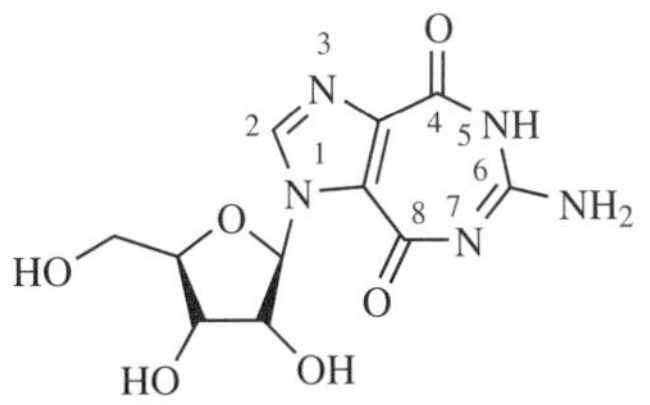

FIGURE 12.3 6-Aminoimidazo[4,5-*e*][1,3]diazepine-4,8-dione.

their interaction with the appropriate substrate through binding to the major or minor groove of the double helix.

REN-5′-triphosphates—unlike their congener substances — do not influence the unwinding reaction, but exert inhibitory effects on the ATPase activity of enzymes. Although most of the RENs are known for their significant toxicity, they could serve as key structures for the development of clinically useful substances.

As an analogue of adenosine, ribavirin appears to interact with the ATP binding site of viral NTPases/helicases and is a classical competitive inhibitor of the ATPase activity of several NTPases/helicases including those of WNV and HCV.[17]

2. Inhibition of NTPase Activity by an Allosteric Mechanism. The unwinding activity of WNV NTPase/helicase is significantly activated by *N*(7)-chloroethyl-guanine and *N*(9)-chloroethylguanine with concentrations of the compounds in the micromolar range.

This effect was not associated with enhanced consumption of ATP. The ATPase activity of the enzyme remained unchanged up to concentrations in the high millimolar range. On the other hand, chemically related O^6-benzyl-*N*(7)-chlor-oethylguanine activated the ATPase activity of the enyzme without affecting its unwinding activity.[22] Similar effects were observed with the HCV and JEV NTPase/helicases. The mechanism of the modulating effects remains unclear. Our kinetic data together with Porter's nucleotide binding studies[16] strongly suggest the existence of a second nucleotide binding site within the NTPase/helicase of the Flaviviridae. One could speculate that the second nucleotide binding site could be occupied by a nucleotide, nucleoside, or even nucleotide base and fulfills a regulatory function with respect to the NTPase and/or helicase activities of the enzyme. In concordance with this hypothesis are our ATP studies performed with the isolated domain 1 of the HCV NTPase/helicase demonstrating that the investigated chloroethylguanine derivatives do not influence the ATP binding to the polypeptide.[22]

3. Inhibition of Coupling of NTP Hydrolysis with the Unwinding Reaction. Compounds intercalating into DNA or RNA structures generally act as inhibitors of enzymes unwinding DNA or RNA structures. Imidazo[4,5-*d*]-pyridazine nucleo-sides interact with double-stranded DNA but paradoxally faciliate the unwinding reaction mediated by WNV NTPase/helicase. These compounds were nevertheless capable of uncoupling ATPase and helicase activities (Figure 12.4).

In the case of 1-(2′-*O*-methyl-β-D-ribofuranosyl)imidazo[4,5-*d*]pyridazine-4,7(5*H*,6*H*)-dione (HMC-HO4), its direct interaction with the enzyme caused

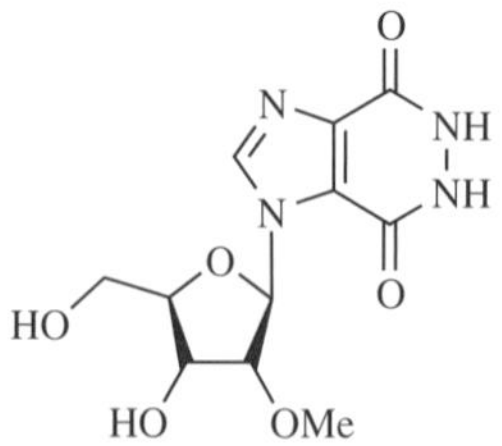

FIGURE 12.4   1-(2′-*O*-methyl-β-D-ribofuranosyl)imidazo[4,5-*d*]pyridazine-4,7(5*H*,6*H*)-dione (HMC-HO4).

inhibition of the helicase activity in both enzyme and viral infection assays with an IC_{50} value of approximately 30 µM. The similar potency of this compound against WNV replication in cell culture and enzyme inhibition assays suggested that inhibition of the helicase activity was responsible for the antiviral activity of HMC-HO4. The activity of this compound seems to be specific for the NS3 of WNV, as it was inactive against hepatitis C virus helicase.[23]

  4. Competitive Inhibition of RNA Binding. Tai and co-workers have demonstrated that polynucleotides increasing the NTPase activity of HCV NTPase/helicase inhibited its unwinding activity.[24] This inhibiting effect results from the competition of the polynucleotides with the RNA or DNA substrates for the nucleic acid binding site(s). Several attempts to develop small molecular inhibitors of the helicase activity acting at the level of the nucleic binding site have been described. Two series of compounds reported only as patents by ViroPharma[25] are composed of two benzimidazoles or aminophenylbenzimidazoles attached to symmetrical linkers of variable lengths.[26] These compounds were reported to inhibit the HCV helicase in low micromolar range, subsequently confirmed and extended by a structure–activity relationship study by Phoon et al.[27] In previous studies, we demonstrated that the lysine-rich histone H1 and the core histones H2B and H4 form stable complexes with the HCV NTPase/helicase.[28] This protein–protein interaction leads to a change of the conformation of the histone molecules, altered their properties as substrates for certain serine/threonine protein kinases, and reduced their DNA binding activity. The binding of the histones resulted in a strong inhibition of the unwinding activity of the HCV NTPase/helicase with IC_{50} values in nanomolar range. One can speculate that the bound histone molecule might affect the mobility of domain 2 and therefore inhibit the march of the enzyme along the double-stranded RNA or DNA structure. Currently running modeling studies should help to find out structurally similar small molecular compounds mimicking the action of histones.

  We have tested a broad range of established, commercially available DNA and RNA binding or intercalating agents as inhibitors of the NTPase/helicase of WNV, HCV, JEV, and DENV. The anthracycline antibiotics mitoxanthrone, doxorubicin, and daunomycin are very effective inhibitors of the helicase activity of the enzymes.[29] Surprisingly, closely related enzymes displayed significantly different IC_{50} values in response to the action of the compounds. Interestingly, none of the antibiotics examined inhibited the NTPase activity of the enzymes up to millimolar concentrations. The high inhibiting potential and selectivity of these substances make them attractive antiviral drugs. However, although widely used in the clinic, their cytotoxicity and weak cell penetration makes the search for less toxic derivatives necessary.

12.8 PROTEASE INHIBITION

The NS3 gene of WNV encodes for a serine protease that requires NS2B as cofactor. The resolution of the three-dimensional structure of the related serine proteases of HCV and DENV made the search for antiviral substances possible. Peptidic compounds mimicking the conserved cleavage sites inhibited the NS3-mediated protease activity of HCV[30] and DENV[31] at micromolar concentrations. Among the standard protease inhibitors only aprotinin showed anti-NS3 activity with an IC_{50} value of 65 nM.[31] The mode of action of this large protein probably consists in preventing the substrate from accessing the protease active site of the enzyme.

12.9 INHIBITION OF VIRAL GLYCOPROTEIN PROCESSING

Endoplasmic reticulum α-glucosidase inhibitors block the trimming stem in the course of *N*-linked glycosylation and eliminate the production of several ER-budding viruses. In a recent study, the iminosugar derivative *N*-nonyl-deoxynojirimycin was found to inhibit the replication of JEV and DENV significantly.[32] This effect was probably mediated by the inhibition of secretion of the viral glycoproteins E and NS1. This latter protein is known to be essential for flavivirus replication.[33] The difficulty to reach therapeutic serum concentrations and adverse side effects have limited the clinical usefulness of these compounds until now.

12.10 OTHER MODES OF INHIBITION OF WNV

12.10.1 Ribavirin

Ribavirin was discovered in 1972 and exhibits antiviral activity against a broad range of RNA viruses. Ribavirin exerts its antiviral effects by different mechanisms of action: In chronic viral infections like HCV infection, the therapeutic effect of ribavirin seems to rely mainly on immunomodulating mechanisms. It could be shown that ribavirin modulated interleukin-10 expression in mice. The combination of interferon and ribavirin is the standard therapy of chronic HCV infection. Acute viral infections like Lassa and RSV infections could be treated efficiently by ribavirin monotherapy.

Ribavirin represents a compound that contains no phosphate groups and may be regarded as an analogue of adenosine in which the C(2)=N(3) fragment of adenosine is removed (Figure 12.5).

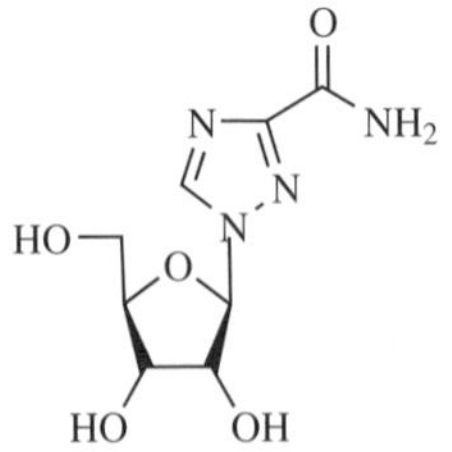

FIGURE 12.5   1-β-D-Ribofuranosyl-1,2,4-triazole-3-caboxamide (ribavirin).

Ribavirin can be incorporated either as ITP or ATP analogue. Interestingly, the L-enantiomer of ribavirin does not have antiviral activity in cell culture but does retain the immunomodulatory properties. Ribavirin is a potent mutagen of poliovirus in cell culture and mutagenic activity correlated directly with its antiviral activity. This observation led to the hypothesis that ribavirin's primary antiviral mechanism of action could be lethal mutagenesis of the viral RNA genomes.[34]

There are reports of significantly higher survival and eradication of WNV from brain in mice after intraperitoneal injection of ribavirin and in vitro studies showing that ribavirin inhibited WNV replication in human oligodendral cells. Recent studies with Vero cells showed that interferon α-2b inhibited viral cytotoxicity when applied after or before cells were infected with WNV. Ribavirin had a protective, but not therapeutic effect in vitro[35]. In vivo, the need to use very high doses of ribavirin in WNV infections proved too toxic to be clinically useful.

12.10.2 Inhibition of NTP Synthesis

Certain known inhibitors of orotidine monophosphate decarboxylase showed activity in viral infection assays against a New York isolate of WNV.[36] Among them, 6-azauridine, 6-azauridine triacetate, pyrazofurin, and 2-thio-6-azauridine had the most significant anti-WNV activity.

Mycophenolic acid and cytopentenylcytosine were found to have antiviral effects as inhibitors of inosine monophosphate dehydrogenase and CTP synthetase, respectively. Interestingly, some differences in drug sensitivities were observed between the New York and the Uganda isolate of WNV.

12.10.3 Neplanocin

(−)-Neplanocin A (NPA) is a naturally occurring carbocyclic nucleoside in which a methylene group replaces the oxygen atom in the furanose ring. The absence of a true glycosidic bond makes carbocyclic nucleosides like NPA chemically more stable, as they are not susceptible to enzymatic cleavage of the glycosidic linkage. Several related substances, among them abacavir and carbovir, have been shown to have antiviral activity and are clinically used for the treatment of HIV infection (Figure 12.6).

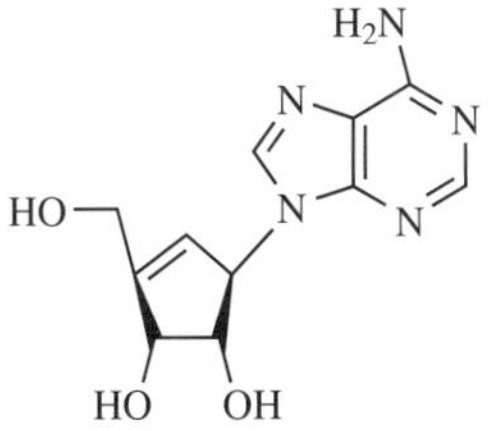

FIGURE 12.6   (−)-Neplanocin A (NPA).

The antiviral effect of NPA seems to be due — at least partially — to inhibition of S-adenosylhomocysteine hydrolase (SAH hydrolase).[37] This enzyme has been studied as an attractive target for the design of antiviral agents for a long time.[38] S-adenosylmethionine acts as a methyl donor in transmethylation reactions. The RNA-dependent RNA polymerase NS5 of flaviviruses presents a characteristic motif of S-adenosyl-L-methionine dependent methyltransferases at its N terminus. The NS5 domain of dengue virus type 2 includes a typical methyltransferase core and exhibits methyltransferase activity on capped RNA.[8]

Cellular and viral methyltransferases are susceptible to inhibition by SAH, and specific SAH inhibitors were able to block the replication of RNA viruses.[39]

However, the therapeutic use of NPA is limited because of its significant cytotoxicity, which could be attributed to the phosphorylation of the primary hydroxyl group at the 6' position by adenosine kinase. The subsequent phosphorylation to the triphosphate may inhibit cellular polymerases. The clinical use of NPA is further reduced by its rapid deamination by adenosine deaminase to its therapeutically inactive inosine congener. Therefore, NPA itself does not seem to be useful as an antiviral agent but may be useful as a lead substance for the development of structurally related antivirals.

Recently, the synthesis and antiviral activity of D- and L-cyclopentenyl nucleosides have been described. D-Cytosine and D-5-fluorocytosine analogues exhibited the most potential antiviral activity against WNV in vitro but also had significant cytotoxicity.[37]

12.11   IDENTIFICATION OF NEW CLASSES OF INHIBITORS

The inhibition of enzymatic activities of viral proteins can be tested by a number of biochemical test systems. We have measured the inhibition of ATP hydrolysis of the NTPase/helicase of Flaviviridae by scintillation counting of ^{32}P resulting from hydrolysis of [γ-^{32}P]-ATP mediated by the viral enzyme.

The helicase activity of the NTPase/helicase was analyzed with a partially double-stranded DNA substrate, the shorter strand being labeled with ^{32}P. After electrophoretic separation of the sample, the ^{32}P radiation was measured as a function of the strand separation activity of the enzyme.

These techniques are labor intensive and the need to screen great amounts of candidate substances for their antiviral activity led to the development of "high-throughput assays." Among the numerous high-throughput assays available, the scintillation proximity assay has gained the most acceptance. This technique is based on emission of light that results from the binding of a radioisotopically labeled molecule to the microsphere where it is brought in close proximity to the scintillant.

Whereas biochemical tests have the advantage that compounds can be tested for their activity against a definite target, genetic approaches, which are usually cell based, often represent a more authentic therapeutic environment. More than one replication target can be analyzed and uptake of the compound into the cell is usually required.

Cell-based assays for WNV inhibitors often rely on the quantification of cytopathic effects or of viral RNA by RT-PCR.

Recently, a genetic test system has been developed using the reporter genes Renilla luciferase (Rluc) and neomycin phosphotransferase (Neo). The reporter genes were engineered into a WNV subgenomic replicon. The efficacy of inhibitors was tested as a function of depression of Rluc activity in the reporting cell lines and was comparable to the inhibition observed in authentic viral infection assays.[40]

12.12 FUTURE PERSPECTIVES

Virally induced cellular responses can be exploited in order to help develop antiviral therapies. The $2'$-$5'$ oligoadenylate synthetase (OAS) /RNase L pathway may be such a candidate. Double-stranded RNA activates the $2'$-$5'$OAS, which synthesizes $2'$-$5'$ oligo(A). The inactive monomeric RNase L dimerizes upon binding to $2'$-$5'$ oligo(A) leading to activation of its endoribonuclease and degradation of single-stranded RNA.

A flavivirus resistance gene in mice has been identified that encodes $2'$-$5'$ OAS, and the $2'$-$5'$ OAS gene has been mapped to the same position as the flavivirus resitance locus.[41]

By coupling the $2'$-$5'$ oligo(A) activator moiety to antisense oligonucleotides with $2'$-$5'$ oligo(A) latent RNase L could be activated to cleave proximal viral RNA. This approach has been successfully explored for therapy of respiratory syncytial virus infection. The fundamental question as to how $2'$-$5'$ OAS confers specific flavivirus resistance although $2'$-$5'$ OAS/RNase L cleaves RNA nonspecifically remains unanswered to date.

Besides novel approaches—like ribozyme and interfering RNA based techniques—progress in antiviral therapy may come from the improvement of current inhibitors by structural optimization.

The crystal structure information of the protease domain of DENV NS3[42] and of the cap methyltransferase domain of DENV NS5 [9] could make the rational design of novel inhibitors possible. These targets are unique to the virus or function differently from their human counterparts, so that specific inhibition of viral replication can be expected.

REFERENCES

1. Burke, D. S.; Monath T. P. Flaviviruses. In *Fields Virology*, Lippincott William & Wilkins, Philadelphia, 2001; pp 1043–1126.

2. Centers for Disease Control and Prevention. Guidelines for surveillance, prevention and control of West Nile virus infection—United States. *MMWR* **2000**, *49*, 25–28.

3. Work, T.; Hurlbut, H.; Taylor, R. Indigenous woldbirds of the Nile Delta as potential West Nile virus circulating reservoir. *Am. Trop. Med. Hyg.* **1965**, *4*, 872–878.

4. Asnis, D. S.; Conetta, R.; Teixeira, A. A.; Waldman, G.; Sampson, B. A. The West Nile virus outbreak of 1999 in New York: the Flushing Hospital experience. *Clin. Infect. Dis.* **2000**, *30*, 413–418.

5. Lindenbach, B. D.; Rice, C. M. Genetic interaction of flavivirus nonstructural proteins NS1 and NS4A as determinant of replicase function. *J. Virol.* **1999**, *73*, 4611–4621.

6. Kummerer, B. M.; Rice, C. M. Mutations in the yellow fever virus nonstructural protein NS2A selectively block production of infectious particles. *J. Virol.* **2002**, *76*, 4773–4784.

7. Tan, B. H.; Fu, J.; Sugrue, R. J.; Yap, E. H.; Chan, Y. C.; et al. Recombinant dengue type 1 virus NS5 protein expressed in *Escherichia coli* exhibits RNA-dependent RNA polymerase activity. *Virology* **1996**, *216*, 317–325.

8. Chu, J. J.; Ng, M. L. Characterization of a 105-kDa plasma membrane associated glycoprotein that is involved in West Nile virus binding and infection. *Virology* **2003**, *312*, 458–469.

9. Egloff, M. P.; Benarroch, D.; Selisko, B.; Romette, J.; Canard, B. An RNA cap (nucleoside-2'-*O*-)-methyltransferase in the flavivirus RNA polymerase NS5: crystal structure and functional characterization. *EMBO J.* **2002**, *21*, 2757–2768.

10. Kim, J. L.; Morgenstern, K. A.; Griffith, J. P.; Dwyer, M. D.; Thomson, J. A.; et al. Hepatitis C virus NS3 RNA helicase domain with a bound oligonucleotide: the crystal structure provides insights into the mode of unwinding. *Structure* **1998**, *6*, 89–100.

11. Lüking, A.; Stahl, U.; Schmidt, U. The protein family of RNA helicases. *Crit. Rev. Biochem. Mol. Biol.* **1998**, *33*, 259–296.

12. Yao, N.; Hesson, T.; Cable, M.; Hong, Z.; Kwong, A.; et al. Structure of the hepatitis C virus RNA helicase domain. *Nat. Struct. Biol.* **1997**, *4*, 463–467.

13. Walker, J. E.; Saraste, M.; Runswick, M. J.; Gay, N. J. Distantly related sequences in the alpha- and beta subunits of ATP sythase, myosin kinases and other ATP-requiring enzymes and a common nucleotide binding fold. *EMBO J* **1982**, *1*, 945–951.

14. Borowski, P.; Lang, M.; Niebuhr, A.; Haag, A.; Schmitz, H.; et al. Inhibition of the helicase activity of HCV NTPase/helicase by 1-β-D-ribofuranosyl-1,2,4-triazole-3-carboxamide-5'-triphosphate (ribavirin-TP). *Acta Biochimi. Pol.* **2001**, *48*, 739–744.

15. Matson, S. W.; Kaiser-Rogers, K. A. DNA helicases. *Annu. Rev. Biochem.* **1990**, *59*, 289–329.

16. Porter, D. J.; Preugshat, F. Strand-separating activity of hepatitis C virus helicase in the absence of ATP. *Biochemistry* **2000**, *39*, 5166–5173.

17. Borowski, P.; Mueller, O.; Niebuhr, A.; Kalitzky, M.; Hwang, L. H.; et al. ATP-binding domain of NTPase/helicase as target for hepatitis C antiviral therapy. *Acta Biochim. Pol.* **2000**, *47*, 173–180.

18. Preugschat, F.; Averett, D.; Clarke, B.; Porter, D. A steady-state and presteady-state kinetic analysis of the NTPase activity associated with the hepatitis C virus NS3 helicase domain. *J. Biol. Chem.* **1996**, *271*, 24449–24457.

19. Kalitzky, M. NTPase/helicase of hepatitis C and West Nile virus: correlation of DNA unwinding activity with NTP hydrolysis. In *Faculty of Medicine, Doctoral Thesis*; University of Hamburg, Hamburg, 2003.

20. Zhang, N.; Chen, H. M.; Koch, V.; Schmitz, H.; Minczuk, M.; et al. Potent inhibition of NTPase/helicase of the West Nile virus by ring-expanded ("fat") nucleoside analogues. *J. Med. Chem.* **2003**, *46*, 4776–4789.

21. Zhang, N.; Chen, H. M.; Koch, V.; Schmitz, H.; Liao, C. L.; et al. Ring-expanded ("fat") nucleoside and nucleotide analogues exhibit potent in vitro activity against Flaviviridae NTPase/helicases, including those of West Nile virus, hepatitis C virus and Japanese encephalitis virus. *J. Med. Chem.* **2003**, *46*, 4149–4164.

22. Borowski, P.; Niebuhr, A.; Mueller, O.; Bretner, M.; Felczak, K.; et al. Purification and characterization of West Nile virus nucleoside triphosphatase (NTPase)/helicase: evidence for dissociation of the NTPase and helicase activities of the enzyme. *J. Virol.* **2001**, *75*, 3220–3229.

23. Borowski, P.; Lang, M.; Haag, A.; Schmitz, H.; Choe, J.; et al. Characterization of imidazo[4,5-*d*]pyridazine nucleosides as modulators of unwinding reaction mediated by West Nile virus nucleoside triphosphatase/helicase: evidence for activity on the level of substrate and/or enzyme. *Antimicrob. Agents Chemother.* **2002**, *46*, 1231–1239.

24. Tai, C. L.; Chi, W. K.; Chen, D. S.; Hwang, L. H. The helicase activity associated with hepatitis C virus nonstructural protein 3 (NS3). *J. Virol.* **1996**, *70*, 8477–8484.

25. Diana, G. D.; Bailey, T. R. Compounds, composition and methods for treatment of hepatitis C. *US Patent No. 6,127,384,* **1996**.

26. Deluca, M. R.; Kervin, S. M. The para-toluenosulfonic acid promoted synthesis of 2-substituted benzoxazoles and benzimidazoles from diacylated precursors. *Tetrahedron* **1996**, *53*, 457–464.

27. Phoon, C. W.; Ng, Y. P.; Ting, A. E.; Yeo, S. L.; Sim, M. M. Biological evaluation of hepatitis C virus helicase inhibitors. *Bioorg. Med. Chem. Lett.* **2001**, *11*, 1647–1650.

28. Borowski, P.; Kühl, R.; Laufs, R.; Schulze zur Wiesch, J.; Heiland, M. Identification and characterization of a histone binding site of the non-structural protein 3 of hepatitis C virus. *J. Clin. Virol.* **1999**, *13*, 61–69.

29. Borowski, P.; Niebuhr, A.; Schmitz, P.; Hosmane, R. S.; Bretner, M.; et al. NTPase/helicase of Flaviviridae: inhibitors and inhibition of the enzyme. *Acta Biochim. Pol.* **2002**, *49*, 597–614.

30. Ingallinella, P.; Altamura, S.; Bianchi, E.; Taliani, M.; Ingenito, R.; et al. Potent peptide inhibitors of HCV NS3 protease are obtained by optimizing the cleavage products. *Biochemistry* **1998**, *37*, 8906–8914.

31. Leung, D.; Schroder, K.; White, H.; Fang, N. X.; Stoermer, M.; et al. Activity of recombinant dengue 2 virus NS3 protease in the presence of a truncated NS2B co-factor, small peptide substrates and inhibitors. *J. Biol. Chem.* **2001**, *276*, 45762–45771.

32. Wu, S. F.; Lee, C. J.; Liao, C. L.; Dwek, R.; Zitzmann, N.; et al. Antiviral effects of an iminosugar derivative on flavivirus infections. *J. Virol.* **2002**, *76*, 3596–3604.

33. Lindenbach, B. D.; Rice, C. M. Trans-complementation of yellow fever virus NS1 reveal a role in early RNA replication. *J. Virol.* **1997**, *71*, 9608–9617.

34. Crotty, S.; Cameron, C.; Andino, R. Ribavirin's antiviral mechanism of action: lethal mutagenesis? *J. Mol. Med.* **2002**, *80*, 86–95.

35. Jordan, I.; Briese, T.; Fischer, N.; Yiu-Nam, J.; Lipkin, W. I. Ribavirin inhibits West Nile virus replication and cytopathic effect in neural cells. *J. Infect. Dis.* **2000**, *182*, 1214–1217.

36. Morrey, J. D.; Smee, D. F.; Sidwell, R. W.; Tseng, C. Identification of active antiviral compounds against a New York isolate of West Nile virus. *Antiviral Res.* **2002**, *55*, 107–116.

37. Song, G. Y.; Paul, V.; Choo, H.; Morrey, J.; Sidwell, R. W.; et al. Enantiomeric synthesis of D- and L- cyclopentyl nucleosides and their antiviral activity against HIV and West Nile virus. *J. Med. Chem.* **2001**, *44*, 3985–3993.

38. De Clercq, E.; Cools, M. Antiviral potency of adenosine analogs: correlation with inhibition of *S*-adenosylhomocysteine hydrolase. *Biochem. Biophys. Res. Commun.* **1985**, *129*, 306–311.

39. De Clercq, E. Antiviral agents: characteristic activity spectrum depending on the molecular target with which they interact. *Adv. Virus Res.* **1993**, *42*, 1–55.

40. Lo, M. K.; Tilgner, M.; Shi, P. Y. Potential high-throughput assay for screening of inhibitors of West Nile virus replication. *J. Virol.* **2003**, *77*, 12901–12906.

41. Perelygin, A. A.; Scherbik, S. V.; Zhulin, I. B.; Stockman, B. M.; Li, Y.; et al. Positional cloning of the murine flavivirus resistance gene. *Proc. Natl. Acad. Sci. U.S.A.* **2002**, *99*, 9322–9327.

42. Murthy, H. M.; Clum, S.; Padmanabhan, R. Dengue virus NS3 serine protease. Crystal structure and insights into interaction of the active site with substrates by molecular modelling and structural analysis of mutational effects. *J. Biol. Chem.* **1999**, *274*, 5573–5580.

43. Leyssen, P.; de Clercq, E.; Neysts, J. Perspectives for the treatment of infections with *Flaviviridae*. *Clin. Microbiol. Rev.* **2000**, *13*, 67–82.

EMERGING
INFECTIOUS DISEASES

EID OnLine

A Peer-Reviewed Journal Tracking and Analyzing Disease Trends   Vol.9, No.3, March 2003

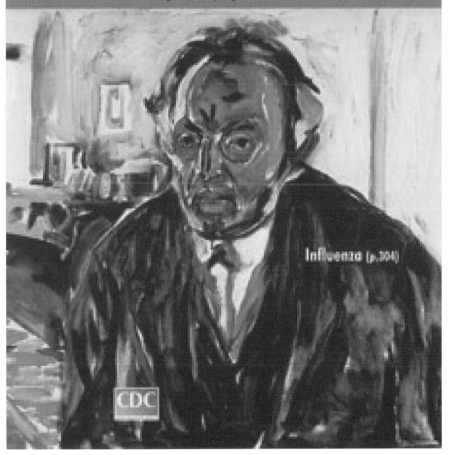

Influenza (p.304)

CDC

CHAPTER 13

The Emergence of Pandemic Influenza A: Bioterrorist Versus Mother Nature

JOHN S. OXFORD, ALISON BOYERS, ALEX MANN, and R. LAMBKIN

Retroscreen Virology Ltd., Centre for Infectious Diseases, Bart's and The London Queen Mary's School of Medicine and Dentistry

Influenza A quite rightly can be viewed as the most threatening virus on our planet. It looks toward us, its human victims, with a two-sided face—the epidemic face and the pandemic face. It could be assumed that the pandemic side of the face is the more important side to avoid, but this is wrong. We must not gaze on either face. When influenza emerges in pandemic mode, probably (but not with certainty) from an avian, pig, or horse ecosystem, it finds a virgin population in our human world, now exceeding six billion. What other virus could spread around the globe and kill 40 million citizens of the world in 18 months? But this was not the end of the effects of the Great Spanish 1918 influenza pandemic: the virus revisited more or less yearly until it was suddenly displaced by another virus, Asian influenza A in 1957 (Table 13.1). A quick totaling of yearly epidemic deaths from 1918 to 1957 gives an astonishing figure of mortality that even exceeds the hammer blow of the dark months at the end of the Great War.[1]

When the influenza A virus first emerged from a presumed avian reservoir at the end of the ice age 10,000 or so years ago, there was a distinct difficulty of finding new human victims. For example, at that time only a few hundred settlers were in the London region near our hospital in a community now containing four million people. At that time a traveler would have to walk 100 miles to find another small settlement perhaps near Salisbury. But today we have a truly global community of six billion people linked so that two million people are moving each day by plane while perhaps 100 million are journeying in their homelands. Influenza, like all viruses, is opportunistic. In 1918 it had the unprecedented opportunity to spread at

Antiviral Drug Discovery for Emerging Diseases and Bioterrorism Threats. Edited by Paul F. Torrence
Copyright © 2005 John Wiley & Sons, Inc.

TABLE 13.1   Global Impact of Pandemic or Potential Pandemics of Influenza in the Nineteenth, Twentieth, and Twenty-first Centuries

Year	Colloquial Name and Subtype	Source	Impact
1889	Russian flu	Emerged in eastern Russia and spread westward	Less than 1918 pandemic; possibly mortality similar to the 1957 H2N2 virus?
1918	"Spanish flu" (H1N1)	Possible emergence from swine or avian host of a mutated H1N1 virus in Europe	Pandemic with 40 million deaths globally.
1957	"Asian flu" (H2N2)	Mixed infection of an animal with human N1N1 and avian H2N2 virus strains in Asia	Substantial pandemic, 5 million deaths; the 1918 H1N1 virus disappeared.
1968	"Hong Kong flu" (H3N2)	Mixed infection of an animal with human H2N2 and avian H3Nx virus strains in Asia	Substantial pandemic, 2 million deaths; the 1957 H2N2 virus disappeared.
1977	"Russian flu" (H1N1)	Source unknown, but virus is almost identical to human epidemic strains from 1950. Reappearance detected at almost the same time in China and Siberia; probably a laboratory escape.	Benign pandemic, primarily involving persons born after the 1950s. H1N1 virus has cocirculated with H3N2 virus in humans since 1977. This combination could prevent a new pandemic but this should not be relied on.
1976	"Swine flu" (H1N1)	United States/New Jersey; virus enzootic in U.S. swine herds since at least 1930.	Localized outbreak in military training camp, with one fatal case.
1986	H1N1	The Netherlands; swine virus derived from avian source.	One adult with severe pneumonia.
1988	"Swine flu" (H1N1)	United States/Wisconsin, swine virus	Pregnant women died after exposure to sick pig.
1993	H3N2	The Netherlands; swine reassortant between "old" human H3N2 (1973/75-like) and avian H1N1.	Two children with mild disease. Father infected by pigs suspected to be the transmitters.
1995	H7N7	United Kingdom, duck virus.	One adult with conjunctivitis.
1997	"Chicken flu" (H5N1)	Hong Kong, poultry.	Eighteen confirmed human cases, six lethal.
1999	H9N2	China, Hong Kong. Quail influenza-like virus	Two human cases with mild disease.
2003	H7N7	Outbreak on chicken farms in the Netherlands	One fatal human case and over 300 cases with conjunctivitis.
2004	H5N1	Outbreaks in chicken farms in twelve countries in Southeast Asia; 200 million chickens killed to abort further outbreaks.	59 fatal human cases (to date March 2005).

the end of the first global war. Ten million soldiers began the move homeward and every steamship was packed as they fanned out from France to England, Europe, the United States, Canada, Australia, India, and Southeast Asia.[2] How perfect for a virus spread by aerosol droplet, close contact, and contamination of towels, cups, and everyday utensils. A virgin population who had never before encountered the virus was on the stage of this theater of infection. Perhaps a billion people were infected in the next 18 months as the virus moved, sometimes silently, across communities and 40 million died.[1,3-5] The 1918 virus may also have caused the subsequent outbreak of encephalitis lethargica (EL, sleepy sickness), although, to date, analysis of EL brains from the time have failed to detect influenza genes.[6]

However, the same happened in the other pandemic years of 1957 and 1968, aided in these two outbreaks by air travel,[7] so why were deaths in these two pandemics restricted to "only" 4 and 2.5 million, respectively? This is the crux of the matter and brings us to the heart of the question about creation. Could a scientist wickedly and with malevolence create a virus like the 1918 virus in the laboratory and thereby use it to threaten the world? The post listing of chemical and biological welfare has shown it to be singularly maladroit. Historians now acknowledge that gas was an unmitigated disaster as a weapon, unpredictable and miniscule in its killing power. In the Great War there were only 91,000 casualties from gas despite the use of 119,000 tons of 24 powerful chemicals (Table 13.2). The second global

TABLE 13.2   Demographics of the Great War of 1914–1918 and the Etaples Army Camp Relevant to Influenza A Emergence and Infection

Total number of soldiers in the war	65×10^6
Total number of soldiers who died in the war	8×10^6
Total number of soldiers who died of disease in the war	2×10^6
Total number of civilian deaths from starvation and disease in the war	6.6×10^6
Quantity of asphyxiating gases used by both sides	119×10^3 metric tons
Number of soldiers who were gassed in the war	1.2×10^6
Number of soldiers who died from gas asphyxiation in the war	91×10^3
Association of pigs, geese, ducks, and chickens with soldiers in and around Etaples 1916–1917	A unique opportunity at Etaples following the experimental establishment of piggeries within the camp itself.
Overcrowded Etaples camp	100,000 soldiers per day.
Asphyxiating gases in the battle of the Somme	1500 tons of phosgene, diphosgene, chloropicrin, xylyl bromide and 21 others used in 1916–1917; some of the gases are mutagenic.

Sources: References 2 and 8.

conflict in the 1940s failed to use these chemical weapons at all. Many nations, including the United Kingdom and the United States, experimented with anthrax and other microbes but the overall conclusion was that their military usefulness would be minute.

So has the military analysis changed in this first decade of the 21st century? Certainly microbes are a threat to humans, but the biggest threat still comes unreservedly from natural outbreaks, often termed Mother Nature.

Nevertheless there are huge long term benefits to society by the interest political analysts are taking in public health. We suspect this focus has not been so urgent since the Victorian time in England when the great sewage and water systems were built in the cities of England and its Empire. A precise example of the curious public health ambiguity we now have, and which needs to be resolved quickly, is the outbreak of monkeypox in the United States.[9] This monkeypox outbreak shows our current vulnerability to emerging viruses. It was not detected with undue haste. This episode reminds us of the power of natural disease and also the urgent need to rebuild and extend our public health infrastructure, which began to be dismantled after apparent reduction of deaths from tuberculosis (TB) in the 1970s and with the advent of a huge range of antimicrobials at the same time. But now TB has appeared again, along with multiply drug-resistant *Staphylococcus aureus* and a strong list of viruses such as severe acute respiratory syndrome (SARS), Nipah virus, West Nile virus, Hendra virus, hepatitis C, chicken influenza A, and Human immunodeficiency virus (HIV): these are known as emergent and resurgent viruses.[10] We will return to the pivotal issue of whether a hyperinfluenza virus could be engineered at present in a laboratory. The answer, at the moment, is probably not, given that we do not understand enough about what makes an influenza virus virulent per se, but the situation could change rapidly in the near future.

13.1 CAN WE DEPEND ON CURRENT VACCINES AND ANTIVIRALS TO PROTECT AGAINST PANDEMIC OR BIOTERRORIST INFLUENZA?

At present the main clinical management of influenza as a disease is centered on the use of prophylactic vaccine, mainly a subunit preparation of hemagglutinin (HA) and neuraminidase (NA) spikes. Most European countries and the United States try to target at least 70% of their "at risk" group. This group is a key to understanding the current approach to the management of influenza as a yearly disease in the community. This would be different for a pandemic or threat situation. No country has a wide immunization strategy across all sectors of the community for two reasons. First, the world production capacity for influenza vaccine (200 million doses) is not large enough at present to cope with the changes to the vaccine required to keep up to date with the yearly antigenic changes of the virus itself and to produce virus for a mass vaccination campaign each year.[11,12] Second, a large-scale vaccination would pressure the virus to change faster antigenically by applying strong selection on the HA and NA proteins of mixed quasispecies. Therefore, the 10–13% or so of persons over the age of 65 (in the E.U., but over the age of 50 in the U.S.) are the targets of vaccinators in normal interpandemic years, as well as persons of any age with asthma or chronic heart disease or diabetes: the so-called "at risk" group because persons in this group more often succumb to postviral complications. It is quite clear that age is by itself a risk factor following an attack of influenza.[13] But this vaccination strategy would be radically different should the world be faced with a pandemic, either natural or deliberate. Also, as noted in 1918, a pandemic virus can target a particular age group. In this latter year people 25–35 years old were at risk. In the reemergence of the H1N1 virus in 1977 people under 25 years old were vulnerable because they had no prior immunity, whereas older persons had experienced the same virus 25 years or so before. The older community group often finds itself more susceptible to virus-induced bronchitis and bronchopneumonia, and hence hospitalization and death.[13,14] In large clinical trials conducted over several seasons,[15] the vaccine clearly reduces both hospitalization and death by all causes including heart attack and stroke.[16] It should also be appreciated that there are large numbers of influenza deaths in most countries of the world in most years in the unvaccinated "at risk" individuals. In the United Kingdom over the millennium period there were nearly 20,000 deaths from pneumonia and bronchitis in a period of 4–5 weeks (Figure 13.1).

There is an alternative management strategy involving influenza vaccine but to date it has been little explored and at first sight seems tenuous in its practicability. There is clear evidence that influenza is predominantly a disease of childhood.[14] An innovative approach, therefore, is to immunize children and thereby break the chain of influenza transmission to parents and grandparents.[17] A reanalysis of such vaccine data from Japan[18] in the 1980s and to a lesser extent from towns in the

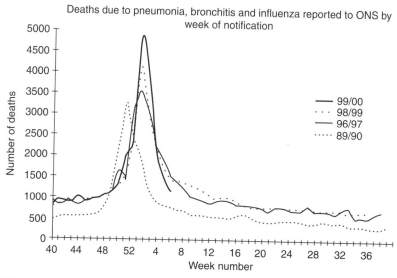

FIGURE 13.1 Excess mortality in the United Kingdom from influenza and bronchitis 1999–2000 reported by the Office of National Statistics (ONS).

United States[19] has shown some validity of this approach. But, in practical terms, could modern parents be persuaded of this benefit and agree to have their child immunized with yet another vaccine? It is possible that an intranasally delivered spray of live-attenuated vaccine[17] or one of the new inactivated vaccines given intranasally[20] could have a comparable effect and at the same time avert parental concerns about conventional vaccines. This could be a public health tactic during a pandemic or threat situation.

Meanwhile, we are left with the clear observation that the 85% or so of the population, which is outside the classical "at risk" group, remain vulnerable to influenza infection each year. Most of these persons will be ill for 5–7 days but there are still many deaths in persons outside the "at risk" groups. It has been estimated that 40–50% of the 20,000 deaths in the United Kingdom at the time of the millennium were in the non- "at risk" groups. Therefore, there is a clear need for an extra intervention with vaccines or antivirals in the wider community. Such increased targeting would simultaneously build up vaccine production capacity and the quantities of antivirals available for an emerging pandemic or threat use. We will return to a discussion of applicability of a new generation of influenza vaccines later. Thus, although the scientific community along with pharmaceutical companies have developed vaccines and antiviral drugs over the last half century, the production and surge capacity to deal with a sudden outbreak could not be coped with.

13.2   X-RAY CRYSTALLOGRAPHY OF THE INFLUENZA VIRUS NA AND THE DEVELOPMENT OF A NEW RANGE OF ANTIVIRAL DRUGS: THE NIs

Concern about the next pandemic has pushed research toward the discovery of new anti-influenza drugs. An anomaly now, however, is how to use these drugs to best advantage. One cannot develop antivirals solely for use in the infrequent pandemics. Conversely, they will be essential at this time to save lives and protect essential workers in the community, particularly during the first wave of the outbreak.

A quarter of a century ago a group of scientists began to explore the much understudied NA protein of influenza. The NA had already been identified as a separate gene product[21] and antibodies to NA were known to reduce viral spread in cell culture.[22] X-ray crystallography revealed the positions of enzyme active sites and the antigenic epitopes of NA.[23,24] The neuraminidase molecule is oriented rather usually for a glycoprotein, its N terminus being anchored in the viral membrane. After the three-dimensional structure of the influenza neuraminidase was established, the positions on the molecule of the catalytic site of the enzyme could be identified and the binding of inhibitory chemicals visualized. But this was not the initial objective of these studies. The NA molecule has a box-shaped head, with a unique folding pattern. Each monomer has six β-sheets and contains four polypeptide strands. Viewed from above, each monomer has the appearance of a flower with the petals somewhat twisted to resemble a pinwheel. The "stem" is considered to span the lipid bilayer of the virus with a hydrophobic stretch of amino acids. The catalytic site of NA was located by difference Fourier analysis of crystals soaked in sialic acid, which is the substrate for the NA enzyme. The site is surrounded by 14 conserved charged residues and contains three hydrophobic residues—Tyr, Trp, and Leu. The new anti-NA drugs bind to 11 of these critical amino acids and knowledge of the crystal structure allowed a design strategy involving the addition of side groups to a "core" inhibitor structure, which would interact with the crucial amino acids in the NA active site (Figure 13.2).

Palese and Schulman[25] were among the first virologists to exploit neuraminidase and its sialic acid (neuraminic acid) substrate as a target for chemical inhibitors. The original neuraminic acid analogues, which had been synthesized a decade before,[26] were carefully reinvestigated for anti-influenza effects on viral replication in mammalian cells. These drugs are transition state analogues active at micromolar levels. They were shown to reduce viral plaque size and cause virus to aggregate at the cell membrane after budding and, therefore, prevent efficient release of progeny virions. Disappointingly, however, the early studies using mouse models of viral infection found the neuraminic acid analogues to have no effect on lung influenza titers after administration via intraperitoneal injection. Essentially, the key molecule, Neu5Ac2en, was a dehydrated neuraminic acid derivative that mimicked the geometry of the transition state during the enzymatic reaction. In retrospect, intranasal or aerosol administration of the drug may have given positive virus

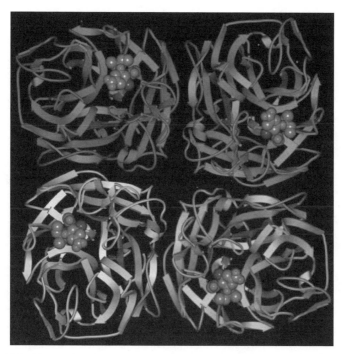

FIGURE 13.2   Interaction of NI (oseltamivir) with the enzyme active site of the viral NA.

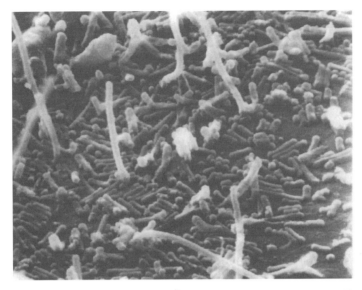

FIGURE 13.3   The NI inhibitor oseltamivir causes virus to aggregate at the cell surface of infected cells. Shown are MDCK cells postinfection with influenza A virus. Note the regular distribution of budding viruses.

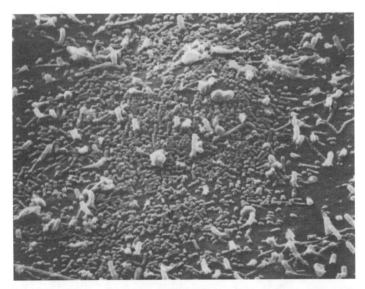

FIGURE 13.4   The NI inhibitor oseltamivir causes virus to aggregate at the cell surface of infected cells. Shown are MDCK cells postinfection with influenza A virus plus oseltamivir. Large clusters of virions are seen as the budding process is interrupted.

inhibitory results in the animal models. However, NA was now identified as a relevant and useful target for new drugs.

A group of chemists actively interested in the discovery of antivirals took Neu5Ac2en as the basic inhibitor and substituted a guanidinyl group for a hydroxyl carbon atom to make zanamivir (Relenza), the first anti-NA drug.[27] Another group of chemists designed a cyclohexene ring and replaced a polar glycerol with lipophilic side chains:[28] this is the drug oseltamivir (Tamiflu). The bioavailable drug is an ethyl ester that is converted into the active carboxylate by esterases in the liver. A third set of chemists designed a cyclopentane derivative with a guanidinyl group and lipophilic chains:[29,30] this drug is RWJ-270201 (also known as BCX-1812 or peramivir). All three drugs (zanamivir, oseltamivir, and peramivir) were shown to be powerful inhibitors of influenza A and B virus NAs in enzyme tests, in viral replication in cell culture, and, importantly, in animal model infections using mice and ferrets[31] and later in humans.[32] As expected, in drug-treated mammalian cell cultures, large viral aggregates can be detected at the cell surface by electron microscopy (Figures 13.3 and 13.4). All nine influenza A NA subtypes including the NA from the 1918 virus and the recent H5N1 chicken flu are inhibited at a micromolar drug level.[33]

13.3 PRACTICAL EXAMPLES OF CLINICAL MANAGEMENT OF INFLUENZA IN AN OUTBREAK USING THE NIs

The original investigations with the first anti-influenza drugs amantadine and rimantadine (now known as M2 blockers) showed clearly that antivirals could be used to prevent infection in the workplace or family[34] or to treat already established infection. The idea that any antiviral drug could abrogate the symptoms of influenza was strongly contested at the time, but it became quite clear that intervention with amantadine 24–48 h after the onset of symptoms could reduce time in bed, cough, and viral titer in the throat. Less controversial at the time were studies showing that judicious use in the family after identification of a member with influenza (index case) could reduce the spread in the family by 80% or more.[34] This sensible intervention is now called postinfection prophylaxis[35] because it is recognized that most family members would have already been infected by the index case even before drug intervention. Undoubtedly, drugs would be used in this way in the face of a pandemic or threat.

Overall, the protective effect of both the zanamivir and oseltamivir drugs, the new NIs, varies between 60% and 90%, suggesting very clearly that these drugs can be used effectively in the community during an influenza outbreak. There is less evidence at present of use in vulnerable settings such as homes for the elderly, but there is no clear reason why the new inhibitors should not be very effective.

Clinical studies in the community showed that administration of inhaled zanamivir within 48 h of natural influenza A or B infection significantly reduced the duration of symptomatic illness by 1 day (4 versus 5 days). The drug reduced the impact of influenza virus infection on a patient's productivity and health status and also the number of contacts made with healthcare professionals.[36–40]

To study the therapeutic effect of zanamivir Monto et al.[40] analyzed the overall intent to treat (ITT) population and showed that the drug reduced the median number of days to alleviation of clinically significant symptoms by 1 day compared with placebo. For patients who began treatment >30 h after onset of symptoms, the difference between zanamivir and placebo groups, although still present, was reduced to 0.5–1 day; this difference was not statistically significant. Zanamivir reduced the time to symptom alleviation in both febrile and nonfebrile patients but had a greater effect on febrile patients. Zanamivir given twice daily reduced the median time for alleviation of symptoms by 0.75 days in the nonfebrile groups ($P = 0.049$) and by 1.5 days in the febrile group ($P = 0.049$). Similar differences were seen when zanamivir was administered four times daily, compared with placebo. Similar benefits regarding symptom alleviation were also seen in the corresponding analyses of the influenza-positive population. A reduction of 1.5 days in the time to symptom alleviation was seen in both the two-times and four-times daily zanamivir groups for the total influenza-positive population, although the differences were not statistically significant.

In comparable studies of oseltamivir in the community,[41] a total of 629 healthy, unimmunized adults aged 18–65 years presenting within 36 h of onset and with a temperature of 38 °C or more plus at least one respiratory symptom and one constitutional symptom were enrolled. Individuals were randomized to one of three treatment groups: oseltamivir 75 mg twice daily, 130 mg twice daily, or placebo for 5 days. A total of 374 participants were confirmed to have influenza (60%). Duration of illness from the initiation of therapy was reduced by approximately 30% in the oseltamivir groups. In the 75 mg twice daily group, the median duration of illness was reduced to 3 days compared with 4.3 days in the placebo group ($P = 0.001$) and in the 150 mg twice daily group the duration was reduced to 2.9 days ($P = 0.001$). There was also a significant decrease in the symptom score AUC as a measure of the severity of illness. Volunteers treated with oseltamivir reported more rapid return to normal health and usual activities. Additionally, the incidence of secondary complications, predefined as pneumonia, bronchitis, sinusitis, and otitis media, in subjects with influenza was reduced from 15% in placebo recipients to 5–9% in the two oseltamivir-treated groups. Antibiotic prescriptions for these complications were also reduced. This is a most important observation for use in a pandemic and bioterrorist threat. It is not known yet whether the NIs prevent death but this would be anticipated by analysis of the strong effects in antiviral animal models.

More recently the clinical data with oseltamivir has been extended in children.[42] Therefore, it is quite clear that the public health community has an armentarium of new anti-influenza drugs. The important practical question is how to use antivirals in the most effective manner. Table 13.3 summarizes the absolute minimum preplanning required for use of these NIs to prevent a serious outbreak pandemic or bioterrorist event. We shall return to this question later in the text.

Drug-resistant mutants can be selected against the NIs[31,43] but, at least to the present day, have been shown to have reduced virulence and transmissibility in animal models and are less likely to spread in the community than the wild-type,

TABLE 13.3   Minimal Preparation for a Pandemic or Bioterrorist Attack Using Antiviral Drugs and Vaccines

An active national plan reviewed and updated yearly.

A thoughtful and coherent priority listing of recipients of vaccine and antiviral prophylaxis if these are in short supply.

A circulating stockpile of NIs and possibly M2 blockers equivalent one-quarter to one-third of the national population (priority use).

A stockpile of vaccines H1–H16, which could be used to immunologically prime health care workers.

A contingency plan for rapid synthesis of NIs and possibly M2 blockers for the remaining two-thirds of the national population.

Increased use of NIs and possibly M2 blockers in the interpandemic years to gain clinical experience with the drugs.

drug-sensitive parent (see below). A European laboratory network has now been established to search for and characterize influenza viruses resistant to NIs or the M2 blockers (www.virgil-net.org).

13.4   PRACTICAL EXAMPLES OF CLINICAL MANAGEMENT OF INFLUENZA USING INHIBITORS OF THE VIRAL M2 PROTON PUMP

As we have seen above to combat influenza, a drug is needed that reaches the respiratory tree and, particularly, the upper regions of the nasal and throat mucosa and trachea, where most influenza infections are thought to begin and thereafter focus.[44] More rarely, the virus descends into the bronchi, bronchioles, and even the alveoli and destroys the cellular lining of the lung. Thus, bronchopneumonia is the hallmark of a serious and life-threatening influenza virus infection, rather than solid consolidation, which more often follows superinfection of the lung with *Streptococcus pneumoniae*.[45,46] Amantadine (also called I-adamantanamine hydrochloride, Symmetrel, or, more recently, Lysovir)[47] has significant antiviral effects against all influenza A viruses in cell culture, including some H5 viruses, in animal model infections in mice, and, most importantly, in humans.[48] The method of action has been well characterized as blocking the viral acidification function of the viral M2 channel.[49] Analysis of rare biopsy material established that the drug was concentrated, to higher levels than simple tissue distribution models predicted, in the upper respiratory tract.[50] However, the most significant discovery was that amantadine, and its molecular relative rimantadine, had prophylactic and therapeutic activity in human infection with influenza A H1N1, H2N2, and H3N2 viruses.[51] At the start of this work 40 years ago, amantadine was most studied in the United Kingdom, Europe, and Japan, while rimantadine was investigated in very large trials in Russia, the United States, and, to a lesser extent, Eastern Europe. These extensive studies will be summarized briefly below and can easily be consulted in reviews.[48] The prophylactic activity, around 80–90%, is similar to that of the recently discovered neuraminidase (NA) inhibitors,[35] as is the therapeutic activity, reducing illness by approximately 1.5 days if the drug is used within 36–48 h of symptoms appearing. In fact, the scientific community did not accept that an anti-influenza drug could have any therapeutic activity until the first studies with amantadine proved otherwise.

In commercial terms, and in view of the investment of some 500 million euros needed to develop any new drug, pharmaceutical companies need to be assured of a market. However, examination of the history of the underuse of amantadine and rimantadine and more recently the NIs illustrates the difficulty of introducing antivirals into the management of influenza in the community in the event of a pandemic. An entirely new plan of approach is required (Table 13.3). Amantadine and rimantadine have been licensed as anti-influenza A drugs for four decades, but their application in the community has been bedeviled by two worries: emergence of drug resistance and fear of toxicity. As regards toxicity, most earlier clinical studies employed a dosage of 200 mg/day of amantadine. Some "jitteriness" was noted in about 10% of patients, particularly the elderly. Subsequent studies indicated that the dose could be halved to 100 mg daily, with continued anti-influenza A activity. At this drug level, no toxicologic problems would be expected, but the dosage can still be adjusted downward for the frail elderly, who could be underweight. We will return to this important low-dose application later.

The problem of drug resistance is more difficult to resolve but is not unique to amantadine. Amantadine-resistant mutants can be generated among experimentally infected mice, but only after the use of very high drug concentrations.[52] It is not known whether these viruses are less pathogenic or virulent than the wild-type virus, like viruses resistant to the NI drugs, but the low frequency of detection in the field does suggest this. Mutations that confer resistance to amantadine can clearly be identified in the viral M2 gene, and such viruses are cross-resistant to all the M2 proton channel inhibitors.

13.5 CLINICAL THERAPEUTIC EFFECTS OF AMANTADINE

Arguably, the most significant discovery for the future development of antivirals against respiratory viruses was that of the therapeutic effect of amantadine. In the initial studies, volunteers were artificially infected with influenza virus and then given amantadine or placebo. Symptoms, including objective parameters such as temperature, subsided more rapidly when amantadine was administered.

Perhaps not surprisingly, the use of the antivirals much later than 48 h after the diagnosis of clinical disease failed to abrogate symptoms of the disease. A similar situation has been documented with the new anti-NA drugs. Surprisingly, few studies have actually been performed on the quantity of influenza virus excreted in the lower respiratory tract of infected humans. Postmortem examination of trachea specimens by immunofluorescence and cytology during the influenza A H2N2 pandemic did show that virus replication was patchy and that many cells remained uninfected.[44] This observation would give credence to the concept that therapeutic intervention with antiviral drugs would prevent the spread of virus further down the respiratory tract. Encouragingly, pharmacologic experiments, in both animals and humans, have shown a preferential accumulation of amantadine in respiratory tissue, including the lung. Therefore, the scientific basis for antiviral therapy with M2 blockers appears firm.

In a typical example of clinical investigations at the time, two therapeutic studies were carried out in the winters of 1972–73 and 1973–74 on general practice in the United Kingdom, when both influenza A and influenza B were circulating. As the influenza A viruses during both winters had essentially the same sensitivity in vitro to amantadine, the authors considered it appropriate to combine the results from the two winters. The mean duration of fever in the drug-treated group was 51.4 h, and that in the controls was 73.4 h ($P < 0.05$). Symptoms cleared completely within 4 days in 53% of patients receiving amantadine, compared with only 23% of controls. Mean days in bed were 2.58 for the amantadine group and 3.44 for the placebo group ($P < 0.01$). In those patients with influenza B, there were no significant differences between active drug and placebo. The appearance of influenza B infection, confirmed only after the clinical recording was completed, illustrated the sensitivity of the trial design, for it had been demonstrated previously that this virus was insensitive to amantadine. No adverse effects were noted in this trial, which employed 200 mg of amantadine each day.

13.6 MODERN USE OF LOW-DOSE (100 mg) AMANTADINE

Because of concern about the mild toxic effects of 200 mg amantadine per day, it is important to briefly review two clinical trials where lower doses of the drug were used, and which demonstrated that most adverse effects could be avoided while antiviral activity was retained. In the event of a new influenza pandemic or deliberate release of virus, both classes of anti-influenza drugs (M2 blockers and NIs) will have vital roles to play.

Younkin et al.[53] treated influenza patients for five days with amantadine 100 mg (16 cases) or 200 mg (14 cases), or 3.25 g of aspirin (17 cases), daily. Although the aspirin treatment group defervesced more rapidly, by the second day the amantadine–100 mg recipients showed greater symptomatic improvements ($P < 0.01$). The 200 mg dose did not show such significance. Bothersome side effects resulted in discontinuation of therapy by 35% of patients on aspirin but only 3% of patients on amantadine. At 100 mg amantadine, the side effects reported were considered to be minimal and consisted of dizziness, loss of concentration, or insomnia. The study also demonstrated that 100 mg/day amantadine had therapeutic efficacy against the virus equal to 200 mg/day.

Sears and Clements[54] induced influenza in 44 healthy volunteers; 22 received 100 mg of amantadine and 22 placebo, once daily for 8 days, with intranasal viral challenge on day 4. Influenza illness was seen in two of 22 volunteers (9%) on amantadine versus nine of 22 (41%) on placebo ($P \leq 0.04$). With amantadine, the illness was mild and tended to consist only of mild transient rhinitis. Infection was seen in 77% of volunteers on amantadine versus 91% of volunteers on placebo. The amount of virus shed was halved by low-dose amantadine treatment, with total days of virus isolation during treatment being 1.2 on amantadine and 3.5 on placebo ($P < 0.03$).

Finally, Reuman et al.[55] carefully investigated the antiviral effects and also toxicity of low-dose (100 mg) amantadine and compared the results with those of a group given 200 mg of the drug. In this direct virus challenge experiment, 100 mg of amantadine reduced the rate of illness from 58% to 15% and the number of volunteers infected from 95% to 60%. Analysis of the three groups for central nervous system and gastroenteritis effects showed no increase in side effects in the low-dose (100 mg) drug group compared to the placebo group.

13.7 NEW MAMMALIAN CELL TECHNIQUES VERSUS ESTABLISHED EGG METHODS TO RAPIDLY CULTIVATE INFLUENZA VIRUS FOR VACCINES IN A THREAT OR PANDEMIC SITUATION

We have defined "at risk" groups in previous sections as those who are the yearly targets of vaccines and recognized that current vaccine production and administration needs to be increased both in the interpandemic years and for a pandemic. Influenza virus for vaccine production has been grown in embryonated hens' eggs for 60 years. The technology is well automated and usually produces one vaccine dose ($3 \times 15\ \mu g$ HA and NA protein) from the virus-containing allantoic fluid of a single embryonated hen's egg. The influenza A viruses are normally reassortant with the HA and NA genes from the wild epidemic strain of H3N2 and H1N1 viruses and the remaining six genes from a classic egg-adapted virus called A/PR/8/34 (H1N1). This latter virus has been extensively passaged in eggs and produces tenfold higher virus yields than a wild-type unadapted virus. Therefore, the new reassortant vaccine virus has the growth capacity in eggs of A/PR/8/34 and the appropriate HA and NA as the wild-type virus. However, the potential problem from the viewpoint of a sudden pandemic or bioterrorist event is lack of production surge capacity using eggs. The eggs are fertilized and have to be ordered six months in advance from specialized farms. Commonly, an influenza vaccine production plant is built to infect 40,000 eggs each time and then, two days later, to harvest allantoic fluid from these eggs. Therefore, the production capacity cannot suddenly be increased five-or tenfold. Obviously, the overall surge would not be necessary if all countries had an interpandemic strategy and therefore vaccinated each year 15% of the 50% of the population at risk of complications, hospitalization, and death following an attack of influenza (mainly those over 65 years old). Should every country produce such a recommended quantity of influenza trivalent vaccine, then a simple calculation would show that producing a monovalent pandemic vaccine rather than a trivalent epidemic vaccine would allow a production of 3×15 or 45% coverage in the same populations. Such a production coverage could be even extended should a whole virus pandemic vaccine be used because this would give a more powerful immune response and could even allow dilution to less than a 15 μg dose, thus extending further the number of potential vaccinees.

But more recent laboratory experience of cultivating influenza viruses in mammalian cells rather than eggs has encouraged two manufacturers at least to invest in cell culture fermenters.[56,57] Here the production capacity can be increased to cope with a surge in demand for pandemic vaccine virus. Moreover, the final vaccine has theoretical advantages of the absence of egg proteins. A minority of the population are allergic to hen's egg protein. The cell culture virus is also easier to purify. Where clinical isolates of influenza viruses are cultivated on mammalian cells and eggs in parallel different antigenic variants are selected.[58] The biological variants have amino acid substitutions in the receptor binding site in proximity to an antigenic site on the HA, and therefore an amino acid change in this region can alter antigenicity. Of the two subpopulations that can be selected, the virus that is grown on MDCK (or Vero) cells rather than in eggs, appears most closely related to the wild-type clinical virus. There is some indication that cell-grown virus vaccines offer greater protection in animal models than the corresponding egg-grown vaccine.[59] Thus, there are powerful arguments in favor of the new generation of influenza vaccines being cultivated in Vero or MDCK cells.

13.8   NEW INFLUENZA VACCINES THAT COULD INDUCE PROTECTION ACROSS THE DIFFERENT SUBTYPES

There are 16 known subtypes of the HA of influenza A virus, distinguished by their antigenicity. Only three subtypes have caused pandemics in humans, namely H1, H2, and H3, while H5, H7, and H9, predominantly circulating in birds, have crossed the species barrier into humans and caused localized outbreaks.[60,61] We do not know whether these latter three subtypes could mutate into human-to-human transmitters and to thereby have pandemic potential. An important question is whether there is any way that a vaccine could be engineered to give so-called heterotypic or cross-subtype immunity. It is well known that the internal proteins of influenza A virus such as M1, M2, and NP are shared by all influenza A viruses. These internally situated proteins are certainly immunogenic (particularly NP) but could the immunity induced, either T cell or antibody, be broadly reacting? To back up the central core of this approach, it has been known for forty years that mice infected with an influenza A H1N1 virus would later resist a lethal challenge with an influenza A H3N2 virus. Given the lack of genetic and antigenic relatedness between the H1 and H3 proteins, or indeed the corresponding N1 and N2 proteins, the strong cross-immunity was attributed to an internal protein such as NP or M. However, it has been difficult to construct a solid database, and there has been a lingering doubt about this so-called cross-protective immunity. Most virologists deduced, by virtual elimination, that a cross-reactive portion of the HA (HA2) could have provided the cross-protection. Furthermore, this cross-protection is particularly seen in the mouse model, leading some to conclude that the mouse recognized cross-protection epitopes that perhaps humans did not.

Fundamental studies to correlate the genetics and immunology of NP established the cytotoxic T cell response to portions of this protein.[62] However, the work clearly showed that M2 could be a cross-reactive immunogen, although a relatively weak one. The M2 protein is an integral membrane protein of influenza A viruses that is expressed at the plasma membrane of virus-infected cells and is also present, in small amounts, on virions. It is some 96 amino acids in length, with a 23 amino acid extracellular domain, a trans domain of 19 amino acids, and a 54 amino acid cytoplasmic tail. The important extracellular domain, potentially targeted by antibodies and T cells, is conserved by virtually all influenza A viruses. Even the 1918 pandemic virus differs only in one amino acid. The first indication that the M2 was immunologically active was the observation that an anti-M2 monoclonal antibody reduced the spread of virus in cell culture. Not unexpectedly, the antibody reacted with the extracellular domain of M2. Even more exciting, the antibody reduced the replication of virus in mouse lung. Immunization studies with M2 constructs, however, have given more mixed results. Immunization of mice with a DNA plasmid of M1 and M2 genes gave protection mainly via T helper cell activity.[63] Neirynck et al.[62] had already showed that a hepatitis B core in M2 fusion protein gave protection in a mouse model. Yegerlehner et al.[64] coupled a peptide of the external portion of M2 to the immunodominant region of the core antigen of hepatitis B virus. The same group later investigated the immunological mechanism and found that the cross-protection resided in antibodies, although the M2-specific antibodies did not neutralize virus in vitro. The authors concluded that the protection was mediated by an indirect mechanism such as complement-mediated cytotoxicity or antibody-dependent cytotoxicity. But importantly, the protection induced in the mouse model was considerably less than that induced by conventional subunit HA/NA vaccine. In a separate series of experiments in pigs Heinen et al.[65] showed that immunisation with an M2 construct offered no protection but actually enhanced the disease. Vaccine-induced enhancement has been noted in the past with experimental chemically inactivated vaccines against measles and RSV but never with influenza. It is possible, of course, that the construct itself is the most important factor and that renewed efforts could identify a more powerful combination immunogen. A series of new viral vectors carrying influenza HA and NA genes including VEE[66] and adenovirus in what are essentially a new generation of genetically modified (GM) vaccines also give expectations of powerfully driven local immune responses with the accompanying cross-immunity.

It could be argued that weak heterotypic immunity may be present already in the community and that this is helping to prevent the emergence of chicken influenza A (H5N1) in Southeast Asia. Certainly with evidence of millions of birds infected since late 2003 in twelve countries in Southeast Asia with only a handful of human infections and no human-to-human transmission, there is a possibility, certainly highly theoretical, that the unique cocirculation since 1977 of two influenza A viruses (H1N1 and H3N2) may have enhanced heterotypic immunity in most communities, which in turn abrogates the emergence of chicken influenza A (H5N1) into humans. It would be foolhardy to take this argument to a fuller conclusion and thereby relax the pressure to prepare for a new pandemic influenza A virus.

13.9 WHO AND NATIONAL PLANNING FOR A PANDEMIC OR DELIBERATE OUTBREAK

The first sections of this chapter represent the crucial points of preventative medicine for influenza using antivirals and vaccines. The communities of the world now have newly developed antivirals and potent vaccines for influenza that would blunt a serious outbreak. But exactly how prevalent are these new influenza viruses and is a pandemic or threat expected? Where will it come from and how long will it take to spread around the world? How long would the warning period be? Table 13.1 summarizes the global outbreaks of influenza during the present and last centuries. It is immediately obvious that these global outbreaks are intermittent and there is an unpredictable time frame.

Influenza is a unique virus in having two epidemiologic forms, epidemics and pandemics, and management of community illness will be different in each case. It is quite clear that effective utilization of antiviral drugs to combat a pandemic virus or bioterrorist threat will depend on the prior widespread use of the drugs during interpandemic years. By definition, most persons of all ages would be vulnerable to infection with a new pandemic or bioterrorist virus. During epidemic years those over 65 years of age are most vulnerable to medical complications. Antivirals can be stored during interpandemic years and only used in a pandemic or in a threat situation. However, in parallel the best approach would be consistent and detailed year-to-year clinical use of antivirals and vaccines to reduce the year-to-year medical and economic impact of influenza. In this manner, physicians and nurses would become familiar with influenza as a unique disease entity, and, at the time of a pandemic or a threat situation considerable clinical expertise in the use of antivirals would have accumulated.

Given the unpredictability of a date for a new reemergent pandemic influenza A virus, there is a tendency, given more pressing medical problems, to forget influenza. The WHO has requested each member state to produce a pandemic plan, but abysmally few governments have responded to date, which is a huge international problem. On a more positive note, several European countries including the UK, France, the Netherlands, and also Australia, the US, Japan, and New Zealand are now considering a strategy of stockpiling anti-influenza drugs; this alongside more clinical use each year of vaccines and antivirals could be a significant investment in future community health care in Europe and the World (Table 13.3).

The essential objectives of a pandemic plan are to alert scientific, medical, and political groups and to reduce the morbidity and mortality from influenza illness, thereby increasing the ability of a community to cope with large numbers of people who are ill and dying, at home and in hospital, and to ensure that essential services

TABLE 13.4 Preparedness Levels for Interpandemic and Postpandemic Periods (WHO Template Plan)

Phase	Characterized by:	Explanation	Action to be Taken by WHO
Interpandemic period, Phase 0	No indications of any new virus type have been reported.		**Coordinate** a program of international surveillance for influenza in humans.
Phase 0, Preparedness Level 1	Appearance of a new influenza strain in a human case	First report(s) of isolation of a novel virus subtype, without clear evidence of spread of such a virus.	**Coordinate** international efforts to assist national and local authorities so as to confirm the infection of human by a novel strain. **Heighten** activities of the laboratory surveillance laboratory network.
Phase 0, Preparedness Level 2	Human infection confirmed	Two or more human infections have occurred with a new virus subtype, but the ability of the virus to readily spread from person-to-person and cause multiple outbreaks of disease leading to epidemics remains questionable.	**Promote** enhanced surveillance activity regionally or internationally and development and evaluation of candidates for production of vaccines against the novel influenza strain. **Recommend** that national health authorities take contingency steps that will facilitate activation of their National Pandemic Preparedness Plans.
Phase 0, Preparedness Level 3	Human transmission confirmed	Clear evidence of person-to-person spread in the general population, such as secondary cases resulting from contact with an index case, with at least one outbreak lasting over a minimum two-week period in one country.	**Facilitate** the distribution to all interested manufacturers of candidate vaccine viruses developed as part of the Preparedness Level 2 activities and **convene** its experts for influenza vaccine composition to develop, disseminate and encourage co-ordinated clinical trials of vaccines against the new strain. **Contact** vaccine manufacturers and national governments about capacity and plans for production and international distribution of a vaccine to the new virus. **Encourage** international coordination for purchase and distribution of vaccine among different countries.

Pandemic Period, Phase 1	Confirmation of onset of pandemic	A virus with a new hemagglutinin subtype compared to recent epidemic strains is beginning to cause several outbreaks in at least one country, and to have spread to other countries, with consistent disease patterns indicating that serious morbidity and mortality are likely in at least one segment of the population.	**Make** recommendations for composition and use (doses and schedules) of vaccines and organize consultations that are intended to facilitate vaccine production and distribution in the most equitable manner possible and **issue** guidance on the best use of available antiviral drugs against the new virus. **National** response measures should be initiated as rapidly as possible according to predetermined national pandemic plans, updated to take account of specific characteristics of the new subtype and knowledge of vaccine availability.
Phase 2	Regional and multiregional epidemics	Outbreaks and epidemics are occurring in multiple countries and spreading region by region across the world.	Organize the distribution of vaccines in the most equitable manner possible and provide **update** guidance on the best use of available antiviral drugs against the new virus. Seek further support in mobilization of resources for countries with limited capacities.
Phase 3	End of first pandemic wave	The increase in outbreak activity in the initially affected countries has stopped or reversed, but outbreaks and epidemics of the new virus are still occurring elsewhere.	
Phase 4	Second or later waves of the pandemic	Based on past experiences, at least a second severe wave of outbreaks caused by the new virus would be expected to occur within 3–9 months of the initial epidemic in many countries.	
Phase 5	End of the pandemic (back to phase 0)	The pandemic period has ended, which is likely to be after 2–3 years.	**Assessment** of the overall impact of the pandemic and **evaluation** of "lessons learned" from the pandemic that will assist in responding to future pandemics. **Update** the WHO Influenza Pandemic Plan.

are maintained. Such a strategy can also be used as a plan for a bioterrorist attack and indeed the U.K. influenza pandemic plan has been modified for a potential outbreak either deliberate or as a reemerged virus such as monkeypox. Tables 13.4 and 13.5 summarize the preparedness levels and some scenarios for vaccine or drug use during a pandemic. A simple mathematical calculation identifies 29, 39, and 10 years between recorded pandemics while 36 years have now elapsed since the 1968 pandemic. The realists could conclude that a new pandemic of influenza A virus is now overdue.

Although a natural influenza pandemic would seem to be almost inescapable, the likelihood of a deliberate terrorist caused outbreak would seem miniscule, at least at present. But of course sensible and urgent preparations for a pandemic would cover both possibilities.

The WHO has issued a consultation document about pandemic influenza, which places the responsibility for management of risk with national authorities and which urges these national committees to take the initiative to discuss new issues such as how scarce supplies of vaccines and antivirals can be shared when the next outbreak comes and whether public gatherings, for example, should be cancelled to slow the spread of infection. The same plan can be modified for a deliberate attack scenario. The document reiterates that in spite of medical and scientific advances since the 1918 pandemic, unparalleled tolls of illness and deaths would be expected in a new influenza A outbreak with air travel speeding up the global spread of influenza infection. There is also the very real problem about build up of fear in a population about even the possibility of an outbreak. To better cope with false alarms and also the public issue of fear, the WHO has designated some warning levels. Possibly the most important part of the NPP is the pre- or interpandemic period designated phase 0 (Table 13.4). Some plans subdivide this phase. Countries must learn to manage the yearly epidemics by vaccinating the "at risk" groups and using antiviral drugs to contain localized outbreaks during this crucial period. Without this experience, there will be less chance of serious and effective clinical management during a pandemic or bioterrorist attack. Another vital aspect of this phase is surveillance, which is now accurate and speedy because of molecular diagnostics. To give two examples, the SARS virus genome was sequenced in a matter of weeks and a diagnostic kit supplied within this time frame to Southeast Asia. Similarly, the 1999 and the recent (2005) outbreak of influenza A H5N1 in Southeast Asia and the H7N7 outbreaks in the Netherlands[67,68] were intensively and very rapidly inves- tigated using PCR-based tests. However, the extreme sensitivity of the test can be a problem itself and lead to overhasty deductions about transfer of virus to other animal or bird species simply by a detection of viral genes in the respiratory tree where they may not be causing overt disease. From the recent experience of the H5 chicken influenza outbreak in Southeast Asia, there is an absence of coordination between human and veterinary virologists. Taubenberger[69] has defined a physician as "a veterinarian who only manages to deal with diseases of one species" and there is more than an element of truth here. One of the problems faced recently is "ownership of new viruses"—patents and general competition between groups of scientists to have hands-on experience with the new virus. Traditionally, a virus emerging from birds or animals is a veterinary virus and in many countries the Ministry of Agriculture may refuse permission for the virus to be brought into the country unless to a veterinary institute. Obviously, a contradictory viewpoint is that once an avian virus is recovered from a human then it could be viewed as a human virus. These apparently small questions of ownership can impede work on the influenza A (H5N1) and other emerging viruses.

Mathematical models can be developed during this viral interpandemic time and these have proved their worth in attempts to avert large outbreaks of SARS. Where countries are contiguous with open borders, such as the E.U., it is most important that national pandemic plans are interchanged. A new factor is the growing recognition by the WHO that it can exert huge economic pressure for countries to take zoonotic outbreaks of influenza seriously. Scientists and virologists took a non-interventionalist approach in the previous pandemics of the twentieth century. However, the WHO is now acting very quickly and the central hypothesis is that unless a pandemic can be stopped very early it will never be stopped. This explains the huge interventions in Southeast Asia in 2003–2005 to kill over 200 million chickens to prevent an emergence of chicken influenza A H5N1 virus and, similarly, the killing of 20 million chickens in Holland to prevent influenza A H7N7. Should a policy of encircling vaccination of chickens also be carried out together with human distancing or quarantine, it is possible that a potential outbreak in humans could be aborted or at least delayed so that enough vaccine could be manufactured. Some scenarios for vaccine and antiviral use in a pandemic or threat situation are summarized in Table 13.5.

Probably the most important contribution to public health is the buildup and stockpiling of antiviral drugs, which can then be used to blunt the effects of the first wave of an outbreak and give opportunities for a new vaccine to be made. It is not widely appreciated that there could be a long delay in the manufacture of a stock of antiviral drugs. The new NIs have a life span, in bulk, of 20 years or more, so chemical stability does not present a problem. The problem is the complex chemical synthesis, and without a designated factory to produce the drug beforehand, the world production capacity will remain miniscule and totally inadequate in a world, or even national, threat situation. It could be argued very strongly that the single biggest investment in public health at present would be the establishment of a reserve of anti-influenza drugs. To give some urgency to planners the situation can be viewed from another direction. When the pandemic or bioterrorist attack arrives and the hospitalizations and deaths begin to mount, who is going to be the messenger that the scientific and medical community knew about the drug and vaccine shortage but failed to act? Some governments including New Zealand, Australia, Japan, the United States, and the European Union are now beginning to stockpile NIs.

Since there are only 16 subtypes of influenza A virus, it would also seem sensible and strategic to prepare this number of experimental vaccines using a representative virus strain of each subtype and to obtain preliminary evidence of immunogenicity. Such vaccine virus could be used, at the very least, as an early release vaccine for health care workers, nurses, and doctors. It could be viewed as a community

TABLE 13.5 Some Selected Scenarios for Vaccine and Antiviral Use in a Pandemic or Threat Situation

Options	BEST CASE SCENARIO The new virus does not spread as much as in serious pandemics or the illness caused overall is not a very severe event in usually vulnerable groups.		WORST CASE SCENARIO The new virus spreads rapidly and widely in the populations, causing illness at least as severe as in most influenza A epidemics.	
	Advantages	Disadvantages	Advantages	Disadvantages
Option 1: No special vaccination or antiviral program against the new virus.	Considerable expenses are avoided.	Potential for the population to feel abandoned by their leaders in the medical care and public health system.	Resources otherwise used for vaccination might be applied to strengthening health care delivery system to dealing with large numbers of severe cases.	Without benefit of antivirals and vaccine, morbidity and probably mortality are high. Strain on the health care services is severe, with reduced staff and increased demand. National economy is seriously affected. Public fear and protest are likely.
Option 2: Vaccinate or protect with antivirals selected groups, considered most important for health care and overall infrastructure of the country. Perhaps 25–30% of the population.	The high costs and social upheaval associated with a large-scale vaccination or antiviral program are avoided.	Potential criticism of process and decisions when identifying "most important" persons to be vaccinated or protected with antivirals.	Disruption of vital community functions, including health care delivery, is minimized.	Impact of virus on most of the population remains severe, and many of the problems expected under *Option 1* would still be expected to occur.

Option 3: Also attempt to vaccinate or protect with antivirals groups considered at high medical risk. Perhaps 15% of the population would be targeted.	Program would be most consistent with normal influenza vaccination activities in many industrialized countries.	The new vaccine will replace at least one component of the traditional one. High-risk populations may remain susceptible to illness if the new virus does not displace the old one.	Overall, there should be a cost–benefit ratio for the vaccination and antiviral program in terms of health care finances, and the impact on critical functions of society will be minimized.	The general populations, including preschool and school-age children and most working-age adults, will be seriously affected. Thus the national economy and many normal noncritical activities will be disrupted, with some of the other problems expected *Option 1* still likely.
Option 4: Attempt to vaccinate or protect with antivirals all (>90% of the population).	Should the new virus evolve into a more serious form, the population will have already been vaccinated.	Such a complicated program draws many resources away from other needs. Major controversy probable. Large-scale vaccination or antiviral use increases chances of adverse events that raise questions about vaccine or drug safety.	The maximum reduction in impact of the pandemic virus would be obtained. National leaders would be acclaimed for their efforts.	There may be lack of understanding of the fact the vaccine or antiviral is not 100% effective, and there will be situations where persons will claim they have been harmed by the vaccine or antiviral.

"priming" vaccine. The practical experience from 1918, 1957, and 1968 influenza pandemics, and more recently the SARS outbreak, showed how vulnerable the health care sector is to infection. An initial vaccine even in small quantities to immunize the most vulnerable 5–10% of the population would ameliorate the otherwise devastating effects in hospitals. Recently, the isolation of a new influenza A H5N1 in humans triggered phase preparedness (PP) at level 2 but no widespread human-to-human transmission was detected. At PP trigger level 3, vaccine manufacturing will start. Experience from the past has shown that phase 3 can last as long as 9–12 months. The objectives during the pandemic phase itself is to organize distribution of vaccines and antivirals (Tables 13.3 and 13.4).

13.10   INCIDENCE OF ILLNESS IN A PANDEMIC OR DELIBERATELY CAUSED OUTBREAK

Analysis of the three global outbreaks of the twentieth century can provide vital information to help plan for the next outbreak. The first observation from the recent past is that pandemic or bioterrorist influenza may appear at any time of the year, not necessarily during the "normal" influenza season (November to March in the northern hemisphere or July to August in the southern hemisphere). In most pandemics, activity can be expected to last 6–8 weeks, although in the 1968–1969 pandemic lower levels of activity continued for 3–4 months. The relatively short period of the outbreak itself, say, 5–6 weeks as in epidemic years, allows prophylactic strategies with antivirals to be implemented.

In 1918, about 23% of the U.K. population developed influenza; in the 1957 Asian influenza pandemic an estimated 17% of the population suffered from influenza illness; and in 1969 the Hong Kong virus produced illness in 8% of the adult population. It could safely be predicted that each clinical case would be accompanied by four nonclinical cases of influenza. In normal years, although most influenza infection occurs in children, the serious morbidity and mortality occurs almost entirely among elderly people with underlying chronic disease. A different pattern may emerge in a pandemic, as it did in 1918. The 1918–1919 pandemic also affected healthy young adults, as well as those at the extremes of life. Similarly, in 1957 the brunt of the outbreak, although not mortality, was suffered by schoolchildren and young adults. Therefore, it is clear that clinical management of influenza with antivirals or vaccines will differ in a pandemic or bioterrorist year compared to the interpandemic period.

13.11   MORTALITY AND MORBIDITY IN A PANDEMIC

Of course, the 1918 pandemic dominates the records of infectious disease during the twentieth century, and indeed for the previous five centuries for both numbers of afflicted persons and deaths. The worst-case scenarios of a new pandemic or deliberate outbreak indicate that, with the current massive world population,

TABLE 13.6   Estimated Death and Hospitalizations, in Population Groups During an Influenza Pandemic or Terrorist Attack

	Total Cases at High Risk (%)	
Category	Age Group (yr)	Mean
Death	0–19	9.0
	20–64	40.9
	65+	34.4
	Total	84.3
Hospitalizations	0–19	4.6
	20–64	14.7
	65+	18.3
	Total	37.6

Source: Reference 70.

rapidity of transport and immunosuppressed persons afflicted with HIV, mortality and hospitalization in a new pandemic could easily exceed that of 1918. In 1957, when the illness was milder compared to the 1918 pandemic, more than 30,000 deaths occurred in England and Wales. Estimates ranged from 1.3 to 3.5 deaths/1000 cases, and two-thirds of the deaths were of people aged over 55 years. Predictions for a new pandemic in the United States also emphasize the disproportionate effect on the 20–64 year age group (Table 13.6). In a pandemic, the number of new general practice consultations for influenza-like illness can be expected to exceed 500/100,000 population per week. A medical practice of 10,000 patients would therefore expect to see at least 50 new patients per week. Pandemics also have a marked effect on hospital admissions. During September and October 1957, between 25,000 and 30,000 more cases of acute respiratory infection were admitted to hospitals in England and Wales than would have been expected at that time of year.

It is easy to see that the health care system of most countries would be quickly overwhelmed in any future outbreak. In recent years, there has been no provision of spare beds for such emergencies and, therefore, as the outbreak of SARS in Southeast Asia and Canada showed, modern health care systems can be more easily disrupted than in the past.

13.12   THE IMPACT OF PANDEMICS ON THE ECONOMY

Not unexpectedly, pandemics have a serious effect on the economy. In 1957 in the United Kingdom, new sickness benefit claims by those working and aged 15–64 years increased by 2.5 million (of 17.5 million insured). Among the uninsured, an additional 1.5 million work absences were estimated. Of the insured population, 8–10% were estimated to have lost 3 working days at home during the epidemic. In

TABLE 13.7   **Direct and Indirect Costs for the United States of an Influenza Pandemic or Terrorist Attack**

Effect	Cost per Gross Attack Rate[a] ($ billion)				
	15%	20%	25%	30%	35%
Deaths:					
Mean	59	79	99	118	138
Hospitalizations:					
Mean	1.9	2.5	3.2	3.8	4.4
Outpatients:					
Mean	5:7	7:6	9:5	11:4	13:3
Ill, no medical care sought[b]:					
Mean	4.2	5.8	7.3	8.8	10.3
Grand totals:					
Mean	71	95	119	143	166

[a]Gross attack rate is the percentage of clinical influenza illness per population.
[b]Persons who become clinically ill due to influenza but do not seek medical care; illness has an economic impact (e.g., half-day off work).
Source: Reference 70.

the pandemic of 1968, just over 1 million excess sickness claims were received in England over 5 months. Modern estimates of cost assuming various attack rates in the community from 15% to 35% are summarized in Table 13.7 and vary between 71 and 166 billion dollars for the United States alone.

13.13   LESSONS TO BE LEARNED FROM THE GREAT SPANISH INFLUENZA OUTBREAK 1916–1919: INFLUENZA PANDEMICS DO NOT ALWAYS START IN SOUTHEAST ASIA AND MAY HAVE A PROLONGED GESTATION PERIOD

A few months in autumn of 1918 saw, among the death of millions of others, those of the U.S. Army private, Private Vaughan, in South Carolina, of "Lucy" at Brevig Mission, Alaska, and of six Norwegian coal miners in Spitsbergen of "Spanish" influenza. Reports of influenza deaths in Norway, Sweden, Finland, Canada, Spain, Britain, France, Germany, Senegal, Tanzania, Nigeria, China, Zimbabwe, South Africa, India, and Indonesia were also recorded within this short time frame. The very wide geographic spread of these deaths in such a short period, in the absence of air travel at that time, suggests that the disease may have spread around the globe before this time and that earlier "seeding" had taken place. Explosive outbreaks of respiratory disease had affected young soldiers in Europe in the winter periods of 1916 to 1918. The clinical descriptions of these epidemics described high mortality with heliotrope cyanosis; these two features characterized the 1918–1919 influenza pandemic. The term "influenza" was not widely used until after the Great Pandemic and these prepandemic outbreaks were called epidemic catarrh, epidemic bronchitis, three day fever, or even pyrexia of unknown origin.

Hammond et al.[71] described an outbreak of such respiratory infection, termed at the time purulent bronchitis, in the huge British army base at Etaples, near the coast town of Boulogne in Northern France, in the winter of 1916 soon after the battle of the Somme (Figures 13.5 and 13.9). This camp housed 100,000 soldiers on any one day and over one million soldiers stayed here en route from England to the Western Front between 1916 and 1918.[72,73] In the 1916–1917 winter outbreak, the soldiers were admitted to the base hospitals, suffering from an acute respiratory infection, high temperature, and cough at a time when recognized influenza was present. Undoubtedly, conditions in the camp, with most soldiers housed in tents or temporary wooden barracks, were ideal for spread of a respiratory virus. This outbreak was further characterized clinically by heliotrope cyanosis, described extensively in the ensuing 1918 outbreak, and very high mortality. Clinical examination showed, in most cases, signs of bronchopneumonia and histology showed an acute purulent bronchitis. Our clinical microbiological review of the report of the outbreak now ranks the description as classic influenza, being essentially similar to the extensive documentation of deaths in 1918–1919.[73]

An almost identical epidemic of so-called purulent bronchitis with bronchopneumonia, with cases showing the peculiar dusky heliotrope cyanosis and mortality rates of 25–50%, was also described in the famous Aldershot barracks near London

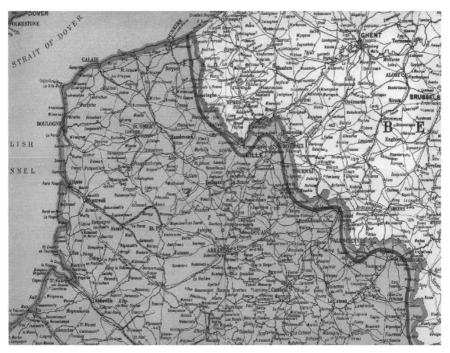

FIGURE 13.5   Map of the most likely origin of the so called Spanish influenza pandemic virus in the U.K. army camp at Etaples in 1917 in northern France and subsequent global spread. Etaples is located near the coast for embarkation of soldiers.

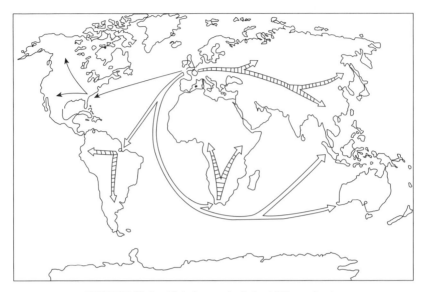

FIGURE 13.6 Global spread of the 1918 pandemic.

in March 1917.[74] The authors of that paper concluded that the unique clinical symptoms together with the pathology delineated a new clinical entity. Very significantly, the same medical team, once they had experienced the 1918–1919 outbreaks, noted in retrospect the similarities in pathology and clinical presentation to the previous Aldershot and Etaples epidemics of 1916.[75] The pathologists in and

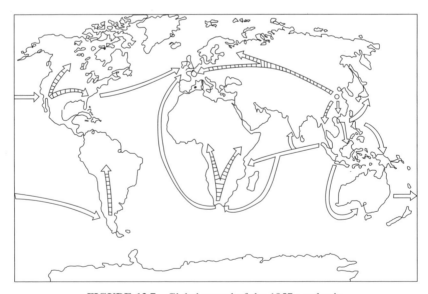

FIGURE 13.7 Global spread of the 1957 pandemic.

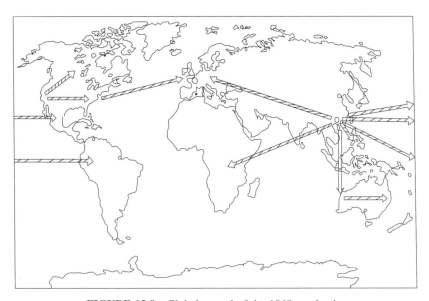

FIGURE 13.8   Global spread of the 1968 pandemic.

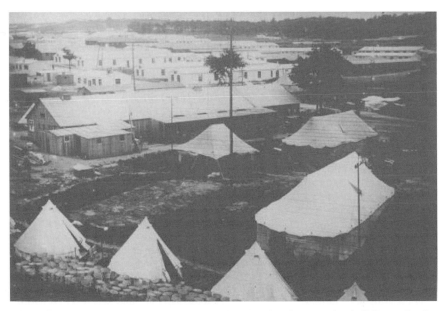

FIGURE 13.9   The U.K. army camp at Etaples, showing the extensive buildings of a city-sized encampment spreading over several miles.

around Etaples carried out transmission experiments in 1918 on macaque monkeys and this group of scientists was perhaps the first to identify the causative agent of the pandemic as a filter-passing virus. The leading pathologist, G Gibson, died as a result of these experiments. Abrahams and his colleagues,[75] once they had experienced the large 1918–1919 outbreak, concluded that both the earlier and 1918 outbreaks had the same causation. "We emphasize our view that in essentials the influenza pneumococcal purulent bronchitis that we and others described in 1916 and 1917 is fundamentally the same conditions as the influenza pneumonia of this recent 1918–1919 pandemic."[75]

Therefore, not only are we considering a forgotten pandemic but a forgotten and overlooked origin. This is not a small point. The unprecedented circumstances of the war on the Western Front, a landscape that was contaminated with over 119,000 tons of respiratory irritants such as mustard gas and phosgene, and characterized by stress and overcrowding, the partial starvation in civilians, and the opportunity for rapid "passage" of influenza in young soldiers, would have provided the opportunity for multiple but small mutational changes throughout the viral genome (see Table 13.2). Such changes could have been important factors in the evolution of the virus into a particularly virulent form, resulting in a pandemic. The origin of the 1918 pandemic is potentially very important because two of the three pandemics of that century (namely, 1957 and 1968) undoubtedly started in Southeast Asia and spread in 1957 by rail, ship, and air, and in 1968 mainly by air travel (Figures 13.7 and 13.8). The 1918 pandemic warns us to search the world for regions where large numbers of young citizens can still contact chickens, ducks, and pigs, much as in Etaples in 1916–1917, and where an avian influenza A virus can emerge, gestate, and then explode into a worldwide pandemic (Figures 13.9 and 13.10). This theoretical epicenter of virus emergence is certainly not restricted to Southeast Asia but would include the E.U., Turkey, the Middle East, South and Central America, and Africa.

The potential lag time in the evolution of a pandemic is a most important parameter. In the well-documented influenza A (H2N2) pandemic of 1957, the first virus was isolated in China in February. Subsequently, the virus spread to Australia and Southeast Asia by June, reaching the rest of Europe and South America by July–September. By December 1957, every continent had been infected, which indicates that a period of 10 months was necessary for global spread. Similarly, in the influenza A (H3N2) pandemic of 1968, the virus spread from China in July but, although the virus was introduced into the rest of Asia by August, the explosive outbreak was delayed by six months. Similarly, in the United Kingdom and Europe, seeding occurred early but explosive outbreaks were delayed for 12–14 months. Early detection of these events would allow a greater lead-time and initiation of general strategies with the new anti-neuraminidase drugs and amantadine as well as the formulation and manufacture of vaccine.

The protracted period that we postulate for the emergence of the Great Pandemic of 1918, almost 18 months, could be explained by the absence of air travel and the effects of restricted travel during the Great War. The new virus mutant could have maintained itself in military camp outbreaks, many of which were like small towns

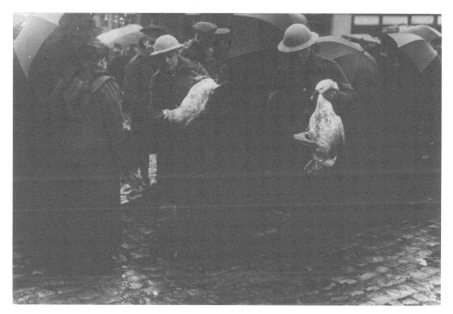

FIGURE 13.10   Near the U.K. army camp at Etaples where soldiers had contact with ducks and geese in the local sector.

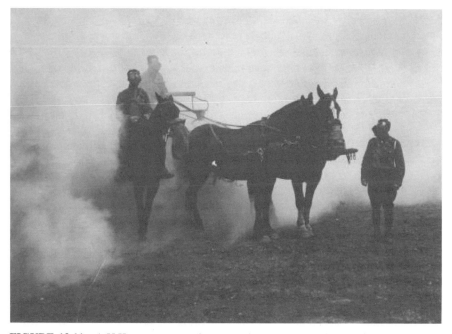

FIGURE 13.11   A U.K. army camp where even horses were equipped with gas masks.

in size, while increasing virulence in a stepwise manner, similar to virus adaptation in animal models where sometimes hundreds of passages are needed to increase virulence of a pneumotropic strain. Several authors refer to "multiple outbreaks" in army camps at this time. Military traffic increased from Europe to the United States in 1917 and it is possible that the new virus was seeded from Europe into the new U.S. army recruiting camps (Figure 13.6, thin line). Demobilization in the autumn of 1918 in Europe would have provided further ideal circumstances for further intimate person-to-person spread and wide dispersion as young soldiers returned home by sea and rail to countries around the globe. Family parties on arrival at home could have further exacerbated the situation. But, as we have noted above, in modern times Asia is only one of many regions where young people live near to chickens, ducks, geese, and pigs.

13.14 COULD A SUPERVIRULENT STRAIN OF INFLUENZA A BE CREATED IN A LABORATORY?

There are only two reports in the literature of unexpected increases in virulence of microbes following genetic manipulation. A strain of mousepox virus became unexpectedly hypervirulent after an extra nonviral gene was inserted. The other example relates to enhanced virulence of TB. Classic studies of microbial passage, since the original studies of Pasteur, indicate clearly that virulence of viruses can be enhanced by rapid animal-to-animal transfer and this is a commonly used method to enhance virulence for animal model experiments. Influenza virus virulence can be increased in mice by so-called skim passage, whereby virus is inoculated intranasally and after 48 h the mouse lungs are removed, ground up in sand and powered glass, and used to reinoculate mice intranasally for the next passage. After 10–15 passages, an essentially benign apathogenic symptomless infection of the mouse begins to turn into a virulent pneumonia. Once established, the virus retains pneumovirulence and can then produce 100% lethality.[76]

However, it is still not clear at the molecular level precisely where in the 12,000 or so nucleotides and eight genes of the influenza virus that the virulence resides. In all probability such virulence mutations are scattered across the eight viral genes. Each new influenza A virus may need to acquire a different set of these mutations before becoming hypervirulent. Furthermore, the eight genes may need to be a perfect interacting fit for maximum virulence. Thus, at least at present, a predetermined pattern of virulence mutations cannot be accessed by a so-called bioterrorist or indeed anyone else; but we could anticipate that within the next few years the rapid advances of molecular virology will unravel this conundrum. For influenza, the techniques of reverse genetics could be used to insert a set of mutations into virulence segments of the genome should these be identified.[77,78]

Earlier work with human influenza A viruses,[79] in quarantine units in Salisbury, established the dominating importance of the HA as a virulence gene and this was confirmed in similar human challenge experiments with influenza B,[80] using influenza viruses where the HA had single amino acid substitutions near the receptor binding site. Obviously, the human volunteer infected in a quarantine unit is the classic model of estimating attenuation or virulence. We have now reestablished such a unit in London, where we can infect up to 100 volunteers in a quarantine building.[20] A laboratory model system to support studies of influenza virus virulence is the ferret and this has demonstrated, for example, that mutants with changes in the NA are less virulent than wild-type viruses.[81]

13.15 VIRULENCE GENES OR GENE SEGMENTS OF PANDEMIC INFLUENZA A VIRUS FROM 1918 HAVE NOT YET BEEN IDENTIFIED

Although sequence analysis of five of the eight genes of 1918 virus has provided the first scientific glimpse of this virus,[82] the most important question that investigators set out to solve, namely, what is the genetic basis of virulence of this virus, remains unanswered. Indeed, the virus may turn out to be not only exceptionally virulent but also unusually infectious. Unlike SARS virus, influenza has a short incubation period of 48 h and a higher R_0 value of five. To enlarge upon this hypothesis, yearly epidemic influenza A viruses have a virulence about tenfold less than the 1918 virus in special groups in the community. Thus, currently, in the United Kingdom 15 million individuals, mainly over the age of 65, are at risk of complications, hospitalization and death following infection with the virus. In the winter of 1999–2000, there were 20,000 deaths in this group (see Figure 13.1). In 1918 the "at risk" group turned out, unexpectedly, to be 25–40 year olds (Figure 13.12), in addition to the very young and old, which would have numbered around 15 million in the United Kingdom. This group suffered 200,000 deaths, a tenfold increase above a normal epidemic year. A combination of a slightly reduced incubation period, a small increase in R_0 value, and a small increase in virulence per se together with the exceptional factor of the war itself could explain the high mortality in 1918.

The quest for the virulence genes of influenza has engaged researchers for over 60 years since Burnet identified the genetic variation of O to D, whereby cultivation of influenza A (H1N1) viruses in the amniotic cavity allowed selection of viruses with different receptor binding properties, and possible changes in virulence.

Extensive studies of natural influenza A infections of poultry identified the virulence contribution of the HA gene.[83] Subsequently, the NA, NP, M, and NS genes have also been shown to affect virulence.[84] More recently, the NSI-encoding gene has been studied most intensively. Among other functions, influenza NSI can block the interferon response of a cell and an influenza virus even marginally more efficient at this activity would be able to replicate at higher titer and spread more widely in the respiratory tree of humans. Nevertheless, transfer of the 1918 NSI to a transfectant influenza A/WSN/33 virus showed reduced virulence rather than enhanced virulence in mice. A possible explanation is that the NSI may not function well in mouse cells.

The viral M gene, which encodes the M1 and M2 proteins, is known to influence virulence of influenza and the rate of viral replication.[76,85–88] M1 is the most

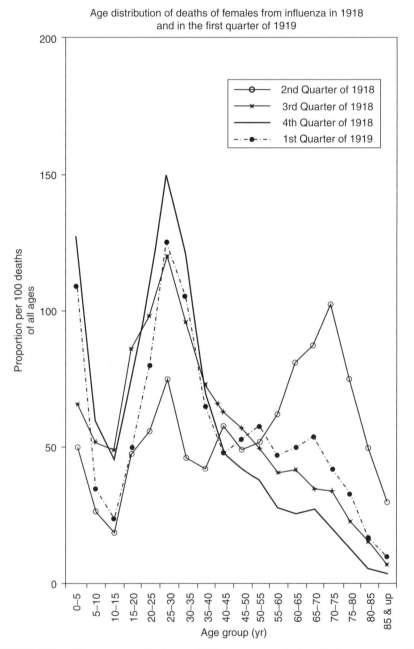

FIGURE 13.12 Skewed mortality in the 1918 pandemic, which included, unexpectedly, younger persons.

TABLE 13.8   In vivo Properties of Recombinant Influenza Viruses Containing Genes of the 1918 Influenza Virus

Virus[a]	Titer[b]-(plaque-forming units/mL)	% Weight Loss[c]	Lung Titers[d]	LD$_{50}$[e]
Parental WSN virus	2.2×10^7	28.4	6.7 ± 0.2	2.5
1918 HA/NA	2.1×10^7	20.9	7.3 ± 0.1	2.75
1918 HA/NA/M	1.4×10^8	28.8	7.9 ± 0.2	2.75
1918 HA/NA/M/ NS	2.1×10^7	23.7	7.3 ± 0.2	3.25
1918 HA/NA/M/NS/NP	1.4×10^8	24.5	7.4 ± 0.2	1.75

[a]All viral genomic segments were derived from the A/WSN/33 virus unless otherwise indicated.
[b]Titer of virus stocks prepared on MDCK cells.
[c]Mean percentage weight loss on day 4 p.i. (five mice per group).
[d]Mean lung titers of four mice on day 4 p.i. expressed as EID$_{50}$/mL $\pm$ SE.
[e]Expressed as the log$_{10}$ plaque-forming units required to give 1 LD$_{50}$.
Source: Adapted from Reference 93.

abundant protein in the viral particle, lines the inner layer of the viral lipid envelope, and is involved in regulating nuclear export of viral RNPs. The M1 protein controls transport of RNPs into the nucleus during infection of the cell and restricts reentry of RNAs into the nucleus at the later stages of infection.[89] M1 may also inhibit viral transcription at a late stage of infection and regulate the switch from replication to virus assembly.[90] An analysis of the M gene from 1918 influenza[91] has not to date identified any amino acid change suggestive of enhanced virulence. Indeed, the 1918 M gene does not code for any of the single amino acid changes that correlate with virulence in previous experimental studies of other influenza A viruses of a high growth phenotype.

More recently, it has been appreciated that balanced HA–NA interactions are crucial for the most efficient replication of influenza, so certain combinations of HA and NA may have to be optimal for virulence.[92] However, biological studies of the HA and NA genes of 1918 influenza failed to demonstrate transfer of intrinsic enhanced virulence in mice[93] (Table 13.8).

13.16   CRYSTAL STRUCTURE OF THE 1918 INFLUENZA HA: THE KEY TO UNDERSTANDING INFLUENZA VIRUS VIRULENCE?

Unexpectedly, the nucleotide sequence of the 1918 virus HA gene[94] failed to show an expected hydrophobic cleavage sequence at the HA1–HA2 junction, or crucial glycosylation patterns and particular receptor binding motifs, which are known virulence factors with some influenza A viruses. Our most recent studies[91] detected nucleotide changes at the receptor binding site sequences extracted from London and U.S. lung samples from 1918 influenza victims, which hinted at the possibility of more than one virus circulating, perhaps with varying biological properties. Receptor binding site substitutions in the HA are known to confer antigenic changes in the important epitope B of the HA[58]: one could speculate that more than one antigenic HA was circulating. Biological analysis of the 1918 HA expressed in vaccinia virus also indicated a 1918 virus with curious receptor binding properties able to agglutinate HAs of chicken, guinea pig, and human origin (A. Elliot, R. Daniels, and J. S. Oxford, in preparation). Thus, our new data indicates that the receptor site on the 1918 HA appeared to have the ability to bind both to 2,3 and 2,6 receptors on sialylated glycoproteins; human and avian influenza viruses are known to bind to 2,6 and 2,3 linkages, respectively. The crystal structure of the uncleaved human H1 HA (HA0) from 1918 influenza virus has been reported by Stevens et al.[95] and Gamblin et al.[96] The 1918 virus A/South Carolina/1/18 was cloned and expressed in a baculovirus expression system. The HA0 was crystallized at pH5.5 and its structure determined by molecular replacement to $3.0\,\text{\AA}$ resolution. The overall structure was similar in many respects to the influenza A H3 HA reported previously.[97]

Superimposition of the 1918 HA2 (H1 subtype) domains with other time-related HAs indicated that the 1918 HA most closely resembles the avian H5 subtype at the receptor. On the other hand, the cleavage site loop of the 1918 HA0 is relatively unique compared to H3 and H5 HAs. There may be an influence of nearby glycosylation sites. Unexpectedly, the 1918 HA0 was not cleaved with trypase from human lung, whereas trypsin cleaved the HA molecule. However, most interest is focused on the receptor binding site, which is situated in a shallow pocket in the HA1 distal domain near the HA tip. As mentioned earlier, in general, avian viruses preferentially bind to receptors that have an α-2,3 linkage, whereas human-adapted viruses prefer the α-2,6 linkage. Unexpectedly, in the 1918 HA the avian type residues Gln[226] and Gly[220] predominate at and around the receptor binding site. Morphologically, the receptor binding site of the 1918 HA is more like that of avian HAs than human HAs. Thus the pocket of 1918 HA is narrower than the corresponding region of the human H3 HA. Overall these features could result in unique cleavage and/or fusion properties as well as receptor binding specificities of the 1918 HA.

In a parallel study, Gamblin et al.[96] concentrated particularly on the receptor binding properties of the 1918 HA as compared to 1934 H1, 1930 swine H1 and avian H1 viruses. Two of the five HAs reported from 1918 have receptor binding sites indistinguishable from 1930 swine HA. The other three 1918 HAs differ at residue 225.[91] Irrespective of the amino acid difference at residue 225, all the sequenced 1918 HAs recognize human receptors and, therefore, they would all be able to infect human cells and presumably spread from human to human.

13.17 COULD A MIXTURE OF PNEUMOCOCCUS AND DRUG-RESISTANT INFLUENZA A VIRUS BE THE BASIS OF A HYPERVIRULENT INFECTION?

During the Edwardian years at the beginning of the twentieth century, pneumonia was a leading cause of death worldwide. Most of these pneumonias were caused by pneumococcus and the bacterium could even cause epidemics in certain communities. When the pandemic of influenza arose and spread between 1917 and 1919, many of the deaths, perhaps one-third, were caused by superinfection of a virus-infected respiratory tree by one or more pneumococcus serotypes. It is also possible that certain patient groups were coinfected with a mixture of virus and bacteria. Many bacterial pneumonias are still untreatable using antibiotics and the situation is even more difficult now with the spread of bacterial drug resistance.

A uniquely difficult scenario would therefore be co-spread of multiple drug-resistant streptococcus or staphylococcus alongside a novel subtype of influenza A virus. In theory, the situation would be even worse if the influenza virus were drug resistant. However, analysis of drug-resistant influenza A virus with mutations in the NA have shown them to be less pathogenic in animal models than wild-type drug-sensitive virus.[81] These observations suggest that drug (NA)-resistant influenza A and B viruses would have a spread disadvantage in the community and would be overtaken by nonresistant viruses.

Selection of drug-resistant virus to NI in vitro is difficult and many passages are required under continual increasing drug pressure. The most common mutation to arise during in vitro selection experiments with either zanamivir, oseltamivir carboxylate, or the RWJ-270201 antiviral is the substitution of the highly conserved arginine at position 292 for lysine. The effect of this R292K substitution, which lies within the NA active site, is to decrease sensitivity to all three drugs of this class and compromise enzyme activity. The R292K mutation in human influenza viruses arises primarily in N2 NA, although it has also arisen in N9 NA (NWS/G70C) (H1N9). This NI-resistant R292K virus is compromised in its ability to replicate in culture and infect animals compared to wild-type virus.

Other resistance mutations to occur within N2 NA are the conserved active site residue glutamic acid 119. E119G or A have been selected in vitro with zanamivir. Changes at position 119 have not been evident during in vitro selections using oseltamivir carboxylate. E119G was also selected by zanamivir in vitro in influenza B, but to date attempts to generate resistance in mutations in influenza B NA using oseltamivir carboxylate in vitro have failed.

In N1 NA, a histidine to tyrosine substitution at position 274 has been selected in vitro in two strains of influenza H1N1 using oseltamivir carboxylate. A single amino acid change H274Y occurred in the NA of A/WS/33, whereas in A/Texas/36/91 the H274Y mutation arose following an earlier I222V substitution. This existed as a mixed population with wild type. The I222V mutation alone afforded only a twofold change on sensitivity of enzyme to oseltamivir carboxylate, whereas sensitivity of the double mutant was reduced more than 1000-fold. To date, there are no reported data on NA mutations selected by zanamivir or RWJ-270201 in H1N1 influenza virus in vitro. However, mutation H274Y, derived in N1 by point mutation gave resistance to zanamivir but not oseltamivir carboxylate.

Decreased susceptibility to NA1 antiviral assays following in vitro selection can also arise due to mutational changes in the hemagglutinin (HA). HA is responsible for viral attachment via sialic acid-rich oligosaccharides on the cell surface and NA cleaves these sialic acid residues, which in turn allows progeny virus to detach from the surface of the infected cell. Resistance mutations in HA that have been identified so far, and which give substantial change in NI drug sensitivity, have been in or around the sialic acid binding site. It is likely that these mutations reduce the affinity of HA for the sialic acid receptors, allowing viruses to detach from the cell surface with less dependence on NA activity. This reduced dependency on NA function results in viruses that are insensitive or less sensitive to NI. Mutations arising in HA can thus lead to cross-resistance to all NIs, even though the NA enzyme remains unaltered.

Consistent with in vitro studies, the emergence of influenza virus resistant to amantadine and rimantadine in a clinical setting has a high incidence (25–38%). In contrast, the emergence of resistant virus in adults with naturally acquired influenza infection treated with oseltamivir phosphate has a low incidence (~1%). The NA mutations that have arisen during NAI use in humans are largely predicted from in vitro selection studies. The exception to this was the identification of E119V with oseltamivir phosphate in influenza A and R152K in influenza B with zanamivir treatment.[98] There have been no mutations to arise during naturally acquired influenza B virus infection in healthy adults or children treated with oseltamivir phosphate. Properties of the clinically derived R292K, E119V, and H274Y NAI resistant viruses generated with oseltamivir phosphate have been found to be severely compromised both in vitro and in vivo and therefore are unlikely to be of clinical significance. For example, the characterization of an oseltamivir-resistant virus with the H274Y mutation in the N1 NA, that arose during a study of efficacy of oseltamivir phosphate in experimental influenza A/Texas/36/91 infection in adults, showed it to be reduced in virulence in vivo in the ferret model.[81]

13.18 ARE THERE LESSONS TO BE LEARNED FROM THE REEMERGENCE OF INFLUENZA A (H1N1) VIRUSES IN 1976 AND 1977?

The world received a shock in 1976 with the emergence of influenza A/swine (H1N1) virus in the Fort Dix army camp in the United States from an infected pig. This virus was obviously lethal because a soldier in the camp died but the virus did not spread outside the camp. We have noted above in 1917 how the pandemic Spanish influenza may have emerged from an army camp in France and, in general, how unique these camps are for viral generation and emergence and yet, at the same time, how difficult it still may be for the new influenza virus to take the next step into a wider world.

The following year (1977) witnessed an even more unprecedented event: namely, a reemergent influenza A virus last seen around 1950. In an extraordinary demonstration of the power of the new science of molecular virology, Nakajima, Desselberger, and Palese[99] were able to prove by nucleotide mapping that the reemerged virus was virtually identical to a virus first isolated 28 years before, namely, A/Fort Worth/50. It was not conceivable then, and still is not, that the virus from 1950 could have continued to circulate for 28 years without mutation in humans or even in pigs or birds. At the time it was described as a virus frozen in time but the alternative explanation is that the virus was a laboratory escape. However, there is absolutely no reason to suppose that it was a deliberate virus release. At the time there was intense interest in using influenza A (H1N1) viruses such as A/PR/8/34 and influenza A (H2N2) viruses such as A/Leningrad/57 or A/ Ann Arbor/63 as a basis for development of a new generation of attenuated influenza vaccine viruses. The idea was to create a master or mistress strain with cold adapted and (ts) mutations, and thereby with attenuated properties and thereafter to reassort new epidemic HA and NA genes into the attenuated parental backbone, giving a gene configuration known as six plus two.

The reemerged influenza A (H1N1) virus quickly spread around the world in 1977–1978. Initially, only those persons born after 1957 were susceptible because this cohort of people had no immunological experience with the H1N1 viruses, which had circulated between 1918 and 1957. Later, the reemerged H1N1 virus mutated and these viruses were then able to also infect more elderly persons. The influenza A H1N1 virus still circulates to this day alongside the influenza A (H3N2) virus. The motality has not been insignificant.

Fortunately, the influenza A (H1N1) virus is not as virulent as the companion influenza A (H3N2) virus, but it has still resulted in hundreds of thousands of deaths in the last 27 years. Most surprisingly, there is, in theory, a potential benefit from the cocirculation of two influenza A viruses simultaneously. It is possible that this cocirculation provides enough opportunity for continued reinfection in the community to boost existing heterotypic cross-immunity, which could prevent the emergence of a third virus, namely, a new pandemic influenza A virus or even a bioterrorist spread virus.

13.19 CONCLUSION

Influenza A virus has a proven record as a bioterrorist virus but driven not by, in Winston Churchill's words, the "evil forces of perverted science"[100] but by the vast unfathomable laws of nature and emergence, reemergence, and resurgence of natural disease. Indeed, the ever inquisitive nature of scientists seems to be poor at present in comparison, although molecular virology is at the edges of important new discoveries using reverse genetics. Information from the human genome project, whereby a significant proportion of the 30,000 active genes are already known to be involved in innate and acquired immunity, provides reassurance that the immune system will continue to provide some protection against new viruses. Gauguin in his last great painting "Who are we, where have we come from, where are we going?" asks crucial questions about the future of humankind. But it was the medieval painter Breugel who asked the major question yet to be answered in the twenty-first century. His medieval painting "The Triumph of Death" shows a horseman on a white charger scything at random and gathering souls for the other world in a sea of Pasteurella pestis and perhaps even of influenza in medieval times. The question haunting the painting is "why some persons survive whilst others die." Even in 1918 in most communities 99% of persons infected with the virus survived. But why did some die and exactly how were they killed by such a minute and fragile form of intermediate life that we know as the orthomyxovirus influenza? Was the immune reaction and ensuing cytokine storm overwhelming or was virus replication in the endothelial cells of the air sacs more important?

Picasso gave us his picture of the caring scientist and doctor in his painting "Science." We would do well to reflect on his vision and abide by the ancient great tradition of science not to be used under any pretext in a harmful way to our potential enemies, or indeed to anyone else. The new technologies of reverse genetics allow RNA viruses to be manipulated for the first time.[78,101–103] Many emergent and threatening viruses such as Ebola, HIV, Lassa, West Nile, influenza, and SARS have RNA genomes. The potential to deliberately, or more likely, to accidentally create a hypervirulent virus is now with us. These observations do not warn us to stop this area of scientific exploration: that would be an absurd conclusion. But there is an extraordinarily clear message emerging, which tells us to build our public health infrastructure and continue and expand our epidemiological vigilance and surveillance against all these infectious viruses and bacteria. For instance for influenza, we need a detailed and practical plan and a supply of antiviral drugs and new vaccines at hand. We would then be "at the end of the beginning"[100] as regards the protection of all citizens of the new world of the twenty-first century. Influenza was the twentieth century's weapon of mass destruction, killing more than the Nazi's, more than the atomic bomb, and more than the First World War. Nature is the greatest bioterrorist of our world and we should concentrate and expand our efforts in public health. Emerging viruses could do for us all, as easily and as quickly, or even more so, than the Great Influenza of 1918.

We can summarize as follows:

1. Influenza A is a global virus with proven ability to cause cataclysmic damage to the health and economy of a country. The virus caused in excess of 60 million deaths in the great natural global outbreaks (pandemics) of 1918, 1957, and 1968.

2. The interpandemic years also bring a very significant toll with large numbers of excess deaths and hospitalizations.

3. There are effective influenza vaccines but the lead-time for manufacture of large quantities of vaccine using the traditional embryonated hen's egg technology extends to 11 months. This would not allow significant vaccine production to combat the first wave of a pandemic or a deliberately caused outbreak.

4. There are new antiviral drugs (the NIs) and the older established M2 blockers but they are not available in large enough quantities at present to be used in a first pandemic wave or threat.

5. Influenza can be viewed as a potential bioterrorist weapon but its use would be very unpredictable compared to the application of traditional high explosives or indeed state terrorism using atomic weapons.

6. It is not possible at present to deduce which genes of influenza govern virulence. It is quite likely that all eight genes contribute to virulence. Additionally, there may need to be an equable fit between particular genes of particular influenza A viruses. Even the virulence of the 1918 pandemic virus is not understood. Therefore, at the present moment, it would not be possible to deliberately construct a hypervirulent influenza A virus.

7. Recent techniques such as reverse genetics could be applied to the construction of a hypervirulent influenza A virus should data become available on precise gene structures causing virus virulence within the next 2–3 years. Until this time, a bioterror scientific program would be restricted to using random gene inserts and subsequent animal passage selection of potentially new hypervirulent viruses. This would entail a large scientific team and extensive facilities and resources. It is unlikely that any country would be able to initiate such a program without leakage of knowledge into the scientific community.

8. The old Greek Hippocratic oath may need to be revisited for scientists to discourage their skills being used under any guise which could result in the construction of hypervirulent influenza or other viruses.

9. The WHO is encouraging every country to produce a pandemic plan dealing with decisions about priority groups for influenza vaccines, antivirals and vaccine stockpiling, and intensive surveillance. These important documents could double as a counter-bioterrorist plan.

10. New technologies of the use of mammalian (Vero and MDCK) cells for influenza vaccine production will increase world capacity very significantly and allow more rapid vaccine production to cope with production surge during the lead up to a pandemic or a deliberate release.

11. New and existing developments with killed intranasally applied vaccines, live attenuated viruses, new adjuvants, or new virus vectors provide extra security against emergence of a novel influenza A virus.

12. Each country should now stockpile anti-influenza A M2 blockers and NIs for one-half of the population for immediate use. Seed vaccine stocks for H1-16 should also be prepared and stockpiled to blunt the first wave with a vaccine that would, at the very least, provide immunological priming even in the absence of detectable HIA antibody.

ACKNOWLEDGMENTS

The authors were supported by a grant from the Wellcome Trust. Retroscan Virology is part of the EU Network of Excellence for Antiviral Drug Reistance (VIRGIL).

REFERENCES

1. Phillips, H.; Killingray, D. The Spanish influenza pandemic of 1918–1919: new perspectives. *Routledge Social History of Medicine Series*, 2002.

2. Churchill, W. S. *The Great War*, Vols. 1 and 2; George Newnes Ltd., London, 1993.

3. Crosby, A. W. *America's Forgotten Pandemic*. Cambridge University Press, New York, 1989.

4. Medical Research Committee. *Special Report Series No 36. Studies of Influenza in Hospitals of the British Armies in France, 1918*, HM Stationary Office, London, 1919, p.112.

5. *Report on the Pandemic of Influenza 1918–1919*. Reports on Public Health and Medical Subjects, No 4. H.M. Stationary Office, London, 1920.

6. Lo, K. C.; Geddes, J. F.; Daniels, R. S.; Oxford, J. S. Lack of detection of influenza genes in archived formalin-fixed, paraffin wax-embedded brain samples of encephalitis lethargica patients from 1916–1920. *Virchows Arch.* **2003**, *442*, 591–596.

7. Oxford, J. S. Influenza A pandemic of the 20th century with special reference to 1918: virology, pathology and epidemiology. *Rev. Med. Virol.* **2000**, *10*, 119–133.

8. Macpherson, W. G.; Herringham, W. P.; Elliott, T. R.; Balfour, A. *Medical Services Diseases of the War. Vol 2. Medical Aspects of Aviation and Gas Warfare and Gas Poisoning*. MSO, London, 1927.

9. Enserink, M. U.S. monkey pox outbreak traced to a Wisconsin pet dealer. *Science* **2003**, *300*, 1639.

10. Collier, L.; Oxford, J. S. *Human Virology: A Text for Students of Medicine*. Oxford University Press, Oxyford, 2002.

11. Wood, J. M. Developing vaccines against pandemic influenza. *Philos. Trans. R. Soc. London* **2001**, *356*(1416), 1953–1960.

12. Fedson, D. S. Pandemic influenza and the global vaccine supply. *Clin. Infect. Dis.* **2003**, *36*(12), 1552–1561.

13. Stuart-Harris, C. H.; Schild, G. C.; Oxford, J. S. *Influenza, the Viruses and the Disease*, Edward Arnold, London, 1983.

14. Betts, R. F.; Treanor, J. J. Approaches to improved influenza vaccination. *Vaccine* **2000**, *18*, 1690–1695.

15. Fedson, D. S.; Wajda, A.; Nichol, J. P.; Hammond, G. W.; Kaiser, D. L.; Roos, L. L. Clinical effectiveness of influenza vaccination in Manitoba. *JAMA* **1993**, *270*, 1956–1961.

16. Nichol, K. L.; Nordin, J.; Mullooly, J.; Lask, R.; Fillbrandt, K.; Iwane, M. Influenza vaccination and reduction in hospitalisations for cardiac disease and stroke among the elderly. *N. Engl. J. Med.* **2003**, *348*, 1322–1332.

17. Belshe, R. B.; Mendelman, P. M.; Treanor, J.; King, J.; Gruber, W. C.; Piedra, P.; Bernstein, D. I.; Hayden, F. G.; Kotloff, K.; Zangwill, K.; Lacuzio, D.; Wolff, M. The efficacy of live attenuated, cold-adapted, trivalent, intranasal influenza virus vaccine in children. *N. Engl. J. Med.* **1998**, *338*, 1405–1412.

18. Reichert, T. A.; Sugaya, N., Fedson, D. S.; Glezen, W. P.; Simonsen, L.; Tashiro, M. The Japanese experience with vaccinating school children against influenza. *N. Engl. J. Med.* **2001**.

19. Monto, A. S.; Davenport, F. M.; Napier, J. A. ; Francis, T. Jr. Effect of vaccination of a school-age population upon the course of an A2-Hong Kong influenza pandemic. *WHO Bull.* **1969**, *41*, 537–542.

20. Fries, L.; Lambkin, R.; Gelder, C.; Burt, D.; Lowe, X. FluInsure: safety immunogenicity and human challenge efficacy of an inactivated trivalent influenza vaccine for intranasal administration. In *Influenza Vaccines for the World*, Lisbon, Portugal, **2004**.

21. Palese, P.; Schulman, J. L. Mapping of the influenza virus genome: identification of the haemagglutinin and neuraminidase genes. *Proc. Nat. Acad. Sci. U.S.A.* **1976**, *73*, 2142–2146.

22. Kilbourne, E. D.; Laver, W. G.; Schulmanm J. L.; Webster, R. G. Antiviral activity of antiserum for an influenza virus neuraminidase. *J. Virol.* **1968**, *2*, 281–288.

23. Colman, P. M.; Varghese, J. N.; Laver, W. G. Structure of the catalytic and antigenic sites in influenza virus neuraminidase. *Nature* **1983**, *303*, 41–44.

24. Varghese, J. N.; Laver, W. G. Colman, Structure of the influenza virus glycoprotein antigen neuraminidase at 2.9 Å resolution. *Nature* **1983**, *303*, 34–40.

25. Palese, P.; Schulman, J. L. Inhibitors of viral neuraminidase as potential antiviral drugs. In *Chemoprophylaxis and Virus Infections of the Respiratory Tract*, Vol. 19, Oxford, J. S. (ed.). CRC Press, Boca Raton, FL, 1977, pp. 189–205.

26. Meindl, P.; Tuppy, H. Desoxy-2,3-dehydrosialinsauren, II, competitive hemmung der vibrio-cholerae-neuraminidase durch 2-desoxy-2,3-dehytro-*N*-acyl-neuramin-sauren. [2-Desoxy-2,3-dehydrosialic acids II. Competitive inhibition of *Vibrio cholerae* neuraminidase by 2-deoxy-2, 3-dehydro-*N*-acylneuraminic acids]. *Hoppe Seyler's Z. Physiol. Chem.* **1969**, *350*, 1088–1092.

27. Von Itzstein, M.; Wu, W. Y.; Kok, G. B.; Pegg, M. S.; Dyason, J. C.; Jin, B.; et al. Rational design of potent sialidase-based inhibitors of influenza virus replication. *Nature* **1993**, *363*, 148–153.

28. Kim, C. U.; Lew, W.; Williams, M. A.; Wu, H.; Zhang, L.; Chen, X.; Escarpe, P. A.; Mendel, D. B.; Laver, W. G.; Stevens, R. C. Structure activity relationship studies of novel carbocyclic influenza neuraminidase inhibitors. *J. Med. Chem.*, **1998**, *41*, 2451–2460.

29. Brouillette, W. J.; Atigadda, V. R.; Luo, M.; Air, G. M.; Babu, Y. S.; Bantia, S. Design of benzoic acid inhibitors of influenza neuraminidase containing a cyclic substitution for the *N*-acetyl grouping. *Bioorg. Med. Chem. Lett.* **1999**, *14*, 1901–1906.

30. Lou, M.; Air, G. M. ; Brouillette, W. J. Design of aromatic inhibitors of influenza virus neuraminidase. *J. Infect. Dis.* **1997**, *176*(Suppl. 1), S62–S65.

31. Ives, J. A. L.; Carr, J. A.; Mendel, D. B.; Tai, C. Y.; Lambkin, R.; Kelly, L.; Oxford, J. S.; Hayden, F. G.; Roberts, W. A. The H274Y mutation in the influenza A NIHI neurominidase action site following aseltamivir phosphate treatment leave virus severely compromised both in vitro and in vivo. *Antiviral Res.* **2002**, *55*, 307–317.

32. Gubareva, L. V.; Kaiser, L.; Hayden, F. G. Influenza virus neuraminidase inhibitors. *Lancet* **2000**, *355*, 827–835.

33. Oxford, J. S.; Lambkin, R. Targeting influenza virus neuraminidase—new strategy for antiviral therapy. *Drug Discov. Today* **1998**, *3*, 448–456.

34. Galbraith, A. W.; Oxford, J. S.; Schild, G. C.; Watson, G. L. Protective effect of 1-adamantanamine hydrochloride on influenza A2 infections in the family environment: a controlled double-blind study. *Lancet* **1969**, *2*, 1026–1028.

35. Welliver, R.; Monto, A. S.; Carewitc, O.; Schatteman, E.; Hassman, M.; Hedrick, J.; Jackson, H. C.; Huson, I.; Ward, P.; Oxford, J. S. Effectiveness of oseltamivir in preventing influenza in household contacts. *JAMA*, **2001**, *285*, 748–754.

36. Elliott, M. Zanamivir: from drug design to the clinic. *Philos. Trans. R. Soc. London B* **2001**, *336*, 1885–1893.

37. Hayden, F. G.; Osterhaus, A. D.; Treanor, J. J. Efficacy and safety of the neuraminidase inhibitor in the treatment of influenza virus infections. *N. Engl. J. Med.* **1997**, *337*, 874–880.

38. Makela, M. J.; Pauksens, K.; Rostila, T.; Fleming, D. M.; Man, C. Y.; Keene, O. N.; Webster, A. Clinical efficacy and safety of the orally inhaled neuraminidase inhibitor zanamivir in the treatment of influenza: a randomised double-blind, placebo-controlled European study. *J. Infect.* **2000**, *40*, 42–48.

39. MIST Study Group. Randomised trial of efficacy and safety of inhaled zanamivir in treatment of influenza A and B virus infections. *Lancet* **1998**, *352*, 1877–1878.

40. Monto, A. S.; Fleming, D. M.; Henry, D.; de Groot, R.; Mekela, M.; Klein, T.; Elliott, M.; Kenne, O. N.; Man, C. Y. Efficacy and safety of the neuraminidase inhibitor zanamivir in the treatment of influenza A and B virus infections. *J. Infect. Dis.* **1999**, *180*, 254–261.

41. Treanor, J. J.; Hayden, F. G.; Vrooman, P. S.; Barbarash, R.; Bettis, R.; Riff, D.; Singh, S.; Kinnersley, N.; Ward, P.; Mills, R. G. Efficacy and safety of the oral neuraminidase inhibitor oseltamivir in treating acute influenza: a randomised controlled trial. U.S. Oral Neuraminidase Study Group. *JAMA* **2000**, *283*, 1016–1024.

42. Whitley, R. J.; Hayden, F. G.; et al. Oral oseltamivir treatment of influenza in children. *Pediatr. Infect. Dis. J.* **2001**, *20*, 127–133.

43. Gubareva, L. V.; Webster, R. G.; Hayden, F. G. Detection of influenza virus resistance to neuraminidase inhibitors by an enzyme inhibition assay. *Antiviral Res.* **2002**, *53*, 47–61.

44. Mulder, J.; Hers, J. F. *Influenza*. Wolters-Noordhoff Publishing, Groningen, 1972.

45. Opie, E. I.; Blake, F. G.; Small, J. C.; Rivers, T. M. In *Epidemic Respiratory Disease: The Pneumonia and Other Infections of the Respiratory Tract Accompanying Influenza and Measles.* Kimpton H., London, 1921, p.402.

46. Winternitz, M. C.; Waton, I. M.; McNamara, F. P. *The Pathology of Influenza*, Yale University Press, New Haven, CT, 1920.

47. Davies, W. L.; Grunert, R. R.; Haff, R. F.; et al. Antiviral activity of 1-ada mantanamine (amantadine). *Science* **1964**, *144*, 826–863.

48. Oxford, J. S.; Galbraith, A. Anti influenza virus activity of amantadine. *Viral Chemother.* **1984**, *1*, 169–252.

49. Hay, A. J.; Wostenholme, A. J.; Skehel, J. J.; Smith, M. H. The molecular basis of the specific anti-influenza action of amantadine. *EMBO J.***1985**, *4* 3021–3024.

50. Aoki, F. Y.; Sitar, D. S. Clinical pharmacokinetics of amantadine hydrochloride. *Clin. Pharmacokinetics* **1988**, *14*, 35–51.

51. Smorodintsev, A. A.; Zlydnikov, D. M.; Kiseleva, A. M.; Romanov, J. A.; Kazantser, A. P.; Rumovsky, V. I. Evaluation of amantadine in artificially induced A2 and B influenza. *JAMA*, **1970**, *213*, 1448–1454.

52. Oxford, J. S.; Logan, L. S.; Potter, C. W. In vivo selection of an influenza A2 strain resistant to amantadine. *Nature* **1970**, *226*, 82–83.

53. Younkin, S. W.; Betts, R. F.; Roth, F. K.; Gordon Douglas R. Reduction in fever in young adults with influenza A/Brazil 78, H1, N1 infection after treatment with aspirin or amantadine. *Antimicrob. Agents Chemother.* **1983**, *23*, 577–582.

54. Sears, S. D.; Clements, M. L. Protective efficacy of low dose amantadine in adults challenged with wild type influenza A virus. *Antimicrob. Agents Chemother.* **1987**, *31*(10), 1470–1473.

55. Reuman, P. D.; Bernstein, D. I.; Keefer, M. C.; Moung, E. C.; Sherwood, J. R.; Schiff, G. M. Efficacy and safety of low dose amantadine hydrochloride as prophylaxis for influenza A. *Antiviral Res.* **1989**, *11*, 27–40.

56. Kistner, O.; Barrett, P. N.; Mundt, W.; et al. Development of a mammalian cell (Vero) derived candidate influenza virus vaccine. *Vaccine* **1998**, *16*, 960–968.

57. Palache, A. M.; Brands, R.; van Scharrenburg, G. Immunogenicity and reactogenicity of influenza subunit vaccines produced in MDCK cells or fertilised chicken eggs. *J. Infect. Dis. (Suppl. 1)* **1997**, S20–S23.

58. Schild, G. C.; Oxford, J. S. de Jong, J. C.; Webster, R. G. Evidence for host-cell selection of influenza virus antigenic variants. *Nature* **1983**, *303*, 706–709.

59. Oxford, J. S.; Al-Jabri, A.; Lambkin, R.; Palache, A. M.; Fleming, D. M. Non-responders to egg grown influenza vaccine seroconvert after booster immunization with MDCK cell grown vaccine. *Vaccine* **2003**, *21*, 2743–2746.

60. Yuen, K. Y.; Chan, P. K.; Peiris, M.; et al. Clinical features and rapid viral diagnosis of human disease associated with avian influenza A H5N1 virus. *Lancet* **1998**, *351*, 467–471.

61. Shortridge, K. F.; Zhou, N. N.; Guan, Y.; Gao, P.; Ito, T.; Kawaoka, Y.; et al. Characterisation of avian H5N1 influenza viruses from poultry in Hong Kong. *Virology* **1998**, *252*(2), 331–342.

62. Neirynck, S.; Deroo, T.; Saelens, X.; Vanlandschoot, P.; Jou, W. M.; Friers, W. A universal influenza A vaccine based on the extracellular domain of the M2 protein. *Nat. Med.* **1999**, *5*, 1157–1163.

63. Okuda, K.; Ihata, A.; Watabe, S.; Okada, X.; Kamakawa, T.; Hamajima, K.; Yang, J.; Ishii, N.; Nakazama, M.; Okuda, K.; Ohnari, K.; Nakajiwa, K.; Yin, K. Q. *Vaccine*, **2001**, *19*, 3681–3691.

64. Yegerlehner, A.; Schmitz, N.; Storni, T.; Bachmann, M. F. Influenza A vaccine based on the extracellular domain of M2: weak protection mediated, via antibody dependent NK cell activity. *J. Immunol.* **2004**, 5598–5605.

65. Heinen, P. P.; Rijsewijk, F. A.; de Boer-Luijtze, E. A.; Bianchi, A. Vaccination of pigs with a DNA construct expressing an influenza virus M2-nucleoprotein fusion protein exacerbates disease after challenge with influenza A virus. *J. Gen. Virol.* **2002**, *83*, 1851–1859.

66. Rayner, J. O.; Dryga, S. A.; Kamrud, K. I. Alpha virus vectors and vaccination. *Rev. Med. Virol.* **2002**, *12*, 279–296.

67. Koopmans, M.; Fouchier, R.; Wilbrink, B.; Meijer, A.; Natrop, G.; Osterhaus, A. D.; et al. Update on human infections with highly pathogenic avian influenza virus A/H7N7 during an outbreak in poultry in the Netherlands. *Eurosurveill. Weekly* **2003**, 7(18).

68. Fouchier, R. A.; Schneeberger, P. M.; Rozendaal, F. W.; et al. Avian influenza A virus (H7N7) associated with human conjunctivitis and a fatal case of acute respiratory distress syndrome. *Proc. Natl. Acad. Sci. U.S.A.* **2004**, *101*, 1356–1361.

69. Taubenberger, J. K. Fixed and frozen flu: the 1918 influenza and lessons for the future. *Avian Dis.* **2003**, *47*, 789–791.

70. Meltzer, M. I.; Cox, N. J.; Fukuda, K. The economic impact of pandemic influenza in the U.S.: priorities for intervention. *Emerging Infect. Dis.* **1999**, *5*, 659–671.

71. Hammond, J. A. R.; Rolland, W.; Shore, T. H. G. Purulent bronchitis: a study of cases occurring amongst the British troops at a base in France. *Lancet* **1917**, *2*, 41–45.

72. Brittain, V. *Testament of Youth*, Penguin Books, London, 1989.

73. Oxford, J. S. The so-called Great Spanish Influenza Pandemic of 1918 may have originated in France in 1916. *Philos. Trans. R. Soc. London* **2002**, *356*, 1857–1859.

74. Abrahams, A.; Hallow, N. F.; Eyre, J. W. H.; French, H. Purulent bronchitis, its influenza and pneumococcal bacteriology. *Lancet* **1917**, *2*, 377–380.

75. Abrahams, A.; Hallow, N.; French, H. A further investigation into influenza pneumo-coccal and influenza-streptococcal septicaemia and epidemic influenzal pneumonia of highly fatal type and its relation to purulent bronchitis. *Lancet* **1919**, *1*, 1–9.

76. Ward, A. C. Virulence of influenza A virus for mouse lung. *Virus Genes* **1997**, *14*, 187–194.

77. Neumann, G.; Kawaoka, Y. Genetic engineering of influenza and other negative strand RNA viruses containing segmented genomes. *Adv. Virus Res.* **1999** *53*, 265–300.

78. Fodor, E.; Devenish, L.; Engelhardt, O. G.; Palese, P.; Brownlee, G. G.; Garcia-Sastre, A. Rescue of influenza A virus from recombinant DNA. *J. Virol.* **1999**, *73*, 9679–9682.

79. Oxford, J. S.; McGeoch, D. J.; et al. Analysis of virion RNA segments and polypeptides of influenza A virus recombinants of defined virulence. *Nature* **1978**, *273*, 778–779.

80. Oxford, J. S.; Schild, G. C.; et al. A host cell-selected variant of influenza B virus with a single nucleotide substitution in HA affecting a potential glycosylation site was attenuated in virulence for volunteers. *Arch. Virol.* **1990**, *X*(1-2), 37–46.

81. Carr, J.; Ives, J.; Kelly, L.; Lambkin, R.; Oxford, J. S.; Mendel, D.; Tai, L.; Roberts, N. Influenza virus carrying neuraminidase with reduced sensitivity to oseltamivir carboxylate has altered properties in vitro and is compromised for infectivity and replicative ability in vivo. Antiviral Res. **2002**, *54*, 79–88.

82. Reid, A. H.; Fanning, T.; Hulktin, J. V.; Taubenberger, J. K. *Proc. Natl. Acad. Sci. U.S.A.* **1999**, *96*, 1651–1656.

83. Bosch, F. X.; Garten, W.; Klenk, H. D.; Rott, R. Proteolytic cleavage of influenza virus hemagglutinins: primary structure of the connecting peptide between HA1 and HA2 determines proteolytic cleavability and pathogenicity of avian influenza viruses. *Virology* **1981**, *113*(2), 725–735.

84. Subbarao, E.; Perkins, M.; Treanor, J.; Murphy, R. The attenuation phenotype conferred by the M gene of the influenza A/Ann Arbor/6/60 cold-adapted virus (H2N2) on the A/Korea/82 (H3N2) reassortant virus results from a gene constellation effect. *Virus Res.* **1993**, *25*, 37–50.

85. Brown, E.; Liu, H.; Kit, I.; Baird, S.; Nesrallah, M. Pattern of mutation in the genome of influenza A virus on adaptation to increased virulence in the mouse lung: identification of functional themes. *Proc. Natl. Acad. Sci. U.S.A.* **2001**, *98*, 6883–6888.

86. Govorkova, E. A.; Gambaryan, A. S.; Clans, E. C.; Smirnov, Y. A. Amino acid changes in the hemagglutinin and matrix proteins of influenza A (H2) viruses adapted to mice. *Acta Virol.* **2002**, *44*, 241–248.

87. Smeenk, C. A.; Wright, K. E.; Burns, B. F.; Thaker, A. J.; Brown, E. G. Mutation in the hemagglutinin and matrix genes of a virulent influenza virus variant. A/FM/147-MA, control different stages in pathogenesis. *Virus Res.* **1996**, *44*, 79–95.

88. Yasuda, J.; Bucher, D. J.; Ishihama, A. Growth control of influenza A virus by M1 protein: analysis of transfectant viruses carrying the chimeric M gene. *J. Virol.* **1994**, *68*, 8141–8146.

89. Bui, M.; Wills, E. G.; Helenius A.; Whittaker, G. R. Role of the influenza virus M1 protein in nuclear export of viral ribonucleoproteins. *J. Virol.* **2000**, *74*, 1781–1786.

90. Zvonarjev, A. Y.;Ghendon, Y. Z. Influence of membrane (M) protein on influenza A virus virion transcriptase activity in vitro and its susceptibility to rimantadine. *J. Virol.* **1980**, *33*, 583–586.

91. Reid, A. H.; Janczewski, T. A.; Lourens, R. M.; Elliot, A. J.; Daniels, R. S.; Berry, C. L.; Oxford, J. S.; Taubenberger, J. K. Influenza pandemic caused by highly conserved viruses with two receptor-binding variants. *Emerging Infect. Dis.* **2003**, *9*, 1249–1253.

92. Mitnaul, L. J.; Matrosovich, M. N.; Castrucci, M. R.; Tuzikov, A. B.; Bovin, N. V.; Kobasa, D.; Kawaoka, Y. Balanced haemagglutinin and neuraminidase activities are critical for efficient replication of influenza A virus. *J. Virol.* **2000**, *74*(13), 6015–6020.

93. Tumpey, T. M.; Garcia-Sastre, A.; Taubenberger, J. K.; Palese, C.; Swayne, D. E.; Baster, C. F. Pathogenicity and immunogenicity of influenza viruses with genes from the 1918 pandemic virus. *Proc. Nat. Acad. Sci.* **2004**.

94. Taubenberger, J. K.; Reid, A. W. The 1918 Spanish influenza pandemic and characteristics of the virus that caused it. In *Influenza*, Potter, C. W. (ed). Elsevier Science, 2002, p. 237.

95. Stevens, J.; Cooper, A. L.; Baster, C. F.; Taubenberger, J. K.; Palese, P.; Wilson, I. A. Structure of the uncleaved human H1 haemogglutinin from the extinct 1918 influenza virus. *Science* **2004**, *303*, 1787–1788.

96. Gamblin, S, J.; Haire, L. F.; Russell, R J.; Stevens, D. J.; Xiao, B.; Ha, Y.; Visishi, N.; Steinhover, D. A.; Daniels, R. S.; Elliott, A.; Wiley, D. C.; Skehel, J. J. The structure and receptor binding properties of the 1918 influenza haemogglutinin. *Science* **2004**, *303*, 1838–1842.

97. Wiley, D. C.; Skehel, J. J. The structure and function of the haemogglutinin membrane glycoprotein of influenza virus. *Ann. Rev. Biochem.* **1987**, *56*, 365–394.

98. Gubareva, L. V.; Matrosovich, M. N.; Brenner, M. K.; Bethall, R. C.; Webster, R. G. Evidence for zanamivir resistance in an immune compromised child infected with influenza B virus. *J. Infect. Dis.* **1998**, 1257–1262.

99. Nakajima, K.; Desselberger, U.; Palese, P. Recent human influenza A (H1N1) viruses are closely related genetically to strains isolated in 1950. *Nature* **1978**, *276*, 334–339.

100. Churchill, Winston S. (Ed.) *The Best of Winston Churchill's Speeches*. Pimlico Press, 2004, p. 524.

101. Hoffman, E.; Neumann, G.; Kawaoka, Y.; Hobom, G.; Webster, R. G. A DNA transfection system for generation of influenza A virus from eight plasmids. *Proc. Natl. Acad. Sci. U.S.A.* **2000** 97(11), 6108–6113.

102. Hoffman, E.; Krauss, S.; Perez, D.; Webby, R.; Webster, R. Eight-plasmid system for rapid generation of influenza virus vaccines. *Vaccine* **2002**, *20*(25-26), 3165–3170.

103. Schickli, J. H.; Flandorfer, A.; Nakaya, T.; Martinez-Sobrido, L.; Garcia-Sastre, A.; Palese, P. Plasmid-only rescue of influenza A virus vaccine candidates. *Philos. Trans. R. Soc. London B* **2001**, *356*(1416), 1965–1973.

EMERGING
INFECTIOUS DISEASES

A Peer-Reviewed Journal Tracking and Analyzing Disease Trends   Vol.8, No.7, July 2002

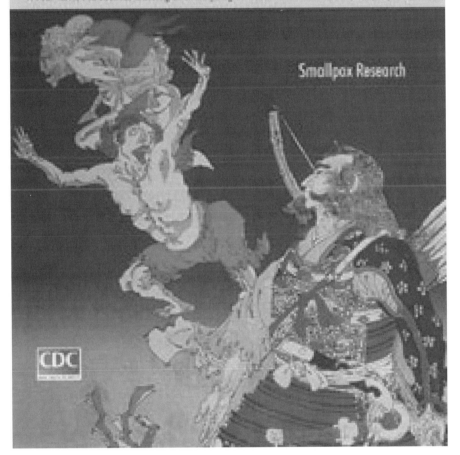

Smallpox Research

CDC

CHAPTER 14

Discovery and Development of New Antivirals for Smallpox

EARL R. KERN

Department of Pediatrics, Division of Infectious Diseases, The University of Alabama at Birmingham

14.1 INTRODUCTION AND BACKGROUND

Smallpox was eradicated worldwide in 1980, and routine vaccination against this dreaded disease was discontinued about the same time, in part due to complications from the vaccine. In recent years there has been increasing concern that variola virus, the causative agent of smallpox or a similar virus, monkeypox virus, may be a potential threat as a weapon of bioterrorism.[1–6] Since these viruses were not previously presumed to be a threat in the past, little efforts were expended in developing new and better vaccines or antiviral therapies. The only well-studied chemotherapeutic agents for treatment of smallpox were the isatin-β-thiosemicar-bazones, particularly the methyl derivative termed methisazone (marboran), which were reported to have activity in animal models[7–9] and in human disease.[10,11] Efficacy was generally considered to be achieved only through prophylaxis and interest in these compounds dwindled over the years. Although there has been only a low level of interest for the past 30 years in developing therapies for smallpox, a few active compounds, including interferon and interferon inducers,[12] and a variety of nucleosides have been reported to have activity against vaccinia virus.[12–19]

The potential use of variola virus or another orthopoxvirus such as monkeypox virus as a bioterrorism weapon, however, has heightened our awareness as to our vulnerability to this disease. This potential threat has resulted in a resurgent effort to identify and develop agents that can be used in an emergency situation to treat these candidate viral diseases. Since there is little incentive for industry to spend hundreds of millions of dollars to develop a drug against a disease that currently

Antiviral Drug Discovery for Emerging Diseases and Bioterrorism Threats. Edited by Paul F. Torrence
Copyright © 2005 John Wiley & Sons, Inc.

does not exist, the emphasis has been on identifying antiviral agents that are already approved for another indication. One such compound, cidofovir (CDV), is approved for intravenous use in the treatment of cytomegalovirus (CMV) retinitis in HIV-infected patients. The drug is very active in tissue culture cells against all the orthopoxviruses that have been tested including vaccinia, cowpox, monkeypox, and variola viruses.[14,15,18–21] The activity of CDV against orthopoxviruses is of particular interest since the compound has been shown to be active in animal models infected with vaccinia virus (VV) and cowpox virus (CV).[16,19,22–26] Importantly, it has recently been reported to be highly effective in treating monkeys infected with variola or monkeypox viruses.[27]

Although CDV is a highly effective inhibitor of orthopoxvirus replication, it is absorbed poorly when administered orally.[28,29] The lack of oral bioavailability is a major limitation to the use of this drug in a large-scale emergency situation such as a smallpox outbreak. While this does not preclude the use of CDV under those conditions, and the drug is approved for use in the treatment of smallpox and complications of vaccination, it does present some challenging logistical problems. Its toxicity and lack of oral activity provide a rationale for the discovery and development of new orally active chemotherapeutic agents for treatment and/or prevention of orthopoxvirus infections whether acquired in a natural setting or through bioterrorism activities.

There are a number of issues that should be considered in the development of a drug for use in a situation such as smallpox when the target population includes all members of society including children and immunocompromised patients. In addition to being active orally, the drug should have a long intracellular half-life so administration can be infrequent and of course have a toxicity profile that is acceptable for all individuals. Additionally, since the drug will need to be stock-piled for a future potential need, it needs to be inexpensive and highly stable under a variety of storage conditions.

The purpose of this chapter is to review recent progress in the development of new agents or modification of existing compounds such as CDV for orthopox-virus infections. The chapter is organized somewhat into nucleoside analogues, cidofovir, nucleoside phosphonate analogues, and the ether lipid ester prodrugs of cidofovir.

14.2   NUCLEOSIDE ANALOGUES

There are numerous nucleoside analogues that have been reported to have antiviral activity against VV.[18] Since there is little incentive to develop a new drug for use in orthopoxvirus infection, we have evaluated most of the antiviral drugs for their activity against VV and CV that have been either licensed for use for some other indication or have been through advanced clinical studies.[30] Those drugs with significant poxvirus activity are listed in Table 14.1 and include drugs approved primarily for herpesvirus or human immunodeficiency virus (HIV) infections. For

TABLE 14.1   Activity of Nucleoside Analogues Against Vaccinia and Cowpox Viruses in HFF Cells

Compound	Cytotoxicity CC_{50} (μM)	Vaccinia Copenhagen		Cowpox Brighton	
		EC_{50}(μM)	SI	EC_{50} (μM)	SI
Cidofovir	>317	31 ± 5.4	>10	42 ± 5.4	>7.5
Idoxuridine	>260	6.0 ± 0.2	>43	2.0 ± 0.2	>130
Trifluridine	>338	1.7	>199	1.5	>225
Vidarabine	>351	12	>29	45	>8
Fialuridine	>269	1.5 ± 0.05	>179	0.2 ± 0.08	>1345
Adefovir dipivoxil	117	5.1 ± 0.7	23	13 ± 8.8	9.0

Source: Adapted from Kern.[30]

the HIV inhibitors, we tested representative compounds for nucleoside reverse transcriptase inhibitors, non-nucleoside reverse transcriptase inhibitors, and protease inhibitors. The compounds that exhibited the greatest activity against the two poxviruses were CDV, idoxuridine, trifluridine, vidarabine, fialuridine, and adefovir dipivoxil. As mentioned previously, CDV is the most promising candidate on this list. Although long-term administration results in significant nephrotoxicity,[31] its use for a smallpox outbreak would be infrequent and short-term and, under these conditions, its toxicity may not be an issue;[32] however its need for parenteral administration remains a logistical limitation. Idoxuridine and trifluridine, which are both approved for topical treatment of herpes simplex virus (HSV) keratitis, do not have a sufficient toxicology database to support parenteral use. Vidarabine, the first parenteral therapy approved for serious herpesvirus infections, is not active orally and was not very active in murine models for VV or CV infections (E.R. Kern, unpublished data).[33]

The results also indicated that adefovir dipivoxil and fialuridine were active candidates. Although fialuridine is very active in tissue culture, its lack of activity in mouse models of VV[33] and its previous toxicity history in treatment of hepatitis in humans probably precludes it as a serious candidate. Adefovir dipivoxil, on the other hand, does appear to be a serious candidate in that it is very active against VV and CV replication in tissue culture, has good oral bioavailability,[34] and has been approved for treatment of hepatitis B. It needs to be evaluated against monkeypox virus and variola virus before its real potential is known. The instability of the compound in mouse plasma has prevented demonstration of activity in VV- or CV-infected mice (E.R. Kern, unpublished data). Another nucleoside analogue, 2-amino-7-[(1,3-dihydroxy-2-propoxy)methyl] purine (S2242), and its orally active prodrug (HOE961) have been reported to be very active against VV and CV in tissue culture and in experimental animal model infections.[35,36] Although these compounds have potential for use in treating orthopoxvirus infections in humans, no clinical studies have been reported.

14.3 CIDOFOVIR

Cidofovir, which is licensed for use in treatment of cytomegalovirus retinitis in AIDS patients, was first reported to have activity against VV in vitro by De Clercq et al.[15] and has been the subject of a number of reviews.[18,32,37,38]

In our studies, we have confirmed the in vitro efficacy of CDV[21,30,39] and utilized CV and VV infections in normal and immunocompromised mice to determine the in vivo efficacy of CDV.[26] Viruses were administered systemically by intraperitoneal (i.p.) inoculation or by the respiratory route using intranasal instillation. Treatments were administered 24–96 h after virus inoculation by using several dosage levels of CDV in order to determine its effectiveness under suboptimal conditions. To determine if CDV could be utilized prophylactically or as postexposure therapy, we evaluated single-dose administration given at various time intervals either prior to infection or postinfection and also determined the efficacy of multiple interval dose administration. In our initial experiments, three-week-old BALB/c mice were inoculated intranasally with CV and treated i.p. once daily for 7 days with 60, 20, or 6.7 mg of CDV/kg of body weight beginning 24, 48, or 72 h after infection. The effect of treatment on the mortality of these mice is summarized in Table 14.2. Placebo-treated animals had a 93% mortality rate and 6.7 mg/kg of CDV significantly reduced mortality even if treatment was delayed until 48–72 h postinfection. When mice were inoculated with VV, results similar to those described above for CV were obtained; however, significant protection against mortality was

TABLE 14.2   Effect of Treatment with CDV on Mortality of BALB/c Mice Inoculated with Cowpox or Vaccinia Virus

Virus	Treatment	Mortality Rate (%)	p	MDD[a]	p
Cowpox	Placebo—saline	14/15 (93)		10.3	
	CDV				
	6.7 mg/kg + 48 h	6/15 (40)	<0.01	12.3	NS[b]
	2.2 mg/kg + 48 h	14/15 (93)	NS	11.2	NS
	6.7 mg/kg + 72 h	8/15 (53)	<0.05	10.8	NS
	2.2 mg/kg + 72 h	10/15 (67)	NS	12.2	<0.05
Vaccinia	Placebo—Saline	15/15 (100)		6.7	
	CDV				
	2.2 mg/kg + 48 h	1/15 (7)	<0.001	7	NS
	0.7 mg/kg + 48 h	6/15 (40)	<0.001	8.3	NS
	2.2 mg/kg + 72 h	6/15 (40)	<0.01	7.3	NS
	0.7 mg/kg + 72 h	10/15 (67)	0.05	7.7	NS
	6.7 mg/kg + 96 h	6/15 (40)	<0.01	8.5	NS
	2.2 mg/kg + 96 h	15/15 (100)	NS	8.3	NS

[a]MDD, mean day of death.
[b]NS, not significant when compared to the placebo control.
Source: Adapted from Quenelle et al.[26]

TABLE 14.3   Effect of Interval Treatment with CDV on Mortality of BALB/c Mice Inoculated with Cowpox Virus

Treatment	Mortality Rate (%)	p	MDD	p
Placebo				
+48 h	14/15 (93)	—	10.1	—
+72 h	14/14 (100)	—	9.3	—
CDV once daily				
6.7 mg/kg+72 h	1/15 (7)	<0.001	11.0	0.07
2 mg/kg+72 h	5/15 (33)	<0.001	15.4	0.001
CDV every 48 h				
6.7 mg/kg+72 h	1/15 (7)	<0.001	15.0	0.07
2 mg/kg+72 h	8/15 (53)	<0.01	11.4	<0.01
CDV every 72 h				
6.7 mg/kg+72 h	0/15 (0)	<0.001	—	—
2 mg/kg+72 h	11/15 (79)	NS[a]	12.8	<0.001

[a]NS, not significant when compared to the placebo control.
Source: Adapted from Quenelle et al.[26]

observed at concentrations of CDV as low as 0.7–6.7 mg/kg. Significant protection could be obtained even if therapy was delayed until 72–96 h postinfection (Table 14.2).

Since daily intravenous administration of CDV under emergency conditions would be logistically difficult and is associated with nephrotoxicity, we also determined if dosing two to three times weekly would be effective. BALB/c mice were inoculated intranasally with CV and treated with CDV either once daily for 7 days, every other day, or every third day to determine the efficacy of interval treatments with lower dosages of CDV. The results in Table 14.3 clearly indicate the protective effects of interval dosing, even with suboptimal levels of CDV and even when delayed up to 72 h postinfection. Since CDV has the unique property of having a long intracellular half-life of about 15–65 h, we next determined how long a single dose of CDV would retain efficacy when given either 5, 3, or 1 day prior to CV infection or if administered 1 or 3 days after infection. The results summarized in Table 14.4 indicate that a single dose of 100 mg of CDV/kg provided significant protection when given any time from day −5 to day +3. The 30 mg/kg dose was highly effective when given at day −3 to day +3. The 10 mg/kg dose was most effective when given at day −1 to day +3, and the 3 mg/kg dose was most effective when given at day 1. Similar results were obtained when mice were infected with VV and treated as described above (Table 14.4). These results indicate that the effectiveness of CDV in these animal models is retained for at least 5 days after a single treatment and is dose related.

Acquisition of smallpox or vaccination with VV in an immunocompromised host can result in serious morbidity and even mortality. As a model for the immuno-compromised host with disseminated orthopoxvirus disease, we have used SCID mice inoculated i.p. with either CV or VV. Groups of 6- to 8-week-old SCID mice

TABLE 14.4 Effect of Single-Dose CDV on Mortality of BALB/c Mice Inoculated with Cowpox or Vaccinia Viruses

	Cowpox Virus		Vaccinia Virus	
Treatment	Mortality Rate (%)	p	Mortality Rate (%)	p
None	12/15 (80)	—	15/15 (100)	—
Placebo	15/15 (100)	—	14/15 (93)	—
Day+1				
CDV				
Day −5				
100 mg/kg	8/15 (53)	<0.01	1/15 (7)	<0.001
Day −3				
100 mg/kg	2/15 (13)	<0.001	2/15 (13)	<0.001
30 mg/kg	3/15 (20)	<0.001	7/15 (47)	0.01
Day −1				
10 mg/kg	5/15 (33)	<0.001	2/15 (13)	<0.001
3 mg/kg	8/15 (53)	<0.01	12/15 (80)	NS[a]
Day+1				
10 mg/kg	7/15 (47)	<0.01	0/15 (0)	<0.001
3 mg/kg	12/15 (80)	NS	4/15 (27)	<0.001
Day+3				
10 mg/kg	4/15 (27)	<0.001	0/15 (0)	<0.001
3 mg/kg	13/15 (87)	NS	8/15 (53)	<0.05

[a]NS, not significant when compared to the placebo control.
Source: Adapted from Quenelle et al.[26]

were inoculated with either CV or VV and treated once daily for 7 days with 20, 6.7, or 2.2 mg of CDV/kg beginning 48, 72, or 96 h after infection. In all the treatment groups, there was essentially 100% mortality; however, the mean day of death (MDD) was significantly prolonged in most groups and particularly for mice infected with VV.[26] To determine if the extended MDD was associated with reduced viral replication in critical target organs, SCID mice were inoculated i.p. with a lethal concentration of CV and treated with CDV three times weekly for 30 days. Treatment was started at 96 h after infection to ensure that viral replication in target organs was maximal prior to initiation of treatment. At various times after infection, tissues were harvested and assayed for the presence of the virus (Figure 14.1). Although there were no alterations of final mortality rates, mice treated with CDV had significantly reduced titers of virus in the four tissues tested. In the lung, peak CV titers were the same in both placebo- and CDV-treated mice; however, virus replication was delayed by about 21 days. There was a dramatic reduction in viral load in liver, spleen, and kidney tissue to low but still detectable levels at 21–31 days in treated mice. These results suggest that to alter poxvirus replication in an immunocompromised host, long-term therapy will be needed to control virus replication. Since there was persistence of CV in all organs and high levels of replication in lung tissue while CDV was being administered, a similar

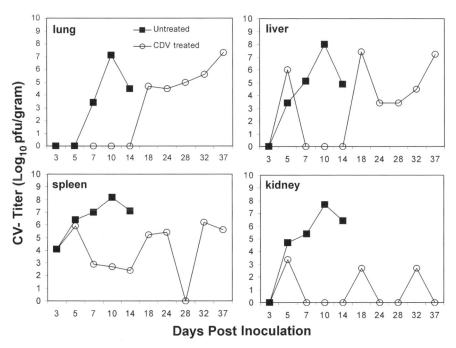

FIGURE 14.1   Alteration of cowpox virus replication in tissues of SCID mice treated with cidofovir.

experiment was conducted to determine if resistance to CDV was developing in these mice. Results indicated that resistance to CDV did not develop during the 30 days of CDV treatment and suggested that failure of CDV to protect against mortality in SCID mice was due to their inability to clear the virus because of their immunodeficient state,[26] and that once therapy was discontinued, virus replication immediately resumed and subsequently killed the animal.

These studies confirm and expand upon previous reports of CDV efficacy in murine models of systemic orthopoxvirus infections.[22–25,40–42] Our results indicated that CDV given systemically as late as 96 h after CV or VV inoculation can protect BALB/c mice from death or delay the time to death in a dose- and time-dependent manner. Since CDV is not effective when given orally, this delay in initiating therapy is necessary for attempting to plan postexposure intravenous treatments for potentially large numbers of people if an actual bioterrorist event occurred. Bray et al.[22] reported similarly that a single treatment with 100 mg of CDV/kg i.p. on day 0, 2, or 4 after aerosol exposure to cowpox virus increased survival of BALB/c mice to 90–100%. Smee et al.[40] reported that a single dose of 10 mg of CDV/kg administered intranasally (i.n.) at +24 h protected mice inoculated i.n. with CV. In our studies, a single dose of 3–100 mg/kg provided protection if given 5 days prior to infection or up to 3 days after infection. Bray et al.[22] also reported that CDV increased the MDD of SCID mice but did not protect them from mortality from CV infections. Our studies confirm these observations and further indicate that viral replication is significantly reduced in target organs of SCID mice while on treatment. Our results with CV mirror those of Neyts and De Clercq,[19] who reported reduced viral titers in lung, kidney, and liver of VV-infected SCID mice treated with CDV. The most appropriate animal model for studying smallpox and monkeypox infections is nonhuman primates inoculated with either variola or monkeypox viruses. In these two experimental infections, cidofovir was highly effective in reducing viral replication and lesion development.[27]

Collectively, these data indicate that CDV is able to significantly reduce mortality in mice exposed to VV or CV when given as late as 96 h postinoculation. For protection from death, CDV can be reduced to one single dose or one to three smaller doses. Protection from infection can also be conferred by pretreatment with CDV as early as 5 days prior to exposure. The results obtained for SCID mice suggest that long-term treatments may be necessary for protecting immunocompromised individuals. These collective results have major implications, as they suggest that CDV, in addition to being effective as a treatment for smallpox or vaccine complications, can be used for pre- or postexposure prophylaxis of smallpox contacts (i.e., ring treatment) and that a single dose may provide significant protection. From these data it is clear that the effect of CDV is long lasting and may translate to short-term or single-dose treatment for smallpox or other orthopoxvirus infections.

14.4 ACYCLIC NUCLEOSIDE PHOSPHONATE ANALOGUES

Since CDV is one of the few well-characterized compounds with good activity against the orthopoxviruses, we have also evaluated a large number of other acyclic nucleoside phosphonates for their activity against VV and CV replication in vitro, and the results are presented in Table 14.5. A number of these compounds have been described previously by De Clercq and his colleagues and are reviewed by

TABLE 14.5 Efficacy and Cytotoxicity of Phosphonate Nucleotides Against Vaccinia and Cowpox Viruses in HFF Cells

Compound	Cytotoxicity CC_{50} (μM)	Vaccinia Virus EC_{50} (μM)	SI^a	Cowpox Virus EC_{50} (μM)	SI
HPMPC (CDV)	278±9.2	33±9.1	8	43±2.5	7
Cyclic HPMPC (cHPMPC)	>302±0	38±11	>8	48±8.0	>6
S-HPMPA	269±21	3.5±2.8	77	5.0±4.7	54
PMEA	>366±0	>366±0	—	>366±0	—
PMEDAP	>339±12	204±15	—	>347±0	—
PMPA	>300	>300	—	>300	—
PMEG	88	4.0±0.7	22	11.4+1.3	8

$^a SI = CC_{50}/EC_{50}$.
Source: Adapted from Kern.[30]

De Clercq.[18] In the CDV series, there are a number of prodrugs that have equal or greater activity against VV and CV than CDV; however, little is known about their toxicity or pharmacokinetics at the present time. The adenine analogue S-HPMPA [(S)-9-(3-hydroxy-2-phosphonylmethoxypropyl)adenine] was about tenfold more active than CDV, an observation that confirms earlier data of De Clercq et al.[15] Of special interest is the fact that S-HPMPA has been reported to have activity against monkeypox and variola viruses at concentrations similar to those reported here for VV and CV.[20] In the PMEA [9-(2-phosphonylmethoxyethyl) adenine] (adefovir) series, PMEA itself was not active. Similarly, the 2-phosphonylmethoxyethyl diaminopurine analogue of PMEA (PMEDAP), and the (R)-9-(2-phosphonylmethoxypropyl)adenine analogue (PMPA) (tenofovir) was inactive against VV and CV. In contrast, the 2-phosphonylmethoxyethyl guanine (PMEG) analogue was very active. From our findings it appears that the compounds that merit additional studies include S-HPMPA, adefovir dipivoxil, and PMEG, as well as additional prodrugs of these nucleoside phosphonates. The major drawback to the development of one of these prodrugs is that little is known about their potential toxicology or their absorption, distribution, metabolism, or excretion in animals or humans and they would require all the same steps necessary for development of a new drug.

The effectiveness of this group of compounds as antiviral agents and the continuing need to discover and develop compounds that may prove useful against orthopoxvirus infections have led to our evaluation of a variety of the prodrugs of CDV, S-HPMPA, PMEA, PMEDAP, or PMPA and/or related substituted analogues against two orthopoxviruses, VV and CV.[39] The results of these studies can provide new information regarding new active compounds that may also be active orally and could be candidates for development as new therapeutic agents for poxvirus infections. In this series of studies, we first determined the activity of a variety of CDV (HPMPC) analogues (Table 14.6). CDV, cyclic CDV (cHPMPC), and 2-(butyl-oxycarbonyl) phenyl cHPMPC had similar 50% effective concentration (EC$_{50}$) and SI values for both VV and CV in HFF cells. As indicated from previous studies,[15,43] S-HPMPA was active against VV and, as determined in our studies, was also effective against CV and was the most active compound in this series. Both (phenethyl L-alaninyl) cHPMPC (mixture of diastereomers) and (butyl L-alaninyl) cHPMPC were five- to sevenfold more active than HPMPC. In the PMEA series, PMEA itself was not active against VV or CV, but an orally active prodrug, bis[(pivaloyl)oxymethyl] PMEA (adefovir dipivoxil), was very active as was bis(butyl L-alaninyl) PMEA, with EC$_{50}$ values of 4.4–13 µM. Similarly, the 2,6-diaminopurine analogue of PMEA (PMEDAP) was inactive, whereas all the prodrugs were efficacious against VV, but less active against CV. Antiviral activity was greatest for bis(butyl L-alaninyl) PME-N6-(cyclopropyl)DAP and (isopropyl L-alaninyl) phenyl PME-N6-(cyclopropyl)DAP. Not unexpectedly, the compounds with the best antiviral activities were generally the most toxic. PMPA and its oral prodrug tenofovir disoproxil fumarate {bis[(isopropoxycarbonyl)oxymethyl]PMPA} were both inactive against VV and CV replication, and the prodrug (isopropyl L-alaninyl) phenyl PMPA was only marginally active.

TABLE 14.6   Efficacy and Cytotoxicity of HPMPC, S-HPMPA, PMEA, PMEDAP, PMPA, and Selected Prodrugs Against Vaccinia and Cowpox Viruses in HFF Cells

Compound	Cytotoxicity	Vaccinia Virus		Cowpox Virus	
	CC_{50} (µM)	EC_{50}(µM)	SI	EC_{50}(µM)	SI
HPMPC (CDV)	278 ± 9.2	33 ± 9.1	8.4	43 ± 2.5	6.5
cHPMPC	$>302 \pm 0$	38 ± 11	>7.9	48 ± 8.0	>6.3
2-(Butyloxycarbonyl)phenylcHPMPC	$>213 \pm 22$	32 ± 13	>6.7	34 ± 4.2	>6.3
(Butyl L-alaninyl)cHPMPC	$>153 \pm 57$	4.6 ± 0.8	>33	8.4 ± 5.3	>18
(Phenethyl L-alaninyl)cHPMPC (mixed iastereomers)	207 ± 18	7.1 ± 0.3	29	6.8 ± 1.8	30
(S)-HPMPA	269 ± 21	3.5 ± 2.8	77	5.0 ± 4.7	54
PMEA	$>366 \pm 0$	$>366 \pm 0$	—	$>366 \pm 0$	—
Bis[(pivaloyl)oxymethyl]PMEA	117 ± 27	5.1 ± 0.7	23	13 ± 8.8	9.0
Bis (butyl L-alaninyl)PMEA	100 ± 27	4.4 ± 0.2	23	10 ± 8.2	10
PMEDAP	$>339 \pm 12$	204 ± 15	1.7	$>347 \pm 0$	—
PME-N6-(cyclopropyl) DAP	$>263 \pm 59$	23 ± 6.9	>11	28 ± 13	>9.4
Bis(butyl L-alaninyl) PME-N6-(cyclopropyl) DAP	49 ± 33	0.08 ± 0.01	613	0.26 ± 0.2	189
(Isopropyl L-alaninyl) phenyl-PME-N6-(cyclopropyl)DAP	$>209 \pm 69$	1.1 ± 0.3	>190	2.6 ± 1.9	>80
PME-N6-(trifluoroethyl)DAP	$>270 \pm 0$	42 ± 11	>6.4	$>270 \pm 0$	—
PME-N6-(dimethyl)DAP	$>316 \pm 0$	35 ± 1.6	>9.0	53 ± 8.3	>6.0
PME-N6-(2-propenyl)DAP	$>305 \pm 0$	25 ± 0.9	>12	115 ± 78	>2.7
PMPA	>300	>300	—	>300	—
Bis[(isopropoxycarbonyl) oxymethyl]PMPA	>157.4	>157.4	—	>157.4	—
(Isopropyl L-alaninyl)phenyl PMPA	>143	23.5	>6.1	98.9	>1.4

[a]$SI=CC_{50}/EC_{50}$
Source: Adapted from Keith, et al.[39]

The results of these studies indicate that many of the acyclic nucleoside phosphonate analogues have potent and selective activity against orthopoxvirus infections. In particular, adefovir dipivoxil, which is active and orally bioavailable and is already approved for use in humans, should be considered a high priority for further evaluation as a treatment for smallpox and complications of VV vaccinations.

14.5   DEVELOPMENT OF ALKOXYALKYL ESTER PRODRUGS OF CDV

Previous studies have shown that alkyglycerol phosphate or alkoxypropyl phosphate esters of acyclovir[44] and ganciclovir[45] have greater oral bioavailability in rodents than the parent compounds. Furthermore, these compounds are active orally in animal models of herpesvirus disease[45] and woodchuck hepatitis.[46] To obtain

TABLE 14.7   Activity[a] of CDV and Alkoxyalkyl Analogues Against Cowpox Virus and Strains of Vaccinia Virus

Compound	CV-BR	VV-COP	VV-WR	VV-Elstree	VV-IHD	VV-NYC
CDV	45 ± 6.3	46 ± 12	46 ± 17	42 ± 22	13 ± 6	10 ± 1
HDP-CDV	0.6 ± 0.3	0.8 ± 0.4	1.1 ± 1.0	1.2 ± 0.8	0.2 ± 0.0	0.4 ± 0.0
ODE-CDV	0.3 ± 0.3	0.2 ± 0.1	0.2 ± 0.2	0.4 ± 0.1	0.1 ± 0.0	0.1 ± 0.0

[a]Values are the mean of two assays.
Source: Adapted from Kern et al.[21]

better oral activity with CDV, a new series of analogues was synthesized using two long-chain alkoxyalkanols, hexadecyloxypropyl (HDP-CDV), and octadecyloxyethyl (ODE-CDV), and their activity compared with that of CDV in HFF cells infected with strains of VV or CV.[21] The activity of CDV and the alkoxyalkyl analogues are presented in Table 14.7. Where CDV required about 10–50 μM to inhibit the replication of either CV or VV by 50%, the alkoxyalkyl analogue, HDP-CDV, was active at about 0.6 and ODE-CDV at 0.3 against CV, respectively. The analogues were 75- to 150-fold more active than CDV against CV. All three of the nucleotides were similarly active against five strains of VV; however, the IHD and NYC strains appeared to be more susceptible than the Copenhagen, WR, or Elstree strain. The EC_{50} values for HDP-CDV ranged from 0.20–1.2 μM, while ODE-CDV EC_{50} values were 0.10–0.40 μM, representing 28- to 209-fold increases in activity versus CDV for these same strains. In cytotoxicity assays, the HDP analogue was about ninefold more toxic than CDV and the ODE analogue nineteen-fold more toxic than CDV. The Selective Index (SI) value for CDV was about 6, whereas that for HDP-CDV was about 30, and for ODE-CDV 40–65, indicating that the analogues, although more toxic than the parent compounds, were more efficacious, which resulted in higher SI values. A similar level of enhanced activity of HDP-CDV and ODE-CDV has been reported for variola and monkeypox viruses[30,47] and ectromelia virus.[48] The in vitro studies summarized above have shown multiple-log increases in antiviral activity against orthopoxvirus replication.[21] Enhanced inhibition of cytomegalovirus, herpes simplex virus, and adenovirus replication by HDP-CDV and ODE-CDV has also been reported.[49,50]

In order to evaluate the importance of chain length or linker type, additional analogues were synthesized by esterification of these compounds with an alkyl chain with or without the propoxy- or ethoxy-linker moieties.[51] As presented in Table 14.8, the most active ether lipid esters of CDV were OLE-CDV, ODBG-CDV, TDP-CDV, OLP-CDV, and ODP-CDV, with 50% effective concentration (EC_{50}) values of 0.06–1.2 μM for VV and 0.07–1.9 μM for CV (a 20- to 600-fold increase compared to the results seen with the parent compound). The majority of the new analogues tested were more active than the parent compounds, and structure–activity analysis revealed that alkoxyalkyl or alkyl esters of CDV having chains shorter than 16 atoms beyond the phosphonate moiety of CDV were less active or inactive. Generally, optimal chain lengths were 20 atoms beyond the phosphonate,

TABLE 14.8 Efficacy and Cytotoxicity[a] of Ether Lipid Esters of Cidofovir (CDV)

Compound	Abbreviation	Cytotoxicity CC$_{50}$ (μM)	Vaccinia Virus EC$_{50}$ (μM)	Vaccinia Virus SI[b]	Cowpox Virus EC$_{50}$ (μM)	Cowpox Virus SI
CIDOFOVIR SERIES						
Cidofovir	CDV	>317±0	31±5.4	>10	42±5.4	>7.5
PROPANEDIOL LINKERS						
Dodecyloxypropyl- (16)[c]	DDP-CDV	>190±0	6.6±0.9	>29	16±1.6	>12
Tetradecyloxypropyl- (18)	TDP-CDV	>100±0	0.5±0.2	>200	0.8±0.5	>125
Hexadecyloxypropyl- (20)	HDP-CDV	29±2.3	0.6±0.4	48	0.5±0.3	58
Octadecyloxypropyl- (22)	ODP-CDV	44±14	1.2±0.5	37	1.9±0.6	23
Oleyloxypropyl- (22:1)[c]	OLP-CDV	87±15	0.4±0.2	218	0.6±0.3	145
Eicosyloxypropyl- (24)	ECP-CDV	92±1.4	2.0±0.9	46	2.4±0.7	38
ETHANEDIOL LINKERS						
Octadecyloxyethyl- (21)	ODE-CDV	21±8.8	0.2±0.1	105	0.2±0.2	105
Oleyloxyethyl- (21:1)	OLE-CDV	56±29	0.06±0.02	933	0.07±0.02	800
GLYCEROL LINKER						
1-O-Octadecyl-2-O-benzyl-glyceryl-	ODBG-CDV	47±24	0.4±0.1	118	0.3±0.01	157
NO LINKER						
Eicosyl- (20)	EC-CDV	45±8.5	1.6±1.3	28	1.5±0.9	30
Docosyl- (22)	DC-CDV	73±8.8	10±1.7	7.3	13±0.1	5.6

[a]Values are the mean of two or more assays ± standard deviation.
[b]Selectivity index (SI)=CC$_{50}$/EC$_{50}$.
[c]Values in parentheses are the number of atoms beyond the phosphonate oxygen; the number after the colon is the number of double bonds in the alkyl chain.
Source: Adapted from Keith et al.[51]

with activity declining sharply at 22 and 24 atoms. The oxyethyl analogues of CDV (ODE- and OLE-CDV) were generally more active than their oxypropyl counterparts (ODP- and OLP-CDV) even though they differ in the overall numbers of atoms by only one methylene. The enhancement in activity of the ether lipid esters appear to be due to their greater uptake into cells, resulting in a significant increase of intracellular levels of CDV.[52] As summarized above, a number of these analogues had significantly enhanced activity and selectivity indices, suggesting that the best of these analogues need to be evaluated for their oral efficacy in animal models of orthopoxvirus disease, particularly since the relative oral bioavailability of HDP-CDV and ODE-CDV ranges from 88% to 97%.[53]

A series of studies were then carried out by Quenelle and co-workers[54] to determine the comparative efficacy of parenteral CDV with oral HDP-CDV and ODE-CDV, on CV and VV infections of mice. Since we have reported previously that CDV is highly active in these models when given as single or multiple doses either prior to or after infection, similar studies were carried out with these analogues. In addition, we also determined the effect of oral treatment with HDP-CDV or ODE-CDV on the replication of CV or VV in important target organs. In initial experiments, HDP-CDV or ODE-CDV were administered once daily for 5 consecutive days by oral gavage to CV- or VV-infected mice beginning 24, 48, or 72 h post viral inoculation. CDV was given i.p. at similar doses and times of initiation of therapy. At the 6.7 mg/kg dose, no toxicity was observed and each compound significantly reduced final mortality in CV-infected mice ($p \leq 0.01$) at one or more times of initiation of therapy (Table 14.9). In mice inoculated with VV, both HDP-CDV and ODE-CDV significantly reduced mortality rates when treatment was initiated as late as 48 h post viral inoculation. Treatment with CDV also resulted in significant protection from mortality and at most times of initiation of treatment. In mice infected with ectromelia virus (mousepox), similar results were obtained to those seen above for VV and CV.[48] At 10 mg/kg both analogues gave complete protection, whereas ODE-CDV was more effective at lower dosages than HDP-CDV.

We have reported previously that CDV can protect mice infected with CV or VV when given as early as 5 days prior to infection.[26] HDP-CDV and ODE-CDV were also evaluated for their prophylactic activity by treating mice by oral gavage beginning 5, 3, or 1 day prior to viral inoculation. The results in Table 14.10 indicated that HDP-CDV and ODE-CDV, as well as CDV, were highly protective against mortality due to CV infection when given 1–5 days prior to infection. CDV has also been reported by us and others to significantly reduce mortality of CV- or VV-infected mice with only one or two doses due to the long intracellular half-life of this drug.[22,25,26] In a similar study, we gave HDP-CDV as a single dose on days −5, −3, or −1 prior to or on days +1 or +3 after intranasal CV inoculation. All regimens used provided significant protection from mortality at all times of initiation with both compounds (Table 14.11). In addition, CDV given as a single dose i.p. was also protective at all times of initiation of treatment.

To determine the effect of treatment with HDP-CDV or ODE-CDV on the replication of VV in target organs of mice, animals were inoculated with VV and

TABLE 14.9 Effect of Oral Treatment with HDP-CDV or ODE-CDV on Mortality of BALB/c Mice Inoculated with Cowpox or Vaccinia Virus

Virus	Treatment	Mortality			MDD[a]	p
		Number	Percent	p		
Cowpox	Placebo					
	Saline + 24 h	15/15	100	—	9.7 ± 0.6	—
	CDV					
	6.7 mg/kg + 24 h	0/15	0	<0.001	—	—
	6.7 mg/kg + 48 h	0/15	0	<0.001	—	—
	6.7 mg/kg + 72 h	5/15	33	<0.001	13.2 ± 3.0	<0.01
	Placebo					
	Water + 24 h	15/15	100	—	9.3 ± 0.6	—
	HDP-CDV					
	6.7 mg/kg + 24 h	6/15	40	0.001	9.5 ± 4.8	NS[b]
	6.7 mg/kg + 48 h	12/14	86	NS	10.5 ± 3.7	NS
	6.7 mg/kg + 72 h	7/15	47	<0.01	12.7 ± 3.3	<0.001
	ODE-CDV					
	6.7 mg/kg + 24 h	3/13	23	<0.001	9.3 ± 6.1	NS
	6.7 mg/kg + 48 h	6/14	43	<0.01	12.7 ± 4.9	0.01
	6.7 mg/kg + 72 h	7/13	54	0.02	11.6 ± 4.1	0.07
Vaccinia	Placebo					
	Saline + 24 h	15/15	100	—	6.8 ± 0.4	—
	CDV					
	5 mg/kg + 24 h	0/15	0	<0.001	—	—
	5 mg/kg + 48 h	4/15	27	<0.001	7.8 ± 0.5	0.01
	5 mg/kg + 72 h	0/15	0	<0.001	—	—
	Placebo					
	Water + 24 h	15/15	100	—	6.8 ± 0.7	—
	HDP-CDV					
	5 mg/kg + 24 h	2/14	13	<0.001	11.0 ± 4.2	<0.05
	5 mg/kg + 48 h	10/15	67	<0.05	8.0 ± 1.2	<0.01
	ODE-CDV					
	5 mg/kg + 24 h	0/15	0	<0.001	—	—
	5 mg/kg + 48 h	6/15	40	0.001	8.0 ± 3.0	0.06

[a]MDD, mean day of death ± standard deviation.
[b]NS, not significant when compared to the placebo control.
Source: Adapted from Quenelle et al.[54]

treated orally with 5 mg/kg of HDP-CDV or ODE-CDV once daily for 5 days beginning 24 h after infection. On various days postinfection, animals were euthanized, and tissues were removed and assayed for VV. All of the treatment regimens resulted in a significant reduction in mortality, and a 3–5 $\log_{10}$ decrease in virus titers in liver, spleen, and kidney. There was little alteration in virus titers in lung; however, all treated control mice survived. Similar results were observed with

TABLE 14.10   Effect of Daily Oral Prophylaxis with HDP-CDV or ODE-CDV on Mortality of BALB/c Mice Inoculated with Cowpox Virus

Treatment	Mortality			MDD[a]	p
	Number	Percent	p		
Day −5					
Placebo (Water)	15/15	100	—	10.1 ± 0.8	—
Day −5					
CDV 5 mg/kg	1/15	7	<0.001	17.0 ± 0	0.07
HDP 5 mg/kg	0/15	0	<0.001	—	—
ODE 5 mg/kg	3/15	20	<0.001	5.7 ± 5.5	NS[b]
Day −3					
CDV 5 mg/kg	6/15	40	<0.01	11.0 ± 4.9	0.05
HDP 5 mg/kg	3/13	23	<0.001	15.0 ± 4.0	<0.01
ODE 5 mg/kg	2/15	13	<0.001	11.0 ± 0	0.07
Day −1					
CDV 5 mg/kg	5/15	33	<0.001	11.4 ± 1.7	0.06
HDP 5 mg/kg	6/15	40	<0.01	10.7 ± 0.5	0.06
ODE 5 mg/kg	0/14	0	<0.001	—	—

[a]MDD, mean day of death ± standard deviation.
[b]NS, not significant when compared to the placebo control.
Source: Adapted from Quenelle et al.[54]

CDV given i.p. (Figure 14.2) and also in mice inoculated with CV (54). Inhibition of virus replication in the liver and spleen was also reported for mice infected with ectromelia virus and treated with HDP-CDV or ODE-CDV.[48] However, as described previously for mice infected with CV or VV, there was little alteration of ectromelia virus titers in lung tissue.

It is interesting that even though orally administered HDP-CDV and ODE-CDV were significantly more active than CDV against orthopoxviruses in vitro and were equally effective in reducing viral replication in the liver, spleen, and kidney, they were no more effective than CDV in reducing replication in the lung. In a study by Bray and co-workers, in which CDV was given subcutaneously at 100 mg/kg, there was significantly reduced virus titers in lung.[23] Similarly, when Smee and co-workers administered CDV directly to the lung via aerosol or intranasal instillation, lung titers were also significantly reduced,[24] further suggesting that oral administration of 5–10 mg/kg of HDP-CDV or ODE-CDV in our studies did not achieve sufficient levels of drug in the lung to reduce viral replication, whereas higher concentrations of CDV itself were more effective in the previous studies.

HDP-CDV and ODE-CDV are both orally bioavailable, have high antiviral efficacy, and persist in tissues for a relatively long period of time.[53,54] The present results comparing i.p. CDV with oral HDP-CDV and ODE-CDV show that these compounds when given orally are at least equivalent to CDV given parenterally. Our results are consistent with pharmacokinetic data indicating oral bioavailability and persistence in tissues of up to 72 h after oral administration of HDP-CDV and

TABLE 14.11   Effect of Oral Pre- or Post-Single Dose Treatment with HDP-CDV or ODE-CDV on the Mortality of BALB/c Mice Inoculated with Cowpox Virus

Treatment	Mortality				
	Number	Percent	p	MDD[a]	p
Placebo					
Saline +24 h	9/15	60	—	12.2±2.8	—
Deionized H$_2$O+24 h	7/15	47	—	11.9±2.9	—
Day −5					
CDV 30 mg/kg	4/15	27	<0.05	11.5±2.5	NS[b]
HDP 12.5 mg/kg	3/15	20	<0.05	10.3±2.1	NS
ODE 10 mg/kg	1/15	7	<0.05	11.0±0	NS
Day −3					
CDV 30 mg/kg	6/15	40	NS	11.7±3.9	NS
HDP 12.5 mg/kg	0/15	0	<0.001	—	—
ODE 10 mg/kg	0/15	0	<0.001	—	—
Day −1					
CDV 30 mg/kg	0/15	0	<0.001	—	—
HDP 12.5 mg/kg	0/15	0	<0.001	—	—
ODE 10 mg/kg	2/15	14	<0.05	10.0±1.4	NS
Day+1					
CDV 30 mg/kg	0/15	0	<0.001	—	—
HDP 12.5 mg/kg	0/15	0	<0.001	—	—
ODE 10 mg/kg	1/15	7	<0.05	21.0±0	NS
Day+3					
CDV 30 mg/kg	1/15	7	<0.05	15.0±0	NS
HDP 12.5 mg/kg	2/15	13	<0.05	11.5±2.1	NS
ODE 10 mg/kg	1/15	7	<0.05	16.0±0	NS

[a]MDD, mean day of death ± standard deviation.
[b]NS, not significant when compared to the combined placebo controls.
Source: Adapted from Quenelle et al.[54]

ODE-CDV and persistence of therapeutic drug levels in critical organs of lung, liver, and kidney after a single oral dose of 10 mg/kg. This translates into oral dosing once or twice weekly instead of daily dosing. Since kidney exposure is reported to be low with oral HDP-CDV or ODE-CDV,[53] one would anticipate reduced nephrotoxic adverse events. Oral HDP-CDV and ODE-CDV are at least equivalent to i.p. CDV in these studies and should be effective when used for prophylaxis, postexposure prophylaxis, or treatment for smallpox and other orthopoxviruses including monkeypox, which has become a problem due to unexpected outbreaks and increasing incidences of natural transmission. The compounds should also be effective in treating complications from vaccination with VV.

Although both HDP-CDV and ODE-CDV appeared to have equivalent activity both in vitro and in vivo, the results of adsorption, distribution, metabolism, and

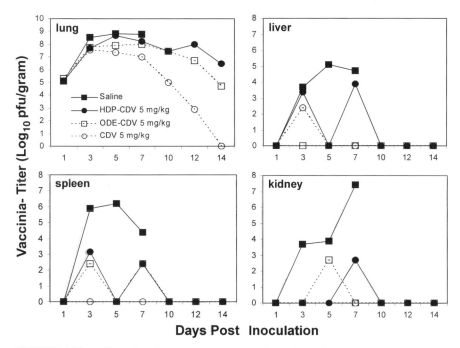

FIGURE 14.2   Effect of oral treatment with HDP-CDV, ODE-CDV, or CDV on pathogenesis of vaccinia virus–IHD infection in mice.

excretion studies have shown a preference for HDP-CDV and this compound should be evaluated in clinical studies in the next few months.

ACKNOWLEDGMENT

The original work performed in the author's laboratory was supported by Contracts NO1-AI-85347 and NO1-AI-15439 from the National Institute of Allergy and Infectious Diseases, National Institutes of Health, Bethesda, Md. The author gratefully acknowledges the excellent assistance of Jena L. Reeves in preparation of the manuscript for this chapter.

REFERENCES

1. Breman, J. G.; Henderson, D. A. Poxvirus delemmas—monkeypox, smallpox, and biological terrorism. *N. Engl. J. Med.* **1998**, *339*, 556–559.

2. Breman, J. G.; Henderson, D. A. Diagnosis and management of smallpox. *N. Engl. J. Med.* **2002**, *346*, 1300–1308.

3. Henderson, D. A. Bioterrorism as a public health threat. *Emerging Infect. Dis.* **1998**, *4*, 488–492.

4. Heymann, D. L.; Szczeniowski, M.; Esteves, K. Re-emergence of monkeypox in Africa: a review of the past six years. *Br. Med. Bull.* **1998**, *54*, 693–702.

5. O'Toole, T. Smallpox: an attack scenario. *Emerging Infect. Dis.* **1999**, *5*, 540–546.

6. Hutin, Y. J.; Williams, R. J.; Malfait, P.; Pebody, R.; Loparev, V. N.; Ropp, S. L.; Rodriguez, M.; Knight, J. C.; Tshioko, F. K.; Khan, A. S.; Szczeniowski, M. V.; Esposito, J. J. Outbreak of human monkeypox, Democratic Republic of Congo, 1996–1997. *Emerging Infect. Dis.* **2001**, *7*, 434–438.

7. Bauer, D. J. The antiviral and synergic actions of isatin thiosemicarbazone and certain phenoxypyrimidines in vaccinia infection in mice. *Br. J. Exp. Pathol.* **1955**, *36*, 105–114.

8. Bauer, D. J.; Sheffield, F. W. Antiviral chemotherapeutic activity of isatin β-thiosemi-carbazone in mice infected with rabbit-pox virus. *Nature* **1959**, *184*(Suppl 19), 1496–1497.

9. Boyle, J. J.; Haff, R. F.; Stewart, R. C. Evaluation of antiviral compounds by suppression of tail lesions in vaccinia-infected mice. *Antimicrob. Agents Chemother* **1966**, *6*, 536–539.

10. Bauer, D. J.; St. Vincent, L.; Kempe, C. H.; Downie, A. W. Prophylactic treatment of smallpox contacts with *N*-methylisatin β-thiosemicarbazone. *Lancet* **1963**, *ii*, 494–496.

11. Bauer, D. J.; St Vincent, L.; Kempe, C. H.; Young, P. A.; Downie, A. W. Prophylaxis of smallpox with methisazone. *Am. J. Epidemiol.* **1969**, *90*, 130–145.

12. De Clercq, E.; De Somer, P. Effect of interferon, polyacrylic acid, and polymethacrylic acid on tail lesions on mice infected with vaccinia virus. *Appl. Microbiol.* **1968**, *16*, 1314–1319.

13. De Clercq, E.; Luczak, M.; Shugar, D.; Torrence, P. F.; Waters, J. A.; Witop, B. Effect of cytosine arabinoside, iododeoxyuridine, ethyldeoxyuridine, thiocyanatodeoxyuridine, and ribavirin on tail lesion formation in mice infected with vaccinia virus. *Proc. Soc. Exp. Biol. Med.* **1976**, *151*, 487–490.

14. De Clercq, E.; Holy, A.; Rosenberg, I.; Sakuma, T.; Balzarini, J.; Maudgal, P. C.. A novel selective broad-spectrum anti-DNA virus agent. *Nature* **1986**, *323*, 464–467.

15. De Clercq, E.; Sakuma, T.; Baba, M.; Pauwels, R.; Balzarini, J.; Rosenberg, I.; Holy, A. Antiviral activity of phosphonylmethoxyalkyl derivatives of purine and pyrimidines. *Antiviral Res.* **1987**, *8*, 261–272.

16. De Clercq, E.; Holy, A.; Rosenberg, I. Efficacy of phosphonylmethoxyalkyl derivatives of adenine in experimental herpes simplex virus and vaccinia virus infections in vivo. *Antimicrob. Agents Chemother.* **1989**, *33*, 185–191.

17. Naesens, L.; Snoeck, R.; Andrei, G.; Balzarini, J.; Neyts, J.; De Clercq, E. HPMPC (cidofovir), PMEA (adefovir) and related acyclic nucleoside phosphonate analogues: a review of their pharmacology and clinical potential in the treatment of viral infections. *Antiviral Chem. Chemother.* **1997**, *8*, 1–23.

18. De Clercq, E. Vaccinia virus inhibitors as a paradigm for the chemotherapy of poxvirus infections. *Clin. Microbiol. Rev.* **2001**, *14*, 382–397.

19. Neyts, J.; De Clercq, E. Efficacy of (*S*)-1-(3-hydroxy-2-phosphonylmethoxypropyl)cy-tosine for the treatment of lethal vaccinia virus infections in severe combined immune deficiency (SCID) mice. *J. Med. Virol.* **1993**, *41*, 242–246.

20. Baker, R. O.; Bray, M.; Huggins, J. W. Potential antiviral therapeutics for smallpox, monkeypox and other orthopoxvirus infections. *Antiviral Res.* **2003**, *57*, 13–23.

21. Kern, E. R.; Hartline, C.; Harden, E.; Keith, K.; Rodriguez, N.; Beadle, J. R.; Hostetler, K. Y. Enhanced inhibition of orthopoxvirus replication in vitro by alkoxyalkyl esters of cidofovir and cyclic cidofovir. *Antimicrob. Agents Chemother.* **2002**, *46*, 991–995.

22. Bray, M.; Martinez, M.; Smee, D. F.; Kefauver, D.; Thompson, E.; Huggins, J. W. Cidofovir protects mice against lethal aerosol or intranasal cowpox virus challenge. *J. Infect. Dis.* **2000**, *181*, 10–19.

23. Bray, M.; Martinez, M.; Kefauver, D.; West, M.; Roy, C. Treatment of aerosolized cowpox virus infection in mice with aerosolized cidofovir. *Antiviral Res.* **2002**, *54*, 129–142.

24. Smee, D. F.; Bailey, K. W.; Wong, M. H.; Sidwell, R. W. Intranasal treatment of cowpox virus respiratory infections in mice with cidofovir. *Antiviral Res.* **2000**, *47*, 171–177.

25. Smee, D. F.; Bailey, K. W.; Sidwell, R. W. Treatment of lethal vaccinia virus respiratory infections in mice with cidofovir. *Antiviral Chem. Chemother.* **2001**, *12*, 71–76.

26. Quenelle, D. C.; Collins, D. J.; Kern, E. R. Efficacy of multiple- or single-dose cidofovir against vaccinia and cowpox virus infections in mice. *Antimicrob. Agents Chemother.* **2003**, *47*, 3275–3280.

27. Huggins, J. W.; Martinez, M. J.; Hartmann, C. J.; Hensley, L. E.; Jackson, D. L.; Refoeven, D. F.; Kuksh, D. A.; Lawson, T.; Miller, D. M.; Mucker, E. A.; Shamblin, J. D.; Tate, M. K.; Whitehour, L. A.; Swiers, S. H.; Jahrling, P. B.. Successful cidofovir treatment of smallpox-like diseases in variola and monkeypox primate models. *Antiviral Res.* **2004**, *62*, A57.

28. Cundy, K. C.; Bidgood, A. M.; Lynch, G.; Shaw, J. P.; Griffin, L.; Lee, W. A. Pharmacokinetics, bioavailability, metabolism, and tissue distribution of cidofovir (HPMPC) and cyclic HPMPC in rats. *Drug Metab. Dispos.* **1996**, *24*, 745–752.

29. Cundy, K. C.; Li, Z. H.; Hitchcock, M. J.; Lee, W. A. Pharmacokinetics of cidofovir in monkeys. Evidence for a prolonged elimination phase representing phosphorylated drug. *Drug Metab. Dispos.* **1996**, *24*, 738–744.

30. Kern, E. R. In vitro activity of potential anti-poxvirus agents. *Antiviral Res.* **2003**, *57*, 35–40.

31. Safrin, S.; Cherrington, J.; Jaffe, H. S. Clinical uses of cidofovir. *Rev. Med. Virol.* **1997**, *7*, 145–156.

32. De Clercq, E. Cidofovir in the therapy and short-term prophylaxis of poxvirus infections. *Trends Pharmacol. Sci.* **2002**, *23*, 456–458.

33. Smee, D. F.; Sidwell, R. W. Anti-cowpox virus activities of certain adenosine analogs, arabinofuranosyl nucleosides, and 2′-fluoro-arabinofuranosyl nucleosides. *Nucleosides Nucleotides Nucleic Acids* **2004**, *23*, 375–383.

34. Barditch-Crovo, P.; Toole, J.; Hendrix, C. W.; Cundy, K. C.; Ebeling, D.; Jaffe, H. S.; Lietman, P. S. Anti-human immunodeficiency virus (HIV) activity, safety, and pharmacokinetics of adefovir dipivoxil (9-[2-(bis-pivaloyloxymethyl) phosphonylmethoxyethyl]adenine) in HIV-infected patients. *J. Infect. Dis.* **1997**, *176*, 406–413.

35. Neyts, J.; De Clercq, E. Efficacy of 2-amino-7-(1,3-dihydroxy-2-propoxymethyl)purine for treatment of vaccinia virus (orthopoxvirus) infections in mice. *Antimicrob. Agents Chemother.* **2001**, *45*, 84–87.

36. Smee, D. F.; Bailey, K. W.; Sidwell, R. W. Treatment of lethal cowpox virus respiratory infections in mice with 2-amino-7-[(1,3-dihydroxy-2-propoxy)methyl]purine and its orally active diacetate ester prodrug. *Antiviral Res.* **2002**, *54*, 113–120.

37. De Clercq, E. In search of a selective antiviral chemotherapy. *Clin. Microbiol. Rev.* **1997**, *10*, 674–693.

38. De Clercq, E. Cidofovir in the treatment of poxvirus infections. *Antiviral Res.* **2002b**, *55*, 1–13.

39. Keith, K. A.; Hitchcock, M. J.; Lee, W. A.; Holy, A.; Kern, E. R. Evaluation of nucleoside phosphonates and their analogs and prodrugs for inhibition of orthopoxvirus replication. *Antimicrob. Agents Chemother.* **2003**, *47*, 2193–2198.

40. Smee, D. F.; Bailey, K. W.; Sidwell, R. W. Treatment of cowpox virus respiratory infections in mice with ribavirin as a single agent or followed sequentially by cidofovir. *Antiviral Chem. Chemother.* **2000**, *11*, 303–309.

41. Smee, D. F.; Bailey, K. W.; Wong, M. H.; Sidwell, R. W. Effects of cidofovir on the pathogenesis of a lethal vaccinia virus respiratory infection in mice. *Antiviral Res.* **2001**, *52*, 55–62.

42. Roy, C. J.; Baker R.; Washburn, K.; Bary, M. Aerosolized cidofovir is retained in the respiratory tract and protects mice against intranasal cowpox virus challenge. *Antimicrob. Agents Chemother.* **2003**, *47*, 2933–2937.

43. Snoeck, R.; Holy, A.; Dewolf-Peeters, C.; Van Den Oord, J.; De Clercq, E.; Andrei, G. Antivaccinia activities of acyclic nucleoside phosphonate derivatives in epithelial cells and organotypic cultures. *Antimicrob. Agents Chemother.* **2002**, *46*, 3356–3361.

44. Hostetler, K. Y.; Beadle, J. R.; Kini, G. D.; Gardner, M. F.; Wright, K. N.; Wu, T. H.; Korba, B. A. Enhanced oral absorption and antiviral activity of 1-*O*-octadecyl-*sn*-glycero-3-phospho-acyclovir and related compounds in hepatitis B virus infection, in vitro. *Biochem. Pharmacol.* **1997**, *53*, 1815–1822.

45. Hostetler, K. Y.; Rybak, R. J.; Beadle, J. R.; Gardner, M. F.; Aldern, K. A.; Wright, K. N; Kern, E. R. In vitro and in vivo activity of 1-*O*-hexadecylpropanediol-3-phospho-ganciclovir and 1-*O*-hexadecylpropanediol-3-phospho-penciclovir in cytomegalovirus and herpes simplex virus infections. *Antiviral Chem. Chemother.* **2001**, *12*, 61–70.

46. Hostetler, K. Y.; Beadle, J. R.; Hornbuckle, W. E.; Bellezza, C. A.; Tochkov, I. A.; Cote, P. J.; Gerin, J. L.; Korba, B. E.; Tennant, B. C. Antiviral activities of oral 1-*O*-hexadecyl-propanediol-3-phosphoacyclovir and acyclovir in woodchucks with chronic woodchuck hepatitis virus infection. *Antimicrob. Agents Chemother.* **2000**, *44*, 1964–1969.

47. Huggins, J. W.; Baker, R. O.; Beadle, J. R.; Hostetler, K. Y. Orally active ether lipid prodrugs of cidofovir for the treatment of smallpox. *Antiviral Res.* **2002**, *53*, A66.

48. Buller, R. M.; Owens, G.; Schriewer, J.; Melman, L.; Beadle, J. R.; Hostetler, K. Y. Efficacy of oral active ether lipid analogs of cidofovir in a lethal mousepox model. *Virology* **2004**, *318*, 474–481.

49. Beadle, J. R.; Hartline, C. B.; Aldern, K. A.; Rodriguez, N.; Harden, E.; Kern, E. R.; Hostetler, K. Y. Alkoxyalkyl esters of cidofovir and cyclic cidofovir exhibit multiple-log enhancement of antiviral activity against cytomegalovirus and herpesvirus replication in vitro. *Antimicrob. Agents Chemother.* **2002**, *46*, 2381–2386.

50. Hartline, C. B.; Gustin, K. M.; Wan, W. B.; Ciesla, S. L.; Beadle, J. R.; Hostetler, K. Y.; Kern, E. R. Ether lipid ester prodrugs of acyclic nucleoside phosphonates: Activity against adenovirus replication in vitro. *J. Infect. Dis.* **2005**, *191*, 396–399.

51. Keith, K. A.; Wan, W. B.; Ciesla, S. L.; Beadle, J. R.; Hostetler, K. Y.; Kern, E. R. Inhibitory activity of alkoxyalkyl and alkyl esters of cidofovir and cyclic cidofovir against orthopoxvirus replication in vitro. *Antimicrob. Agents Chemother.* **2004**, *48*, 1869–1871.

52. Aldern, K. A.; Ciesla, S. L.; Winegarden, K. L.; Hostetler, K. Y. Increased antiviral activity of 1-O-hexadecyloxypropyl-[2-(14)C]cidofovir in MRC-5 human lung fibroblasts is explained by unique cellular uptake and metabolism. *Mol. Pharmacol.* **2003**, *63*, 678–681.

53. Ciesla, S. L.; Trahan, J.; Wan, W. B.; Beadle, J. R.; Aldern, K. A.; Painter, G. R.; Hostetler, K. Y. Esterification of cidofovir with alkoxyalkanols increases oral bioavailability and diminishes drug accumulation in kidney. *Antiviral Res.* **2003**, *59*, 163–171.

54. Quenelle, D. C.; Collins, D. J.; Wan, W. B.; Beadle, J. R.; Hostetler, K. Y.; Kern, E. R. Oral treatment of cowpox and vaccinia virus infections in mice with ether lipid esters of cidofovir. *Antimicrob. Agents Chemother.* **2004**, *48*, 404–412.

CHAPTER 15

Viral Countermeasures to the Host Interferon Response: Role of the Vaccinia Virus E3L and K3L Genes

JEFFREY O. LANGLAND, VANESSA LANCASTER, and BERTRAM L. JACOBS

School of Life Sciences/Biodesign Institute, Arizona State University

15.1 INTERFERON RESPONSE

To establish an infection in a host organism, viruses must overcome the forceful nature of the immune response. In 1957 A. Isaacs and J. Lindenmann found that chicken cells exposed to inactivated influenza virus secreted a substance that interfered with the infection of live influenza virus in other chicken cells. This inhibitor was subsequently called interferon. Most cells produce interferon when infected by viruses and evolutionarily, interferons can be found in mammals, birds, fish, and reptiles. Interferons are grouped into the cytokine family of genes, which include secreted protein signaling molecules, and interferon is, in fact, the oldest known cytokine. Interferons are grouped into two major classes, interferon-α/β and interferon-γ. Both major classes of interferon, also know as type I and type II interferons, respectively, mediate diverse and potent roles in the defense against virus infection although there is no obvious structural similarity between the interferon types.

Cells do not induce the synthesis of interferon unless exposed to some type of interferon-inducing agent. Biologically, viruses are the most common agent inducing interferon agent; however, bacteria, mycoplasma, and protozoa can also have profound effects on the interferon response. The primary viral agent responsible for the induction of interferon is double-stranded RNA (dsRNA). Within the cytoplasm of an uninfected cell, the presence of dsRNA molecules is minute, if present at all. Cellular RNAs with significant secondary structures are present, but the length of the dsRNA structure and/or accessibility of the RNA likely prevents activation of

---

Antiviral Drug Discovery for Emerging Diseases and Bioterrorism Threats. Edited by Paul F. Torrence
Copyright © 2005 John Wiley & Sons, Inc.

the interferon response. Most viruses induce the synthesis of dsRNA at some point during their replication cycle. This fact exemplifies the power, specificity, and effectiveness of this portion of the host immune response toward virus infection. For viruses with dsRNA genomes, activation of the interferon defense is likely due to minute amounts of the viral genome becoming incorrectly uncoated or packaged during the replication process.[1] For single-stranded RNA viruses, the obvious source of dsRNA is the replicative intermediate present in infected cells. For DNA viruses, like poxviruses, dsRNA accumulation appears to result from overlapping convergent transcription. At intermediate and late times after infection with vaccinia virus, viral transcripts fail to terminate at discrete sites at the ends of genes.[2] This results in the synthesis of complementary RNAs produced from genes transcribed in opposing directions.[3,4] Subsequent annealing of these complementary RNAs will result in the formation of molecules with a high degree of dsRNA character. The vaccinia virus A18R gene product modulates the termination of transcription, thereby altering the level of dsRNA accumulation in the infected cell.[5,6]

The biological activities of interferon occur after binding of the secreted interferon to their cognate receptors on the surface of surrounding cells. Subsequent signal transduction results in the activation of distinct signaling pathways involving the Jak/STAT cascade.[7,8] The decisive effect of this signal transduction cascade is the activation of transcription of target genes, which are normally quiescent or expressed at low basal levels within the cell. Two of the most well-characterized cellular genes whose transcriptional expression is clearly regulated by the presence of interferon are the protein kinase PKR and the enzyme 2′5′-oligoadenylate synthetase (OAS) (Figure 15.1). After induction by interferon, both of these enzymes remain inactive until subsequent virus infection. Since activation of either of these enzymes leads to dramatic and destructive effects within the cell, this regulation at the level of activation ensures cell viability until the ensuing virus infection. Again, once this cell becomes infected, viral dsRNA is the apparent cofactor recognized by these enzymes leading their activation. Both enzymes can bind to and be potently activated at this post-translational step by dsRNA. In the case of PKR, activation appears to occur concomitantly with protein homodimerization and intermolecular phosphorylation.[9–12] The PKR enzyme is composed of two well-characterized domains consisting of an N-terminal regulatory domain involved in binding dsRNA and a C-terminal catalytic domain that contains conserved motifs for protein kinase activity.[13] Activation of PKR is dependent on the dsRNA structure, rather than the nucleotide sequence, and approximately 50 base pairs of duplexed RNA are required for activation.[14] Activated PKR is involved in a number of cellular regulatory roles. Most well characterized is PKR's involvement in the phosphorylation of eukaryotic initiation factor eIF2.[15,16] In the initial step of translation, the initiator Met-tRNA is recruited to the 40S ribosomal subunit due to interaction with eIF2-GTP. This complex subsequently interacts with mRNA, additional initiation factors, and the 60S ribosomal subunit, resulting in the formation of the preinitiation complex. The formation of this complex results in the hydrolysis of the GTP bound to eIF2 and the release of eIF2-GDP. For another round of translation

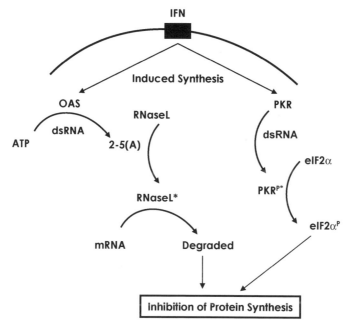

FIGURE 15.1 Schematic of the interferon-induced antiviral mechanisms: dsRNA protein kinase (PKR) and 2′5′-oligoadenylate synthetase (OAS). Asterisk (*) indicates activated form of enzyme.

initiation to begin, the GDP bound to eIF2 must be exchanged for GTP. This exchange reaction is catalyzed by eIF2B. The phosphorylation of eIF2 on the α subunit leads to a higher affinity interaction between eIF2B and eIF2-GDP, thereby preventing the GDP:GTP exchange reaction from occurring. Therefore, the phosphorylation of eIF2 by PKR during virus infection ultimately leads to an inhibition in protein synthesis and a block in viral replication.

PKR also plays a role in regulating several signal transduction cascades in the cell. The transcription factor NF-κB, which leads to expression of many pro-inflammatory genes, is activated indirectly by PKR via association with TRAF and activation of the I kappa B kinase (IKK) complex[17]. PKR has also been shown to play a role in the activation of p38 MAP kinases and the stress-activated protein kinase (SAPK)/c-Jun amino-terminal kinases (JNKs).[18] Interestingly, the activation of transcription factors IRF-3 and IRF-7, which lead to the expression of interferon-β, can occur in the presence of dsRNA, but this induction does not appear to require PKR, suggesting the presence of additional dsRNA-responsive enzymes present in the cell.[19]

Activation of OAS by dsRNA is likely not a consequence of post-translational modification, but a conformational change in the enzyme due to dsRNA binding. Once activated, OAS can polymerize ATP and other nucleotides in novel 2′5′-linkages.[20] These 2′5′-oligoadenylates can bind with high affinity and activate an endogenous ribonuclease, RNaseL, that can cleave ssRNAs including mRNA and rRNA.[21,22] The cleavage of the 28S rRNA by RNaseL has been shown to lead to ribosomal inactivation and a subsequent block in translation.

The effectiveness of the interferon response has led to the development of resistance mechanisms to counteract and overcome the production or actions of interferons by numerous viruses. Given that most, if not all, viruses synthesize dsRNA, which can lead to efficient activation of the interferon-induced, dsRNA-dependent enzymes, it is not surprising that many viruses have evolved elaborate mechanisms to block these defenses. Due to the complexity of the interferon response, a variety of steps at which a virus can intervene are available. African swine fever virus encodes a homologue of IκB that inhibits the activation of NF-κB, which normally acts to induce expression of immunomodulatory genes including interferons.[23,24] Other viruses use similar strategies to inhibit interferon production (see Table 15.1), including human papillomavirus type 16, which encodes the E6 protein that functions to bind IRF-3 and again block the transcriptional activation role of IRF-3, including induction of interferon-β.

Still other viruses have evolved mechanisms to block the downstream signaling pathway of interferon. Blocking of the interferon signaling pathways can occur at various steps and viruses have evolved mechanisms to block most, if not all, of these steps (Table 15.1). Poxviruses have devoted a large portion of their genome with the overall goal of interrupting the host defense system. Several poxviruses are known to encode soluble interferon-receptor homologues that function to bind to and sequester interferons and block their activity. Secreted interferon-γ receptors have been identified for vaccinia virus, as well as myxoma virus, ectromelia virus, cowpox virus, and camelpox virus. Likewise, interferon-α/β receptors are encoded by most orthopoxviruses including vaccinia virus.[25–28] Loss of the interferon-α/β receptor leads to a highly attenuated virus supporting the importance of this protein in viral pathogenesis and the importance of the host interferon response.[29]

Interferon signaling can also be disrupted by altering the activity of intracellular components involved in the signal transduction cascade following interferon binding to the cellular receptor (Table 15.1). Human cytomegalovirus induces degradation of the Jak1 and p48 proteins, while murine polyomavirus encodes a protein that functionally binds to and blocks the signal transduction activity of Jak1.[30,31] Further downstream, the STAT proteins are additional targets for viral activity. Simian virus 5 and mumps virus induce proteasome-mediated degradation of STAT1, while Sendai virus and human parainfluenza virus 3 likely block phosphorylation of STAT1, thereby preventing subsequent activation.[32–35] Similarly, vaccinia virus appears to block interferon-γ signal transduction by encoding a viral phosphatase to reverse STAT1 activation.[36]

By far, the most widespread cellular defense proteins targeted during viral infection are the interferon-induced antiviral enzymes, PKR and OAS. Given the importance of PKR activity in blocking viral replication, it is not surprising that viruses have developed a multitude of mechanisms to counteract this defense pathway. VAI RNA and EBER RNA from adenovirus and Epstein-Barr virus, respectively, have the ability to bind to PKR but fail to lead to activation.[14]

TABLE 15.1   Viral Proteins Involved in Evading the Interferon Response

Virus	Protein Name	Mechanism
		I. dsRNA Binding Proteins/PKR and OAS Inhibition
Vaccinia virus	E3L	dsRNA binding protein, masks dsRNA, preventing activation of PKR and OAS antiviral systems, dsRNA-dependent apoptosis
Vaccinia virus	K3L	Poxviruses analogue to eIF2α, inhibits eIF2α phosphorylation
Influenza virus	NS1	dsRNA binding protein
	p58	Influenza virus cellular PKR inhibitor
Group C rotavirus	NSP3	dsRNA binding protein
Baculovirus	PK2	Blocks phosphorylation of eIF2α by binding and inhibiting PKR
Reovirus	σ3	Binds dsRNA, inhibiting activation of PKR and OAS
Herpes simplex virus	γ34.5	Activates cellular eIF2α phosphatase
Hepatitis C	E2/NS5A	Binds PKR, prevents dimerization and activation
Adenovirus	VAI RNA	Binds PKR, preventing activation
Epstein-Barr virus	EBER RNA	Binds PKR, preventing activation

TABLE 15.1 (*Continued*)

Virus	Protein Name	Mechanism
	II. Inhibition of Jak/STAT Pathway	
Paramyxoviruses (e.g., simian virus 5)	V protein	Sequesters STAT proteins in the cytoplasm and targets them for proteosome-mediated degradation
Adenovirus	E1A	Decreases levels of STAT1 and p48 by sequestering the transcriptional coactivator CBP/p300, as well as direct interaction with STAT1
Human papillomavirus type 16	E7	Binds p48, blocking IFN-α/β signaling
Murine polyoma virus	T antigen	Binds and inactivates Jak1
	III. Other	
African swine fever virus (ASFV)	IκB homologue	Inhibits activation of NF-κB
Human papillomavirus type 16	E6 protein	Binds IRF-3, blocking its transcriptional activation functions
Poxviruses	B18R	Soluble IFN-α/β receptor
	B8R	Soluble IFN-γ receptor
Ebola virus	VP35	Blocks IRF-3 activation

Hepatitis C virus takes advantage of the fact that PKR requires dimerization for activation and encodes a protein, NS5A, which binds to PKR and prevents this event.[37] Other viruses utilize cellular PKR regulatory components including herpes simplex virus, which redirects the cellular phosphatase 1 to dephosphorylate eIF2α, and influenza virus, which induces a cellular inhibitor of PKR, P58IPK.[38,39] The most common mechanism thus far characterized for inhibition of the PKR and OAS pathway involves viral synthesis of dsRNA binding proteins. Since dsRNA is a danger signal that the cell uses to recognize the presence of the virus, many viruses synthesize excessive amounts of dsRNA-binding proteins, which function to bind to and sequester any free dsRNA molecules. Such proteins include the σ3 protein of reovirus, the NSP3 protein of rotaviruses, the NS1 protein of influenza virus, and the E3L protein of vaccinia virus.[40–42] Interestingly, vaccinia virus has evolved redundant mechanisms to evade PKR activity and encodes the K3L protein, which functions as a competitive pseudosubstrate blocking eIF2α phosphorylation.[43,44]

15.2 VACCINIA VIRUS

Poxviridae compose a diverse group of large DNA viruses that replicate solely within the cytoplasm of infected cells. Although eradicated in 1977, smallpox has been one of humankind's greatest scourges, affecting humankind like no other disease in history and having a pivotal role in the destruction of at least three empires.[45]

The genome of poxviruses is composed of a linear double-stranded DNA molecule of 130–300 kilobase pairs with a hairpin loop at each end forming a covalently continuous polynucleotide chain. Inverted terminal repeat sequences, which are identical but oppositely oriented, are present at each end of the genome. The Poxviridae family is divided into two subfamilies based on host range, Chordopoxviridae (vertebrates) and Entomopoxviridae (insects). The Chordopox-viridae is composed of eight genera, *Orthopoxvirus, Parapoxvirus, Avipoxvirus, Capripoxvirus, Leporipoxvirus, Suipoxvirus, Molluscipoxvirus,* and *Yatapoxvirus.* Of the *Orthopoxviruses,* vaccinia virus and variola, the causative agent of smallpox, typically have been the most significant members in the scientific community. Although the origin of vaccinia virus is unknown, more than 90% sequence identity exists between vaccinia virus and variola. However, of the orthopoxviruses, horse-pox appears to be most closely related to vaccinia, suggesting that our current vaccine was derived from horsepox and not directly from the cowpox originally described by Jenner.[46]

Upon infection of cells with vaccinia virus, intense cytopathic effects are observed, leading to changes in membrane permeability and an inhibition of cellular DNA, RNA, and protein synthesis.[2] After a few hours postinfection, the majority of mRNA present in the infected cell is of viral origin. This likely accounts for the predominant shift in protein synthesis from cellular to viral.

For decades, vaccinia virus has been utilized as an invaluable tool for studying a multitude of cellular phenomenon. This has come about due to the usefulness of

TABLE 15.2 Poxviral Immune Evasion Genes

Protein	Mechanism
E3L	Masks dsRNA, preventing activation of PKR and OAS antiviral systems, dsRNA-dependent apoptosis, induction of IFN-α/β
K3L	Poxviruses analogue to phosphorylated eIF2-α, inhibits shutdown of protein synthesis
B18R	Soluble IFN-α/β receptor
B8R	Soluble IFN-γ receptor
VCP	Inhibitor of complement binding protein
CKBP-II	Binds β chemokines
B13R	Inhibits apoptosis
VGF	Stimulates growth of surrounding uninfected cells to facilitate the spread of viral infection
IL-10	(Orf) Impairs the initiation of the acquired immune response and subsequent immune memory, allowing reinfection
TNFR	(Myxoma) Tumor necrosis factor receptor
B15R	IL-1β receptor
N1L	Disrupts signaling from toll-like receptors to NF-κB by inhibiting IKK
VH1 phosphatase	Dephosphorylates STAT1

vaccinia virus as a live recombination vector. Vaccinia virus attributes—including the capacity to accommodate large quantities of DNA, high levels of gene expression, and a wide host range—have directed many of these efforts. Furthermore, many methodologies have been developed to allow easy and direct screening or selection of recombinant virus constructs. These include color screening, antibiotic resistance, host range, plaque morphology, antibody interaction, and DNA hybridization.

Given the size and long evolutionary history of poxviruses, they have acquired a large variety of genes to counteract host defenses and devote a large portion of their genome to achieve this goal (Table 15.2). As mentioned before, most of these immune counteractive proteins are directed toward the early, nonspecific host responses including interferons and other cytokines. In addition to those proteins described, many poxviruses are able to block MHC class I presentation, apoptosis induction through the synthesis of serpins, and complement activation via complement binding proteins.[26]

One of the key viral factors recognized by the host cell during vaccinia virus infection is viral dsRNA synthesized at intermediate and late times postinfection. For vaccinia virus, termination of early viral transcription is dramatically different from termination of intermediate or late transcription. Early transcription termination occurs 20–50 base pairs downstream of the sequence T T T T T N T.[47] This results in early transcripts having reasonably precise 3′ ends near the end of the gene. In contrast, most intermediate and late transcription results in imprecise termination and transcripts having extremely heterogeneous 3′ ends.[48] This terminal heterogeneity, along with genes encoded in convergent orientations, results in the formation of transcripts having the ability to anneal and form a dsRNA product. Temporally, the presence of dsRNA during a vaccinia virus infection is not detectable until approximately 4 hours postinfection, in agreement with dsRNA formation being dependent on intermediate/late transcription.[49]

Due to the sensitivity and impact of dsRNA within a cell, it is not surprising that poxvirus evolution has led to the acquisition of genes to counteract these effects. The first, and apparently most important, gene encoded by vaccinia virus to cope with the presence of viral dsRNA is the E3L gene. This gene encodes a full-length protein of 190 amino acids. A second E3L gene product, deleted of the first 37 amino acids, is also observed in virus-infected cells, which is thought to be synthesized due to leaky scanning to the second start codon present on the mRNA. Two distinct domains have been identified on E3L linked together by an acidic linker region: a C-terminal dsRNA-binding domain that is required for both replication in many cells in culture and for pathogenesis in mice, and an N-terminal domain that is dispensable for replication in cells in culture but is required for pathogenesis in mice. A second gene, the K3L gene, also regulates the cellular response to dsRNA, but instead of interacting with the dsRNA molecule itself, the K3L gene product regulates the activity of PKR, one of the cellular proteins involved in the recognition of dsRNA. Results suggest that both genes may have distinct roles dependent on the stage in the replication cycle and/or the type of cell infected. Nonetheless, virus deleted for E3L has a more dramatically attenuated phenotype in most cells investigated. However, deletion of K3L appears to affect viral translation at very early times postinfection and decrease the host range of vaccinia virus.[50,51]

Both the E3L and K3L genes are highly conserved among the *Orthopoxvirus* genera, supporting the importance of these genes to the virus replication and, likely, in immune evasion. Furthermore, homologues of these genes have also been identified in *Capripoxviruses, Leporipoxviruses, Suipoxviruses,* and *Yatapoxviruses* (Table 15.3). An E3L homologue is present in *Parapoxviruses,* but a K3L

TABLE 15.3 Homologues of E3L and K3L of Vaccinia Virus

Virus	Host	E3L Homologue	K3L Homologue
Orthopoxvirus	Mammals	+[a]	+[b]
Capripoxvirus	Sheep, goat, buffalo	+	+
Leporipoxvirus	Rabbit, squirrel	+[c]	+
Suipoxvirus	Swine	+	+
Yatapoxvirus	Monkey, rodents	+	+
Parapoxvirus	Sheep	+	—
Avipoxvirus	Birds	—	—
Molluscipoxvirus	Humans	—	—

[a] All known orthopoxviruses have full-length E3L with the exception of monkeypox, which is E3LΔ37N.
[b] Interrupted in monkeypox and ectromelia.
[c] This E3L homologue is Δ58N when compared to vaccinia virus E3L.

homologue is missing. Neither gene has been found in *Avipoxvirus* or *Mollusci-poxvirus* genera. A few members of these genera contain partial deletions and/or insertions in these genes, which may or may not alter function. In particular, monkeypox virus, an *Orthopoxvirus,* contains a deletion in the C terminus of K3L and an N-terminal deletion in the E3L gene (Table 15.3).

15.3   THE K3L GENE

The K3L gene of vaccinia virus functions as a pseudosubstrate competitive inhibitor of PKR, thereby blocking PKR phosphorylation of eIF2α. Evidence also suggests that K3L can inhibit the autophosphorylation and, therefore, activation of PKR itself.[51] Functionally, K3L has been shown to form a physical interaction with PKR and this interaction leads to the inhibition of PKR activity.[44] The K3L gene encodes a relatively small gene product of 88 amino acids in length and is 28% identical to the N-terminal third of eIF2α (Figure 15.2).[52] The sequence of eIF2α is perfectly conserved from yeast to humans over a region of 19 amino acids surrounding the phosphorylation site recognized by PKR, Ser-51. As would be expected for a competitive inhibitor, a corresponding phosphorylation site is not present in K3L. However, somewhat surprisingly, there is also no homology between K3L and eIF2α in the amino acids flanking Ser-51. This suggests that this

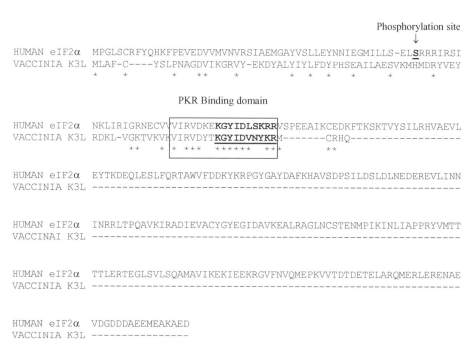

FIGURE 15.2   Homology of VV WR K3L protein sequence, with human eIF2α.

region of eIF2α is not required for PKR recognition. Instead, the greatest homology between eIF2α and K3L resides in a 12 amino acid sequence located approximately 30 amino acids from Ser-51 (residues 72–83). This suggests that PKR substrate recognition occurs through interactions with sequences that are located distal from the actual phosphorylation site.

Structurally, PKR is composed of two N-terminal dsRNA binding domains (amino acids 55–75 and 145–166) and a C-terminal catalytic domain containing eleven conserved kinase subdomains characterizing PKR as a serine/threonine kinase.[13] Between subdomains IV and V there is a 24 amino acid kinase insert and a highly conserved LFIQMEFCD motif. This LFIQMEFCD motif is indispensable for kinase activity and is found in all known eIF2α kinase family members.[53] As expected, K3L binding to PKR does not require the dsRNA binding domains present on PKR. Somewhat unexpected, the kinase insert domain of PKR is also dispensable for K3L interaction.[54] However, K3L does have the ability to inhibit eIF2α phosphorylation by all the known eIF2α kinases, including GCN2, HRI, and PEK.[44,55,56] Mutational analysis of PKR suggests that amino acids 367–415 of PKR contain the minimal K3L binding site. This region lies between kinase domains V and VI and forms an α-helical structure between two β-sheets.[57]

Recently, the X-ray crystal structure of K3L has been elucidated.[58] The resulting crystal structure suggests that K3L consists of a monomeric five-strand, antiparallel β barrel. Strands β1–β3 form the larger of two β sheets, while strands β4 and β5 form the smaller sheet. The interaction angle between sheets is approximately 90°. Inserted between β strands 3 and 4 is a single turn 3_{10} helix followed by a structured connecting segment of four amino acids and then an eleven residue right-hand α helix. This region between β strands 3 and 4 is the area of greatest sequence dissimilarity between K3L and eIF2α and has been suggested to function *directly* as a PKR inhibitor rather than a competitive eIF2α substrate.[58] Consistent with this is data suggesting that a $His_{47}Arg$ mutation in this region increases K3L inhibitory activity.[59] Interestingly, this region of K3L corresponds to the Ser-51 phosphoacceptor site in eIF2α This noncompetitive mode of PKR inhibition appears to require PKR dimerization with K3L. Inhibitory activity affects PKR autophosphorylation and phosphorylation of an additional, unrelated histone substrate.[58]

The conserved region between eIF2α and K3L (amino acids 72–83 of K3L) includes residues Lys74, Tyr76, and Asp78, which forms a highly structured epitope on the β barrel. Mutations in this region reduce PKR–K3L interaction, supporting the role of this epitope in high-affinity binding to PKR.[58]

In the context of a virally infected cell, the competitive inhibitor role of K3L is likely involved in blocking PKR activation and eIF2α phosphorylation in order to maintain active translation even in the presence of dsRNA molecules. PKR has also been shown to have a pivotal role in additional cellular cascades including the induction of apoptosis and the transcriptional upregulation of proinflammatory genes. Since PKR substrates involved in these additional cascades are unrelated to eIF2α, the ability of K3L to noncompetitively inhibit PKR activation may have relevance toward efficiency of viral replication.

15.4 THE E3L GENE

In the early 1980s vaccinia virus was shown to produce an inhibitor of PKR.[60–62] This inhibitor was reported to be proteinaceous and to interact with dsRNA. Nearly ten years later, the viral gene encoding this inhibitor was identified as the vaccinia virus E3L gene.[63] The E3L gene encodes a dsRNA binding protein containing one copy of a highly conserved dsRNA binding motif in the C terminus. This dsRNA binding domain is essential for the replication of vaccinia virus in a wide range of host cells and necessary for the interferon resistance phenotype of the virus (see Figure 15.3).[50,64] The full-length protein exists as a dimer in solution and this protein–protein interaction appears to contribute to high-affinity binding to dsRNA.[65] Vaccinia virus constructs expressing dsRNA binding proteins in place of the E3L gene maintain the phenotypic characteristics of the wild-type virus in cells-in-culture.[40,50,66] This rescue phenotype was observed even with the expression of a functional dsRNA binding protein that has no apparent sequence homology to E3L.[50]

The amino-terminal half of the E3L protein is highly conserved among distantly related poxviruses, but the functional role of this region has been less well characterized (see Figure 15.3). Loss of the N terminus does not affect viral host range or the interferon resistance phenotype.[64,67] The E3L gene products have been shown to be subcellularly distributed in both the cytoplasm and nucleus. Poxviruses are unusual among DNA-containing viruses in that replication occurs solely in the cytoplasm of the infected cell. Therefore, it was unexpected that viral gene products should be present in the nucleus during vaccinia virus replication. To date, the only known vaccinia virus gene product shown to localize to the nucleus is the E3L protein.[68] Nuclear localization of E3L maps to the N-terminal region of the protein, although the role of this subcellular localization remains unclear. PKR and several translation initiation factors have been found to be present in both the cytoplasm and nucleus of cells, possibly suggesting a role of E3L nuclear translocation.[69–76]

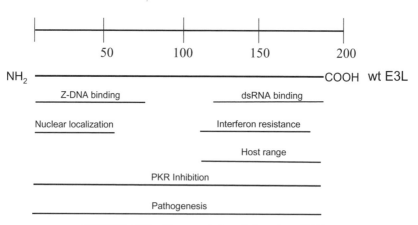

FIGURE 15.3 Characteristics of domains of E3L.

```
                  ^    ^         ^  ^   ^   *    *  ^*  ^      ^      ** *
Variola      YIDERSDAEIVCEAIKNIGLEGVT-AVQLTRQLNMEK-REVNKALYDLQRSAMVYSSDDIPPRW 62
Vaccinia     YIDERSDAEIVCAAIKNIGIEGAT-AAQLTRQLNMEK-REVNKALYDLQRSAMVYSSDDIPPRW 62
Monkeypox    ----------------------------------MEK-REVNKALYDLQRSTMVYSSDDTPPRW 25
ADAR-1 Zβ    -------KEKICDYL--FNVSDSS-ALNLAKNIGLTKARDINAVLIDMERQGDVYRQGTTPPIW 58
ADAR-1 Zα    LSIYQDQEQRILKFLEELGEGKATTAHDLSGKLGTPK-KEINRVLYSLAKKGKLQKEAGTPPLW 63
DLM Zα       LSTGDNLEQKILQVLSDDG--GPVKIGQLVKKCQVPK-KTLNQVLYRLKKEDRVSSPE--PATW 59
CaPKR Zα     MSAETQMERKIIDFLRQNG---KSIALTIAKEIGLDK-STVNRHLYNLQRSNQVFNSNEKPPVW 58
```

FIGURE 15.4   Z-DNA binding motifs. Shown are Z-DNA binding motifs from variola, vaccinia, and monkeypox E3L proteins, and for the cellular proteins ADAR1 (Zα and Zβ domains), DLM, and the *Carassius auratus* PKR. Caret ($\Diamond$), indicates conserved hydrophobic residues in the core of ADAR1 Zα, and asterisk (*) indicates conserved residues that contact Z-DNA.

Hinnebusch et al.[77] has suggested that the N terminus of E3L functions to directly interact with PKR. Indeed, the N terminus of E3L is required for full inhibition of PKR activity. Viral constructs expressing E3L deleted of the N terminus lead to PKR activation and subsequent eIF2α phosphorylation to levels similar to that of viruses containing a full E3L deletion. However, these phosphorylation events occur much later in the replication cycle and the phosphorylation of eIF2α does *not* lead to an inhibition in protein synthesis.[49] As with nuclear localization, these results tend to lead to more questions regarding the role of the N terminus of E3L in the vaccinia virus life cycle.

Finally, the amino terminus of E3L shares homology to other known cellular proteins including an RNA-specific adenosine deaminase, ADAR1, the murine tumor stroma and activated macrophage protein, DLM-1, and a novel PKR-like gene isolated from fish cells (Figure 15.4).[78–80] For ADAR1 and DLM-1, this domain of homology has been shown to bind to Z-form DNA. The E3L-like proteins from orf, lumpyskin, swinepox, and yaba-like disease poxviruses all demonstrate specificity for binding to Z-DNA, suggesting that Z-DNA binding is a common feature of E3L gene products in poxviruses.[81] Construction of a chimeric virus where the N terminus of E3L was replaced with the Zα domain from ADAR1 or DLM1 resulted in a virus construct that retained wild-type pathogenesis after intracranial inoculation of mice.[81] Based on the crystal structure of the ADAR1 Zα domain, mutations in the $Z\alpha_{ADAR1}$-E3L chimera, which specifically disrupted Z-DNA binding affinity, directly correlated with a reduction in pathogenesis. When analogous putative Z-DNA binding residues were mutated in the wild-type E3L protein, a direct correlation between putative Z-DNA affinity and pathogenesis was observed. For ADAR1, which binds to Z-DNA with a K_d of 40 nM, the mutation of Y177F reduces the K_d to 350 nM, and Y177A reduces the K_d further to 700 nM. When the analogous tyrosine in E3L (Y48) was mutated to phenylalanine, an ~ 1 $\log_{10}$ loss of pathogenesis was observed compared to wild-type virus and when mutated to an alanine, an ~3 $\log_{10}$ reduction in pathogenesis was observed.[81] In addition, viruses expressing alanine substitutions of proline 63 or proline 64 in E3L result in a reduction in pathogenesis, with a more dramatic loss of pathogenesis

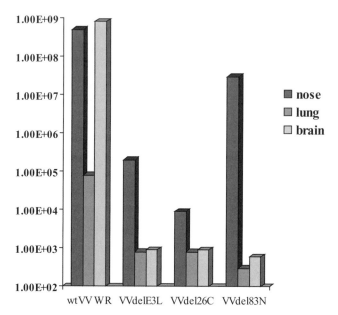

FIGURE 15.5 Titers of VV WR in tissues after intranasal inoculation: 4-week-old C57BL/6 mice were infected with 10^6 pfu of VV WR. Tissues were harvested 5 days postinfection and titered on RK-13 cells.

observed with the P63A mutation. Corresponding residues in ADAR1 result in a reduced affinity for Z-DNA. Of the two prolines, the ADAR1 equivalent residue to E3L P63 is more essential for high-affinity Z-DNA binding, therefore reinforcing the correlation of Z-DNA binding with pathogenicity of vaccinia virus.

As shown with the Z-DNA binding mutants, what is known about the N terminus of E3L is the requirement of this domain, as well as the C-terminal dsRNA binding domain, in viral pathogenesis. In C57Bl6 mice, wild-type vaccinia virus replicates to high titers in nasal tissue upon intranasal inoculation and then spreads to the lungs and brain (Figure 15.5). Animals apparently die of encephalitis 5–8 days postinfection. Vaccinia virus deleted of E3L or of the dsRNA binding domain replicate poorly in the nasal tissue, no virus is detected in the lungs or brain, and infected animals show no signs of illness. Virus that still encodes the dsRNA domain but is deleted for the N terminus of E3L replicates to wild-type levels in the nasal mucosa but fails to spread. This virus is more pathogenic than a full E3L deletion but is at least 1000-times less pathogenic than wild-type virus.

As mentioned before, the dsRNA binding activity associated with E3L is much more well understood. More than 20 functionally distinct proteins containing the conserved dsRNA binding motif have been identified.[82] Over the years, mutational analysis of E3L and other proteins containing this conserved motif of 65–68 amino acids has revealed many of the residues required for high-affinity binding to

```
PKR-1      -FFMEELNTYRQKQGVVLKYQELPNSGPPHDRRFTFQVIIDGREFPEGEGRSKKEAKNAAAKLAVEILN
VV WR E3L  -NPVTVINEYCQITRRDWSFR-IESVGPSNSPTFYACᵥDIDGRVFDKADGKSKRDAKNNAAKLAVDKLL
ADAR-1     -NPISGLLEYAQFASQTCEFNMIEQSGPPHEPRFKFQVVINGREFPPAEAGSKKVAKQDAAMKAMTILL
RNASE III  -QLQEIVQRDRDVL---IEYDILGETGPAHNKAFDAQVIVNGQVLGKGSGRTKKQAEQSAAQFAINKLI
STAUFEN-2  -SEISQVFEIALKRNLPVNFEVARESGPPHMKNFVTKVSV-GEFVGEGEGKSKKISKKNAAIAVLEELK
TN RNA BP  -NPVSALHQFAQMQRVQLDLKETVTTGNVMGPYFAFCAVVDGIQYKTGLGQNKKESRSNAAKLALDELL
Consensus   NP    NEYCQ T R    F      G  H P F   V I G  F A G SKK A   AA A     LL
```

FIGURE 15.6 dsRNA binding domain homology of E3L to select cellular dsRNA binding proteins. PKR: human dsRNA-dependent protein kinase (domain 1); VV WR-E3L: vaccinia virus E3L; ADAR1: human RNA-specific adenosine deaminase (domain 1); RNase III: *Listeria monocytogenes*; Staufen-2: human Staufen-2 (domain 2); TN RNA BP: testis nuclear dsRNA binding protein from *Mus musculus*.

dsRNA. The E3L protein binds dsRNA molecules in a sequence-independent manner with a $K_d \sim$ 7–9 nm.[82] The dsRNA binding domain of E3L shares significant homology to dsRNA domains identified on many cellular proteins (Figure 15.6). This domain on E3L shares the greatest homology with the ADAR protein, followed by the testis nuclear RNA binding protein and PKR. Substitutions at six conserved residues present on the same face of the binding motif, Glu-124, Phe-135, Phe-148, Lys-167, Arg-168, and Lys-171, greatly reduce dsRNA affinity, and are therefore likely part of the RNA binding site.[82] Although the structure of E3L has not yet been elucidated, relevance regarding the structure of the E3L dsRNA binding motif can be inferred based on structural data from similar domains present on other proteins. F or PKR, which contains two tandem motifs, the structure reveals a dumb-bell shape with each motif having an $\alpha–\beta–\beta–\beta–\alpha$ fold.[83] Similar motif folds were demonstrated for Staufen and RNase III.[84–86] The dsRNA recognition mechanism involves interactions with the 2′-OH groups present in the minor groove of the RNA duplex and the dsRNA binding domain.[87] When bound to the 2′-OH groups through hydrogen bonding, positively charged residues (equivalent to Lys-167 in E3L) likely make electrostatic interactions with the negatively charged phosphate backbone on the RNA duplex. For PKR, the linker region between the dsRNA binding motifs is highly flexible, which allows the two motifs to wrap around the RNA duplex for cooperative and high-affinity binding.[83] For E3L, two RNA binding motifs are presented after protein dimerization.

In recent years, the structure of the dsRNA binding motif complexed with dsRNA has been resolved. The structure reveals that an RNA duplex of 12–16 base pairs is necessary for binding.[88,89] Interaction involves recognition of two successive minor grooves and spanning across the intervening major groove on one face of the RNA duplex. This manner of interaction explains the nonsequence-specific recognition of dsRNA and lack of binding to ssRNA or dsDNA. Of the $\alpha–\beta–\beta–\beta–\alpha$ motif, the N terminus of $\alpha1$ and the loop between $\beta1$ and $\beta2$ interact with the adjacent minor grooves on the RNA duplex and $\alpha2$ interacts with the intervening major groove.[89,90] Considering corresponding conserved residues in E3L, it is likely that Glu-122 in $\alpha1$, and Lys-167 and Lys-171 in $\alpha2$ are involved in direct interaction with the RNA duplex.

15.5 VACCINE EFFICACY OF VACCINIA VIRUS E3L MUTANTS

Currently the only commercially approved smallpox vaccine available for limited use in the United States is Wyeth Dryvax. This vaccine is derived from the New York City Board of Health (NYCBH) strain that underwent 22–28 heifer passages.[91] This live-virus vaccine is very effective but can lead to serious adverse reactions. These safety concerns, along with the threat of biological terror agents, have spearheaded a push toward development of improved smallpox vaccine agents. Modified vaccinia virus Ankara (MVA) and NYVAC are two attenuated strains currently being developed. MVA was attenuated through multiple passages in chicken cells and does not grow productively in cells of human origin.[92,93] Compared to Dryvax, MVA produces equivalent antibody neutralizing titers and T-cell responses and has been deemed safe for use in immunocompromised individuals.[94,95] NYVAC as well is highly attenuated due to the precise deletion of 18 open reading frames from the viral genome but does not produce ulceration at the site of inoculation, which is a generally accepted indicator of vaccine "take."[96]

Given the role of the vaccinia virus E3L gene in viral pathogenesis, the gene is a logical target toward the construction of a novel attenuated vaccine vector. Indeed, recent research suggests that vaccinia virus constructs expressing mutations in E3L are highly attenuated yet are capable of inducing a highly protective immune response. By either scarification or intranasal inoculation of mice with the vaccinia virus constructs expressing mutations in E3L, mice were protected against subsequent challenge with wild-type virus. With virus expressing E3L deleted of the N terminus, vaccination with as little as 100 plaque forming units (pfu) intranasally was sufficient to protect against a wild-type vaccinia virus challenge of 10^6 pfu. For virus deleted of E3L completely or deleted of the dsRNA binding motif, 1000 pfu was able to provide an equivalent level of protection against wild-type virus challenge. Thus, these mutants can produce a mucosal or dermal protective response even though they are at least 5 $\log_{10}$ units less virulent than wild-type virus. For virus deleted of E3L, the 1000 pfu inoculum provides effective protection yet the virus does not replicate efficiently in the nasal tissue reaching maximal titers around 1000 pfu/g tissue. With the loss of the N terminus of E3L, the 100 pfu inoculation required for effective protection leads to efficient virus replication in the nasal turbinates with virus titers reaching 1×10^6 pfu/g of tissue. This increase in virus titer is *required* for the protective response, since when mice are inoculated with 10 pfu of the E3L N-terminally deleted virus protection against a wild-type vaccinia virus challenge is not achieved even though virus titers reach levels of 1×10^5 pfu/g. These results suggest that vaccinia virus containing a full deletion of E3L may be the most effective vaccine since protection does not appear to require an increase in virus titers.

15.6 CONCLUSION

Of the weapons of mass destruction, biological weapons are the most feared,[97] in part because many biological weapons are infectious and can spread to large parts of the community after release. The fear of biological weapons is even greater with terrorist groups, since biological agents are easily hidden, have high potency, and are relatively easy to make and deliver.[97] As Pearson points out,[98] "biological weapons are sometimes referred to as the poor man's atomic bomb." While numerous biological organisms could potentially be used as weapons, the Working Group on Civilian Biodefenses has identified only a few organisms that could cause disease and deaths in sufficient numbers to cripple a city or region.[99] Of the potential biological agents available for use as weapons, smallpox is considered to be among the most dangerous threats.[100] Variola virus, the virus that causes smallpox, is extremely lethal, is infectious by aerosol, and can be produced in large quantities in a stable form. While there are only two acknowledged repositories for smallpox, it is thought that several "rogue" nations have clandestine stocks of smallpox.

Smallpox is a highly communicable, often fatal disease (approximately 30% mortality in susceptible individuals[101]). While immunization with vaccinia virus can provide good protection against exposure to variola virus, the current vaccine is far from optimal. Overall reportable complications occur in 1/1000 to 1/10,000 vaccinees, with at least one death per million vaccinees likely, with the strains of vaccinia virus currently available for use.[101]

Attempts are being made to develop smallpox vaccines with fewer complications. Inactivated vaccinia virus does not provide adequate protection[101] and many current attenuated strains provide inadequate protection or are difficult to grow in large quantities. It is well known that poxviruses encode a multitude of proteins that function by blocking the host antiviral and immune responses. These data imply that vaccinia virus infection leads to the activation of these host responses to which the virus must respond in order to maintain efficient replication. An alternative approach to preparing safer vaccine strains of vaccinia virus is to prepare replication competent strains that are attenuated for pathogenesis. Targets for attenuation include viral genes known to be involved in blocking the cellular immune or antiviral response. Viruses containing mutations in the vaccinia virus E3L gene are candidates for such vaccine vectors.[1] Mutations in E3L render the virus attenuated but yield a virus that is otherwise fully replication competent in cells-in-culture. These viruses are drastically reduced in terms of pathogenesis in mouse model systems[102] and since these viruses do not disseminate from the site of infection, the major complications associated with wild-type virus vaccination should be greatly reduced, if not completely eliminated.

Given the importance of dsRNA and possibly Z-DNA (or Z-RNA) in controlling viral replication, the E3L gene, in many ways, is the optimal target for developing attenuated vaccinia virus strains and as a possible target for novel anti-poxvirus compounds. The future holds great promise in these regards with many directions of research being conducted. One day, the foreseen threat of smallpox as a bioterror agent that could once again wreak havoc on the human population may be a peril of the past.

REFERENCES

1. Jacobs, B. L.; Langland, J. O. When two strands are better than one: the mediators and modulators of the cellular responses to double-stranded RNA. *Virology* **1996**, *219*, 339–349.

2. Moss, B. Poxviridae and their replication. *In Virology*, 2nd Ed., Fields, B.N.; Knipe, D. M. (eds.). Raven Press, New York, **1990**, pp. 2079–2111,

3. Colby, C.; Jurale, C.; Kates, J. R. Mechanism of synthesis of vaccinia virus double-stranded ribonucleic acid in vivo and in vitro. *J. Virol.* **1971**, *7*, 71–76.

4. Boone, R. F.; Parr, R. P.; Moss, B. Intermolecular duplexes formed from polyadenylated vaccinia virus RNA. *J. Virol.* **1979**, *30*, 365–374.

5. Bayliss, C. D.; Condit, R. C. Temperature-sensitive mutants in the vaccinia virus A18R gene increase double-stranded RNA synthesis as a result of aberrant viral transcription. *Virology* **1993**, *194*, 254–262.

6. Simpson, D. A.; Condit, R. C. The vaccinia virus A18R protein plays a role in viral transcription during both the early and the late phases of infection. *J. Virol.* **1994**, *68*, 3642–3649.

7. Stark, G. R.; Kerr, I. M.; Williams, B. R. G.; Silverman, R. H.; Schreiber, R. D. How cells respond to interferon. *Ann. Rev. Biochem.* **1998**, *67*, 227–264.

8. Goodbourn, S.; Didcock, L.; Randall, R. E. Interferons: cell signaling, immune modulation, antiviral responses and virus countermeasures. *J. Gen. Virol.* **2000**, *81*, 2341–2364.

9. Kostura, A. E.; Mathews, M. B. Purification and activation of the double-stranded RNA-dependent eIF-2 kinase DAI. *Mol. Cell. Biol.* **1989**, *9*, 1576–1586.

10. Langland, J. O.; Jacobs, B. L. Cytosolic double-stranded RNA-dependent protein kinase is likely a dimer of partially phosphorylated Mr = 66,000 subunits. *J. Biol. Chem.* **1992**, *267*, 10729–1073.

11. Patel, R. C.; Stanton, P.; McMillan, N. M.; Williams, B. R.; Sen, G. C. The interferon-inducible double-stranded RNA-activated protein kinase self-assembles in vitro and in vivo. *Proc. Natl. Acad. Sci. U.S.A.* **1995**, *92*, 8283–8287.

12. Thomis, D. C.; Samuel, C. E. Mechanism of interferon action: Characterization of the intermolecular autophosphorylation of PKR, the interferon-inducible, RNA-dependent protein kinase. *J. Virol.* **1995**, *69*, 5195–5198.

13. Meurs, E. F.; Chong, K.; Galabru, J.; Thomas, N. S.; Kerr, I. M.; Williams, B. R.; Hovanaessian, A. G. Molecular cloning and characterization of the human double-stranded RNA-activated protein kinase induced by interferon. *Cell* **1990**, *62*, 379–390.

14. Robertson, H. D.; Mathews, M. B. The regulation of the protein kinase PKR by RNA. *Biochimie* **1996**, *78*, 909–914.

15. Meurs, E. F.; Watanabe, Y.; Kadereit, S.; Barber, G. N.; Katze, M. G.; Chong, K.; Williams, B. R. G.; Hovanessian, A. G. Constitutive expression of human double-strnaded RNA-activated p68 kinase in murine cells mediates phosphorylation of eukaryotic initiation factor 2 and partial resistance to encephalomyocarditis growth. *J. Virol.* **1992**, *66*, 5805–5814.

16. Clemens, M. J.; Elia, A. The double-stranded RNA-dependent protein kinase PKR: structure and function. *J. Interferon Cytol. Res.* **1997**, *17*, 503–524.

17. Gil, J.; Garcia, M. A.; Gomex-Puertas, P.; Guerra, S.; Rullas, J.; Nakano, H.; Alcami, J.; Esteban, M. TRAF family proteins link PKR with NF-kappa B activation. *Mol. Cell. Biol.* **2004**, *24*, 4502–4512.

18. Goh, K. C.; deVeer, M. J.; Williams, B. R. G. The protein kinase PKR is required for p38 MAPK activation and the innate immune response to bacterial endotoxin. *EMBO J.* **2000**, *19*, 4292–4297.

19. Smith, E. J.; Marie, I.; Prakash, A.; Garcia-Sastre A.; Levy, D. E. IRF3 and IRF7 phosphorylation in virus-infected cells does not require double-stranded RNA-dependent protein kinase R or Ikappa B kinase but is blocked by Vaccinia virus E3L protein. *J Biol Chem* **2001**, *276*, 8951–8957.

20. Kerr, I. M.; Brown, R. E.; pppA2′p5′A2′p5′A2′p5′A: an inhibitor of protein synthesis synthesized with an enzyme fraction from interferon-treated cells. *Proc. Natl. Acad. Sci. USA* **1978**, *75*, 256–260.

21. Silverman, R. H.; Jung, D. D.; Nolan-Sorden, N. L.; Dieffenbach, C. W.; Kedar, V. P.; Sengupta, D. N. Purification and analysis of murine 2-5A-dependent RNase. *J. Biol. Chem.* **1988**, *263*, 7336–7341.

22. Bisbal, R. A.; Salehzada, T.; Lebleu, B.; Bayard, B. Characterization of two murine (2′-5′) (A)n-dependent endonucleases of different molecular mass. *Eur. J. Biochem.* **1989**, *179*, 595–602.

23. Powell, P. P.; Dixon, L. K.; Parkhouse, R. M. An IkB homolog encoded by Africa swine fever virus provides a novel mechanism for downregulation of proinflammatory cytokine responses in host macrophages. *J. Virol.* **1996**, *70*, 8527–8533.

24. Revilla, Y.; Callejo, M.; Rodriguez, J. M.; Culabras, E.; Nogal, M. L.; Salas, M. L.; Vinuela, E.; Fresno, M. Inhibition of nuclear factor kB activation by a virus-encoded IkB-like protein. *J. Biol. Chem.* **1998**, *273*, 5405–5411.

25. Mossman, K.; Upton, C.; Buller, R. M. L.; McFadden, G. Species specificity of ectromelia virus and vaccinia virus interferon-g binding proteins. *Virology* **1995**, *208*, 762–769.

26. Alcami, A.; Smith, G. L. Receptors for gamma-interferon encoded by poxviruses: implication for the unknown origin of vaccinia virus. *J. Virol.* **1995**, *69*, 4633–4639.

27. Symons, J. A.; Alcami. A.; Smith, G. L. Vaccinia virus encodes a soluble type I interferon receptor of novel structure and broad species specificity. *Cell* **1995**, *81* (4), 551–560.

28. Colamonici, O. R.; Domanski, P.; Sweitzer, S. M.; Larner, A.; Buller, R. M. L. Vaccinia virus B18R gene encodes a type I interferon-binding protein that blocks interferon a transmembrane signaling. *J. Biol. Chem.* **1995**, *270*, 15974–15978.

29. Ronco, L. V.; Karpova, A. Y.; Vidal, M.; Howley, P. M. Human papillomavirus 16 E6 oncoprotein binds to interferon regulatory factor-3 and inhibits its transcriptional activity. *Genes and Dev.* **1998**, *12*, 2061–2072.

30. Miller, D. M.; Rahill, B. M.; Boss, J. M.; Lairmore, M. D.; Durbin, J. E.; Waldman, J. W.; Sedmak, D. D. Human cytomegalovirus inhibits major histocompatibility complex class II expression by disruption of the Jas/STAT pathway. *J. Exp. Med.* **1998**, *187*, 675–683.

31. Weihua, X.; Ramanujam, S.; Lindner, D. J.; Kudaravalli, R. D.; Freund, R.; Kalvakolanu, D. V. The polyoma virus T antigen interferes with interferon-inducible gene expression. *Proc. Natl. Acad. Sci. USA* **1998**, *95*, 1085–1090.

32. Didcock, L.; Young, D. F.; Goodbourn, S.; Randall, R. E.; The V protein of simian virus 5 inhibits interferon signaling by targeting STAT1 for proteasome-mediated degradation. *J. Virol.* **1999**, *73*, 9928–9933.

33. Yokosawa, N.; Kubota, T.; Fujii, N. Poor induction of interferon-induced 2′-5′-oligoa-denylate synthetase (2-5 AS) in cells persistently infected with mumps virus is caused by decrease of STAT1a. *Achives Virol.* **1998**, *143*, 1985–1992.

34. Young, D. F.; Didcock, L.; Goodbourn, S.; Randall, R. E. Paramyxoviridae use distinct virus-specific mechanisms to circumvent the interferon response. *Virology* **2000**, *269*, 383–390.

35. Komatsu, T.; Takeuchi, K.; Yokoo, J.; Tanaka, Y.; Gotoh, B. Sendai virus blocks alpha interferon signaling to signal transducers and activators of transcription. *J. Virol.* **2000**, *74*, 2477–2480.

36. Najarro, P.; Traktman, P.; Lewis, J. A. Vaccinia virus blocks gamma interferon signal transduction: viral VH1 phosphatase reverses Stat1 activation. *J. Virol.* **2001**, *75*, 3185–3196.

37. Gale, M. J.; Korth, M. J.; Tang, N. M.; Tan, S. L.; Hopkins, D. A.; Dever, T. E.; Polyak, S. J.; Gretch, D. R.; Katze, M. G.; Evidence that hepatitis C virus resistance to interferon is mediated through repression of the PKR protein kinase by the nonstructural 5A protein. *Virology* **1997**, *230*, 217–227.

38. Melville, M. W.; Hansen, W. J.; Freeman, B. C.; Welch, W. J.; Katze, M. G. The molecular chaperone hsp40 regulates the activity of P58IPK, the cellular inhibitor of PKR. *Proc. Natl. Acad. Sci. U.S.A.* **1997**, *94*, 97–102.

39. He, B.; Gross, M.; Roizman, B. The g34.5 protein of herpes simplex virus 1 complexes with protein phosphatase 1a to dephosphorylate the a subunit of the eukaryotic translation initiation factor 2 and preclude the shutoff of protein synthesis by double-stranded RNA-activated protein kinase. *Proc. Natl. Acad. Sci. U.S.A.* **1997**, *94*, 843–848.

40. Langland, J. O.; Pettiford, S.; Jiang, B.; Jacobs, B. L. Products of the porcine group C rotavirus NSP3 gene bind specifically to double-stranded RNA and inhibit activation of the interferon-induced protein kinase PKR. *J. Virol.* **1994**, *68*, 3821–3829.

41. Jacobs, B. L.; Langland, J. O. Characterization of viral double-stranded RNA-binding proteins. *Methods* **1998**, *15*, 225–232.

42. Chien, C. Y.; Xu, Y.; Xiao, R.; Aramini, J. M.; Sahasrabudhe, P. V.; Krug, R. M.; Montelione, G. T. Biophysical characterization of the complex between double-stranded RNA and the N-terminal domain of NS1 protein from influenza A virus: evidence for a novel RNA-binding mode. *Biochemistry* **2004**, *43*, 1950–1962.

43. Davies, M. V.; Elroy-Stein, O.; Jagus, R.; Moss, B.; Kaufman, R. J.; The vaccinia virus K3L gene product potentiates translation by inhibiting double-stranded RNA-activated protein kinase and phosphorylation of the alpha subunit of eukaryotic initiation factor 2. *J. Virol.* **1992**, *66*, 1943–1950.

44. Carroll, K.; Elroy-Stein, O.; Moss, B.; Jagus, R. Recombinant vaccinia virus K3L gene product prevents activation of double-stranded RNA-dependent initiation factor 2 alpha-specific protein kinase. *J. Biol. Chem.* **1993**, *268*, 12837–12842.

45. Barquet, N; Domingo, P. Smallpox: the triumph over the most terrible of the ministers of death. *Ann. Intern. Med.* **1997**, *127*, 635–642.

46. Tizard, I. Grease, anthraxgate, and kennel cough: a revisionist history of early veterinary vaccines. *Adv. Vet. Med.* **1999**, *41*, 7–24.

47. Yuen, L.; Moss, B. Oligonucleotide sequence signaling transcriptional termination of vaccinia virus early genes. *Proc. Natl. Acad. Sci. USA* **1987**, *84*, 6417–6421.

48. Mahr, A.; Roberts, B. E. Arrangement of late RNAs transcribed from a 7.1 kilobase Eco RI vaccinia virus DNA fragment. *J. Virol.* **1984**, *49*, 510–520.

49. Langland, J. O.; Jacobs, B. L. Inhibition of PKR by vaccinia virus: role of the N- and C-terminal domains of E3L. *Virology* **2004**, *324*, 419–429.

50. Beattie, E.; Paoletti, E.; Tartaglia, J. Distinct patterns of IFN sensitivity observed in cells infected with vaccinia K3L- and E3L- mutant viruses. *Virology* **1995**, *210*, 254–263.

51. Langland, J. O.; Jacobs, B. L. The role of the PKR-inhibitory genes, E3L and K3L, in determining vaccinia virus host range. *Virology* **2002**, *299*, 133–141.

52. Beattie, E.; Tartaglia, J.; Paoletti, E. Vaccinia virus encoded eIF-2a homolog abrogates the antiviral effects of interferon. *Virology* **1991**, *183*, 419–422.

53. Koromilas, A. E.; Roy, S.; Barber, G. N.; Katze, M. G.; Sonenberg, N. Malignant transformation by a mutant of the IFN-inducible dsRNA-dependent protein kinase. *Science* **1992**, *257*, 1685–1689.

54. Craig, A. W. B.; Cosentino, G. P.; Donze, O.; Sonenberg, N. The kinase insert domain of interferon-induced protein kinase PKR is required for activity but not for interaction with the pseudosubstrate K3L. *J. Biol. Chem.* **1996**, *271*, 24526–24533.

55. Qian, W.; Zhu, S.; Sobolev, A. Y.; Wek, R. C. Expression of vaccinia virus K3L protein in yeast inhibits eukaryotic initiation factor-2 kinase GCN2 and the general amino acids control. *J. Biol. Chem.* **1996**, *271*, 13202–13207.

56. Sood, R.; Porter, A. C.; Ma, K.; Quilliam, L. A.; Wek, R. C.; Pancreatic eukaryotic initiation factor-2 alpha kinase (PEK) homologues in humans, *Drosophila melanogaster* and *Caenorhabditis elegans* that mediate translational control in response to endoplasmic reticulum stress. *Biochem J.* **2000**, *346*, 281–293.

57. DeBondt, H. L.; Rosenblatt, J.; Jancarik, J.; Jones, H. D.; Morgan, D. O.; Kim, S. H. Crystal structure of cyclin-dependent kinase 2. *Nature* **1993**, *363*, 595–602.

58. Dar, A. C.; Sicheri, F. X-ray crystal structure and functional analysis of vaccinia virus K3L reveals molecular determinants for PKR subversion and substrate recognition. *Mol. Cell* **2002**, *10*, 295–305.

59. Kawagishi-Kobayashi, M.; Silverman, J. B.; Ung, T. L.; Dever, T. E. Regulation of the protein kinase PKR by the vaccinia virus pseudosubstrate inhibitor K3L is dependent on residues conserved between the K3L protein and the PKR substrate eIF2alpha. *Mol. Cell. Biol.* **1997**, *17*, 4146–4158.

60. Paez, E.; Esteban, M. Resistance of vaccinia virus to interferon is related to an interference phenomenon between the virus and the interferon system. *Virology* **1984**, *134*, 12–28.

61. Rice, A. P.; Kerr, I. M. Interferon-mediated, double-stranded RNA-dependent protein kinase is inhibitied in extracts from vaccinia virus-infected cells. *J. Virol.* **1984**, *50*, 220–228.

62. Whitaker-Dowling, P.; Youngner, J. S. Vaccinia rescue of VSV from interferon-induced resistance: reversal of translation block and inhibition of protein kinase activity. *Virology* **1983**, *131*, 128–136.

63. Chang, H. W.; Watson, J. C.; Jacobs, B. L. The E3L gene of vaccinia virus encodes an inhibitor of the interferon-induced, double-stranded RNA-dependent protein kinase. *Proc. Natl. Acad. Sci. U.S.A.* **1992**, *89*, 4825–4829.

64. Chang, H. W.; Uribe, L. H.; Jacobs, B. L.; Rescue of vaccinia virus deleted for the E3L gene by mutants of E3L. *J. Virol.* **1995**, *69*, 6605–6608.

65. Romano, P. R.; Zhang, F.; Tan, S.; Garcia-Barrio, M. T.; Katze, M. G.; Dever, T. E.; Hinnebusch, A. G. Inhibition of double-stranded RNA-dependent protein kinase PKR by vaccinia virus E3: role of complex formation and the E3 N-terminal domain. *Mol. Cell. Biol.* **1998**, *18*, 7304–7316.

66. Shors, T.; Kibler, K. V.; Perkins, K. B.; Seidler-Wulff R.; Banaszak, M. P.; Jacobs, B. L. Complementation of vaccinia virus deleted of the E3L gene by mutants of E3L. *Virology* **1997**, *239*, 269–276.

67. Shors, S. T.; Beattie, E.; Paoletti, E.; Tartaglia, J.; Jacobs, B. L. Role of the vaccinia virus E3L and K3L gene products in rescue of VSV and EMCV from the effects of IFN-α. *J. Interferon and Cytokine Res.* **1998**, *18*, 721–729.

68. Yuwen, H.; Cox, J. H.; Yewdell, J. W.; Bennink, J. R.; Moss, B. Nuclear localization of a double-stranded RNA-binding protein encoded by the vaccinia virus E3L gene. *Virology* **1993**, *195*, 732–744.

69. DeGarcia, D. J.; Sullivan, J. M.; Neumar, R. W.; Alousi, S. S.; Hikade, K. R.; Pittman, J. E.; White, B. C.; Rafols, J. A.; Krause, G. S. Effect of brain ischemia and reperfusion on the localization of phosphorylated eukaryotic initiation factor 2α. *J. Cerebral Blood Flow Metab.* **1997**, *17*, 1291–1302.

70. Goldstein, E. N.; Owen, C. R.; White, B. C.; Rafols, J. A. Ultrastructural localization of phosphorylated eIF2α [eIF2α(P)] in rat dorsal hippocampus during reperfusion. *Acta Neuropathol.* **1999**, *98*, 493–505.

71. Jeffrey, I. W.; Kadereit, S.; Meurs, E. F.; Metzger, T.; Bachmann, M.; Schwemmle, M.; Hovanessian, A. G.; Clemens, M. J. Nuclear localization of the interferon-induced protein kinase PKR in human cells and transfected mouse cells. *Exp. Cell. Res.* **1995**, *218*, 17–27.

72. Lobo, M. V.; Alonso, F. J.; Rodriguez, S.; Alcazar, A.; Martin, E.; Munoz, F.; G-Santander, R.; Salinas, M.; Fando, J. L.; Localization of eukaryotic initiation factor 2 in neuron primary cultures and established cell lines. *Histochem. J.* **1997**, *29*, 453–468.

73. Martin, M. E.; Alcazar, A.; Fando, J. L.; Garcia, A. M.; Salinas, M. Translational initiation factor eIF2 subcellular levels and phosphorylation status in the developing brain. *Neurosci. Letters* **1993**, *156*, 109–112.

74. Takizawa, T.; Tatematsu, C.; Watanabe, M.; Yoshida, M.; Nakajima, K. Three leucine-rich sequences and the N-terminal region of double-stranded RNA-activated protein kinase (PKR) are responsible for its cytoplasmic localization. *J. Biochem. (Tokyo)* **2000**, *128*, 471–476.

75. Ting, N. S. Y.; Kao, P. N.; Chan, D. W.; Lintott, L. G.; Lees-Miller, S. P. DNA-dependent protein kinase interacts with antigen receptor response element binding proteins NF90 and NF45. *J. Biol. Chem.* **1998**, *273*, 2136–2145.

76. Strudwick, S.; Borden, K. L. B. The emerging roles of translation factor eIF4E in the nucleus. *Differentiation* **2002**, *70*, 10–22.

77. Romano, P. R.; Zhang, F.; Tan, S. L.; Garcia-Barrio, M. T.; Katze, M. G.; Dever, T. E.; Hinnebusch, A. G. Inhibition of double-stranded RNA-dependent protein kinase PKR by vaccinia virus E3: role of complex formation and the E3 N-terminal domain. *Mol. Cell Biol.* **1998**, *18*(12), 7304–7316.

78. Liu, Y.; Herbert, A.; Rich, A.; Samuel, C. E. Double-stranded RNA-specific adenosine deaminase: nucleic acid binding properties. *Methods* **1998**, *15*, 199–205.

79. Rothenburg, S.; Shwartz, T.; Korch-Nolte, F.; Haag, F. Complex regulation of the human gene for the Z-DNA binding protein DLM-1. *Nucleic Acids Res.* **2002**, *30*, 993–1000.

80. Hu, C.; Zhang, Y.; Huasng, G.; Zhang, Q.; Gui, J. Molecular cloning and characterization of a fish PKR-like gene from cultured CAB cells induced by UV-inactivated virus. *Fish Shellfish Immun.* **2004**, *17*, 353–366.

81. Kim, Y. G.; Muralinath, M.; Brandt, T.; Pearcy, M.; Hauns, K.; Lowenhaupt, K.; Jacobs, B. L.; Rich, A. A role for Z-DNA binding in vaccinia virus pathogenesis. *Proc. Natl. Acad. Sci. U.S.A.* **2003**, *100*, 6974–6979.

82. Ho, C. K.; Shuman, S. Mutational analysis of the vaccinia virus E3 protein defines amino acid residues involved in E3 binding to double-stranded RNA. *J. Virol.* **1996**, *70*, 2611–2614.

83. Nanduri, S.; Carpick, B. W.; Yang, Y.; Williams, B. R. G.; Qin, J. Structure of the double-stranded RNA-binding domain of the protein kinase PKR reveals the molecular basis of its dsRNA-mediated activation. *EMBO J.* **1998**, *17*, 5458–5465.

84. Bycroft, M.; Grunert, S.; Murzin, A. G.; Proctor, M.; St. Johnston, D. NMR solution structure of a dsRNA binding domain from *Drosophila staufen* protein reveals homology to the N-terminal domain of ribosomal protein S5. *EMBO J.* **1995**, *14*, 3563–3571.

85. Doyle, M.; Jantsch, M. F. New and old roles of the double-stranded RNA-binding domain. *J. Struct. Biol.* **2002**, *140*(1–3), 147–53.

86. Wu, H.; Henras, A.; Chanfreau, G.; Feigon, J. Structural basis for recognition of the AGNN tetraloop RNA fold by the double-stranded RNA-binding domain of Rnt1p RNase III. *Proc. Natl. Acad. Sci. USA* **2004**, *101*, 8307–8312.

87. Bevilacgua, P. C.; Cech, T. R. Minor-groove recognition of double-stranded RNA by the double-stranded RNA-binding domain from the RNA-activated protein kinase PKR. *Biochemistry* **1996**, *35*(31), 9983–9994.

88. Ryter, N. M.; Schultz, S. C. Molecular basis of double-stranded RNA-protein interactions: structure of a dsRNA-binding domain complexed with dsRNA. *EMBO J.* **1998**, *17*(24), 7505–7513.

89. Ramos, A.; Bayer, P.; Varani, G. Determination of the structure of the RNA complex of a double-stranded RNA-binding domain from *Drosophila staufen* protein. *Biopolymers* **2001**, *52*, 181–196.

90. Fierro-Monti, I.; Mathews, M. B. Proteins binding to duplexed RNA: one motif, multiple functions. *TIBS* **2000**, *25*, 241–246.

91. Rosenthal, S. R.; Merchlinsky, M.; LKleppinger C.; Goldenthal K. L. Developing New Smallpox Vaccines 2001. http://www.cdc.gov/ncidod/EID/eid.htm

92. Carroll, M. W.; Moss, B. Host range and cytopathogenicity of the highly attenuated MVA strain of vaccinia virus: propagation and generation of recombinant viruses in a nonhuman mammalian cell line. *Virology* **1997**, *238*, 198–211.

93. Ramirez, J. C.; Gherardi, M. M.; Rodriguez, D.; Esteban, M. Attenuated modified vaccinia virus Ankara can be used as an immunizing agent under conditions of preexisting immunity to the vector. *J. Virol.* **2000** *74*(16), 7651–7655.

94. Earl, P. L.; Americo, J. L.; Wyatt, L. S.; Eller, L. A.; Whitbeck, J. C.; Cohen, G. H.; Eisenberg, R. J.; Hartmann, C. J.; Jackson, D. L.; Kulesh, D. A.; Martinez, M. J.; Miller, D. M.; Mucker, E. M.; Shamblin, J. D.; Zwiers, S. H.; Huggins, J. W.; Jahrling, P. B.;

Moss, B. Immunogenicity of a highly attenuated MVA smallpox vaccine and protection against monkeypox. *Nature* **2004**, *428*, 182–185.

95. Stittelaar, K. J.; Kuiken, T.; de Swart, R. L.; van Amerongen, G.; Vos, H. W.; Niesters, H. G.; van Schalkwijk, P.; van der Kwast, T.; Wyatt, L. S.; Moss, B.; Osterhaus, A. D. Safety of modified vaccinia virus Ankara (MVA) in immune-suppressed macaques. *Vaccine* **2001**, *19*, 3700–3709.

96. Tartaglia, J.; Cox, W. I.; Taylor. J.; Perkus. K.; Riviere, M.; Meignier, B.; Paoletti, E. Highly attenuated poxvirus vectors. *AIDS Res. Hum. Retroviruses* **1992**, *8*(8), 1445–1447.

97. Danzig, R.; Berkowsky, P. B. Why should we be concerned about biological warfare? *JAMA* **1997**, *278*, 431–432.

98. Pearson, G. S. The complementary role of environmental and security biological control regimes in the 21st century. *JAMA* **1997**, *278*, 369–372.

99. Inglesby, T. V.; Henderson, D. A.; Bartlett, J. G.; Ascher, M. S.; Eitzen, E.; Friedlander, A. M.; Hauer, J.; McDade, J.; Osterholm, M. T.; O'Toole, T.; Parker, G.; Perl, T. M.; Russell, P. K.; Tonat, K. Anthrax as a biological weapon: medical and public health management. Working Group on Civilian Biodefense. *JAMA* **1999**, *281*, 1735–1745.

100. Henderson, D. A. The looming threat of bioterrorism. *Science* **1999**, *283*, 1279–1282.

101. Fenner, F.; Henderson, D. A.; Arita, I.; Jezek, Z.; Ladnyi, I. D. *Smallpox and Its Eradication*. World Health Organization, Geneva, 1988.

102. Brandt, T. A; Jacobs, B. L. Both carboxy- and amino-terminal domains of the vaccinia virus interferon resistance gene, E3L, are required for pathogenesis in a mouse model. *J. Virol.* **2001**, *75*, 850–856.

103. Saunders, L. R.; Barber, G. N. The dsRNA binding protein family: critical roles, diverse cellular functions. *FASEB* **2003**, *17*, 961–983.

EMERGING

EID
OnLine

INFECTIOUS DISEASES

A Peer-Reviewed Journal Tracking and Analyzing Disease Trends   Vol. 12, No. 4, April 2006

Arthropod-borne Infections

CDC

Broad-Spectrum Antiviral Prophylaxis: Inhibition of Viral Infection by Polymer Grafting with Methoxypoly(ethylene glycol)

LORI L. McCOY and MARK D. SCOTT

Canadian Blood Services and Department of Pathology and Laboratory Medicine, University of British Columbia

16.1   INTRODUCTION

Previous bioterrorism research on viruses centered on agents characterized by rapid onset and high mortality.[1,2] These agents typically included the smallpox, encephalitis, and hemorrhagic fever viruses.[3–5] However, these specific agents also pose significant, long-term risks to the individuals or nations utilizing them. Consequently, considerable interest has developed in easily transmissible viral agents that are characterized by rapid onset and significant, often immobilizing morbidity but that are of less long-term concern to the parties employing them.[6]

Nature itself has demonstrated significant versatility in designing such agents as evidenced by the annual cold and flu epidemics and more recently by the severe acute respiratory syndrome (SARS) and avian flu viruses.[7–9] Indeed, analysis of the transmissibility traits of respiratory viruses (e.g., rhino, adeno, corona, and picornaviruses) clearly indicates that virulent and/or bioengineered strains could function as potent bioterrorism vectors without the serious long-term concerns of a smallpox-like agent. More importantly, these viruses are characterized by high mutation rates, making development of an antiviral cocktail difficult. Indeed, current prophylactic options (versus disease treatment) to viral bioterrorism agents are almost exclusively focused on vaccine development.[10,11] An inherent fallacy/presumption of the vaccine approach is that it requires an informed guess as to the agent to be used, including any newly engineered genetic changes. As demonstrated

Antiviral Drug Discovery for Emerging Diseases and Bioterrorism Threats. Edited by Paul F. Torrence
Copyright © 2005 John Wiley & Sons, Inc.

by the efficacy of the annual flu vaccine, this approach has been only partially effective.[12] To this end, a broad-spectrum antiviral prophylactic agent would be of significant benefit. To date no such agent exists.

Previous research from our laboratory has clearly demonstrated that the covalent grafting of methoxypoly(ethylene glycol) (mPEG) to cell surfaces sterically obscures membrane epitopes and obscures surface charge, leading to the immuno-camouflage of the modified cell.[13–26] The resultant immunocamouflage globally inhibits receptor–ligand interactions, which result in decreased/absent red blood cell agglutination, loss of red cell sedimentation, attenuated allorecognition and T cell proliferation, and diminished antibody recognition of membrane surface anti-gens. Because of the importance of receptor–ligand interactions to viral entry and infection, we hypothesized that the covalent grafting of mPEG to host cells and/or the virus particles would provide a potent, broad-spectrum antiviral effect.[27–30] This hypothesis is diagrammatically shown in Figure 16.1 using the nasal passage epithelium as an example. In normal viral pathogenesis, the virus is introduced into the local environment, whereupon it recognizes cellular receptors (e.g., ICAM-1 for 80–90% of rhinoviruses) and is taken up by receptor-mediated endocytosis.[31] The virus then uncoats and undergoes replication within the host cell and eventually packages and releases progeny virus into the nasal cavity, which infect naive epi-thelial cells. As proposed in Figure 16.1, covalent grafting of mPEG to either the virus (direct viral inactivation) or host cells (indirect viral inactivation) interferes with receptor–ligand interactions, thereby preventing viral entry and disease induc-tion. The same protective mechanism also functions with viruses whose entry is mediated by cell fusion.

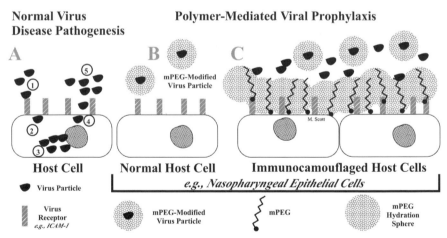

FIGURE 16.1 Effects of immunocamouflage on viral pathogenesis. (A) Virus recognizes, binds to cell receptor ①, is internalized ② undergoes multiple rounds of replication ③, progeny virus is packaged and shed ④ into the extracellular environment ⑤, whereupon it infects new host cells ①. mPEG grafting to either the *free virus* (B) or *host cells* (C) interrupts the disease cycle.

16.2 IMMUNOCAMOUFLAGE OF CELLS AND VIRUSES

Over the last several years, our laboratory has focused on the prevention of allorecognition of donor tissues (erythrocytes, lymphocytes, endothelial cells, and pancreatic islets) by the application of cellular *immunocamouflage*.[13–30] The immunocamouflage of cells is mediated by the covalent grafting of cell surfaces with poly(ethylene glycol) [PEG; $HO—(CH_2CH_2O)_n—CH_2CH_2OH$]. To chemically graft the PEG to proteins, a chemical linker compound is attached to one of the terminal hydroxyl (—OH) residues. Chemical linkers commonly employed include cyanuric chloride, succinimidyl proprionate, and benzotriazolylcarbonate. To further diminish any residual reactivity of the grafted PEG, the remaining —OH group is substituted with a methyl (—CH_3) group to produce activated methoxypoly(ethylene glycol) [mPEG; $CH_3—(CH_2CH_2O)_n—CH_2CH_2$ linker chemistry].

Biophysically, the grafted mPEG confers its immunoprotective effects due to the rapid mobility and intramolecular flexibility of the heavily hydrated PEG chains. As shown in Figure 16.2, rigid linear molecules lack any significant radius of gyration (R_g), resulting in poor or absent camouflaging of membrane antigens. In contrast, mPEG, while a linear molecule, exhibits a high degree of intrachain flexibility due to the repeating, highly mobile, ethoxy units. Based on this intrachain mobility, its R_g is very close to its linear length (L). As a result of this intrachain mobility, as

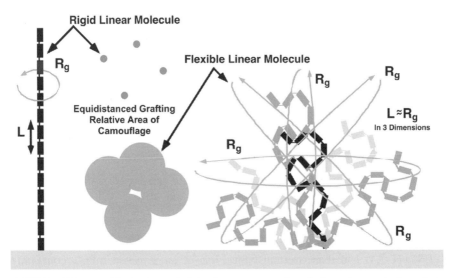

FIGURE 16.2   The biophysics underlying immunocamouflage is dependent on the intrachain molecular flexibility of the mPEG polymer. Rigid linear molecules have a small radius of gyration (R_g) and fail to effectively camouflage the cell surface. In contrast, the linear, but highly flexible, mPEG polymer yields a large zone of steric occlusion. The size of the area of protection is dependent on the length (L) of the polymer and its resultant R_g. As noted, the immunocamouflaged area produced by the flexible mPEG effectively covers a large surface area relative to the very small number of grafted polymers.

well as the heavy hydration of the polymer chain itself, a small number of grafted mPEG sterically occupies and occludes a large three-dimensional volume, thereby giving rise to the immunocamouflage of membrane proteins and carbohydrates (Figure 16.2).

The potential utility of immunocamouflage was apparent from the early work by Abuchowski and Davis on the pegylation of purified proteins, which resulted in improved solubility, in vivo longevity, vascular retention, and decreased/absent in vivo immunogenicity even after repeated administration of PEG-conjugated xenogeneic proteins.[32,33] As a consequence of these attributes, a number of pegylated proteins are clinically used for enzyme-replacement therapy.[34–38] Similarly, polymerized PEG-hydrogels have been investigated as immunoprotective barriers for transplanted cells.[39–43] However, only recently has mPEG grafting to intact, viable cells and tissues been explored. To date, the majority of these studies have focused on the prevention of allorecognition.[13–30,44–46] These intact cell studies have clearly demonstrated that mPEG grafting dramatically reduces cell–cell (e.g., T cell–antigen presenting cell and erythrocyte Rouleaux formation) and receptor–ligand interactions (e.g., CD28–CD80 costimulatory pathway) consequent to the steric hindrance and cell surface charge occlusion by the heavily hydrated neutrally charged polymer. More importantly, the grafted polymer does not affect either the function or viability of the modified cells. This is most dramatically demonstrated by normal in vivo survival of pegylated murine erythrocytes and the establishment of normoglycemia in diabetic rats transplanted with pegylated pancreatic islets.

Based on these findings, we proposed that immunocamouflage of either the virus (direct viral inactivation) or host cell (indirect viral inactivation) would prevent viral entry and subsequent infection. Furthermore, because mPEG grafting results in the global immunocamouflage of the virus or host cell, we hypothesized that mPEG derivatization should be capable of preventing infection by a broad spectrum of viruses—including those that enter via receptor-mediated endocytosis or via membrane fusion. To test the antiviral efficacy of immunocamouflage, multiple viral families were examined. These families include Picornaviridae, Adenoviridae, and Coronaviridae (all representative of common human respiratory viruses), as well as Papovaviridae and Herpesviridae (Table 16.1).

To experimentally test these hypotheses, mPEG derivatization of virus or host (target) cells (CV-1, BHK-21, L2, BALB/3T3, and MRC-5 cell lines) was preformed as previously described, with slight modifications due to cell type.[13–30] Cells were split into either 35 or 60 mm petri dishes and were grown until 75–100% confluent. The cells were briefly washed with phosphate buffered saline (PBS, pH 7.4) and then overlaid with 1 mL of an activated mPEG containing solution (PBS, pH 8.4) and incubated at room temperature for 30 minutes. Following this incubation, the cells were washed with complete media to remove any excess mPEG prior to viral challenge. The activated mPEG chemistries used in these studies all targeted exposed lysine residues. As shown in Table 16.2, the known viral cell surface receptors are characterized by an abundance of potential lysine target residues. More importantly, as demonstrated in our previous studies, it should be noted that mPEG grafting does not specifically target these receptors but

TABLE 16.1 Viral Models that Include Enveloped and Nonenveloped Viruses Utilizing Both Receptor-Mediated Endocytosis and Cell Fusion Modes of Cell Entry

Virus, Family	Receptor	Mode of Entry	Particle Size	Target Cell Line, Cell Lineage and Morphology
Mouse adenovirus (MAV), Adenoviridae	Murine homologue of coxsackie and adenovirus receptor (mCAR)	Receptor-mediated endocytosis	70–90 nm	BALB/3T3 (ATCC CCL-163), mouse embryo fibroblast
Rat coronavirus (RCV), Coronaviridae	Not yet identified	Fusion	80–160 nm	L2 (ATCC CCL-149), rat lung epithelial
Theiler's murine encephalo-myelitis virus (TMEV), Picornaviridae	Not yet identified	Receptor-mediated endocytosis	~20 nm	BHK-21 (ATCC CCL-10), hamster kidney fibroblast
Simian virus 40 (SV40), Papovaviridae	Major histocompatibility molecule-1 (MHC-1)	Receptor-mediated endocytosis	~45 nm	CV-1 (ATCC CCL-70), monkey kidney fibroblast/epithelial
Cytomegalovirus (CMV), Herpesviridae	Epidermal growth factor receptor (EGFR)	Fusion	~200 nm	MRC-5 (ATCC CCL-171), human lung fibroblast

will covalently bind lysine residues of any membrane protein, which may, in turn, effectively camouflage all or part of the viral receptor.[13–30]

Direct immunocamouflage of viruses was examined using SV40. The capsid of SV40 is primarily composed of viral protein 1 (VP1), which contains 25 lysine residues (Table 16.3). The entire capsid consists of 72 VP1 pentamers, thereby providing a suitable substrate for mPEG grafting.[47] Viral lysates were combined with activated mPEG in PBS at a pH of 8.0 at room temperature for 30 minutes. In order to separate unmodified and mPEG-modified virus, an aqueous polymer two-phase system of PEG and Dextran was used.[48] PEG 8 kDa (43%, Sigma) was layered over 5% Dextran T500 (Pharmacia) in 150 mM NaCl and 10 mM sodium phosphate buffer, and the viral sample was added. The layers were mixed and allowed to separate for 1 hour at room temperature. In the two-phase system, unmodified virus had a greater affinity for the Dextran phase and the interface while modified virus separated to the PEG phase. Host cell modification was done by the direct overlay of activated BTCmPEG (5 or 20 kDa polymer at concentrations of 0–15 mM) in phosphate buffered saline (pH 7.8) at room temperature for

TABLE 16.2   Protein Sequences of Virus Receptors[a]

A. MHC-1 (Cercopithecus aethiops) [Protein ID: AAL34325]

LTKTWAGSHS LKYFHTSVSR PGRGEPRFIS VGYYDDTQFV RFDSDAASPRMQPRAP
WVEQ EGPEYWDQET RSARDTAQTF RVNLNTLRGY YNQSEGGSHTLQWMYG-
CDLG PDGRFLRGYE QFAYDGKDYL TLNEDLRSWS AVDTAAQISE QKSNDGSEAE-
HQRAYL EDTC VEWLRRYLEN GKETLQRSEP PKT

*B. CAR [Coxsackie and Mouse Adenovirus (MAV) Receptor
(Mus musculus)] [Protein ID: AAH16457]*

MARLLCFVLL CGIADFTSGL SITTPEQRIE KAKGETAYLP CKFTLSPEDQGPLDI-
EWL IS PSDNQIVDQV IILYSGDKIY DNYYPDLKGR VHFTSNDVKS GDASINVT-
MLQLSDIG TYQC KYKKAPGVAN KKFLLTYLVK PSGTRCFYDG SEEIGNDFKL
KCEPKEGSLPLQ FEWQKLSD SQTMPTPWLA EMTSPVISVK NASSEYSGTY
SCTVQNRVGSDQCMLRLD VV PPSNRAGTIA GAVIGTLLAL VLIGAILFCC HRKRR-
EEKYEKEVHHDIREDVPPPKS RT ST ARSYIGSNHS SLGSMSPSNM EGYSKTQYNQ
VPSEDFERAP QSPTLAPAKFKY AYKTDGIT VV

C. EGFR [Epdermal Growth Factor Receptor (Mus musculus)] [Protein ID: AAH23729]

MRPSGTARTT LLVLLTALCAAGGALEEKKV CQGTSNRLTQ LGTFEDHFLSLQR-
MYN NCEV VLGNLEITYV QRNYDLSFLK TIQEVAGYVL IALNTVERIP LENLQIIRG-
NALYE NTYALA ILSNYGTNRT GLRELPMRNL QEILIGAVRF SNNPILCNMD
TIQWRDIVQNV FMSNMSMDL QSHPSSCPKC DPSCPNGSCW GGGEENCQKL TKII-
CAQQCSHRCRGRS PSDCCHNQCAAGCTGPRESDCLVCQKFQDEATCKDTCPPLM-
LYNPTTYQMDVNPEG KYSFGAT CVKKCPRNYV VTDHGSCVRA CGPDYYEVEE
DGIRKCKKCDGPCRKVC NGI GIGEFKDTLSINATNIKHFKYCTAISGDLH ILP-
VAFKGDSFTRTPPLDPRELEILKTV KE ITGFLLIQAW PDNWTDLHAF ENLEIIRGRT
KQHGQFSLAV VGLNITSLGL RSLKEI SDGD VIISGNRNLC YANTINWKKL
FGTPNQKTKI MNNRAEKDCK AVNHVCNPLCSS EGCWGPEP RDCVSCQNVS
RGRECVEKCN ILEGEPREFV ENSECIQCHPECLPQAMNI TCTGRGPDNCIQCA-
HYIDGPHCVKTCPAQIMGENNTLVWKYADANNVCHLC   HANCT   YGCAG
PGLQGCEVWP SGYVQWQWIL KTFWI

[a]Each viral receptor has several lysine residues (K) that can be modified by mPEG. In addition, it should be noted that many other membrane proteins are also modified during mPEG grafting and direct modification of the receptor is neither essential nor crucial in the generation of the immunocamouflage barrier.

TABLE 16.3   Protein Sequence of SV40 VP1[a] **[Protein ID: NP043126]**

MKMAPTKRKG SCPGAAPKKPKEPVQVPKLV IKGGIEVLGV KTGVDSFTEV ECFL-
NPQMGN PDEHQKGLSK SLAAEKQFTD DSPDKEQLPC YSVARIPLPN LNEDLTC-
GNI LMWEAVTVKT EVIGVTAMLN LHSGTQKTHE NGAGKPIQGS NFHFFAVGGE
PLELQGYLAN YRTKYPAQTV TPKNATVDSQ QMNTDHKAVL DKDNAYPVEC
WVPDPSKNEN TRYFGTYTGG ENVPPVLHIT NTATTVLLDE QGVGPLCKAD SLYV-
SAVDIC GLFTNTSGTQ QWKGLPRYFK ITLRKRSVKN PYPISFLLSD LINRRTQRVD
GQPMIGMSSQ VEEVRVYEDT EELPGDPDMI RYIDEFGQTT TRMQ

[a]VP1 is the dominant capsid protein of SV40 and is also lysine (K) rich, resulting in an abundance of potential sites for the covalent grafting of mPEG.

3–30 minutes. Viral entry and infection was determined by either immunostaining for virus-specific viral products (SV40, T antigen; CMV, IE72) or by plaque assays.

Viral infection was determined by plaque assays (SV40, TMEV, MAV, and RCV) or by intracellular immunostaining for early virus-specific antigens [T antigen for SV40 and the immediate early 72 kDa protein (IE72) for CMV]. For plaque assays, host cells were grown until 75–90% confluent in 35 mm petri dishes overlaid with 1 mL of the viral stock dilution (10^{-3}–10^{-8} of viral stocks) for 2 hour incubation at room temperature. Following removal of the remaining viral lysate, the monolayer was overlaid with 4 mL of the plaque overlay media [equal parts 0.6% melted Bacto-Agar and 2× MEM (without phenol red, Gibco) with 10% FBS]. On day 5 to 9 (virus-dependent), the agar was removed from each plate and 1 mL of ice cold methanol was added and incubated for 10 minutes. The methanol was removed and 1 mL of neutral red was added and incubated for 30 minutes. Following removal of the neutral red solution, the plates were dried overnight for visualization of the plaques. Plaques appeared as clear areas where infected cells had died, while living cells stained red.[49]

16.3 IMMUNOCAMOUFLAGE: BROAD-SPECTRUM ANTIVIRAL PROPHYLAXIS

As hypothesized in Figure 16.1, only covalently grafted mPEG was capable of preventing viral infection (Figure 16.3). Indeed, as demonstrated in Figure 16.3B, the presence of soluble (noncovalently bound) mPEG did not inhibit viral (SV40) entry or propagation over the 72 hour time course as demonstrated by T antigen immunodetection. In contrast, pegylation of either the virus (SV40; Figure 16.3A) or host cell (CV-1; Figure 16.3C) resulted in a dose-dependent decrease in viral infection as determined by T antigen expression. This antiviral prophylaxis was highly effective even at very low (e.g., 0.2 mM) derivatization concentrations.

Similar findings were observed using a rat coronavirus (RCV) model. As shown in Figure 16.4, even very low levels of mPEG grafting (0.2 mM BTCmPEG) to the host cell (L2 rat lung epithelial cells) resulted in an almost complete prevention of viral entry and propagation as determined by plaque assays. Furthermore, at derivatization concentrations ≥5 mM BTCmPEG, a complete abrogation of viral entry was observed. Photomicrographs further document the effectiveness of mPEG grafting. As shown in Figure 16.4, plaques are readily identified in the control infections while the mPEG modified L2 monolayers remain uninfected following viral challenge. Importantly, RCV is a member of the same viral family as the SARS virus, thus suggesting that mPEG grafting to nasopharyngeal epithelium may similarly prove to be an effective prophylactic approach.

In contrast to existing antiviral prophylactic approaches, mPEG grafting proved surprisingly effective against a broad spectrum of viral families. As shown in Table 16.1 and Figure 16.5, pegylation of the host cells provides potent prophylactic protection against adeno (MAV), picorna (TMEV), papova (SV40), and corona (RCV) viruses. Using a grafting concentration of 5 mM BTCmPEG (5 kDa)

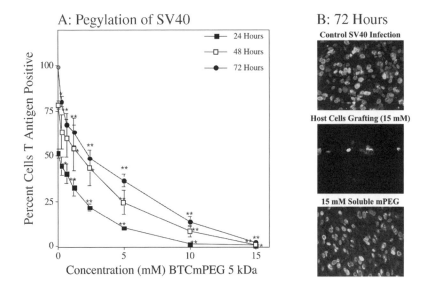

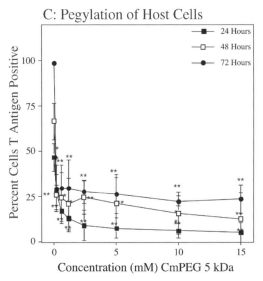

FIGURE 16.3 Covalent grafting of BTCmPEG (5 kDa) is essential for antiviral activity. (A) Covalent grafting of mPEG directly to SV40 results in a mPEG dose-dependent decrease in viral entry and T antigen expression at 24, 48, and 72 hours post viral challenge. (B) Large T antigen immunostaining of SV40-infected CV-1 cells 72 hours postchallenge. As noted, nearly 100% of cells in the control infection are T antigen positive while challenge of mPEG-grafted CV-1 cells results in low T antigen expression at 72 hours postchallenge. The presence of high concentrations (15 mM) of soluble mPEG exhibits no antiviral effect. (C) Covalent grafting of mPEG to the host cell prevents SV40 entry and T antigen expression in a mPEG dose-dependent manner. Data presented are the mean ± SD of a minimum of three independent experiments.

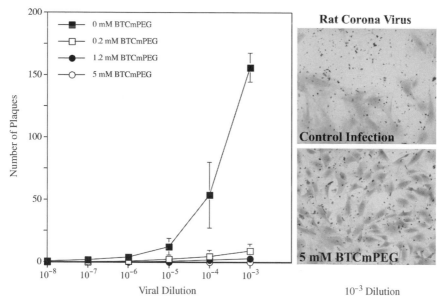

FIGURE 16.4 Covalent grafting of mPEG to host cells exerts a potent antiviral prophylaxis as demonstrated by an RCV infection model. As shown, even very low grafting concentrations (e.g., 0.2 mM BTCmPEG, 5 kDa) of mPEG resulted in an almost complete inhibition of viral entry and plaque formation relative to control infections. This is further demonstrated in photomicrographs of control infections versus host (L2) cells modified with 5 mM BTCmPEG. The data presented are the mean $\pm$ SD of a minimum of three independent experiments.

resulted in >99%, 79%, 84%, and 99% reduction in plaque formation for RCV, MAV, TMEV, and SV40, respectively ($p < 0.0001$ in all cases). Of the viruses shown, TMEV demonstrated the highest absolute plaque formation subsequent to host cell modification with 5 mM BTCmPEG. This may relate to the fact that it is also the smallest ($\sim$20 nM) virus examined. To determine if the density and composition of the mPEG brush border could further decrease TMEV entry, BTCmPEG dose–response curves were conducted using 5 and 20 kDa polymers as well as an equimolar combination (5 + 20 kDa) of the two species. As shown in Table 16.4, polymer size and derivatization concentration both dramatically affect the efficacy of protection against TMEV plaque formation. While all polymer species demonstrated a strong BTCmPEG dose dependency, the equimolar combination of the 5 and 20 kDa BTCmPEGs yields clearly superior ($p < 0.0001$) protection. Indeed, at host cell derivatization concentrations as low as 0.2 mM BTCmPEG, an 82% reduction in plaque formation was noted. At the 5 mM grafting concentration shown in Table 16.4, the 5 + 20 kDa combination yielded a >99% reduction in plaque formation versus a decrease of 84% noted with the 5 mM concentration of the 5 kDa polymer alone.

mPEG-mediated antiviral prophylaxis was also demonstrated in a cytomegalovirus (CMV; herpesvirus) model as determined by IE72 expression at 24, 48, and

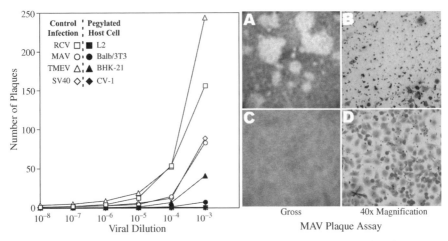

FIGURE 16.5 mPEG grafting (5 mM BTCmPEG 5 kDa) results in a broad-spectrum antiviral prophylaxis as demonstrated by the inhibition of plaque formation following challenge with RCV, MAV, TMEV, and SV40 viruses. The viruses shown infect cells via either receptor-mediated endocytosis (SV40, MAV, and TMEV) or membrane fusion (RCV). Host cells were covalently derivatized in the presence of 5 mM BTCmPEG for 5 minutes. Photomicrographs of MAV plaque assay are also presented at the gross (A, C) and at the microscopic (B, D) levels. As shown, control MAV infections result in extensive plaque formation at both the gross (A) and microscopic (B) levels. In contrast, pegylation of the BALB/3T3 cells with 5 mM BTCmPEG prevents plaque formation at both the gross (C) and microscopic (D) levels. The data presented are the mean ± SD of a minimum of three independent experiments.

72 hours (Figure 16.6). Furthermore, propagation of CMV was dramatically reduced in host cells covalently modified with mPEG. For example, in control CMV infections at 24 hours approximately 50% of the cells were infected. Consequent to viral propagation and infection of adjacent cells, by 48 and 72 hours >70% and >90% of the MRC-5 cells were IE72 positive. In contrast, when the host cells

TABLE 16.4 Effect of BTCmPEG Concentration and Polymer Size on TMEV Infection[a]

BTC mPEG[b]	Control Infection Plaque Number	Percent Control Infection					
		0.2 mM	1.2 mM	2.4 mM	5 mM	10 mM	15 mM
5 kDa	244 (100%)	54%	35%	28%	16%	11%	5%
20 kDa	216 (100%)	44%	29%	13%	6%	2%	1%
5 + 20	316 (100%)	18%	5%	2%	<1%	<1%	<1%

[a]The average number of plaques for $n = 3$ independent experiments from the 10^{-3} TMEV dilution are shown in Figure 13.5.
[b]$p < 0.0001$ for all BTCmPEG concentrations. $p < 0.0001$ for the 5 + 20 kDa combination relative to the 5 kDa polymer at all concentrations and for the 20 kDa polymer at derivatization concentration <10 mM.

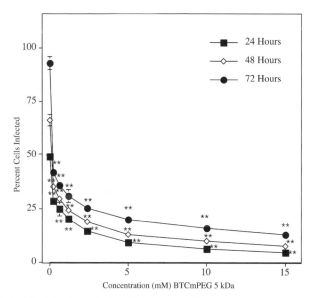

FIGURE 16.6 Modification of the CMV host MRC-5 cells with BTCmPEG (5 kDa) prevents viral fusion and entry. Viral infection was determined by immunostaining for IE72. As shown, an mPEG dose-dependent antiviral response is noted. Both the initial cell entry and secondary entry by progeny virus are blocked by the grafted mPEG as noted by the 24, 48, and 72 hour timepoints. Shown are the mean $\pm$ SD of a minimum of three independent experiments. $**p < 0.001$; $*p < 0.05$ from positive control.

were modified with 10 mM BTCmPEG, an initial infection rate of only $6 \pm 1.4\%$ is noted ($p < 0.0001$) at 24 hours. However, propagation of the infection secondary to this initial infection rate is subsequently abrogated. At 48 and 72 hours the IE72 positive population is only $9.9 \pm 1.9\%$ and $15.9 \pm 2.0\%$ ($p < 0.0001$), clearly suggesting that progeny virus are unable to propagate the infection. This loss of infectivity likely arises as a consequence of the presence of pegylated host proteins on the viral envelope (occurring during viral shedding) and/or the continued existence of the protective mPEG brush border on surrounding cells.

Thus, as evidenced by multiple viral models, pegylation of either the virus or target cells blocks viral entry. The antiviral effect of grafted mPEG is noted for viruses gaining entry to the host cell by either receptor-mediated endocytosis or membrane fusion. Most importantly, this unique approach results in a broad-spectrum antiviral effect.

16.4 IMPLICATIONS OF IMMUNOCAMOUFLAGE TO BIOTERRORISM

Viruses constitute an emerging bioterrorism threat in today's world. In general, previous viral biologics focused initially on highly lethal, native agents (e.g., smallpox) and subsequently on genetically modified agents that would circumvent existing vaccines. However, these agents were difficult to work with and typically required highly sophisticated research and production facilities as well as complex delivery and decontamination mechanisms. Because of these limitations, as well as the traditional governmental powers developing them, viral weapons have not been employed in *modern* warfare, although it must be mentioned that humankind has historically harnessed nature's own terrors to inflict injury upon one's enemies. Historical examples of biowarfare include the trading/donation of blankets from smallpox victims to native North Americans by Lord Jeffrey Amherst and the catapulting of bubonic plague victims over parapet walls.[50]

Modern terrorism is not, however, modern warfare. The most successful terrorist actions are often the most simplistic in approach as demonstrated by 9/11 and suicide bombings. These attacks, while gruesome, are in effect small in scale and have the primary goal of imparting mass hysteria and fear within a population. The "terror" needed to accomplish this public hysteria is surprisingly small as evidenced by the world reaction to the 2003/2004 SARS virus.[51,52] The SARS virus in reality had a very limited public health effect in terms of morbidity and mortality but had a highly exaggerated public health/governmental/public response in terms of airport screening, implementation of new, expensive, and unproved technologies (i.e., body temperature scanners at airports), and mass hysteria as evidenced by cancellations of flights to, and conferences in, affected cities (e.g., Toronto), the wearing of facial masks (despite the ineffective nature of the majority of these masks) by the general population, shunning of individuals returning from SARS hotspots (e.g., Hong Kong), as well as the avoidance of all people and even food of the "wrong" ethnicity (e.g., Chinese).[53,54] Similar examples can be cited with regard to cruise ship epidemics hit by the Norwalk-like viruses.[55] While often treated in the press as a new emerging disease, Norwalk viruses are not a new problem to the cruise industry.[56]

In light of these findings, it is reasonable to assume that virus-mediated bioterrorism is likely to expand in the future. However, in contrast to the complex weapon-grade organisms such as smallpox, today's terrorists are more likely to focus on easily transmitted agents that can be readily propagated in culture or in vivo (e.g., martyrdom). Primary among these possibilities will be respiratory viruses that can be efficiently spread in public locations such as shopping malls, airline flights, and subways. Many of these viruses are characterized by a degree of longevity (several hours) within the environment as well as easy transmissibility via hand-to-mouth or inhalational routes. Furthermore, many of these viruses can easily be cultured and expanded within the laboratory and, in some cases, enhanced pathogenicity can be selected for via either tissue culture or laboratory animals. But perhaps more importantly, for the majority of these agents neither a suitable vaccine nor herd immunity exists due to the rapid mutations noted in respiratory viruses.

Thus, a broad-spectrum prophylactic antiviral agent would be of significant benefit. To date, no such agent exists. This deficit exists primarily because our current approach to viral prevention is focused primarily on vaccine development and secondly on the treatment of viral diseases once infected. Some pseudoprophylactic agents do exist such as amantadine, which prevents the uncoating of the influenza A virus, but it is only effective during the very early stages of viral infection.[57,58] Within cells, amantadine specifically inhibits viral uncoating by blocking the activity of the proton channel of the influenza A M2 protein.[59] In addition to its very small window of clinical efficacy, amantadine therapy also has serious toxic side effects. For example, amantadine affects the nervous system and approximately 10% of people using the drug experience nervousness, depression, anxiety, difficulty concentrating, and lightheadedness.[60] But most importantly, amantadine is highly specific to influenza A virus and is not effective against other influenza strains, much less different viral families.

More analogous to the approach described here is Zicam, an over-the-counter preparation consisting of a highly concentrated zinc gel (zincum gluconicum), which interacts with rhinovirus capsid proteins.[61,62] Crystallographic evidence suggests the surface of rhinovirus-14 contains binding sites for at least 360 Zn^{2+} ions. When bound, zinc ions physically block the ICAM-1 (intracellular adhesion molecule-1) binding pocket of the rhinovirus capsid, thereby interfering with the rhinovirus–cell receptor interactions necessary for cell entry.[61,63–66] Importantly, ICAM-1 is the receptor for approximately 80–90% of rhinovirus strains.[31] Clinical studies have demonstrated that nasal administration of Zicam within 24–48 hours of symptom onset is effective in shortening the length and severity of illness.[61] This effect is most likely due to the prevention of secondary invasion by progeny virus. However, the zinc treatment is only effective for rhinoviruses that use ICAM-1 for cell invasion and has no beneficial effect on other common cold viruses such as adenoviruses and coronaviruses.

In summary, the immunocamouflage of either the virus itself or host cell is multivalent and capable of inhibiting cell entry by a very broad range of viruses as evidenced by Table 16.1 and Figures 16.3–16.6. This finding is in stark contrast to the current univalent (e.g., Zicam and strain-specific vaccination) approaches to preventing viral entry and disease. While mPEG grafting will not replace vaccinations against known pathogens, it may prove to be a highly effective approach in the prevention of ill-defined respiratory viruses during flu season or, potentially, viruses unleashed to promote public panic. The application of this immunoprotective barrier is surprisingly simple, requiring only a 3–5 minute application of the activated mPEG compound as either a nasal gel or throat spray. Our studies demonstrate that near maximal protection by a single application lasts a minimum of 24 hours and still has significant protective benefits up to 48 or even 60 hours postapplication. Indeed, the immunocamouflage of host cells or multiple viral families represents perhaps the only broad-spectrum antiviral approach described to date.

ACKNOWLEDGMENTS

This work was completed in partial fulfillment of a doctoral thesis (by L.L.M.) to fulfill the requirements of the Graduate Program in Pathology and Laboratory Medicine at the University of British Columbia. This work was supported by the Canadian Blood Services and the Canadian Institutes of Health Research.

REFERENCES

1. Ales, N. C.; Katial, R. K. Vaccines against biologic agents: uses and developments. *Respir. Care Clin. N. Am.* **2004**, *10*, 123–146.

2. Venkatesh, S.; Memish, Z. A. Bioterrorism—a new challenge for public health. *Int. J. Antimicrob. Agents* **2003**, *21*, 200–206.

3. Utrup, L. J.; Frey, A. H. Fate of bioterrorism-relevant viruses and bacteria, including spores, aerosolized into an indoor air environment. *Exp. Biol. Med. (Maywood)* **2004**, *229*, 345–350.

4. Hilleman, M. R. Overview: cause and prevention in biowarfare and bioterrorism. *Vaccine* **2002**, *20*, 3055–3067.

5. Pennington, H. Smallpox and bioterrorism. *Bull. World Health Organ.* **2003**, *81*, 762–767.

6. Tucker, J. B.; Zilinskas, R. A. The 1971 smallpox outbreak in the Soviet city of Aralsk: implications for variola virus as a bioterrorist threat. *Crit. Rev. Microbiol.* **2003**, *29*, 81–95.

7. Longini, I. M. Jr.; Halloran, M. E.; Nizam, A.; Yang, Y. Containing pandemic influenza with antiviral agents. *Am. J. Epidemiol.* **2004**, *159*, 623–633.

8. Fleck, F. Avian flu virus could evolve into dangerous human pathogen, experts fear. *Bull. World Health Organ.* **2004**, *82*, 236–237.

9. Shurtleff, A. C. Bioterrorism and emerging infectious disease—antimicrobials, therapeutics and immune-modulators. SARS coronavirus. *IDrugs* **2004**, *7*, 91–95.

10. Titball, R. W.; Williamson, E. D. Vaccine development for potential bioterrorism agents. *Curr. Drug Targets Infect. Disord.* **2003**, *3*, 255–262.

11. Bronze, M. S.; Greenfield, R. A. Preventive and therapeutic approaches to viral agents of bioterrorism. *Drug Discov. Today* **2003**, *8*, 740–745.

12. Gerdil, C. The annual production cycle for influenza vaccine. *Vaccine* **2003**, *21*, 1776–1779.

13. Scott, M. D.; Murad, K. L.; Koumpouras, F.; Talbot, M.; Eaton, J. W. Chemical camouflage of antigenic determinants: "stealth" erythrocytes. *Proc. Natl. Acad. Sci. U.S.A.* **1997**, *94*, 7566–7571.

14. Scott, M. D.; Murad, K. L.; Eaton, J. W. The other blood substitute: antigenically inert erythrocytes. In *Advances in Blood Substitutes: Industrial Opportunities and Medical Challenges*, Winslow, R. M.; Vandegriff, K. D.; Intaglietta, M. (eds.). Birkhäuser, Boston, 1997, pp. 133–150.

15. Scott, M. D.; Murad, K. L. Cellular camouflage: fooling the immune system with polymers. *Curr. Pharm. Des.* **1998**, *4*, 423–438.

16. Murad, K. L.; Mahany, K. L; Kuypers, F. A.; Brugnara, C.; Eaton, J. W.; Scott, M. D. Structural and functional consequences of antigenic modulation of red cells with methoxypoly(ethylene glycol). *Blood* **1999**, *93*, 2121–2127.

17. Murad, K. L.; Gosselin, E. J.; Eaton, J. W.; Scott, M. D. Stealth cells: prevention of MHC class II mediated T cell activation by cell surface modification. *Blood* **1999**, *94*, 2135–2141.

18. Scott, M. D; Bradley, A. J.; Murad, K. L. Camouflaged red cells: low technology bioengineering for transfusion medicine? *Transfusion Med. Rev.* **2000**, *14*, 53–63.

19. Chen, A. M.; Scott, M. D. Current and future applications of immunologic attenuation via PEGylation of cells and tissues. *BioDrugs* **2001**, *15*, 833–847.

20. Bradley, A. J.; Test, T. T.; Murad, K. L.; Mitsuyoshi, J.; Scott, M. D. Complement inter-actions with methoxypoly(ethylene glycol)-modified human erythrocytes. *Transfusion* **2001**, *41*, 1225–1233.

21. Bradley, A. J.; Murad, K. L.; Regan, K. L.; Scott, M. D. Biophysical consequences of linker chemistry and polymer size on stealth erythrocytes: size does matter. *Biochim. Biophys. Acta* **2002**, *1561*, 147–158.

22. Chen, A. M.; Scott, M. D. Immunocamouflage: prevention of transfusion-induced graft-versus-host disease via polymer grafting of donor cells. *J. Biomed. Mater. Res.* **2003**, *67A*, 626–636.

23. Scott, M. D.; Bradley, A. J.; Murad, K. L. Stealth erythrocytes: effects of polymer grafting on biophysical, biological and immunological parameters. *Blood Transfusion* **2003**, *1*, 245–266.

24. Scott, M. D.; Chen, A. M. Beyond the red cell: pegylation of other blood cells and tissues. *Transfusion Clin. Biol.* **2004**, *11*, 40–46.

25. Bradley, A. J.; Scott, M. D. Separation and purification of methoxypoly(ethylene glycol) grafted red blood cells via two-phase partitioning. *J. Chromatogr. B* **2004**, *807*, 163–168.

26. U.S. Patent No. 5,908,624 (June 1, 1999), Scott, M. D; Eaton, J. W. *Antigenic Modulation of Cells.* Assignee: Albany Medical College.

27. U.S. Patent No. 6,524,586 (February 25, 2003), Scott, M. D. *Enhancement of Oligomeric Viral Immunogenicity.* Assignee: Albany Medical College.

28. U.S. Patent No. 6,699,465 (March 3, 2004), Scott, M. D. *Covalent Attachment of Polymer to Cell to Prevent Virus Bonding to Receptor.* Assignee: Albany Medical College.

29. Mizouni, S. K.; Lehman, J. M.; Cohen, B.; Scott, M. D. Viral modification with methoxypoly(ethylene glycol): implications for gene therapy and viral inactivation. *Blood* **1998**, *92*(Suppl. 1), 4627.

30. McCoy, L. L; Scott, M. D. Prevention of viral invasion by immunocamouflage of target cells. *Antiviral Res.* **2004**, *62*, A53 (67).

31. Marlin, S. D.; Staunton, D. E.; Springer, T. A.; Stratowa, C.; Sommergruber, W.; Merluzzi, V. J. A soluble form of intercellular adhesion molecule-1 inhibits rhinovirus infection. *Nature* **1990**, *344*, 70–72.

32. Abuchowski, A.; van Es, T.; Palczuk, N. C.; Davis, F. F. Alteration of immunological properties of bovine serum albumin by covalent attachment of poly(ethylene glycol). *J. Biol. Chem.* **1977**, *252*, 3578–3581.

33. Abuchowski, A.; McCoy, J. R.; Palczuk, N. C.; van Es, T.; Davis, F. F. Effect of covalent attachment of poly(ethylene glycol) on immunogenicity and circulating life of bovine liver catalase. *J. Biol. Chem.* **1977**, *252*, 3582–3586.

34. Jackson, C-J.; Charlton, J. L.; Kuzminski, K.; Lang, G. M.; Sehon, A. H. Synthesis, isolation, and characterization of conjugates of ovalbumin with monomethoxypoly(ethy-lene glycol) using cyanuric chloride as the coupling agent. *Anal. Biochem.* **1987**, *165*, 114–127.

35. Beckman, J. S.; Minor, R. L.; White, C. W.; Repine, J. E.; Rosen, G. M.; Freeman, B. A. Superoxide dismutase and catalase conjugated to polyethylene glycol increases endo-thelial enzyme activity and oxidant resistance. *J. Biol. Chem.* **1988**, *263*, 6884–6892.

36. Abuchowski, A.; Kazo, G. M.; Verhoest, C. R. Jr.; Van Es, T.; Kafkewitz, D.; Nucci, M. L.; Viau, A. T.; Davis, F. F. Cancer therapy with chemically modified enzymes. I. Antitumor

properties of poly(ethylene glycol)-asparaginase conjugates. *Cancer Biochem. Biophys.* **1984**, *7*, 175–186.

37. Herschfield, M. S.; Buckley, R. H.; Greenberg, M. L.; Melton, A. L.; Schiff, R.; Hatem, C.; Kurtzber, J.; Markert, M. L.; Kobayashi, R. H.; Kobayashi, A. L. Treatment of adenosine deaminase deficiency with polyethylene glycol-modifed adenosine deaminase. *N. Engl. J. Med.* **1987**, *316*, 589–596.

38. Kimura, M.; Matsumura, Y.; Konno, T.; Miyauchi, Y.; Maeda, H. Enzymatic removal of bilirubin toxicity by bilirubin oxidase in vitro and excretion of degradation products in vivo. *Proc. Soc. Exp. Biol. Med.* **1990**, *195*, 64–69.

39. Lyman, M. D.; Melanson, D.; Sawhney, A. S. Characterization of the formation of inter-facially photopolymerized thin hydrogels in contact with arterial tissues. *Biomaterials* **1996**, *17*, 359–364.

40. Nagaoka, S.; Mori, Y.; Takiuchi, H.; Yokata, K.; Tanzawa, H.; Nishiumi, S. Interaction between blood components and hydrogels with poly(oxyethylene) chains. In *Polymers as Biomaterials*, Shalaby, S. W.; Hoffman, A. S.; Ratner, B. D.; Horbett, T. A. (eds.). Plenum Press, New York, 1985, pp. 361–374.

41. Lim, F. Microencapsulated islets as bioartificial endocrine pancreas. *Science* **1980**, *210*, 908–910.

42. Sawhney, A. S.; Pathak, C. P.; Hubbell, J. A. Modification of islet of Langerhans surfaces with immunoprotective poly(ethylene glycol) coatings via interfacial photopolymeriza-tion. *Biotechnol. Bioeng.* **1994**, *44*, 383–386.

43. Lacy, P. E.; Hegre, O. D.; Gerasimidi-Vazeou, A.; Gentile, F. T.; Dionne, K. E. Mainte-nance of normoglycemia in diabetic mice by subcutaneous xenografts of encapsulated islets. *Science* **1991**, *254*, 1782–1794.

44. Jeong, S. T.; Byun, S. M. Decreased agglutinability of methoxy-polyethylene glycol attached red blood cells: significance as a blood substitute. *Artif. Cells Blood Substit. Immobil. Biotechnol.* **1996**, *24*, 503–511.

45. Hortin, G. L.; Lok, H. T.; Huang, S. T. Progress toward preparation of universal donor red cells. *Artif. Cells Blood Substit. Immobil. Biotechnol.* **1997**, *25*, 487–491.

46. Armstrong, J. K.; Meiselman, H. J.; Fisher, T. C. Covalent binding of poly(ethylene glycol) (PEG) to the surface of red blood cells inhibits aggregation and reduces low shear blood viscosity. *Am. J. Hematol.* **1997**, *56*, 26–28.

47. Fields, B. N.; Knipe, P. M.; Howley, X. Papovaviridae. In *Fundamental Virology*, 2nd ed., Lippincott-Raven Publishers, Philadelphia, **1998**, pp. 1997–2041.

48. Mizouni, S. K.; Bradley, A. J.; Scott, M. D. Use of a two-phase partitioning system to purify an immunologically attenuated viral vector. *Blood* **1999**, *94*(Suppl. 1) 5081.

49. Tremblay, J. D.; Sachsenmeier, K. F.; Pipas, J. M. Propagation of wild-type and mutant SV40. In *Methods in Molecular Biology, Vol. 165: SV40 Protocols.* Humana Press, Totowa, NJ, 2001, pp. 1–7.

50. Christopher, G. W; Cieslak, T. J.; Pavlin, J. A.; Eitzen, E. M. Jr. Biological warfare. A historical perspective. *JAMA* **1997**, *278*, 412–417.

51. Levett, J. Severe acute respiratory syndrome (SARS): loud clang of the Leper's bell. *Croat. Med. J.* **2003**, *44*, 674–680.

52. Schwartz, N. D.; Creswel, J. Flying scared. Seven ways to make air travel safer. *Fortune* **Apr 28, 2003**, *147*, 72–76.

53. Chang, I. Fear of SARS, fear of strangers. *New York Times*, May 21, 2003, Section A, Column 2, p. 31.

54. Person, B.; Sy, F.; Holton, K.; Govert, B.; Liang, A. National Center for Infectious Diseases/SARS Community Outreach Team. Fear and stigma: the epidemic within the SARS outbreak. *Emerging Infect. Dis.* **2004**, *10*, 358–363.

55. Levine, S. Sick cruise ships. Cleaning vessels. *U.S. News World Rep.* **Dec 16, 2002**, *133*, 50.

56. Gunn, R. A.; Terranova, W. A.; Greenberg, H. B.; Yashuk, J.; Gary, G. W.; Wells, J. G.; Taylor, P. R.; Feldman, R. A. Norwalk virus gastroenteritis aboard a cruise ship: an outbreak on five consecutive cruises. *Am. J. Epidemiol.* **1980**, *112*, 820–827.

57. McKinlay, M. A.; Pevear, D. C. Treatment of the picornavirus common cold by inhibitors of viral uncoating and attachment. *Annu. Rev. Microbiol.* **1992**, *46*, 635–654.

58. Flint, S. J.; Enquist, L. W.; Krug, R. M.; Racaniello, V. R.; Skalka, A. M. Prevention and control of viral diseases. In *Principles of Virology: Molecular Biology, Pathogenesis, and Control*, ASM Publishing, New York, **2000**, pp. 662–712.

59. Kandel, R.; Hartshorn, K. L. Prophylaxis and treatment of influenza virus infection. *BioDrugs* **2001**, *15*, 303–323.

60. Osondu-Alilonu, N.; Gross, P. A. Influenza: the recurring, re-emerging infection. *Curr. Treatment Options Infect. Dis.* **2003**, *5*, 129–136.

61. Hirt, M.; Nobel, S.; Ernesto, B. Zinc nasal gel for the treatment of common cold symptoms: a double blind, placebo-controlled trial. *ENT J.* **2000**, *79*, 778–782.

62. Mossad, S. B. Effect of zincum gluconicum nasal gel on the duration and symptom severity of the common cold in otherwise health adults. *QJM* **2003**, *96*, 35–43.

63. Novick, S. G.; Godfrey, J. C.; Godfrey, N. J.; Wilder, H. R. How does zinc modify the common cold? Clinical observations and implications regarding mechanisms of action. *Med. Hypotheses* **1996**, *46*, 295–302.

64. Eby, G. A.; Davis, D. R.; Halcomb, W. W. Reduction in duration of common colds by zinc gluconate lozenges in a double blind study. *Antimicrob. Agents Chemother.* **1984**, *25*, 20–24.

65. Godfrey, J. C.; Conant-Sloane B.; Smith, D. S.; Turco, J. H.; Mercer, N.; Godfrey, N. J. Zinc gluconate and the common cold: a controlled study. *J. Int. Med. Res.* **1992**, *20*, 234–246.

66. Korant, B. D.; Butterworth, B. E. Inhibition by zinc of rhinovirus protein cleavage: interaction of zinc with capsid polypeptides. *J. Virol.* **1976**, *18*, 298–306.

CHAPTER 17

Viral Evasion of the Interferon System: Novel Targets for Drug Discovery

PAUL F. TORRENCE and LINDA POWELL

Department of Chemistry and Biochemistry, Northern Arizona University

The paradigms of antiviral drug discovery have resulted in the pursuit of the classical targets of virus replication known to all students of virology; namely, attachment, penetration, uncoating, replication, maturation, and release. Yet, the ongoing battles of evolution have produced a host of other potential antiviral drug targets that to date have not been exploited to alter the course of virus-induced disease.

Viruses and their hosts have coevolved and therefore have developed the means to contain and/or to evade one another. Vertebrate hosts have complex immune systems. In order for a virus to survive, it must replicate amidst the onslaught of the host immune defenses. Interferons (IFNs) play a key role in establishing this armament that triggers the activation of interferon-stimulated genes and elicits an antiviral state to curb viral infections. In response, viruses have evolved mechanisms to circumvent the interferon-induced defenses. Nearly fifty years ago, Isaacs and Lindenmann identified and described the antiviral and cytostatic properties of interferons.[1] These pathways are increasingly more complex. The dynamic process of viral evasion of the host IFN system can be attributed to the many years of coevolution and adaptation of viruses to produce proteins that downregulate IFN production, or block the actions of the products of this pathway. This is a rapidly expanding research arena and yields an array of potential targets for therapeutic intervention with viral infections. We do not pretend to review this field exhaustively, but simply point out here some findings of relevance to the domain of emerging diseases and biodefense concerns.

Antiviral Drug Discovery for Emerging Diseases and Bioterrorism Threats. Edited by Paul F. Torrence
Copyright © 2005 John Wiley & Sons, Inc.

17.1 THE INTERFERON REGULATORY PATHWAY

There are hundreds of interferon-stimulated genes (ISGs).[2] While involved in host antiviral defense, the products of ISGs are also potent regulators of cell growth and have increasingly complex immunomodulatory activities. Numerous interferon-induced genes are involved in innate immunity.[3]

The complex cross-signaling of cellular regulatory pathways involved in apoptosis, inflammation, and the stress response all are linked to the interferon pathway. Cellular signaling pathways involved in the antiviral response have adapted due to the presence of viruses. This observation illuminates a host repertoire for dealing with viral infection that is intriguingly complex.

There are two main types of interferon (IFN), type I and type II. Type I IFNs include IFN-α, IFN-β, IFN-ω, and IFN-τ and are primarily produced in leukocytes. These interferons are commonly called "viral interferons" and are a group of antiviral cytokines induced during viral infection by the viral replication processes. A new recently described[4] IFN-λ and its class II cytokine receptor system may contribute to antiviral or other defenses by a mechanism similar to, but independent of, type I IFNs. Type II IFN is IFN-γ, which is produced only by certain cells involved in the immune response such as natural killer (NK), cytotoxic T cells (CD8$^+$), and CD4$^+$ T helper 1 (T$_h$1) cells. Not produced in direct response to the presence of virus, these IFNs are secreted when an infected cell is recognized as a part of the host's acquired immune response.

Type I and II IFNs share no obvious structural homology and have separate cell membrane receptors.[2] These receptors activate signal transduction pathways, which ultimately lead to the transcription of hundreds of interferon-stimulated genes (ISGs). There exists an overlap in the ISGs triggered by type I and type II IFNs.

Type I IFNs activate the JAK/STAT signal transduction pathway by binding to the IFN-α/β receptor (IFNAR). The cytoplasmic tails of IFNAR are associated with tyrosine kinases (JAK and TYK), which phosphorylate signal transducers and activators of transcription (STAT).[5] STATs are latent transcription factors that, upon phosphorylation, dimerize and form complexes with interferon response factors (IRFs). These complexes move to the nucleus and bind to interferon-stimulated regulatory elements (ISRE).[6] Several genes are then transcriptionally stimulated. Of these gene products, many contribute to the antiviral actions of the host immune response.

PKR is a double-stranded RNA (dsRNA)-dependent serine/threonine kinase. In the presence of dsRNA, most likely produced from the viral genome itself or formed from its replication or convergent transcription, PKR phosphorylates the α subunit of the eukaryotic initiation factor eIF-2. When eIF-2α is phosphorylated, it is unable to recycle and the translation of proteins is arrested, thereby inhibiting viral reproduction.

Also, activation of PKR results in the phosphorylation of substrates necessary to initiate the transcription factor NF-κB. Once freed from restraint, NF-κB can enter the nucleus of the cell and bind to the IFN-β promoter.[7]

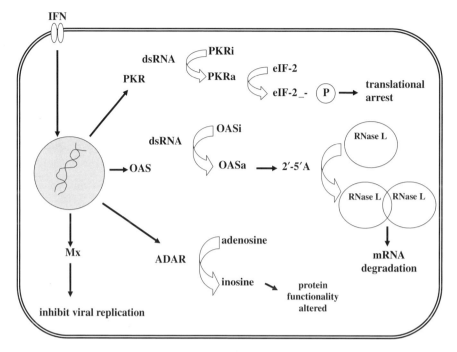

Figure 17.1 Interferon defense pathway. Interferons (IFNs) bind to cell surface receptors and trigger intracellular IFN signaling pathways, which stimulate the transcription of numerous genes. Translation of these gene products yields inactive precursors for the RNA-dependent protein kinase (PKR) and oligoadenylate synthetase (OAS). In the presence of dsRNA, PKR phosphorylates the a subunit of eukaryotic initiation factor 2 and prevents translation of proteins. Upon activation, OAS produces $2'$-$5'$A, an oligonucleotide of adenosines linked in a $2'$-$5'$ manner, which in turn binds to the endoribonuclease L (RNase L), causing the formation of an active RNase L dimer that degrades mRNA. Translation of the adenosine deaminase that acts on RNA (ADAR) yields a product that deaminases adenosine to inosine. An altered protein as inosine is treated like a guanosine. Myxovirus-resistance proteins (Mx) are interferon-induced GTPases that bind to nucleocapsids of certain viruses and prevent replication.

The $2'$-$5'$ oligoadenylate synthetases (OAS, 2-5A synthetases) also are produced in a latent state and activated by dsRNA. Upon activation, OAS catalyzes the production of $2'$-$5'$-oligoadenylates [2-5A, $(pp)p5'A2'(p5'A2')_np5'A$,]. The 2-5A then binds to the latent endoribonuclease RNase L, which then dimerizes to an active ribonuclease that degrades mRNA, thus inhibiting viral replication and/or inducing apoptosis in infected cells (Figure 17.1).

Adenosine deaminases that act on RNA (ADAR) are another group of enzymes that are induced by type I IFNs and can contribute to antiviral activity. Post-translational conversions of adenosine to inosine have the potential to alter proteins and their functions, as inosine behaves like a guanosine. Thus, the number of mutant proteins in virus-infected cells is increased.[8]

Yet another class of proteins with antiviral activity induced by type I IFNs is the Mx proteins. Mx proteins are GTPases with enzymatic function, existing in multiple forms (cytoplasmic and nuclear). These proteins appear to associate with viral nucleocapsids from different virus families and inhibit their biological and transport properties, thus blocking viral replication.[9]

Whereas PKR and Mx genes are induced by type I IFNs, 2-5A synthetase (OAS) and RNase L are also induced by type II IFN, known as IFN-γ.[8] IFN-γ has been shown to stimulate the production of nitric oxide and inhibit replication of ectromelia, vaccinia, and herpes simplex type-1 viruses in mouse macrophages.[8] Inhibition of viral replication directly correlated to levels of nitric oxide synthetase.

17.2 VIRUS COUNTERMEASURES FOR HOST DEFENSE MECHANISMS

All of the preceding host defense mechanisms utilize cellular machinery in order to interfere with the replicative process of the virus. Translational arrest, induction of apoptosis, and introduction of mutations in proteins target the necessary replication of the virus vital to the establishment of infection.

Evolving under these pressures from the host, viruses have developed an impressive arsenal to nullify these defenses. With high rates of evolution and packaging limitations, viruses have pirated host genes, modified and retained them to successfully propagate. The main focus of this piracy is to ensure production of viral proteins and reproduction of genetic material for the manufacture of viral progeny. With many products of the interferon system having a role in numerous cell pathways involved in apoptosis and translation of proteins, these pathways are the police and the prize of viral infection. What is this conundrum? The virus must defeat the cell's machinery attempting to stop the production of viral proteins, yet parts of the cellular apparatus may be required for virus multiplication. At the same time, the cell must use its pathways that regulate cell proliferation to stop viral proliferation. Viruses vary in their ability to circumvent the host interferon response. In general, DNA viruses produce less dsRNA and initially are therefore less potent inducers of IFN.[10] However, viral evasion tactics exist at much more sophisticated levels.

Bray established the key role of type-1 IFN in the resistance of mice to the Ebola virus infection, showing that significant compromise of the interferon response gave rise to disease progress resembling that in primates.[11] In line with these latter observations, Harcourt et al.[12] found that induction of the major histocompatibility complex class I family of genes, OAS, interleukin-6 (IL-6), PKR, interferon (IFN) regulatory factor-1, and intercellular adhesion molecule-1 (ICAM-1) by dsRNA in human umbilical vein endothelial cells was suppressed by infection with the filovirus Ebola-Zaire. Likewise, Ebola and Marburg viruses each could infect dendritic cell cultures and support exponential viral replication without releasing

TABLE 17.1 **Virus Inhibition of IFN Signaling and Transcription of ISGs**

Target of Inhibition	Virus/Viral Product
ISG transcription	Human herpesvirus 8 IRF homologue (Ref. 16) human papillomavirus type 16 E7 protein (Ref. 17)
IFNs binding to receptors	Poxvirus soluble IFN receptor homologue (Refs. 18–21)
JAK and/or p48 expression	Human cytomegalovirus (Refs. 22,23), murine polyomavirus T antigen (Ref. 24)
IRF 3	Ebola virus VP35 (Ref. 15)
STAT and/or p48	Dengue virus (Refs. 11–15), paramyxovirus, simian virus 5 V protein (Refs. 25, 26), mumps virus (Ref. 27), human parainfluenza virus 2 (Ref. 28), adenovirus E1A protein (Ref. 29)
Induction of MxA gene	Hepatitis B virus nucleocapsid protein (Ref. 30)

interferon-α (IFN-α).[13] In addition, such cultures were impaired in IFN-α production if treated with dsRNA that normally should lead to IFN production.[13] Basler et al.[14] reported that Ebola virus protein VP35 blocked dsRNA- and virus-mediated induction of the IFN-stimulated response element reporter gene and also inhibited dsRNA- and virus-mediated induction of the IFN-β promoter. Moreover, Ebola virus VP35 protein inhibits activation of the interferon regulatory factor-3 (IRF-3), a key component in the initiation of the host cell interferon response, through inhibition of IRF-3 phosphorylation.[15] IRF-3 subsequently cannot dimerize and translocate to the nucleus.

Dengue virus nonstructural proteins NS2A, NS4B, and NS4A have been shown to downregulate IFN-β-stimulated gene.[19] Table 17.1 shows the mechanism of action and inhibition for some viruses that target the signaling and transcriptional responses of IFNs.

Viruses have evolved mechanisms that target products of the IFN pathway and render them ineffective. Two products that have been extensively researched are PKR and OAS. Table 17.2 lists some viruses that inhibit PKR and OAS and are able to reproduce in the face of the host cell's defenses. These processes are discussed below.

The importance of PKR in mounting an antiviral defense can be attested to by the numerous viral mechanisms devoted to inhibit this activity. Viruses that encode proteins to bind to and sequester dsRNA prevent the activation of PKR indirectly. Poxviruses (vaccinia, ectromelia, cowpox, and camelpox) encode a gene product E3L that contains a dsRNA binding domain and inhibits PKR.[8,31,33,34,36,39–43,60–65] The orf virus OV20.0L gene product is 33% homologous to E3L and presumably contributes to interferon evasion by the same mechanism.[38,66,67] Many viruses also encode products that actively bind to PKR and thus inhibit its activity. Adenovirus (AV), Epstein-Barr virus (EBV), and human immunodeficiency virus type 1 (HIV-1) all encode small RNA transcripts that bind to the active site for dsRNA binding.[20,45,53,54] Influenza virus NS1 protein binds directly to PKR but has also

TABLE 17.2 Virus Inhibition of PKR and OAS

Target of Inhibition	Virus/Viral Product
dsRNA binding/sequestering	Poxvirus E3L gene product (Refs. 10, 31–44), influenza virus NS1 protein (Refs. 45–49), reovirus σ3 and rotavirus NSP3 (reviewed in Ref. 20)
PKR binding	Adenovirus VA1 transcript (reviewed in Ref. 20, hepatitis C virus NS5Aand E2 proteins (Refs. 50, 51), baculovirus PK2 protein (Ref. 52), poxvirus E3L [also OV20.0L (Ref. 38)], influenza NS1, poxvirus K3L (Refs. 32, 34, 35), Epstein-Barr virus EBER1 and EBER2 transcripts (Ref. 45), HIV Tat protein, and TAR (Refs. 53, 54)
PP1 (cellular protein phosphatase 1α)	Herpes simplex virus ICP34.5 protein (Ref. 55)
RNase L	Herpes simplex virus 2′5′A derivatives (Ref. 56), HIV-1 and encephalomyocarditis virus (Refs. 56, 57)
PKR degradation	Poliovirus (Refs. 58, 59)

been reported to induce p58IPK, a cellular inhibitor of PKR.[63–65,68] Poliovirus degrades PKR, possibly through transcriptional control,[59] and herpes simplex virus (HSV) indirectly evades PKR by encoding the γ_1 ICP34.5 protein that interacts with cellular PP1 (protein phosphatase 1α).[55] ICP34.5 redirects PP1 to phosphorylate and the eukaryotic initiation factor eIF2α subunit is able to be recycled and translation of proteins continues. All of the above viruses that encode products that are able to sequester dsRNA are also inhibitors of OAS, as dsRNA is required to activate this enzyme as well.

17.3 MODIFICATION OF 2′,5′-OLIGOADENYLATES (2-5A) BY VIRAL DEFENSES AND OTHER EVASIONS OF RNase L

The potency of 2-5A in inhibition of translation through activation of RNase L would seem to be a critical target for a virus to neutralize in some fashion. There appear to be at least two distinct mechanisms that can be teased out presently from existing studies. One involves the covalent modification of the highly active ppp5′(A2′p)$_n$5′pA molecules. Another may be the generation of a protein inhibitor of RNase L. The latter molecule may or may not possess other virus-related functions.

Of particular relevance to the discovery and development of poxvirus counter-measures would be the past observations from Ian Kerr's laboratory. Thus, Rice et al.[69] found that vaccinia virus replication was relatively insensitive to the antiviral effects of interferon in mouse L929 and HeLa cells. Nonetheless, high concentrations of 2-5A (up to 5 µM) of 2-5A were found during vaccinia infection of all of these types of cells treated at interferon concentrations too low to inhibit significantly the virus growth. High levels of 2-5A (up to 5 µM) also were found in non-interferon-treated HeLa cells (which have a high constitutive level of 2-5A synthetase) in which vaccinia virus replicates perfectly well. Rice et al.[69] concluded that high levels of 2-5A per se have no necessary antiviral effect on vaccinia virus in these systems. HPLC analysis of the extracts of such cells revealed the presence of authentic 2-5A dimer, trimer, and tetramer 5'-triphosphates, 5'-dephosphorylated "cores" of the general formula $A2'(5'pA2')_n5'pA$ ($n = 0-2$), and a considerable number of unidentified compounds, some of which activated RNase L and some that did not. The role of these unidentified molecules in the insensitivity of vaccinia virus to interferon remains unknown.

Paez and Estaeban[70] also noted the resistance of vaccinia virus to interferon but obtained evidence that resistance was related to inhibition of the 2-5A system by intervention of a vaccinia viral ATPase (that would block production of 2-5A from the synthetase) and a viral phosphatase that would 5'-dephosphorylate biologically active 2-5A 5'-mono-, di-, and triphosphates.

Similarly, novel oligoadenylates of unknown structure and unable to activate RNase L accumulate in interferon-treated SV-40 virus-infected monkey CV-1 cells.[71] Some of the 2',5'-oligoadenylates corresponded to nonphosphorylated "cores," $(A2'p)_nA$, but a considerable amount eluted in the HPLC at retention times intermediate between $ppp(A2'p)3A$ and cores. The unknown peaks did not seem to be changed upon digestion with alkaline phosphatase, implying the lack of terminal phosphate residues. Poly(I)·poly(C) addition to interferon-treated CV-1 cells gave high levels of authentic biologically active 2-5A.

In yet another apparent virus-related evasion of the 2-5A pathway, Cayley et al.[56] noted that in human Chang cells herpes simplex viruses 1 and 2 (HSV-1 and HSV-2) were much more resistant to interferon's antiviral action than was encephalo-myocarditis virus. In all the above cases of interferon virus (HSV-1, HSV-2 or EMCV)-infected cells, similar amounts of 2',5'-oligoadenylates were synthesized, but in the instances of HSV-1 and HSV-2 infections, these oligoadenylates did not produce the characteristic RNase L activation footprints of ribosomal RNA cleavage. HPLC analysis of extracts from interferon, virus-infected cells showed that while RNase L-activating trimer $ppp(A2'p)_2A$ and tetramer $ppp(A2'p)_3A$ were present, there were also present apparent 2',5'-oligoadenylates that competed with the above 2-5A activators, but themselves were only weak activators of RNase L. These inhibitory compounds of unknown structure could account for the poor activation of RNase L and the relative resistance of HSV-1 and HSV-2 to interferon in Chang cells.

One past observation is of special interest because the experiment was done in intact animals and involved an RNA virus—rabies. IFN administered intravenously, subcutaneously, or intraperitoneally to mice crosses the blood–brain barrier to cause enhanced levels of the two double-stranded RNA-dependent enzymes, the protein kinase and 2',5'-oligoadenylate (2-5A) synthetase in the brain.[72,73] However, in spite of this effect, interferon seems to be unable to prevent the evolution of rabies disease in immunocompetent and immunosuppressed mice. This may be related to the subsequent observation that neither virus infection nor interferon treatment after virus infection is able to generate the same spectrum of $2',5'$-oligoadenylates that are formed when mice are treated with both interferon and poly(I)·poly(C) dsRNA. The products that accumulated during virus infection alone were mostly RNase L-inactive phosphorylated dimers; however, during combined interferon and poly(I)·poly(C) treatment, the entire spectrum of RNase L-active phosphorylated molecules (dimer to pentamer) was present. These data implied that infection of mice with rabies virus causes both the induction and the activation of 2-5A synthetase, as does interferon and poly(I)·poly(C) treatment.[72,73] However, the intracellular products were different under different conditions. Virus-induced 2-5A synthetase seemed quite capable of synthesis of the longer 2-5A oligomers when evaluated in cell extracts, yet it was not able to bring about the synthesis of longer oligomers in the infected animal. This could be related simply to a difference in the 2-5A synthetase isoform present in the two conditions since it is now well-established that four isoforms (p40, p44, p69, p100) of IFN have been described,[74] and they differ in response to dsRNA, salt, divalent cation, and soon in terms of the 2-5A product spectrum they generate. They are also differentially induced in vivo versus in vitro conditions.

Schroder and co-workers[75,76] reported that the nuclear matrix of HIV-infected as well as uninfected H9 (human T cells) contained 2-5A synthetase, which was increased by a factor of 7.7 in the HIV-infected cells. This latter increase was accompanied by a five- to ten fold increase in 2-5A oligonucleotides in nuclei from HIV-1-infected H9 cells. Also increased in HIV-infected cells was an exonuclease activity that degraded 2-5A. The 2-5A-dependent RNase activity also underwent an increase to coincide with the time of maximum 2-5A synthetase activity. The RNase was also associated with the nuclear matrix as determined by photochemical cross-linking and probably was responsible for degradation of HIV transcripts. Failure of infected H9 cells to release HIV was correlated with the presence of high concentrations of 2-5A and high levels of the 2-5A-dependent RNase. When 2-5A concentration decreased, the cells began to release HIV. Treatment of cells with AZT ($3'$-azido-$3'$-deoxythymidine) extended the duration of time during which HIV transcript degradation occurred. Schroder et al.[75,76] suggested that a useful approach to screen for potential chemotherapeutic agents for HIV would be to search for compounds that would act to stabilize the concentration of 2-5A in order to extend degradation of HIV transcripts. Thus, productive strategies for treating HIV infection using the 2-5A system may include the development of dsRNA analogues that increase 2-5A production, and nuclease-stable, phosphatase-stable, more potent 2-5A analogues. It remains to be established that this is a viable strategy that could be applied to HIV or any other RNA virus.

In the absence of IFN treatment and when cells are infected with encephalo-myocarditis virus (EMCV), a considerable decrease in RNase L occurs, but this decrease is prevented by pretreatment of the cells with IFN.[57,77] Semliki Forest virus infection also results in inactivation of RNase L activity also by an unknown mechanism. This clearly represents a viral defense against one arm of the 2-5A system. The mechanism of this loss of RNase L activity is unknown and its occurrence in other RNA virus infections is largely unexplored, but probably is not related to the activity described below as RLI.

Bisbal et al.[78–83] isolated a polypeptide inhibitor (termed RLI) of the 2-5A system based on their screening of an expression library assayed by binding to radioactive 2-5ApCp. This protein was proposed as a regulator that would inhibit the binding of 2-5A to RNase L, thereby blocking activation of RNase L and its nuclease activity. Although RLI had a poor affinity for RNase L, it may associate directly but noncovalently with the enzyme to alter its activation potential by 2-5A. Overexpression of RLI in HeLa cells partly antagonized the anti-picornaviral effects of interferon, whereas RLI antisense constructs partly blocked downregulation of the 2-5A/RNase L pathway in EMCV-infected cells. RLI increased during human immunodeficiency virus type 1 (HIV-1) infection. This might be related to the downregulation of RNase L activity that has been described previously. Overexpression of RLI caused a decrease in RNase L activity and a twofold enhancement of HIV production. The HIV replication increase correlated with enhancement of levels of HIV RNA and proteins. To the contrary, reduction of RLI levels in RLI antisense cDNA-expressing clones reversed the inhibition of RNase L activity associated with HIV multiplication and led to a threefold diminution in the viral load and a decrease in HIV RNA and proteins. ABCE homologues, subfamilies of ATP binding cassette (ABC) transporters, have been identified in 37 species that apparently lack an RNase L.[84] ABCE is the proposed inhibitor of RNase L identified by Bisbal and co-workers. Thus, RNase L inhibition must not be the only functional role of ABCE. Indeed, it has been postulated that the ABCE protein may be necessary for the assembly of Gag polypeptides into immature HIV-1 capsids.[85] The role, if any, of ABCE proteins in other virus's replications and their interaction with elements of the interferon system remains unknown.

17.4   RNA VIRUS NONSTRUCTURAL PROTEINS AS ANTAGONISTS OF INTERFERON ACTION

The influenza virus can express the NS1 protein, which binds double-stranded RNA.[86] The NS1 protein represses the host cell antiviral response by several different mechanisms.[86–93] These mechanisms include the inhibition of the IFN-inducible double-stranded RNA-activated kinase PKR (protein kinase RNA-regulated) and the blocking of IFN-β production by preventing NF-κB, IFN regulatory factor (IRF) 3, and IRF-7 activation. Indeed, the nonstructural (NS) gene segment of the 1918 influenza virus has been evaluated to test the hypothesis that the enhanced virulence in 1918 could have been due to type I interferon inhibition by the NS1 protein. Most significantly, a virus containing the 1918 pandemic NS1 gene was more efficient at blocking the expression of IFN-regulated genes than its parental influenza A/WSN/33 virus.[94,95]

Bovine respiratory syncytial virus (BRSV) nonstructural proteins NS1 and NS2 cooperate to antagonize IFN-mediated antiviral mechanisms.[96,97] Furthermore, introduction of BRSV NS1 and NS2 into rabies virus also evoked resistance to interferon.

In distinct contrast to wild-type BRSVs, recombinant BRSVs (rBRSVs) without the NS proteins, and those lacking NS2 in particular, are strong inducers of IFN-α/β in bovine nasal fibroblasts and bronchoalveolar macrophages. In addition, although the NS deletion mutants grew to wild-type rBRSV levels in cells lacking a functional IFN-α/β system, their replication was severely inhibited in IFN-competent cells.[98] These results suggested that the NS proteins block induction of IFN-α/β gene expression.

Wild-type human respiratory syncytial virus (HRSV) is a poor inducer of α/β interferons (IFN-α/β). In accord with the results seen with BRSV, recombinant HRSV lacking the NS1 and NS2 genes was able to induce high levels of IFN-α and IFN-β in epithelial cells and macrophages.[99] The two proteins can function independently or coordinately. Alphaviruses including Venezuelan (VEEV), eastern (EEEV), and western equine encephalitis viruses (WEEV) are potential agents of biological warfare and terrorism and important, naturally emerging zoonotic viruses. A representative virus of this group is Sindbis virus, which possesses a nonstructural protein nsP2 that is a significant regulator of Sindbis virus–host cell interactions. This protein not only is a component of the replicative enzyme complex required for replication and transcription of viral RNAs but also plays a role in suppressing the antiviral response in Sindbis virus-infected cells. nsP2 may act by decreasing interferon (IFN) production.[100,101] In another study, White and co-workers[102] found that a single change (G to A) at nucleotide 3 of the 5' untranslated region (UTR) of the Venezuelan equine encephalitis virus (VEEV) V3000 virulent strain genome resulted in a virus that was avirulent in mice. This mutant showed no growth disadvantage compared to the wild-type virus in cells derived from IFN-α/βR($-$/$-$)mice. Induction of IFN-α/β was the same for avirulent and virulent viruses; however, the avirulent mutant virus was more sensitive than the virulent strain to the antiviral actions of IFN-α/β. Thus, increased sensitivity to IFN-α/β must play a major role in the in vivo attenuation.

Virus zoonoses causing hemorrhagic fevers include the Bunyaviridae. Thomas et al.[103] found that bunyaviruses activate PKR but are only marginally sensitive to its antiviral effect. In addition, NSs appeared to be different from other IFN antagonists, since it inhibited dsRNA-dependent IFN induction but had no effect on the dsRNA-activated PKR and RNase L systems. Bunyamwera virus, of the family Bunyaviridae, possesses a nonstructural protein NSs that is a virulence factor that inhibits IFN-β gene expression in the mammalian host. In an unconventional mechanism of interferon antagonism, NSs targets the RNA polymerase II (RNAP II) complex.[103–106]

Rift Valley fever virus (RVFV), a phlebovirus of the family Bunyaviridae, is a major public health threat in Egypt and sub-Saharan Africa. Bouloy and co-workers[107] could show that the ability of RVFV to inhibit IFN-α/β production correlated with viral virulence, thereby suggesting that the accessory protein NSs is an interferon antagonist.

The nonstructural protein 5A (NS5A) of hepatitis C virus (HCV) has been implicated in inhibition of antiviral activity of IFN—through both an interaction between NS5A and the double-stranded RNA-dependent protein kinase (PKR), as well as the 2′,5′-oligoadenylate synthetase (OAS).[108,109]

Both Newcastle disease virus (NDV) and Nipah virus possess interferon evasion proteins. The Nipah virus proteins V, W, and C all act to sequester STAT1, but V and P proteins act by retaining STAT1 in the cytoplasm while the W protein sequesters STAT1 in the nucleus.[110,111]

Dengue virus nonstructural proteins NS2A, NS4B, and NS4A have been shown to downregulate IFN-β-stimulated genes. NS4B at least may block IFN signaling during dengue virus infection by interference with STAT1 signaling.[19]

17.5 ASPECTS OF POXVIRUS ESCAPE FROM INTERFERONS

Poxviruses, of intense interest for bioterrorism potential or as emerging natural infections (monkeypox), have devised at least six separate mechanisms to evade the interferon system.

1. Poxvirus infections lead to secretion of proteins that bind to type I or II IFNs.[18,21,43,112–116] The IFN-binding proteins of myxoma virus and vaccinia have a sequence similar to the extracellular domain of the IFN-γ receptor and bind to IFN-γ. A type I IFN inhibitor has been reported in the supernatants and on the surface of cells infected with vaccinia and other orthopoxviruses. Mutant vaccinia viruses with a deletion of the type I IFN binding gene were attenuated in mice.

2. Orthopoxviruses contain a gene for a double-stranded RNA binding protein (E3L gene of vaccinia virus) that can block activation of PKR. Vaccinia virus E3L deletion mutants exhibit host range restriction, apoptosis, enhanced RNA degradation, and interferon sensitivity.[31–34] This same dsRNA binding protein, since it soaks up dsRNA, can also block 2-5A synthesis by the dsRNA-activated 2-5A synthetase enzyme family.

3. Orthopoxviruses also can express an eIF-2 homologue (the K3L gene of vaccinia virus), deletion of which may enhance the interferon sensitivity of vaccinia virus. K3L acts as an eIF-2 decoy, thereby inhibiting eIF-2 phosphorylation and activation of PKR.[35–37]

4. IL-18 induced IFN-γ production in macrophages and was able to protect mice from the pathological effects of vaccinia virus infection. An IL-18 binding protein (IL-18BP) is a soluble, secreted inhibitor of IL-18 produced by humans and mice presumably for regulatory purposes. Orthopoxviruses encode IL-18BP homologues that bind IL-18 and block IFN-γ production.[117]

5. Vaccinia virus invokes several mechanisms to negate the effects of the RNase L activator, 2-5A (discussed above).

6. Poxvirus protein N1L inhibited NF-κB and interferon regulatory factor-3 (IRF-3) signaling.[118]

17.6 CONCLUSION

Virus interferon-evasion strategies have been shown to play key roles in virulence. We have presented examples here of factors that determine virulence in infections with influenza virus, dengue virus, bunyaviruses, respiratory syncytial virus, and orthopoxviruses, to name a few. Surely, there is no a priori reason to expect that this diverse group of viral gene products should not be as rich a source of antiviral agents as has been the group of more classical targets.

REFERENCES

1. Isaacs, A.; Lindenmann, J. Virus interference. I. The interferon. *Proc. R. Soc. London B* **1957**, *147*, 258.

2. Katze, M. G.; He, Y.; Gale, M. Jr. Viruses and interferon: a fight for supremacy. *Nat. Rev. Immunol.* **2002**, *2*(9), 675–687.

3. Decker, T.; Stockinger, S.; Karaghiosoff, M.; Muller, M.; Kovarik, P. IFNs and STATs in innate immunity to microorganisms. *J. Clin. Invest.* **2002**, *109*(10), 1271–1277.

4. Kotenko, S. V.; Gallagher, G.; Baurin, V. V.; Lewis-Antes, A.; Shen, M.; Shah, N. K.; Langer, J. A.; Sheikh, F.; Dickensheets, H.; Donnelly, R. P. IFN-λs mediate antiviral protection through a distinct class II cytokine receptor complex. *Nat. Immunol.* **2003**, *4*, 69–77.

5. Garcia-Sastre, A. Mechanisms of inhibition of the host interferon α/β-mediated antiviral responses by viruses. *Microbes Infect.* **2002**, *4*(6), 647–655.

6. Stark, G. R.; Kerr, I. M.; Williams, B. R. G.; Silverman, R. H.; Schreiber, R. D. How cells respond to interferons. *Annu. Rev. Biochem.* **1998**, *67*, 227–264.

7. Israel, A. The IKK complex: an integrator of signals that activate NF-KB? *Cell Biol.* **2000**, 10, 129–133.

8. Liu, Y.; Wolff, K. C.; Jacobs, B. L.; Samuel, C. E. Vaccinia virus E3L interferon resistance protein inhibits the interferon-induced adenosine deaminase A-to-I editing activity. *Virology* **2001**, *289*, 378–387.

9. Weber, F.; Haller, G.; Kochs, A. Mx, GTPase blocks reporter gene expression of reconstituted Thogoto virus ribonucleoprotein complexes. *J. Virol.* **2000**, *74*, 560–563.

10. Jacobs, B. L.; Langland, J. O. When two strands are better than one: the mediators and modulators of the cellular responses to double-stranded RNA. *Virology,* **1996**, *219*, 339–349.

11. Bray M. The role of the type I interferon response in the resistance of mice to filovirus infection. *J. Gen. Virol.* **2001**, *82*(Pt. 6), 1365–1373.

12. Harcourt, B. H.; Sanchez, A.; Offermann, M. K. Ebola virus inhibits induction of genes by double-stranded RNA in endothelial cells. *Virology* **1998**, *252*(1), 179–188.

13. Bosio, C. M.; Aman, M. J.; Grogan, C.; Hogan, R.; Ruthel, G.; Negley, D.; Mohamadzadeh, M.; Bavari, S.; Schmaljohn, A. Ebola and Marburg viruses replicate in monocyte-derived dendritic cells without inducing the production of cytokines and full maturation *J. Infect. Dis.* **2003**, *188*(11), 1630–1638.

14. Basler, C. F.; Wang, X.; Muhlberger, E.; Volchkov, V.; Paragas, J.; Klenk, H. D.; Garcia-Sastre, A.; Palese, P. The Ebola virus VP35 protein functions as a type I IFN antagonist. *Proc. Natl. Acad. Sci. U.S.A.* **2000**, *97*(22), 12289–12294.

15. Basler, C. F.; Mikulasova, A.; Martinez-Sobrido, L.; Paragas, J.; Muhlberger, E.; et al. The Ebola virus VP35 protein inhibits activation of interferon regulatory factor 3. *J. Virol.* **2003**, *77*, 7945–7956.

16. Zimring, J. C.; Goodbourn, S.; Offermann, M. K. Human herpesvirus 8 encodes an interferon regulatory factor (IRF) homolog that represses IRF-1-mediated transcription. *J. Virol.* **1998**, *72*, 701–707.

17. Barnard, P.; McMillan, N. A. The human papillomavirus E7 oncoprotein abrogates signaling mediated by interferon-α. *Virology* **1999**, *259*, 305–313.

18. Alcami, A.; Smith, G. L. Vaccinia, cowpox, and camelpox viruses encode soluble gamma interferon receptors with novel broad species specificity. *J. Virol.* **1995**, *69*, 4633–4639.

19. Munoz-Jordan, J.; Sanchez-Burgos, G. G.; Laurent-Rolle, M.; Garcia-Sastre, A. Inhibition of interferon signaling by dengue virus. *Proc. Natl. Acad. Sci. U.S.A.* **2003**, *100*, 14333–14338.

20. Goodbourn, S.; Didcock, L.; Randall, R. E. Interferons: cell signalling, immune modulation, antiviral response and virus countermeasures. *J. Gen. Virol.* **2000**, *81*, 2341–2364.

21. Upton, C.; Mossman, K.; McFadden, G. Encoding of a homolog of the IFN-γ receptor by myxoma virus. *Science* **1992**, *258*, 1369–1372.

22. Miller, D. M.; Rahill, B. M.; Lairmore, M. D.; Durbin, J. E.; Waldman, J. W.; et al. Human cytomegalovirus inhibits major histocompatibility complex class II expression by disruption of the JAK/STAT pathway. *J. Exp. Med.* **1998**, *187*, 675–683.

23. Miller, D. M.; Zhang, Y.; Rahill, B. M.; Waldman, W. J.; Sedmak, D. D. Human cytomegalovirus inhibits IFN-α-stimulated antiviral and immunoregulatory responses by blocking multiple levels of IFN-α signal transduction. *J. Immunol.* **1999**, *162*, 6107–6113.

24. Weihua, X.; Ramanujam, S.; Lindner, D. J.; Kudaravalli, R. D.; Freund, R.; et al. The polyoma virus T antigen interferes with interferon-inducible gene expression. *Proc. Natl. Acad. Sci. U.S.A.* **1998**, *95*, 1085–1090.

25. Didcock, L.; Young, D. F.; Goodbourn, S.; Randall, R. E. The V protein of simian virus 5 inhibits interferon signalling by targeting STAT1 for proteasome-mediated degradation. *J. Virol.* **1999**, *73*, 9928–9933.

26. Didcock, L.; Young, D. F.; Goodbourn, S.; Randall, R. E. Sendai virus and simian virus 5 block activation of interferon-responsive genes. *J. Virol.* **1999**, *73*, 3125–3133.

27. Yokosawa, N.; Kubota, T.; Fujii, N. Poor induction of interferon-induced 2′,5′-oligoadenylate synthetase (2-5 AS) in cells persistently infected with mumps virus is caused by decrease of STAT1-α. *Arch. Virol.* **1998**, *143*, 1985–1992.

28. Young, D. F.; Didcock, L.; Goodbourn, S.; Randall, R. E. Paramyxoviridae use distinct virus-specific mechanisms to circumvent the interferon response. *Virology* **2000**, *269*, 383–390.

29. Leonard, G. T.; Sen, G. C. Effects of adenovirus E1A protein on interferon-signaling. *Virology* **1996**, *224*, 25–33.

30. Rosmurduc, O.; Sirma, H.; Soussan, P.; Gordien, E.; Lebon, P.; et al. Inhibition of interferon-inducible MxA protein expression by hepatitus B virus capsid protein. *J. Gen. Virol.* **1999**, *80*, 1253–1262.

31. Brandt, T. A.; Jacobs, B. L. Both carboxy- and amino-terminal domains of the vaccinia virus interferon resistance Gene, E3L, are required for pathogenesis in a mouse model. *J. Virol.* **2001**, *75*(2), 850–856.

32. Carroll, K.; Elroy-Stein, O.; Moss, B.; Jagus, R. Recombinant vaccinia virus K3L gene product prevents activation of double-stranded-RNA-dependent initiation factor 2 alpha-specific protein kinase. *J. Biol. Chem.* **1993**, *268*, 12837–12842.

33. Chang, H.-W.; Watson, J. C.; Jacobs, B. L. The E3L gene of vaccinia virus encodes an inhibitor of the interferon-induced, double-stranded RNA-dependent protein kinase. *Proc. Natl. Acad. Sci. U.S.A.* **1992**, *89*, 4825–4829.

34. Davies, M. V.; Chang, H.-W.; Jacobs, B. L.; Kaufman, R. J. The E3L and K3L vaccinia virus gene products stimulate translation through inhibition of the double-stranded-RNA-dependent protein kinase by different mechanisms. *J. Virol.* **1993**, *67*, 1688–1692.

35. Davies, M. V.; Elroy-Stein, O.; Jagus, R.; Moss, B.; Kaufman, R. J. The vaccinia virus K3L gene product potentiates translation by inhibiting double-stranded-RNA-activated protein kinase and phosphorylation of the alpha subunit of eukaryotic initiation factor 2. *J. Virol.* **1992**, *66*, 1943–1950.

36. Dunlop, L. R.; Oehlberg, K. A.; Reid, J. J.; Avci, D.; Rosengard, A. M. Variola virus immune evasion proteins. *Microbes Infect.* **2003**, *5*, 1049–1056.

37. Fang, Z.-Y.; Limbach, K.; Tartaglia, J.; Hammonds, J.; Chen, X.; et al. Expression of vaccinia E3L and K3L genes by a novel recombinant canarypox HIV vaccine vector enhances HIV-1 psuedovirion production and inhibits apoptosis in human cells. *Virology* **2001**, *291*, 272–284.

38. Haig, D. M.; McInnes, C.; Thomson, J.; Wood, A.; Bunyan, K.; et al. The orf virus OV20.0L gene product is involved in interferon resistance and inhibits an interferon-inducible, double-stranded RNA-dependent kinase. *Immunology* **1998**, *93*, 335–340.

39. Ho, C. K.; Shuman, S. Mutational analysis of vaccinia virus E3 protein defines amino acid residues involved in E3 binding to double-stranded RNA. *J. Virol.* **1996**. *70*(4), 2611–2614.

40. Kibler, K. V.; Shors, T.; Perkins, K. B.; Zeman, C. C.; Banaszak, M. P.; et al. Double-stranded RNA is a trigger for apoptosis in vaccinia virus-infected cells. *J. Virol.* **1997**, *71*, 1992–2003.

41. Moss, B.; Shisler, J. L. Immunology 101 at poxvirus U: immune evasion genes. *Semin. Immunol.* **2001**, *13*, 59–66.

42. Shors, S. T.; Beattie, E.; Paoletti, E.; Tartaglia, J.; Jacobs, B. L. Role of vaccinia virus E3L and K3L gene products in rescue of VSV and EMCV from the effects of IFN-α. *J. Interferon Cytokine Res.* **1998**, *18*, 721–729.

43. Smith, V. P.; Alcami, A. Inhibition of interferons by ectromelia virus. *J. Virol.* **2002**, *76*(3), 1124–1134.

44. Xiang, Y.; Condit, R. C.; Vijaysri, S.; Jacobs, B. L.; Williams, B. R. G.; et al. Blockade of interferon induction and action by the E3L double-stranded RNA binding proteins of vaccinia virus. *J. Virol.* **2002**, *76*, 5251–5259.

45. Sharp, T. V.; Schwemmle, M.; Jeffrey, I.; Laing, K.; Mellor, H.; et al. Comparative analysis of the regulation of the interferon-inducible protein kinase PKR by Epstein-Barr

virus RNAs EBER-1 and EBER-2 and adenovirus VAI RNA. *Nucleic Acids Res.* **1993**, *21*, 4483–4490.

46. Lu, Y.; Qian, X. Y.; Krug, R. M. The influenza virus NS1 protein: a novel inhibitor of pre-mRNA splicing. *Genes Dev.* **1994**, *8*, 1817–1828.

47. Li, W.-X.; Li, H.; Lu, R.; Li, F.; Dus, M.; et al. Interferon antagonist proteins of influenza and vaccinia viruses are suppressors of RNA silencing. *Proc. Natl. Acad. Sci. U.S.A.* **2004**, *101*, 1350–1355.

48. Hatada, E.; Saito, S.; Fukuda, R. Mutant influenza viruses with a defective NS1 protein cannot block the activation of PKR in infected cells. *Virology* **1999**, *73*, 2425–2433.

49. Fortes, P.; Beloso, A.; Ortin, J. Influenza virus NS1 protein inhibits pre-mRNA splicing and blocks mRNA nucleocytoplasmic transport. *EMBO J.* **1994**, *13*, 704–712.

50. Gale, M. J.; Korth, M. J.; Tang, N.; Tan, S. L.; Hopkins, D. A.; et al. Evidence that hepatitis C virus resistance to interferon is mediated through repression of the PKR protein kinase by the nonstructural 5A protein. *Virology* **1997**, *230*, 217–227.

51. Taylor, D. R.; Shi, S. T.; Romano, P. R.; Barber, G. N.; Lai, M. M. Inhibition of the interferon-inducible protein kinase PKR by HCV E2 protein. *Science* **1999**, *285*, 107–110.

52. Dever, T. E.; Sripriya, R.; McLachlin, J. R.; Lu, J.; Fabian-Matcher, J. R.; et al. Disruption of cellular translational control by a viral truncated eukaryotic translation initiation factor 2-α kinase homolog. *Proc. Natl. Acad. Sci. U.S.A.* **1998**, *95*, 4164–4169.

53. McMillan, N. A.; Chun, R. F.; Siderovski, D. P.; Galabru, J.; Toone, W. M.; et al. HIV-1 Tat directly interacts with the interferon-induced, double-stranded-RNA-dependent kinase PKR. *Virology* **1995**, *213*, 413–424.

54. Brand, S. R.; Kobayashi, R.; Mathews, M. B. The Tat protein of human immunodeficiency virus type 1 is a substrate and inhibitor of the interferon-induced, virally activated protein kinase, PKR. *J. Biol. Chem.* **1997**, *272*, 8388–8395.

55. He, B.; Gross, M.; Roizman, B. The gamma1 34.5 protein of herpes simplex virus 1 complexes with protein phosphatase 1a to dephosphorylate the alpha subunit of the eukaryotic translation initiation factor 2 and preclude the shutoff of protein synthesis by double-stranded RNA-activated protein kinase. *Proc. Natl. Acad. Sci. U.S.A.* **1997**, *94*, 843–848.

56. Cayley, P. J.; Davies, J. A.; McCullagh, K. G.; Kerr, I. M. Activation of the ppp(A2′p)$_n$A system in interferon-treated, herpes simplex virus-infected cells and evidence for novel inhibitors of the ppp(A2′p)$_n$A-dependent RNase. *Eur. J. Biochem.* **1984**, *15*, 165–174.

57. Cayley, P. J.; Knight, M.; Kerr, I. M. Virus-mediated inhibition of the ppp(A2′p)$_n$A system and its prevention by interferon. *Biochem. Biophys. Res. Commun.* **1982**, *104*, 376–382.

58. Black, T. L.; Barber, G. N.; Katze, M. G. Degradation of the interferon-induced 68,000-Mr protein kinase by poliovirus requires RNA. *J. Virol.* **1993**, *67*, 791–800.

59. Black, T. L.; Safer, B.; Hovanessian, A. G.; Katze, M. G. The cellular 68,000Mr protein kinase is highly autophosphorylated and activated yet significantly degraded during poliovirus infection: implications for translational regulation. *J. Virol.* **1989**, *63*, 2244–2251.

60. Sharp, T. V.; Moonan, F.; Romashko, A.; Joshi, B.; Barber, G. N.; et al. The vaccinia virus E3L gene product interacts with both the regulatory and the substrate binding regions of PKR: implications for PKR autoregulation. *Virology* **1998**, *250*, 302–315.

61. Romano, P. R.; Zhang, F.; Tan, S.-L.; Garcia-Barrio, M. T.; Katze, M. G.; et al. Inhibition of double-stranded RNA-dependent protein kinase PKR by vaccinia virus E3:

role of complex formation and the E3 N-terminal domain. *Mol. Cell. Biol.* **1998**, *18*, 7304–7316.

62. Rivas, C.; Gil, J.; Melkova, Z.; Esteban, M.; Diaz-Guerra, M. Vaccinia virus E3L protein is an inhibitor of the interferon (IFN)-induced 2-5A synthetase enzyme. *Virology* **1998**, *243*, 406–414.

63. Lee, T. G.; Tomita, J.; Hovanessian, A. G.; Katze, M. G. Characterization and regulation of the 58,000-dalton cellular inhibitor of the interferon-induced, dsRNA-activated protein kinase. *J. Biol. Chem.* **1992**, *267*, 14238–14243.

64. Lee, T. G.; Tomita, J.; Hovanessian, A. G.; Katze, M. G. Purification and partial characterization of a cellular inhibitor of the interferon-induced protein kinase of Mr 68,000 from influenza virus-infected cells. *Proc. Natl. Acad. Sci. U.S.A.* **1990**, *87*, 6208–6212.

65. Lee, T. G.; Tang, N.; Thompson, S.; Miller, J.; Katze, M. G. The 58,000-dalton cellular inhibitor of the interferon-induced double-stranded RNA-activated protein kinase (PKR) is a member of the tetratricopeptide repeat family of proteins. *Mol. Cell. Biol.* **1994**, *14*, 2331–2342.

66. Haig, D. M. *Subversion and piracy: DNA viruses and immune evasion. Res. Vet. Sci.* **2001**, *70*, 205–219.

67. Haig, D. M.; Thomson, J.; McInnes, C.; McCaughan, C.; Imlach, W.; et al. Orf virus immuno-modulation and the host immune response. *Vet. Immunol. Immunopathol.* **2002**, *87*, 395–399.

68. Melville, M. W.; Hansen, W. J.; Freeman, B. C.; Welch, W. J.; Katze, M. G. The molecular chaperone hsp40 regulates the activity of P58IPK, the cellular inhibitor of PKR. *Proc. Natl. Acad. Sci. U.S.A.* **1997**, *94*, 97–102.

69. Rice, A. P.; Roberts, W. K.; Kerr, I. M. 2-5A accumulates to high levels in interferon-treated, vaccinia virus-infected cells in the absence of any inhibition of virus replication. *J. Virol.* **1984**, *50*(1), 220–228.

70. Paez, E.; Esteban, M. Nature and mode of action of vaccinia virus products that block activation of the interferon-mediated ppp(A2′p)$_n$A-synthetase. *Virology* **1984**, *134*(1), 29–39.

71. Hersh, C. L.; Brown, R. E.; Roberts, W. K.; Swyryd, E. A.; Kerr, I. M.; Stark, G. R. Simian virus 40-infected, interferon-treated cells contain 2′,5′-oligoadenylates which do not activate cleavage of RNA. *J. Biol. Chem.* **1984**, *259*(3), 1731–1737.

72. Laurence, L.; Roux, D.; Cailla, H.; Riviere, Y.; Marcovistz, R.; Hovanessian, A. Comparison of the effects of rabies virus infection and of combined interferon and poly(I)·poly(C) treatment on the levels of 2′,5′-adenyladenosine oligonucleotides in different organs of mice. *Virology* **1985**, *143*(1), 290–299.

73. Marcovistz, R.; Germano, P. M.; Riviere,Y.; Tsiang, H.; Hovanessian, A. G. The effect of interferon treatment in rabies prophylaxis in immunocompetent, immunosuppressed, and immunodeficient mice. *J. Interferon Res.* **1987**, *7*(1), 17–27.

74. Witt, P. L.; Marie, I.; Robert, N.; Irizarry, A.; Borden, E. C.; Hovanessian, A. G. Isoforms p69 and p100 of 2′,5′-oligoadenylate synthetase induced differentially by interferons in vivo and in vitro. *J. Interferon Res.* **1993**, *13*, 17–23.

75. Schroder, H. C.; Wenger, R.; Kuchino, Y.; Muller, W. E. G. Modulation of nuclear matrix-associated 2′,5′-oligoadenylate metabolism and ribonuclease L activity in H9 cells by human immunodeficiency virus. *J. Biol. Chem.* **1989**, *264*, 5669–5673.

76. Schroder, H. C.; Wenger, R.; Rottman, M.; Muller, W. E. G. Alteration of nuclear (2′-5′)oligoriboadenylate synthetase and nuclease activities preceding replication of human immunodeficiency virus in H9 cells. *Biol. Chem. Hoppe-Seyler* **1988**, *369*, 985–995.

77. Silverman, R. H.; Cayley, P. J.; Knight, M.; Gilbert, C. S.; Kerr, I. M. Control of the ppp(a2′p)$_n$A system in HeLa cells. Effects of interferon and virus infection. *Eur. J. Biochem.* **1982**, *124*(1), 131–138.

78. Bisbal, C.; Martinand, C.; Silhol, M.; Lebleu, B.; Salehzada, T. Cloning and characterization of a RNAse L inhibitor. A new component of the interferon-regulated 2-5A pathway. *J. Biol. Chem.* **1995**, *270*(22), 13308–13317.

79. Martinand, C.; Salehzada, T.; Silhol, M.; Lebleu B.; Bisbal, C. RNase L inhibitor (RLI) antisense constructions block partially the downregulation of the 2-5A/RNase L pathway in encephalomyocarditis-virus-(EMCV)-infected cells. *Eur. J. Biochem.* **1998**, *254*(2), 248–255.

80. Martinand, C.; Montavon, C.; Salehzada, T.; Silhol, M.; Lebleu, B.; Bisbal, C. RNase L inhibitor is induced during human immunodeficiency virus type 1 infection and down regulates the 2-5A/RNase L pathway in human T cells. *J Virol.* **1999**, *73*(1), 290–296.

81. Martinand, C.; Salehzada, T.; Silhol, M.; Lebleu, B.; Bisbal, C. The RNase L inhibitor (RLI) is induced by double-stranded RNA. *J. Interferon Cytokine Res.* **1998**, *18*(12), 1031–1038.

82. Bisbal, C.; Salehzada, T.; Silhol, M.; Martinand, C.; Le Roy, F.; Lebleu, B. The 2-5A/ RNase L pathway and inhibition by RNase L inhibitor (RLI). *Methods Mol. Biol.* **2001**, *160*, 183–198.

83. Le Roy, F.; Bisbal, C.; Silhol, M.; Martinand, C.; Lebleu, B.; Salehzada, T. The 2-5A/ RNase L/RNase L inhibitor (RLI) [correction of (RNI)] pathway regulates mitochondrial mRNAs stability in interferon alpha-treated H9 cells. *J. Biol. Chem.* **2001**, *276*(51), 48473–48482.

84. Kerr, I. D. Sequence analysis of twin ATP binding cassette proteins involved intranslational control, antibiotic resistance, and ribonuclease L inhibition. *Biochem. Biophys. Res. Commun.* **2004**, *315*(1), 166–173.

85. Zimmerman, C.; Klein, K. C.; Kiser, P. K.; Singh, A. R.; Firestein, B. L.; Riba S. C.; Lingappa, J. R. Identification of a host protein essential for assembly of immature HIV-1 capsids. *Nature* **2002**, *415*, 88–92.

86. Garcia-Sastre, A. Inhibition of interferon-mediated antiviral responses by influenza A viruses and other negative-strand RNA viruses. *Virology* **2001** *279*(2), 375–384.

87. Tan, S. L.; Katze, M. G. Biochemical and genetic evidence for complex formation between the influenza A virus NS1 protein and the interferon-induced PKR protein kinase. *J Interferon Cytokine Res.* **1998**, *18*(9), 757–766.

88. Bergmann, M.; Garcia-Sastre, A.; Carnero, E.; Pehamberger, H.; Wolff, K.; Palese, P.; Muster, T. Influenza virus NS1 protein counteracts PKR-mediated inhibition of replication. *J. Virol.* **2000**, *74*(13), 6203–6206.

89. Hatada, E.; Saito, S.; Fukuda, R. Mutant influenza viruses with a defective NS1 protein cannot block the activation of PKR in infected cells. *J. Virol.* **1999** *73*(3), 2425–2433.

90. Wang, X.; Li, M.; Zheng, H.; Muster, T.; Palese, P.; Beg, A. A.; Garcia-Sastre, A. Influenza A virus NS1 protein prevents activation of NF-κB and induction of α/β interferon. *J. Virol.* **2000**, *74*(24), 11566–11573.

91. Talon, J.; Horvath, C. M.; Polley, R.; Basler, C. F.; Muster, T.; Palese, P.; Garcia-Sastre, A. Activation of interferon regulatory factor 3 is inhibited by the influenza A virus NS1 protein. *J. Virol.* **2000**, *74*(17), 7989–7996.

92. Donelan, N. R.; Basler, C. F.; Garcia-Sastre, A. A. Recombinant influenza A virus expressing an RNA-binding-defective NS1 protein induces high levels of beta interferon and is attenuated in mice. *J. Virol.* **2003**, *77*(24), 13257–13266.

93. Dauber, B.; Heins, G.; Wolff, T. The influenza B virus nonstructural NS1 protein is essential for efficient viral growth and antagonizes beta interferon induction. *J. Virol.* **2004** *78*(4), 1865–1872.

94. Taubenberger, J. K.; Reid, A. H.; Janczewski, T. A.; Fanning, T. G. Integrating historical, clinical and molecular genetic data in order to explain the origin and virulence of the 1918 Spanish influenza virus. *Philos. Trans. R. Soc. London B Biol. Sci.* **2001**, *356*(1416), 1829–1839.

95. Geiss, G. K.; Salvatore, M.; Tumpey, T. M.; Carter, V. S.; Wang, X.; Basler, C. F.; Taubenberger, J. K.; Bumgarner, R. E.; Palese, P.; Katze, M.; Garcia-Sastre, A. Cellular transcriptional profiling in influenza A virus-infected lung epithelial cells: the role of the nonstructural NS1 protein in the evasion of the host innate defense and its potential contribution to pandemic influenza. *Proc. Natl. Acad. Sci. U.S.A.* **2002**, *99*(16), 10736–10741.

96. Schlender, J.; Bossert, B.; Buchholz, U.; Conzelmann, K. K. Bovine respiratory syncytial virus nonstructural proteins NS1 and NS2 cooperatively antagonize α/β interferon-induced antiviral response. *J. Virol.* **2000**, *74*(18), 8234–8242.

97. Bossert, B.; Conzelmann, K. K. Respiratory syncytial virus (RSV) nonstructural (NS) proteins as host range determinants: a chimeric bovine RSV with NS genes from human RSV is attenuated in interferon-competent bovine cells. *J. Virol.* **2002**, *76*(9), 4287–4293.

98. Valarcher, J. F.; Furze, J.; Wyld, S.; Cook, R.; Conzelmann, K. K.; Taylor, G. Role of α/β interferons in the attenuation and immunogenicity of recombinant bovine respiratory syncytial viruses lacking NS proteins. *J. Virol.* **2003**, *77*(15), 8426–8439.

99. Spann, K. M.; Tran, K. C.; Chi, B.; Rabin, R.; Collins, P. L. Suppression of the induction of alpha, beta, and lambda interferons by the NS1 and NS2 proteins of human respiratory syncytial virus in human epithelial cells and macrophages. *J. Virol.* **2004**, *78*(8), 4363–4369.

100. Frolova, I.; Frolova, E. I.; Fayzulin, R. Z.; Cook, S. H.; Griffin, D. E.; Rice, C. Roles of nonstructural protein nsP2 and α/β interferons in determining the outcome of Sindbis virus infection. *J. Virol.* **2002**, *76*(22), 11254–11264.

101. Frolov, I. Persistent infection and suppression of host response by alphaviruses. *Arch. Virol. Suppl.* **2004**, *18*, 139–147.

102. White, L. J.; Wang, J. G.; Davis, N. L.; Johnston, R. E. Role of α/β interferon in Venezuelan equine encephalitis virus pathogenesis: effect of an attenuating mutation in the 5' untranslated region. *J. Virol.* **2001**, *75*(8), 3706–3718.

103. Thomas, D.; Blakqori, G.; Wagner, V.; Banholzer, M.; Kessler, N.; Elliott, R. M.; Haller, O.; Weber, F. Inhibition of RNA polymerase II phosphorylation by a viral interferon antagonist. *J. Biol. Chem.* **2004**, *279*, 31471–31477.

104. Weber, F.; Dunn, E. F.; Bridgen, A.; Elliott, R. M. The Bunyamwera virus nonstructural protein NSs inhibits viral RNA synthesis in a minireplicon system. *Virology* **2001**, *281*(1), 67–74.

105. Streitenfeld, H.; Boyd, A.; Fazakerley, J.; Bridgen, A.; Elliott, R. M.; Weber, F. Activation of PKR by Bunyamwera virus is independent of the viral interferon antagonist NSs. *J. Virol.* **2003**, *77*(9), 5507–5511.

106. Bridgen, A.; Weber, F.; Fazakerley, J. K.; Elliott, R. M. Bunyamwera bunyavirus nonstructural protein NSs is a nonessential gene product that contributes to viral pathogenesis. *Proc. Natl. Acad. Sci. U.S.A.* **2001**, *98*(2), 664–669.

107. Bouloy, M.; Janzen, C.; Vialat, P.; Khun, H.; Pavlovic, J.; Huerre, M.; Haller, O. Genetic evidence for an interferon-antagonistic function of Rift Valley fever virus nonstructural protein NSs. *J. Virol.* **2001**, *75*(3), 1371–1377.

108. Gale, M. J. Jr.; Korth, M. J.; Katze, M. G. Repression of the PKR protein kinase by the hepatitis C virus NS5A protein: a potential mechanism of interferon resistance. *Clin. Diagn. Virol.* **1998**, *10*(2-3), 157–162.

109. Taguchi, T.; Nagano-Fujii, M.; Akutsu, M.; Kadoya, H.; Ohgimoto, S.; Ishido, S.; Hotta, H. Hepatitis C virus NS5A protein interacts with 2',5'-oligoadenylate synthetase and inhibits antiviral activity of IFN in an IFN sensitivity-determining region-independent manner. *J. Gen. Virol.* **2004**, *85*(Pt. 4), 959–969.

110. Park, M. S.; Shaw, M. L.; Munoz-Jordan, J.; Cros, J. F.; Nakaya, T.; Bouvier, N.; Palese, P.; Garcia-Sastre, A.; Basler, C. F. Newcastle disease virus (NDV)-based assay demonstrates interferon-antagonist activity for the NDV V protein and the Nipah virus V, W, and C proteins. *J. Virol.* **2003**, *77*(2), 1501–1511.

111. Shaw, M. L.; Garcia-Sastre, A.; Palese. P.; Basler, C. F. Nipah virus V and W proteins have a common STAT1-binding domain yet inhibit STAT1 activation from the cytoplasmic and nuclear compartments, respectively. *J. Virol.* **2004**, *78*(11), 5633–5641.

112. Mossman, K.; Upton, C.; Buller, R. M.; McFadden, G. Species specificity of ectromelia virus and vaccinia virus interferon-γ binding proteins. *Virology* **1995**, *208*, 762–769.

113. Mossman, K.; Nation, P.; Macen, J.; Garbutt, M.; Lucas, A.; McFadden, G. Myxoma virus M-T7, a secreted homolog of the interferon-γ receptor, is a critical virulence factor for the development of myxomatosis in European rabbits. *Virology* **1996**, *215*, 17–30.

114. Essani, K.; Chalasani, S.; Eversole, R.; Beuving, L.; Birmingham, L. Multiple anti-cytokine activities secreted from tanapox virus-infected cells. *Microb. Pathog.* **1994**, *17*, 347–353.

115. Symons, J. A.; Alcami, A.; Smith, G. L. Vaccinia virus encodes a soluble type 1 interferon receptor of novel stucture and broad species specificity. *Cell* **1995**, *81*, 551–560.

116. Colamonici, O. R.; Domanski, P.; Sweitzer, S. M.; Larner, A.; Buller, R. M. Vaccinia virus B18R gene encodes a type I interferon-binding protein that blocks interferon α transmembrane signaling. *J. Biol. Chem.* **1995**, *270*, 15974–15978.

117. Symons, J. A.; Adams, E.; Tscharke, D. C.; Reading, P. C.; Waldmann, H.; Smith, G. L. The vaccinia virus C12L protein inhibits mouse IL-18 and promotes virus virulence in the murine intranasal model. *J. Gen. Virol.* **2002**, *83*(Pt. 11), 2833–2844.

118. DiPerna, G.; Stack, J.; Bowie, A. G.; Boyd, A.; Kotwal, G.; Zhang, Z.; Arvikar, S.; Latz, E.; Fitzgerald, K. A.; Marshall, W. L. Poxvirus protein N1L targets the I-κ B kinase complex, inhibits signaling to NF-κ B by the tumor necrosis factor superfamily of receptors, and inhibits NF-κ B and IRF3 signaling by toll-like receptors. *J. Biol. Chem.* **2004**, *279*, 36570–36578.

Antiviral Drug Discovery for Emerging Diseases and Bioterrorism Threats. Edited by Paul F. Torrence
Copyright © 2005 John Wiley & Sons, Inc.